Essentials of
Breast Imaging

Essentials of
Breast Imaging

(Late) Smiti Sripathi MBBS DNB Radiology
Professor
Department of Radiodiagnosis and Imaging
Kasturba Medical College
Manipal University
Manipal, Karnataka, India

Aron Sraj Medical Diploma CCST Radiology
Clinical Lead Breast Radiologist
Specialized Medical Solutions, WLL
Primary Healthcare Corporation
Doha, Qatar

Foreword
Sabita Desai

JAYPEE

JAYPEE BROTHERS MEDICAL PUBLISHERS
The Health Sciences Publisher
New Delhi | London

JAYPEE **Jaypee Brothers Medical Publishers (P) Ltd**

Headquarters
Jaypee Brothers Medical Publishers (P) Ltd
4838/24, Ansari Road, Daryaganj
New Delhi 110 002, India
Phone: +91-11-43574357
Fax: +91-11-43574314
Email: jaypee@jaypeebrothers.com

Overseas Office
J.P. Medical Ltd
83, Victoria Street, London
SW1H 0HW (UK)
Phone: +44 20 3170 8910
Fax: +44 (0)20 3008 6180
E-mail: info@jpmedpub.com

Website: www.jaypeebrothers.com
Website: www.jaypeedigital.com

Essentials of Breast Imaging

First Edition: **2021**

Reprint 2024

ISBN: 978-93-89587-48-7

Printed at Replika Press Pvt. Ltd.

Dedicated to

My dear sister *Rashmi* who is a breast cancer survivor and to all the breast cancer patients who have fought this disease and given hope to others.

Dr Smiti Sripathi

Message

I had the privilege of spending a little over nine years with Dr Smiti, initially as a junior colleague, and later, as a close friend. From the eyes of someone who got to know her really well over those years, I can say this much:

If there was one word that could describe her
most accurately, it had to be 'passionate.'

Absolutely nothing in her life was unaffected by that passion—whether it was her work as a radiologist, her approach to academics, her strong desire to 'do more' for the public than merely as a doctor, or her dedication towards her friends, relatives and students.

Breast Radiology was the subject she was the most passionate about. And to publish a book on it was her enduring dream. It is worth recalling that hers was not merely a desire to write an informative book, but a book that would inspire radiology students and young radiologists to venture into the rather complex and often perturbing field of breast radiology with confidence and understanding.

No wonder then that the same passion reflects in this labor of love, the *Essentials of Breast Imaging*. While the ideas and the material for this book were collected over many years, her last three years were involved in tireless and extensive brainstorming with her co-author (Dr Aron), her husband (Dr Sripathi) and some colleagues—and all this, while physically and emotionally battling an insidiously progressing cancer.

It is profoundly unfortunate then, that the book could be completed only after her untimely demise. Had she been with us today, it would have been the single most gratifying experience for her to see it published and duly appreciated by her peers and students.

Each line, each illustration, each chapter of this book is infused with the same passion that represented her, and I sincerely hope and wish that this book will be remembered as the crowning glory of her legacy.

We miss you Smiti ma'am ... Always will.

Anurag Ayachit
Ex-Associate Professor of Radiology
Kasturba Medical College
Manipal, Karnataka, India

Foreword

Being a busy consultant in metropolis like Mumbai always keeps you on your toes, yet at the same time gives you ample opportunities to meet more academically oriented people pursuing your field. I first met Dr Smiti around seven years back when she was an observer in breast imaging and interventions at Tata Memorial Hospital, Mumbai. Subsequently we have met at several academic meets and it has always been a pleasure to see her diligently pursue the field of breast imaging and grow substantially as a breast radiologist. I have seen her rise to the role of a senior faculty at one of the most prestigious universities in the country, and later, following her passion, as a Commonwealth Academic Fellow at the Southend University Hospital, United Kingdom.

Breast imaging is an upcoming and rapidly growing radiologic subspecialty in India, with an increasing number of radiologists opting to specialize in this field. This book is unique not only because it effectively covers the entire gamut of breast pathologies as contributed by Dr Smiti's Indian experience, but also because of the valuable inputs stemming from Dr Aron Sraj's vast experience in breast imaging from different countries including Hungary, United Kingdom and Qatar—all having regional differences in disease patterns and clinical approach.

Breast radiologists will certainly be pleased with this comprehensive new book on breast imaging that will prove to be the need of the hour in the context of the Indian population. It will serve to educate, and simultaneously, empower both budding and established breast radiologists with the *Essentials of Breast Imaging*. The sections on mammography covering techniques and positioning and a separate chapter on quality assurance will also be useful for the radiographers. Breast ultrasound has now become a part of mainstream breast imaging, making it imperative that radiologists be familiar with the ultrasound machine and the technical parameters optimized for evaluating the breast.

The section on self-evaluation with cases arranged in a graded manner will certainly give a new perspective to all learners in developing a thorough case-based approach. Inflammatory breast diseases, including granulomatous mastitis and tuberculosis that are particularly common in the Indian subcontinent and often cause a diagnostic dilemma have been covered well. The imaging evaluation of postoperative breast in patients having undergone breast conservative therapy is often a nightmare for any beginner and related key concepts have been adequately explained and clarified with the help of line diagrams. The chapter on breast screening briefly describes the scenario of breast screening around the world, putting emphasis on the fact that we in India still have a long way to go in this extremely important aspect of breast imaging.

To conclude, this book is a brave attempt at comprehensively covering all aspects of the vast field of breast imaging, including technical advances and complex case studies for the experts, while also succinctly unraveling the fundamentals and essentials to the young radiologists interested in pursuing this field. I congratulate Dr Smiti and Dr Aron for collaborating and combining their knowledge and experiences in the form of this book and wish them all the success they deserve.

Sabita Desai MD DMRE
Consultant Radiologist
Breach Candy Hospital and Trust
Mumbai, Maharashtra, India

Preface

Breast imaging is a rapidly expanding radiologic subspecialty and this book, the *Essentials of Breast Imaging*, is our first combined venture to cover the entire spectrum of breast diseases. It comprehensively discusses the basics and essentials of imaging modalities including mammography, ultrasound and MRI. Chapters are well laid out and profusely illustrated with figures integrating a broad array of images, line diagrams and illustrations encompassing mammography, ultrasound and MRI. The last section named 'Self-evaluation based on Case Discussions' discusses 48 cases graded in order of complexity, helping the reader to learn how to ask the right questions. We hope that this book will prove extremely useful to both young budding breast radiologists and established breast radiologists with expertise in the field of breast imaging.

Dr Aron's passion for breast imaging and rich experience of more than 20 years in the field of breast imaging in Europe, UK and now Qatar, has helped us in including topics which are practically more useful and enabling the correct approach towards diagnosis of breast disorders.

The key feature of our book is that it deals with the basic and key concepts of breast imaging with simplicity and clarity without compromising relevant details. The use of self-explanatory line diagrams and illustrations simplifies important concepts making them easier to grasp. The inclusion of high quality images helps the readers to understand the disease process and interpret the findings they are likely to see in practice. The chapter on positioning is dealt with in detail, and addresses the problems faced in positioning by both radiographers and radiologists.

Reporting of postoperative mammograms is always a challenge, and especially so for budding radiologists, therefore we have discussed chronological changes in patients with breast conservative therapy in detail. Breast implants, not dealt in detail by earlier authors, is a bonus chapter in our book. Common conditions encountered in the male breast are covered in an exclusive chapter while the chapter on 'Breast Cancer Screening' discusses the status of major screening programs all over the world and its relevance in the Indian scenario.

This book is our attempt to systematically discuss all aspects of breast imaging and condense it into a nutshell for the benefit of both the budding breast radiologist and the established radiologist. We look forward for your valuable suggestions and inputs.

(Late) Smiti Sripathi
Aron Sraj

Acknowledgments

I would like to express my gratitude to my friends and colleagues who saw me through this journey; to those who discussed and talked things over and above all, to those who patiently read the drafts, offered suggestions and a patient listening.

I am thankful to Dr Aron, my co-author and dear friend who had confidence and trust in me and who agreed to collaborate with me in this daunting task. He has shared his rich experience of 25 years in the field of breast imaging and together we have tried to make certain concepts simple for the budding breast radiologists.

I would especially like to thank Dr Anurag Ayachit for critically evaluating the book right from its inception through all its stages, proof reading and commenting on various chapters. I thank Dr Rajagopal KV for his constant encouragement and support in pursuing the field of breast imaging.

I am grateful to all my other colleagues and faculty who were co-travellers in this journey, especially Dr Samir, Dr Lakshmikanth, Dr Deepika, Dr Anand, Dr Grieselda, Sravya and Winnecia. Their views, opinions and discussions helped me in further simplifying and clarifying concepts, especially since this book targets not just the beginners in breast radiology but also practicing breast radiologists. Dr Samir Parthikunnan's contribution to the chapter on Breast MRI was particularly invaluable. I am really appreciative of work done by Deepika and Griselda in helping me compile the section on case studies.

Proper follow-up of cases and immaculate data collection is essential for any academic work and I thank my postgraduate students not only for their immense help in this regard but also for always doing it with a smile! I would specially like to thank Shiva, my postgraduate student without whose help I would have been unable to create the line diagrams and figures extensively illustrating this book.

I thank the radiographers doing mammography in my department at Kasturba Medical College, Manipal. I would also like to thank the breast radiologists, radiographers and assistant practitioners of Breast unit at Southend University Hospital, United Kingdom for their support during my Commonwealth Academic Fellowship which further nurtured my passion for breast imaging.

I extend my thanks to the Indian Breast Imaging family group. The extensive discussions on the forum proved to be a common platform for sharing experience and clinical problems.

I acknowledge, with immense gratitude, the love and support of my family: my mother for her warmth appreciation and her confidence in me, my sisters Rashmi & Alka, and brother Arun who kept me going through these challenging times.

I am ever thankful to Dr Sripathi, my husband for providing emotional support and relentless inspiration. Standing by me like a rock he made sure I never gave up, thus making it possible for me to achieve this dream.

Last but not the least, I thank all my patients who kept me going.

Above all I would like to thank God Almighty—the reason behind everything.

I would like to thank Shri Jitendar P Vij (Group Chairman), Mr Ankit Vij (Managing Director), Mr MS Mani (Group President), Ms Chetna Malhotra Vohra (Associate Director—Content Strategy), Ms Pooja Bhandari (Production Head), Ms Prerna Bajaj (Development Editor) and the publishing staff at M/s Jaypee Brothers Medical Publishers (P) Ltd, New Delhi, India, for their work in completing this book.

Contents

Abbreviations

DCIS	Ductal carcinoma in situ
IDC	Invasive ductal carcinoma
ILC	Invasive lobular carcinoma
LCIS	Lobular carcinoma in situ
DBT	Digital breast tomosynthesis
DM	Digital mammography
FFDM	Full-field digital mammography
CC	Craniocaudal
MLO	Mediolateral oblique
BI-RADS	Breast imaging reporting and data system
PASH	Pseudoangiomatous stromal hyperplasia
FNAC	Fine needle aspiration cytology
TDLU	Terminal ductolobular unit
AMF	Anterior mammary fascia
PMF	Posterior mammary fascia
ALH	Atypical lobular hyperplasia
ADH	Atypical ductal hyperplasia

Anatomy of Breast and Pathophysiology of Breast Diseases

CHAPTER 1

ANATOMY

The breasts, or mammary glands, are derived from apocrine glands and consist of parenchyma, stroma and covering skin containing the nipple-areola complex (Fig. 1).

These are located on the anterior thoracic wall extending from the lateral border of the sternum to the midaxillary line horizontally and between the second and sixth intercostal spaces vertically. The base of the breast lies on the pectoral fascia, which is a flat sheet of connective tissue associated with the pectoralis major muscle acting as an attachment for the suspensory ligaments. There is an axillary tail of Spence that extends into axilla. There may be accessory breast tissue present along the milk line (axilla → anterior chest wall → pubis → upper thighs).

Breast Parenchyma

It is made up of glandular and ductal tissue consisting of 15–20 lobes arranged like a pyramid with apex toward the nipple. Each lobe consists of a number of lobules that contain approximately 10-100 acini or blind ending sacs. These lobules and lobes are drained by interlobular, intralobar and interlobar ducts that unite to form a lactiferous duct. Each duct (about 15–20) converges toward the nipple and dilates into an ampulla or lactiferous sinus (Fig. 2) before terminating at the nipple. The number of lobules per lobe and the number of acini per lobule vary according to age, parity and other individual factors.

The terminal ductolobular unit or (TDLU) is the functional unit and basic building block of lobule and consists of extralobular duct, intralobular duct and acini or ductules (Fig. 3).

Connective tissue stroma: It is a supporting structure that surrounds the mammary gland and has a fibrous and a fatty component. The fibrous stroma condenses to form suspensory ligaments of Cooper that attach and secure the breast to the dermis and underlying pectoral fascia thereby seperating the secretory lobules of the breast. The stroma in the interlobular region surrounds large ducts and TDLU and is composed of mature adipose tissue, fibroconnective tissue, blood vessels, lymphatics and nerves. The intralobular stroma surrounds the acini in TDLU and is composed of myxoid tissue and is loose in appearance. The fatty stroma is distributed all over the breast except beneath the nipple-areolar complex.

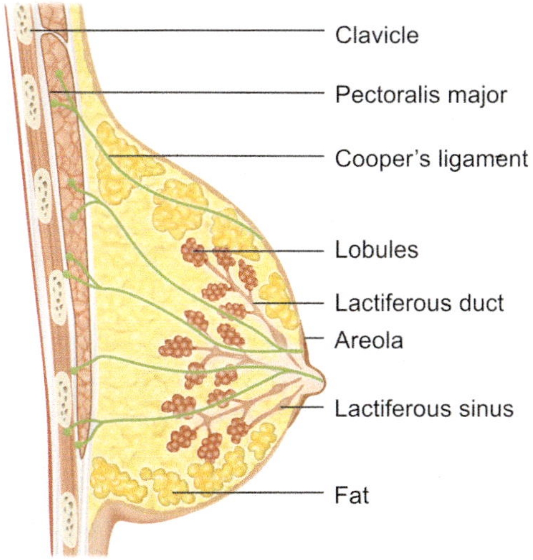

Fig. 1: Anatomy of normal female breast.

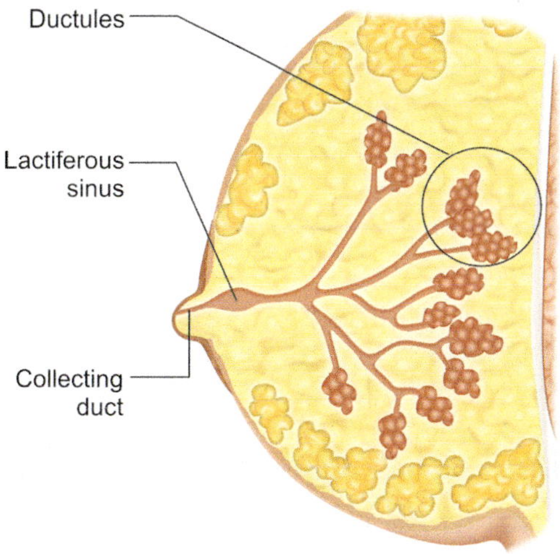

Fig. 2: Magnified view of breast showing normal anatomy.

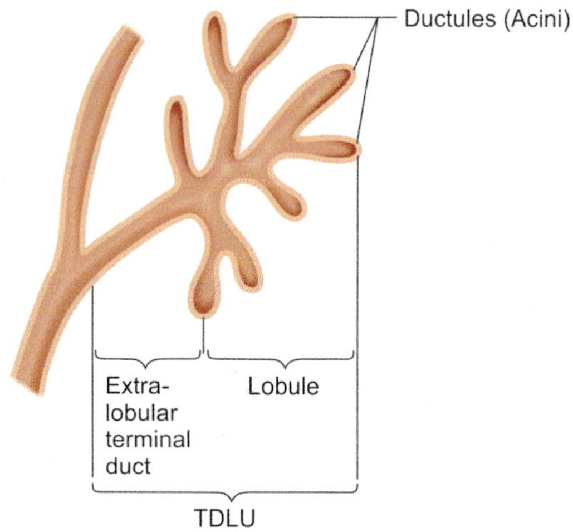

Fig. 3: Anatomy of terminal ductolobular unit (TDLU).

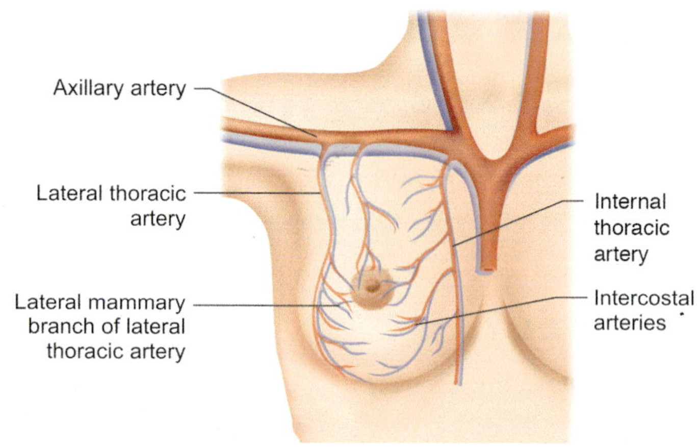

Fig. 4: Arterial supply of breast.

Nipple–Areolar Complex

The nipple is located inferomedially at fourth intercostal space and is pierced by 15–20 lactiferous ducts.

It is a cone-shaped protuberance that has an average height of 10–12 mm, mean nipple diameter of 11–13 mm and mean areolar diameter of approximately 4 cm. The Montgomery tubercles are areolar protuberances (about 10 to 20 in number) that are composed of ducts and sebaceous glands and become more prominent during pregnancy.

Most of the breast lies in the superficial fascia with a small part called, axillary tail of Spence, that extends superolaterally and pierces the deep fascia in axilla. The retromammary space is loose connective tissue that separates the mammary gland from deep fascia covering pectoralis.

VASCULAR SUPPLY

Arterial supply (Fig. 4) to the medial part of the breast is via the internal thoracic artery that is a branch of the subclavian artery. The lateral part of the breast receives blood supply from four vessels:

1. Lateral thoracic and thoracoacromial branches from the axillary artery
2. Branches of lateral thoracic artery (sometimes called external mammary artery) which supply the lateral aspect of the breast in the second, third and fourth intercostal spaces
3. Mammary branch of the anterior intercostal artery.

Venous supply: The veins of the breast correspond with the arteries, draining into the axillary and internal thoracic veins.

LYMPHATIC DRAINAGE

With the introduction of lymphatic mapping and sentinel lymph node biopsy, there is an increased interest in studying the lymphatic drainage of breast.[1]

There are three groups of lymph nodes that receive lymph from breast tissue. These are axillary nodes (75%), internal mammary nodes (20%) and posterior intercostal nodes (5%). There are two groups of lymphatics in breast-superficial and deep. The superficial lymphatics drain the skin over the breast except nipple and areola, while the deep lymphatics drain the breast parenchyma, nipple and areolar region.

Axillary lymph nodes: The axillary lymph nodes are 20–30 in number and drain lymphatics of breast, pectoral region, upper abdominal wall and upper limb. They are arranged into five groups that lie in axillary fat (Fig. 5A):

1. *Anterior or pectoral group*: lies on the pectoralis minor along lateral thoracic vessels.
2. *Posterior group*: Lies on posterior wall of axilla on lower border of subscapularis along subscapular vessels.
3. *Lateral group*: Lies on lateral wall of axilla along third segment of axillary vessels.
4. *Central group*: Lies in axillary fat at the base of axilla.
5. *Apical group*: Lies at apex of axilla.

The central and lateral parts of the breast (75%) drain into anterior or pectoral group of axillary lymph nodes, while upper part of the breast drains into apical group of axillary lymph nodes (Fig. 5B). The medial part of the breast drains into internal thoracic (parasternal) lymph nodes forming a chain along the internal thoracic vessels.

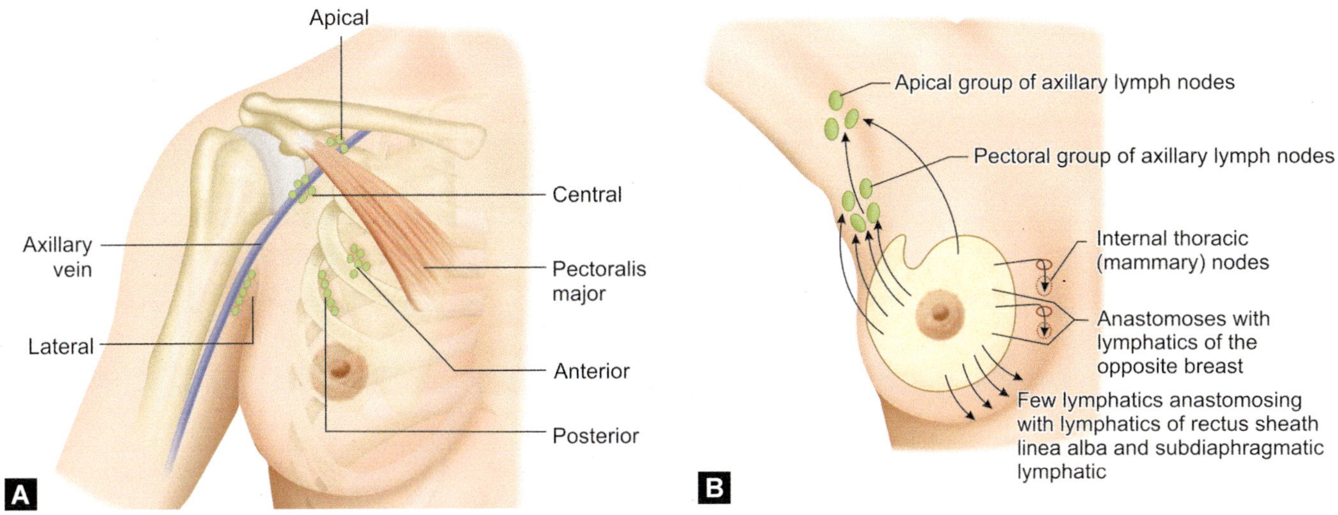

Figs. 5A and B: (A) Group of axillary lymph nodes draining the breast; (B) Lymphatic drainage of breast.

Some lymphatics from the medial part of the gland pass across the front of sternum to anastomose with that of the opposite side. Because of this, carcinoma of one breast can spread to contralateral breast and the opposite axillary lymph nodes. The lymphatics from the inferomedial part anastomose with lymphatics of rectus sheath and linea alba and some vessels pass deep to anastomose with the subdiaphragmatic lymphatics. Internal mammary lymph nodes drain the lymph not only from inner half of breast but from outer half also.

The skin of the breast drains to the axillary, inferior deep cervical and infraclavicular nodes. The nipple and areola drains into the subareolar lymphatic plexus.

NERVE SUPPLY

The breast is innervated by the anterior and lateral cutaneous branches of the fourth to sixth intercostal nerves that contain both sensory and autonomic nerve fibers.

RADIOLOGICAL ANATOMY OF BREAST

Mammogram

Zonal anatomy of breast: The breast is divided in three zones (Figs. 6A and B) from superficial to deep as follows:

Anterior one-third or premammary zone: This is the superficial zone whose anterior margin is defined by skin and posterior margin by anterior mammary fascia (AMF). It contains subcutaneous fat, blood vessels, Cooper ligaments and provides support to the breast. It is a part of integument and lesions arising from here are not true breast lesions but lesions of skin and subcutaneous tissue, for example sebaceous cyst.

Middle one-third or mammary zone: This is the middle zone that is defined anteriorly by AMF and posteriorly by posterior mammary fascia (PMF). It contains majority of lobar ducts and their branches, TDLUs, stromal fat and stromal connective tissue.

Posterior one-third or retromammary zone: This is the posterior zone, defined anteriorly by PMF and posteriorly by chest wall. It contains fat, blood vessels, lymphatics and posterior supportive ligaments that attach PMF with chest wall.

The retromammary zone is appreciated better on mammogram as retromammary fat is pulled away from the chest wall and expands in anteroposterior direction. It is not visualized adequately on ultrasound as it gets compressed against the chest wall when the patient lies in supine position during ultrasound examination.

Factors influencing mammographic appearance of breast: There is a wide variation in the normal appearance of mammographic images due to variable composition of breast elements.

The mammographic appearance is marginally influenced by degree of hydration of the intra- /extracellular spaces.

Hormonal Effects on the Breast

Breast tissue is responsive to hormone changes, some of which influence the degree of hydration of the adult breast. Estrogen levels are higher in younger women as compared to the elderly. After menopause, the estrogen

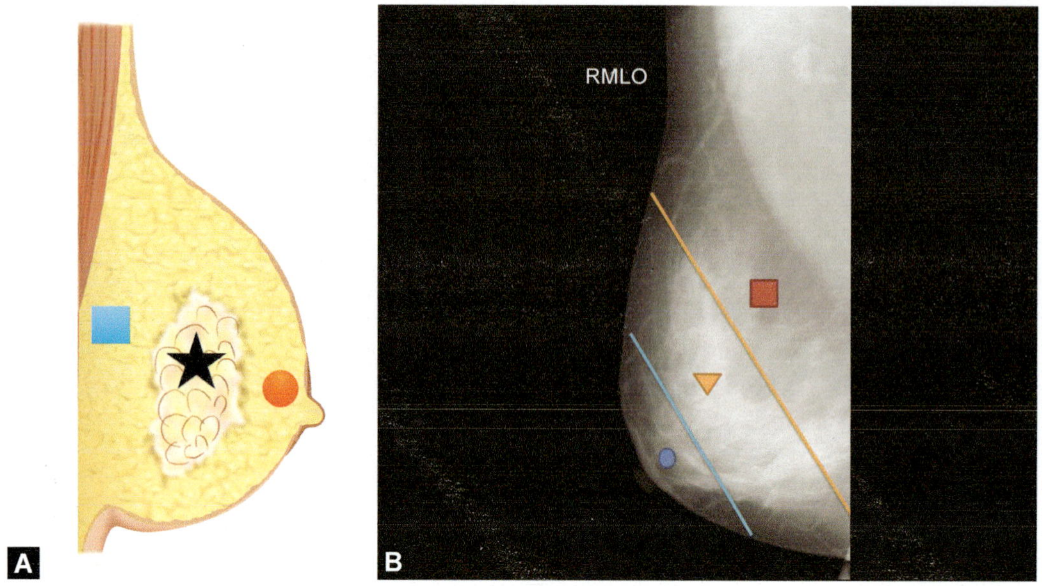

Figs. 6A and B: (A) Zonal anatomy of breast on line diagram: circle—premammary zone, star—mammary zone, square—retromammary zone; (B) Various zones on mammogram: circle—anterior one-third or premammary zone, triangle—middle one third or mammary zone and square—posterior one third or retromammary zone.

levels diminish and cause the breast lobules to regress, which causes fatty replacement of the parenchyma and decrease in breast density.

Younger women have a better contrast in the preovulatory phase of the menstrual cycle. Pregnancy and lactation increase breast density due to glandular and connective tissue hypertrophy caused by hormonal influence.

Ultrasound Anatomy of Normal Breast

The skin is usually 1–3 mm thick and is seen as two echogenic lines with a very thin hypoechoic zone between them. The fat within the breast is relatively hypoechoic, whereas the parenchymal or fibroglandular tissue is more echogenic or of mixed echogenicity.

The three zones present structurally (Fig. 7A): Subcutaneous (premammary), mammary and retromammary zones are well seen on ultrasound. The subcutaneous fat lobules are interrupted by echogenic Cooper ligaments that insert on the undersurface of the dermis.

Breast parenchyma is echogenic with fibrous tissue giving stronger echoes than glandular tissue. The curvilinear bands of connective tissue or Cooper ligaments traverse through the breast parenchyma. Intramammary ducts are usually not visible when normal in caliber; however, they may be seen as branching anechoic/hypoechoic tubular structures when dilated.

A zone of hypoechoic retromammary fat is seen deep to the breast parenchyma. Posterior to the retromammary fat is pectoral muscle fibers that are fibrillar and hypoechoic in appearance and are covered by the echogenic pectoralis fascia. Costal cartilages are seen medially as well-defined oval hypoechoic structures or curvilinear hypoechoic bands, while ribs are seen laterally casting posterior acoustic shadowing. Deeper to the ribs lies the echogenic chest wall/pleura/lung interface.

The anterior and posterior mammary fascia, stromal fibrous tissue, Cooper ligaments and skin appear echogenic on ultrasound Fig. 7B.

The AMF is tough and is resistant to spread of invasive cancer as compared to loose stromal fibrous tissue. AMF is continuous with Cooper ligaments and courses superficially through the subcutaneous fat, attaches to skin and then courses down through the fat again and continues as PMF.

Most of the true breast pathologies arise in the mammary zone as TDLUs and ducts are present in this zone. The anterior TDLUs are more numerous compared to posterior TDLUs, and regress over a period of time; hence, most pathology arising from TDLUs occur in superficial half of mammary zone just deep to AMF.

The echogenicity of both normal and pathologic anatomic structures is compared to the intramammary fat before terming them as "hypoechoic," "hyperechoic" and "isoechoic" in nature.

Breast development–ultrasound imaging: There are two phases in development of breast anatomically: initial fetal phase and later thelarche or puberty. At the time of birth, bilateral subareolar nodules develop and during thelarche

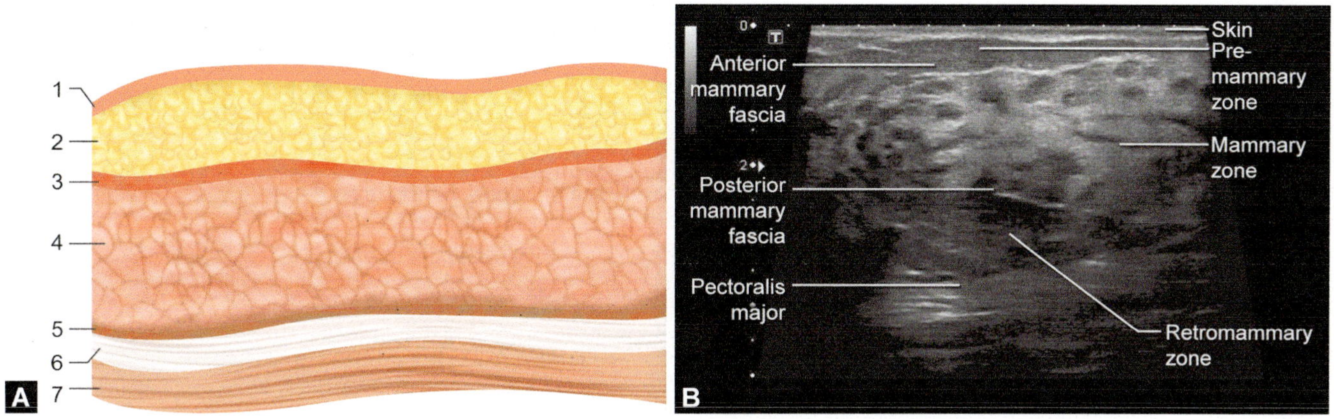

Figs. 7A and B: (A) Line diagram showing ultrasound anatomy of breast: 1-skin; 2-premammary zone; 3-anterior mammary fascia; 4-mammary zone; 5-posterior mammary fascia; 6-retromammary zone; 7-pectoralis muscle; (B) Normal anatomy of breast on ultrasound.

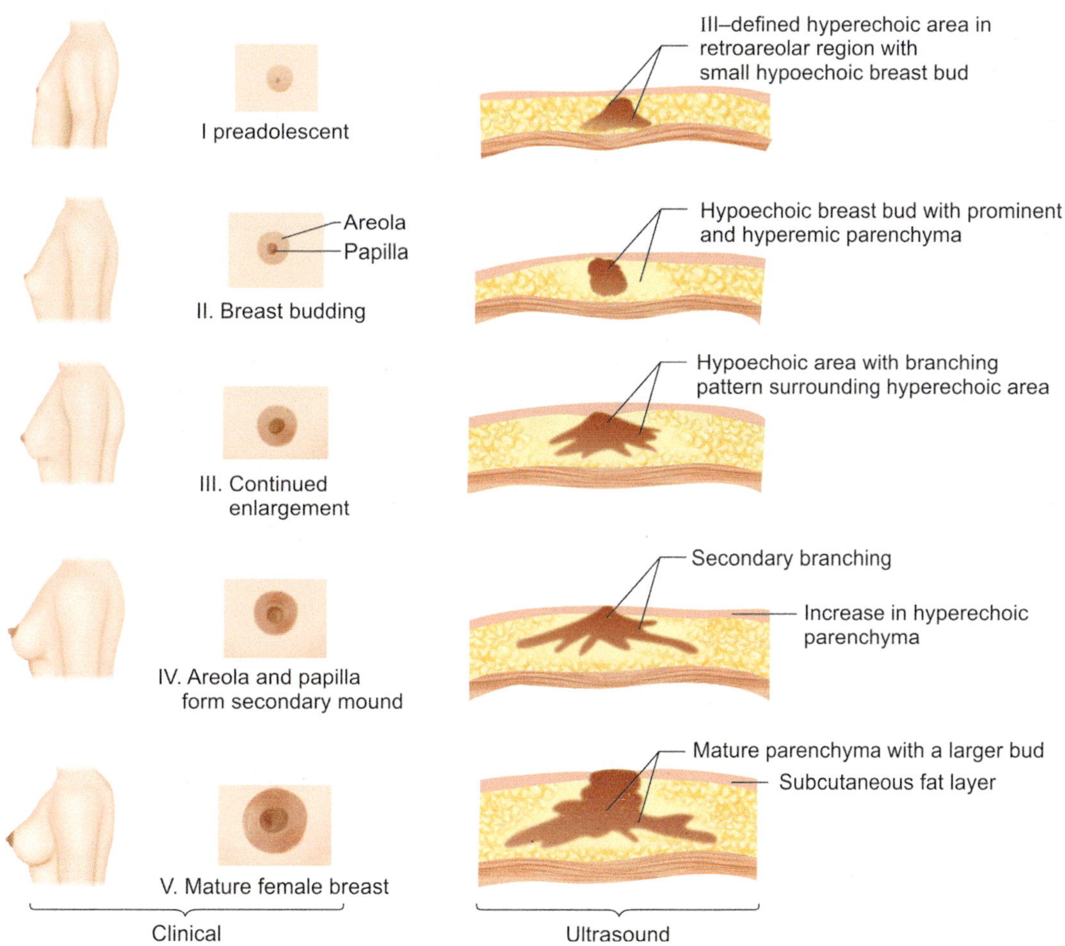

Fig. 8: Tanner classification for breast development and its correlation with ultrasound findings.

phase, there is development of breast bud. Under the influence of estrogen, duct elongation and differentiation occurs while progesterone leads to terminal lobule development.

There are five stages of breast development according to Tanner (Fig. 8) which can be correlated with the ultrasound findings[2] with an overlap in ultrasound findings from stages II to IV. It is generally accepted that rising estrogen levels correlate with maturation of breast tissue.[3] García et al. described ultrasound features of each Tanner stage in a normally developing breast (Table 1).[4]

Table 1: Tanner classification of breast development.

Breast stage	*Clinical findings*	*Ultrasound findings*
Stage I	Elevation of papilla above chest wall (Approx. 8 years)	Small focus of subareolar echogenic tissue Breast bud is absent
Stage II	Breast budding stage: elevation of breast and papilla with a small mound Palpable subareolar nodule	Subareolar hypoechoic nodule
Stage III	Further enlargement of breast and areola Initial conical shape that becomes round There is no separation of contours	Enlargement of hypoechoic bud Linear projections in a spider-like shape
Stage IV	Projection of areola and papilla to form a secondary mound	Echogenic tissue fans out The hypoechoic bud becomes elongated Subcutaneous fat present (estrogen causes deposition of fat)
Stage V	Projection of papilla and recession of areola	Mature breast tissue having hypoechoic fat lobules and echogenic glandular component

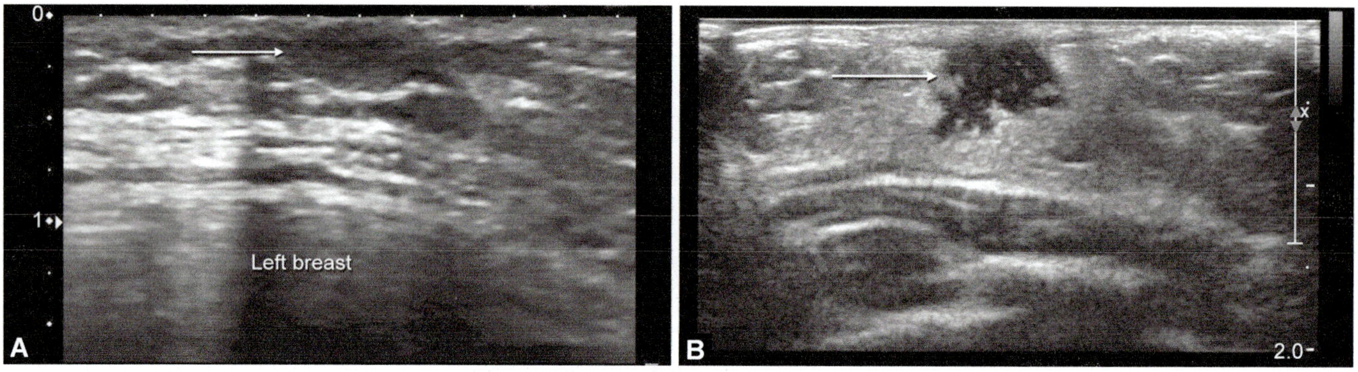

Figs. 9A and B: Ultrasound of breast in two young girls: (A) A 6-year-old girl showing development of breast bud (Tanner stage II); (B) An 8-year-old girl showing hypoechoic area with branching pattern (Tanner stage III).

Sometimes beginners performing ultrasound of breast in a child mistake it for a mass which can lead to dire consequences and should be avoided at all costs (Figs. 9A and B)

In premature thelarche, there is isolated early breast development without bone maturation in girls up to 8 years of age and no treatment is required.[5] In precocious puberty, there is early activation of hypothalamic-pituitary gonadal axis leading to development of secondary sexual maturation with rapid somatic growth.[6] Usually there is a difference of more than a year between bone age and chronological age in precocious puberty.

PATHOPHYSIOLOGY OF BREAST DISEASES

As a radiologist, one must know the origin of various pathologies of breast including benign and malignant lesions.

The TDLU is extremely important as it is the functional unit of breast and all epithelial cancers arise from this. Apart from cancers and fibroadenomas, most components of fibrocystic disease including cysts and all forms of fibroadenosis also arise from the TDLU. Benign papillomas and malignant papillary tumors arise from large ducts, while sarcomas begin in muscle, fat or connective tissues.

PATHOLOGIC CLASSIFICATION OF BENIGN BREAST DISEASES

Nonproliferative Lesions

- Cysts and apocrine metaplasia
- Mild ductal epithelial hyperplasia
- Calcifications
- Fibroadenoma and related lesions.

Proliferative Lesions without Atypia

- Sclerosing adenosis
- Radial and complex sclerosing lesions
- Florid ductal epithelial hyperplasia
- Intraductal papillomas

Atypical Proliferative Lesions

- Atypical lobular hyperplasia (ALH)
- Atypical ductal hyperplasia (ADH)

BENIGN DISEASES

The lobule has epithelial (ductal) and stromal components, which when acted upon by hormones such as estrogen, progesterone and prolactin undergoes development, maturation and differentiation.

Aberrations of normal development and involution (ANDI): Most of the benign breast disorders are essentially minor aberrations in the normal development process, hormonal response and involution of the breast, which occur throughout life (Table 2).

The most common changes (Fig. 10) are (1) cyst formation, (2) adenosis-increase in glandular tissue, (3) fibrosis, (4) epitheliosis due to proliferation of epithelium lining the ducts and acini and (5) papillomatosis due to extensive epithelial hyperplasia.

Cyst formation is due to cystic lobular involution with formation of lobular microcysts that coalesce to form macrocyst. It is because of obstruction to lobular outflow and is associated with hyperestrogenism.

Fibroepitheal lesions are composed of stromal and epithelial components. These fibroepithelial lesions with

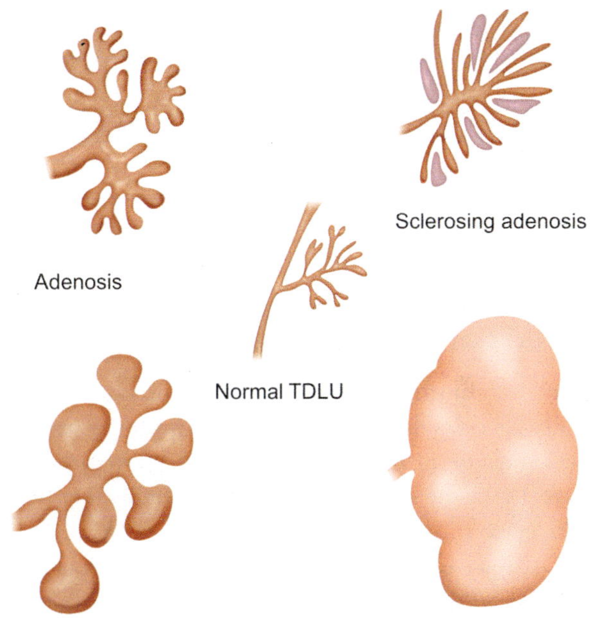

Fig. 10: Development and pathophysiology of benign breast diseases. TDLU: terminal ductolobular unit

Table 2: Spectrum of benign breast diseases.

Age	*Component*	*Normal process*	*Aberration*	*Disease*
Early reproductive years (15–25)	Glandular	Cyclical mastalgia	Fibroadenoma	Giant/multiple fibroadenomas
	Ductal	Normal	Normal	Normal
	Stromal	Normal	Juvenile hypertrophy	Gigantomastia
Mature reproductive years (25–35)	Glandular	Cyclical mastalgia	Cyclical mastalgia and nodularity	Incapacitating mastalgia
	Ductal	Normal	Normal	Normal
	Stromal	Normal	Areas of fullness on physical examination	Firm discrete areas which may require biopsy
Late age (35–55 years)	Glandular	Cyclical mastalgia, Microcysts	Multiple microcysts Sclerosing adenosis Lobular hyperplasia	Lobular carcinoma in situ
	Ductal	Normal	Duct ectasia Macrocysts	Multiple macrocysts Periductal mastitis Atypical ductal hyperplasia
	Stromal	Normal	Periductal fibrosis Nipple retraction	Lumps requiring biopsy

cellular stroma may turn out to be a fibroadenoma or phyllodes tumor at excision. Stromal proliferation indices are higher in phyllodes tumor in comparison to fibroadenoma. Assessment of stromal cellularity, mitoses and proliferation indices helps one to determine the probability of phyllodes.

Papilloma arises from the epithelium lining the ducts. Solitary papillomas are seen in subareolar region, while multiple papillomas are peripheral and have a malignant potential.

MALIGNANT DISEASES

Pathologically, epithelial breast cancers are of two types: noninvasive and invasive. These are further subdivided as in Table 3.

Ductal Carcinoma In Situ

Ductal carcinoma in situ (DCIS) a noninvasive cancer, in which the cells have not invaded through the walls of the ducts (basement membrane) into the surrounding breast tissue. Once the cells invade through the wall, it becomes an invasive cancer (Fig. 11).

- **Comedo** type is a high-grade subtype of DCIS, which completely fills and dilates the ducts with plugs of high-grade tumor cells with central necrosis or "comedonecrosis." It is the most aggressive of intraductal carcinomas and in 30% of cases it can be multicentric and/or multifocal.
- The **noncomedo** type of DCIS (Fig. 12) is less aggressive and has low nuclear grading pathologically. It is of three types: cribriform**, micropapillary** and **solid types** and these can often coexist.

Table 3: Pathological classification of epithelial malignancies.

Noninvasive	*Invasive*
1. Ductal carcinoma in situ a. Comedo b. Noncomedo - Cribriform - Micropapillary - Solid	1. Invasive ductal carcinoma a. Not otherwise specified b. Special types - Medullary - Mucinous - Tubular - Metaplastic
2. Lobular carcinoma in situ.	2. Invasive lobular carcinoma

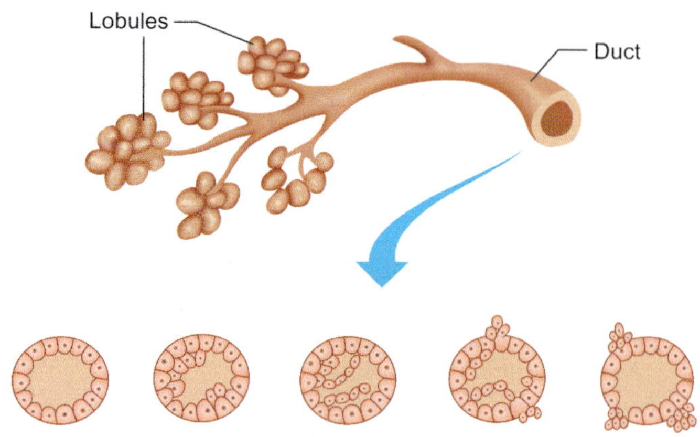

Fig. 11: Pathology of development of breast carcinoma.

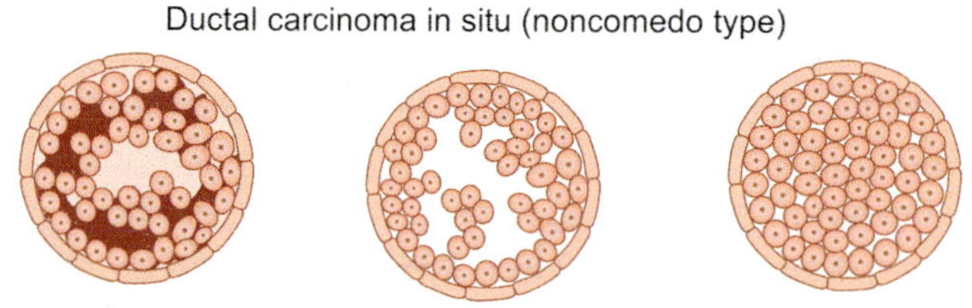

Fig. 12: Ductal carcinoma in situ-noncomedo type.

- In the **cribriform type**, the cancer cells grow in the duct but do not fill the duct completely. The fluid in between these cells petrifies and later calcifies.
- In the **micropapillary type**, there are fern-like extensions that produce secretory material which petrifies and calcifies. In both these types, crushed stone-like calcifications are seen on mammograms.
- In the **solid type**, it fills the duct completely and does not produce any calcifications.

Mammographically casting types of calcifications are seen more commonly in comedo type, which is more aggressive as compared to the noncomedo type that shows granular calcifications.

Lobular Carcinoma In Situ (LCIS)

It originates in the acini of terminal TDLU. The malignant cells fill and distend the lobular acini without invading the basement membrane. One must remember that approximately 20% of cases diagnosed as LCIS at core needle biopsy will be upgraded to invasive cancer at surgical excision.

Invasive Ductal Carcinoma

Not Otherwise Specified (NOS)

This is the most common type of infiltrative breast carcinoma (75%–80%) which lacks features of any other subtypes (i.e., a diagnosis of exclusion) and arises from TLDU.

Special Types

- **Medullary carcinoma** is a rare subtype of infiltrative ductal carcinoma accounting for 3–5% of these cancers. It arises in the ducts and is called "medullary" because pathologically it appears as grayish soft tissue in the medulla. It is a triple negative cancer and though the cells look aggressive histopathologically, it does not metastasize to lymph nodes and has a better prognosis.
- **Mucinous carcinoma** arises in the ducts and the tumor is made up of abnormal cells that "float" in pools of mucin. It is a less aggressive type that is seen in postmenopausal women and responds well to treatment.
- **Tubular carcinomas** are usually small (about ≤1 cm) and arise from the ducts of TDLU. They are made up of tube-shaped structures called "tubules." These tumors are low-grade, grow slowly, do not involve lymph nodes and have a good prognosis.
- **Metaplastic carcinoma:** A rare (<1%) aggressive malignant neoplasm, it exhibits a variety of histopathologic patterns and appears to be both epithelial and mesenchymal in origin. It has poorer prognosis compared to general invasive ductal carcinoma (IDC) and triple negative IDC.

Invasive Lobular Carcinoma

This accounts for approximately 10% of cancers and is the second most common cancer after IDC. This invades the wall of lobules and spreads into surrounding tissues.

Since there is a large amount of glandular tissue in upper outer quadrant, most of the cancers develop here.

Lymphovascular invasion is presence of cancer cells in lymphatic vessels and blood vessels and is an important process in spread of cancer.

One must be aware of the normal anatomy of breast and its appearance in various imaging modalities to interpret the findings correctly. The knowledge of pathophysiology of various breast diseases gives an added confidence and is essential in making a correct diagnosis.

REFERENCES

1. Tanis PJ, Nieweg OE, Valdés Olmos RA, Kroon BB. Anatomy and physiology of lymphatic drainage of the breast from the perspective of sentinel node biopsy. J Am Coll Surg. 2001;192(3):399-409.
2. Chung EM, Cube R, Hall GJ, et al. From the archives of AFIP: breast masses in children and adolescents: radiologic-pathologic correlation. Radiographics. 2009;29:907-31.
3. Weinstein SP, Conant EF, Orel SG, et al. Spectrum of ultrasound findings in paediatric and adolescent patients with palpable breast masses. Radiographics. 2000;20:1613-21.
4. García CJ, Espinoza A, Dinamarca V, et al. Breast US in children and adolescents. Radiographics 2000;20:1605-12.
5. Della Manna T, Setian N, Damiani D, Kuperman H, Dichtchekenian V. Premature thelarche: identification of clinical and laboratory data for the diagnosis of precocious puberty. Rev Hosp Clin Fac Med Sao Paulo. 2002;57:49-54.
6. Pescovitz OH, Hench KD, Barnes KM, Loriaux DL, Cutler Jr. GB. Premature thelarche and central precocious puberty: the relationship between clinical presentation and the gonadotropin response to luteinizing hormone-releasing hormone. J Clin Endocrinol Metab. 1988;67:474-9.

Mammography

CHAPTER 2

2.1 Technique and Positioning

INTRODUCTION

Mammography has been long the imaging modality of choice for early detection of breast cancer all over the world as it is the most common malignancy in women.[1]

It is important to obtain good quality images including maximum tissue so that accurate diagnosis can be made. A complete clinical history with a good quality mammogram is a prerequisite for proper interpretation of the images.

With the increased number of breast cancer's cases in India, we do not need only breast radiologists but also trained technologists to obtain optimal quality mammograms so that early breast cancer can be detected. It is imperative that budding breast radiologists also learn techniques and positioning of mammography properly to guide their radiographers.

There is tremendous improvement in both hardware and software of mammography over the last few years, thereby improving image quality. The factors that need to be taken care of are adequate compression and correct positioning and therefore a good technologist is a must.

It is worth remembering what Dr Eklund said, "Bad mammography cannot be perceived without the knowledge of good mammography." One must follow the standards of positioning to get good quality mammograms so that "the cancer is not left behind in the mammography room." A badly taken mammogram can result in a blurred image, whereas a properly taken mammogram shows a detailed map of breast, which will prove to be a huge difference between life and death. One must not forget that sometimes subtle changes in breast architecture can be the only sign of cancer. Remember, no matter how many mammograms are done that day, the patient is receiving her first and only mammogram of the year.

Screen Film Mammography

This has been used for a long time all over the world. It helps in detecting early breast cancer as microcalcifications are seen well because of high spatial resolution.[2] Contrast resolution is a limitation and especially so in women with dense breasts. Because of this, it has a lower sensitivity (62.9%) in dense breast as compared to fatty breast (87%).[3]

It is extremely important that dedicated equipment for mammography should be used.

Those with computed radiography (CR)-based system should use high-resolution cassettes (20 pixel/mm) and CR reader.

Full-field Digital Mammography

Digital radiography began once the transfer of images to digital format started. Slowly the digital technology started getting adopted by other imaging modalities. The first full-field digital mammography (FFDM) unit was approved for sale by the Food and Drug Administration in 2000.[4]

Digital mammography has several advantages over screen film mammography that include:

- Easier access to images and computer-assisted diagnosis
- Better transmission, retrieval and storage of images
- Lower average radiation dose without a compromise in diagnostic accuracy.

The workflow in digital mammography is more effective[5] and the time taken to perform it is reduced.[6] The storage space required is also less as compared to screen film mammography. In women with dense breast and in younger women, digital mammography is more accurate.[7]

This may be because of dynamic range of digital mammography as it captures contrasting densities and displays them without compromising the contrast resolution very much.

TECHNIQUE AND POSITIONING: AN OVERVIEW

Patient preparation: Mammogram should be done after the menstrual phase. There is no specific preparation required for a mammography, but it is always better if the patient is told about the procedure beforehand to reduce apprehension. The patient should be asked to avoid using talcum powder on the day of examination as it can produce artifacts. A proper clinical history and indication for mammogram is mandatory. The patient should be asked to bring previous mammograms for comparison.

Positioning: Proper positioning of breast is very important for optimum mammogram quality and maximizes the amount of tissue obtained. Proper attention during positioning eliminates most of the artifacts and increases the diagnostic accuracy of mammography. Since body habitus of each individual is different, adjustments have to be made in positioning for maximum tissue visualization. For example, the head should be turned for craniocaudal (CC) view, arm should be raised for mediolateral oblique (MLO) view and any injury to shoulder and arm should be avoided.

Two of the most important principles of breast positioning are (1) the mobile tissues have to be moved toward fixed tissue and (2) the compression paddle should not be moved against fixed tissue; hence, these principles should be adhered to during mammography positioning. One should remember that inferior and lateral portions of breast are mobile and medial and superior portion are fixed.

Role of breast compression: Breast compression is very important during mammography as it improves image quality by preventing overlapping of structures and produces sharper images.

This is because of the following reasons:

- The breast thickness is reduced during compression that reduces ratio of scatter radiation to primary radiation, thereby improving subject contrast
- The structures in breast are brought closer to image receptor; hence, geometric blurring is reduced
- The uniform breast thickness results in even penetration and uniform radiographic density
- Compression causes immobilization of breast and reduces motion blur
- The spreading of the breast tissue during compression reduces superimposition of breast tissue enabling suspicious lesions to be more easily identified
- Both image unsharpness and radiation dose are reduced.

The failure in optimal positioning and compression are operator dependent and can be avoided by proper training.

Standard mammographic views: There are two standard views:

1. Craniocaudal view
2. Mediolateral Oblique (45 degrees) view

Additional views

- Extended CC view
- True lateral view
- Axillary view (Cleopatra view)
- Cleavage view/valley view
- Spot compression view
- Magnification view
- Rolled view
- Tangential view
- Caudocranial or from below view
- Eklund view for implants.

STANDARD MAMMOGRAPHIC VIEWS

Craniocaudal View

This view is one of the standard views and guidelines for positioning must be followed while doing it (Fig. 1A).

Technique

- Technologist should stand on medial side of patient and film tray should be raised to the height of inframammary crease/fold. The patient should be asked to take half step away from the receptor or film tray and breast should be placed on the image receptor
- The patient is then asked to lean forward toward receptor—chest forward and hip backward and head is brought around side of a tube
- The breast is pulled laterally and nipple is centered and placed in profile
- The breast tissue is pulled toward nipple and taut compression is applied at the same time
- Wrinkles and folds on the skin should be smoothened out
- Marker should be placed at axilla

Once the above steps are done, a good quality CC view is produced (Fig. 1B).

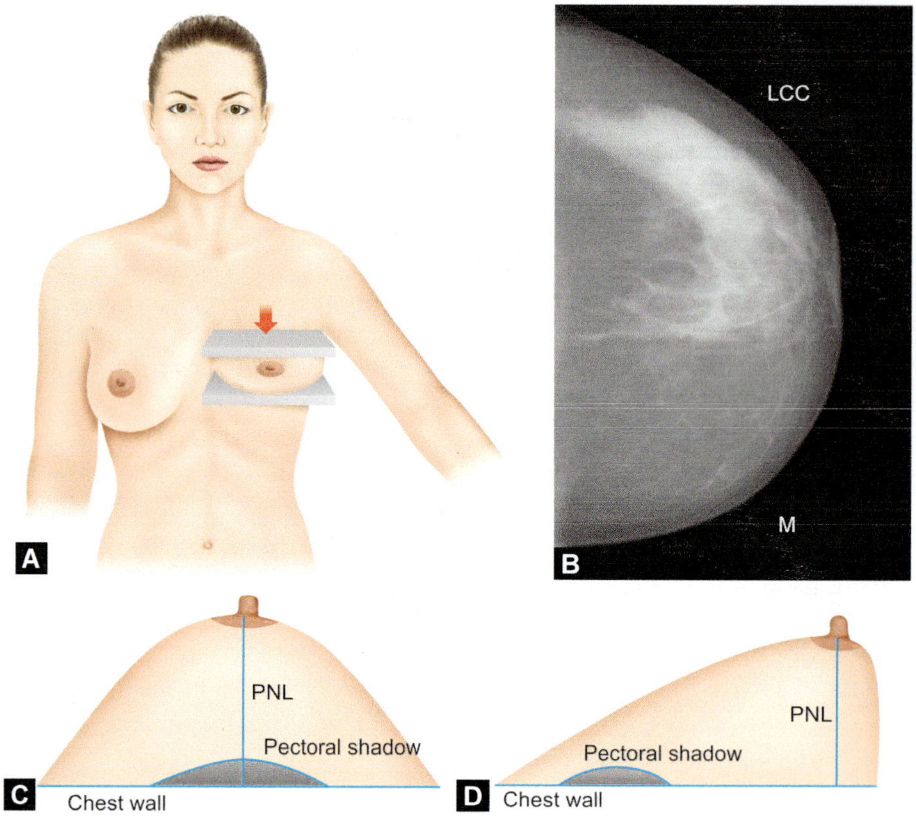

Figs. 1A to D: (A) Positioning for CC view; (B) Mammogram image showing correctly positioned CC view; (C) PNL on a correctly positioned CC view; (D) PNL on a badly positioned CC view. (CC: craniocaudal; PNL: posterior nipple line).

CHECKLIST FOR A PROPER CRANIOCAUDAL VIEW

1.	Uniform tissue thickness
2.	Visualization of central, subareolar and medial aspect of breast
3.	Posterior most extent of breast are covered adequately
4.	Retroglandular fat is well seen
5.	No skin folds are present
6.	No artifacts are present
7.	Pectoral muscle is seen in 30–40% cases
8.	Posterior nipple line (PNL) is within 1 cm on mediolateral oblique (MLO) view

Posterior nipple line is a line drawn posteriorly from the nipple towards the pectoral muscle on mammogram. In an adequately positioned breast, the difference in measurement of this line in CC and MLO view should be <1 cm (Figs. 1C and D).

Mediolateral Oblique (MLO) or Lundgren's View

This is the second standard view (Fig. 2A) done on mammogram.

Technique

- The plane of the image receptor is between 30 and 60° to the horizontal so that it is parallel to pectoralis muscle. The angle can differ depending upon the built of the patient.
  - For average height and built patients: 40-50°
  - For tall and thin patients: 50-60° (steeper angle)
  - For short patients: 30-40°.
- The top of image receptor should be kept at axilla, following which the breast should be lifted and both pectoralis muscle and breast should be pulled anteriorly and medially. The breast should be held away from the chest wall and compression should be then applied. The upper corner of the compression paddle should be just below the clavicle. It is important to ensure that nipple is in profile and marker is kept at axilla. While the hand is moved out

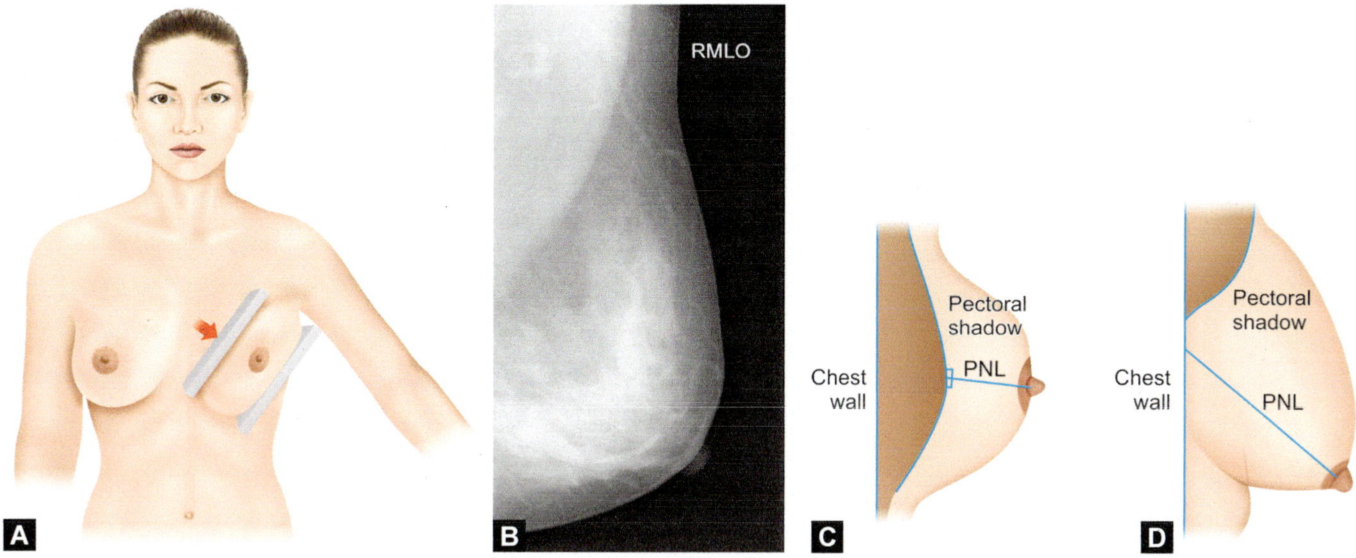

Figs. 2A to C: (A) Positioning for MLO view; (B) Mammogram image showing correctly positioned MLO view; (C) PNL on a correctly positioned MLO view; (D) PNL on a badly positioned MLO view. (MLO: mediolateral oblique; PNL: posterior nipple line).

of the field, anterior portion of the breast should be supported and at the same time abdominal tissue should be pulled down to open inframammary fold. The entire breast from infra mammary fold to the axilla must be centered on the image receptor. The patient is asked to hold on to the bar with the ipsilateral arm.

Once the above steps are followed, a properly taken MLO view is obtained (Fig. 2B).

CHECKLIST FOR PROPER MEDIOLATERAL OBLIQUE VIEW

1.	Breast supported up and away from thorax and perpendicular to chest wall
2.	Visualization of retroglandular fat
3.	Inframammary fold should open out
4.	Nipple should be in profile
5.	Pectoralis muscle should be well seen. It is wide superiorly with a convex anterior border extending to or below the posterior nipple line
6.	No artifacts
7.	No skin folds

ADDITIONAL MAMMOGRAPHIC VIEWS

Lateral View

This is the most commonly done additional view. It is a 90° true lateral view and can be mediolateral (Figs. 3A and B) or lateromedial view (Fig. 4).

It is done commonly before stereotactic biopsy to decide upon the approach.

It is used to triangulate the exact location of lesion in the breast.

To see calcification due to milk of magnesia (tea-cup calcification).

Technique (90° Mediolateral View)

- The image receptor is at 90° to horizontal
- Confirm true lateral (90°) position
- Compression is applied
- Nipple should be in profile
- Marker should be placed at axilla.

Extended CC View

This view depicts lesions in deeper outer portion of breast including the axillary tail (Figs. 5A and B). The nipple should be in profile. Sometimes pectoralis muscle may be seen.

Technique

The patient should be positioned as in CC view after which the inframammary fold should be elevated and the patient is rotated till lateral aspect of breast is positioned on the receptor. A 5° lateral rotation should be given to remove the shoulder from the way. Both the shoulders should be at the same level.

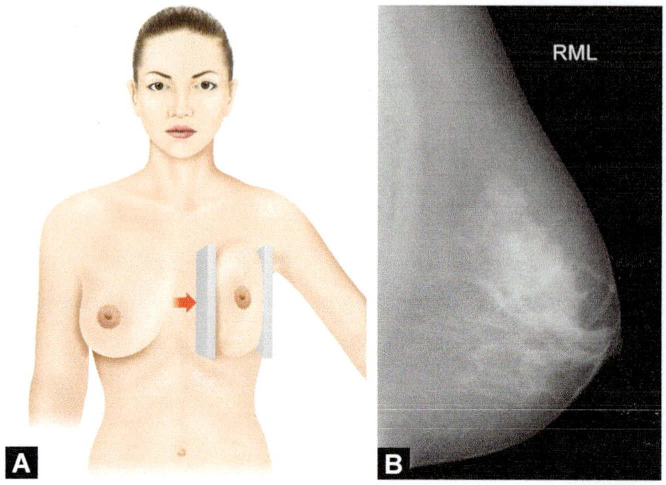

Figs. 3A and B: (A) Positioning for 90° mediolateral view; (B) Mammogram showing correctly positioned ML (Mediolateral view). (MLO: mediolateral oblique).

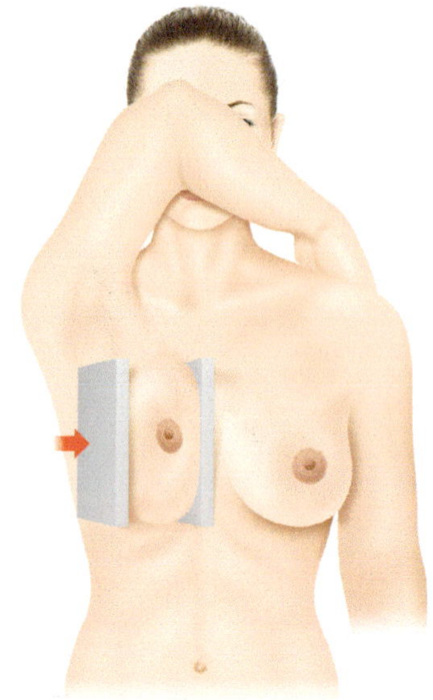

Fig. 4: Positioning for 90° lateromedial view.

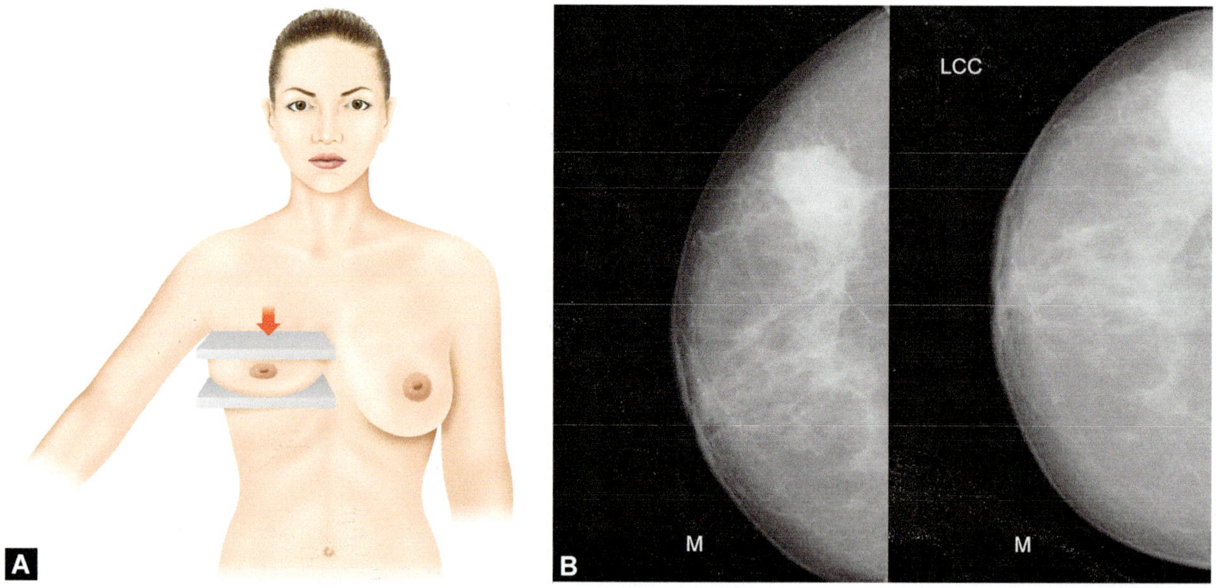

Figs. 5A and B: (A) Positioning for extended CC view; (B) Mammogram showing inadequate coverage of laterally placed mass in routine CC view that would be covered properly in the extended CC view. (CC: craniocaudal).

Axillary Tail View (Cleopatra View)

This view is done to look for abnormalities in axillary tail region and most lateral portion of breast.

The C arm should be raised at 25–30° and breast should be comfortably positioned on bucky.

The axillary aspect of the breast should be gently pulled out away from the chest wall and placed on the image receptor while applying compression (Figs. 6A and B) mass.

Cleavage View or Valley View

This view is taken for demonstration of mass at medial aspect of breast (Figs. 7A and B) which is not adequately covered in CC view.

Technique

The radiographer should stand behind the patient and wrap her arm around the patient to reach her breast at the

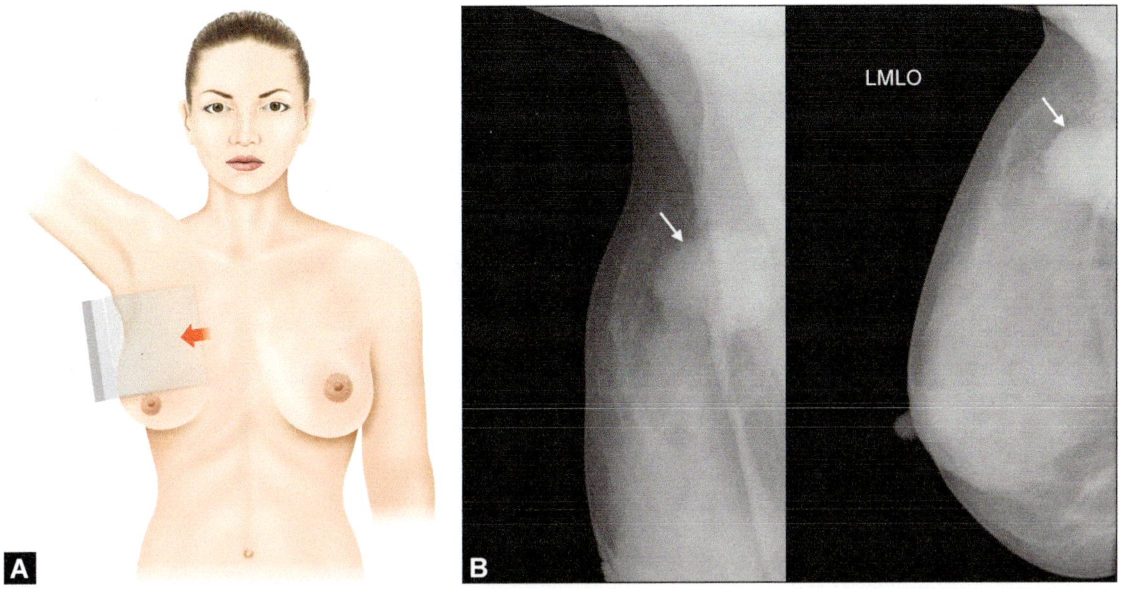

Figs. 6A and B: (A) Positioning for axillary tail (Cleopatra view); (B) Mammogram MLO view shows an inadequately covered mass in axillary tail region that was seen better on the axillary tail view. (MLO: mediolateral oblique).

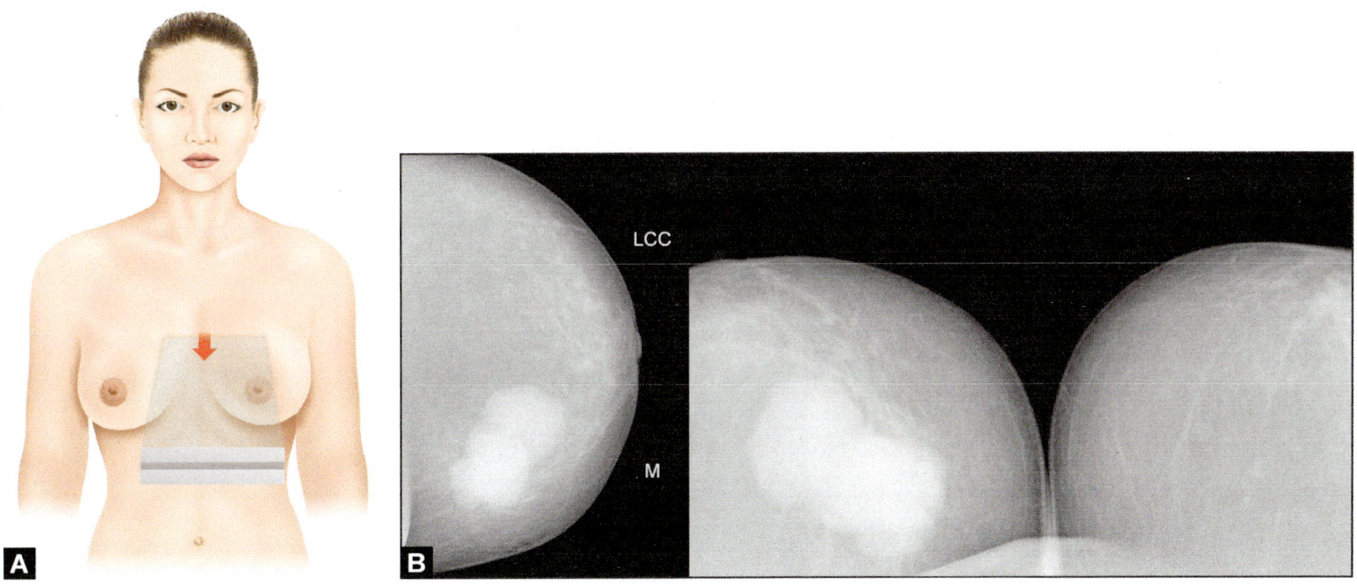

Figs. 7A and B: (A) Positioning for cleavage view also called as valley view; (B) CC view shows a mass in the medial quadrant that is seen well on cleavage view. (CC: craniocaudal.)

same time pulling the medial aspect of both the breasts anteriorly and position them on the image receptor. This way the cleavage area will be positioned adequately.

Spot Compression View

Spot compression is also known as compression mammogram, spot view, cone view or focal compression view.

Spot compression is used to evaluate focal asymmetries and any obscured areas or equivocal findings in dense breast. The basis of this technique is to spread out the breast tissue to decrease overlap so that underlying abnormality is seen well. This is done with the help of a small paddle or cone that provides localized and intense focal compression (Figs. 8A and B).

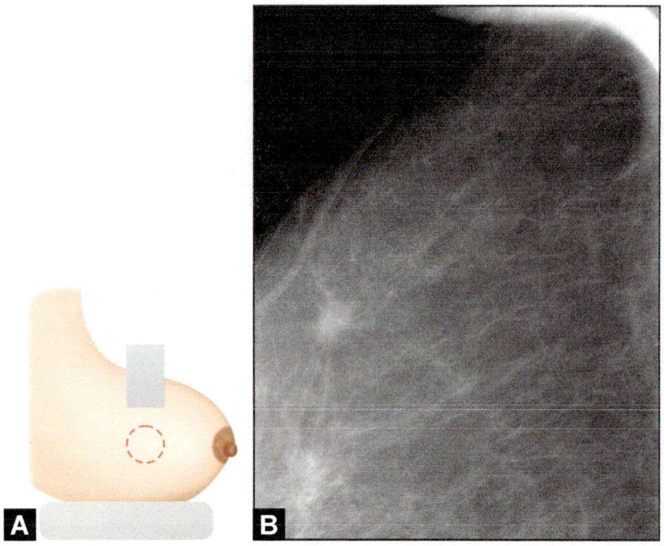

Figs. 8A and B: (A) Spot compression view showing a small paddle compressing the mass in question; (B) Mammogram with spot compression view shows a well-defined spiculated mass with morphological features appreciated well.

How to Determine the Location of the Lesion for Spot Compression?

Technique

To determine the location of lesion to take a spot compression view, it is important to decide in which standardized view (CC or MLO) has to be done. For example, if it is CC view then, on the film first draw a line posteriorly from the nipple and measure the distance of the lesion from this line. In addition, draw a line from the skin surface to the lesion that gives the depth of lesion. The patient is then repositioned and compression given with hand and the same measurements are transferred to breast and a marker put on the breast to identify the lesion location. A spot compression device is then applied over the lesion and the requisite view is taken

Magnification View

This view can be done with or without compression.

It is often used to evaluate microcalcifications to assess their number, location and morphology (Figs. 9A and B) or to delineate the margins of an irregular mass or suspicious mass/area.

Technique

To do this view, an X-ray tube with a microfocal spot to offset geometric sharpness is required along with a magnification platform. This separates the compressed breast from the image receptor for 1.5–2 times magnification.

During the exposure, the patient has to hold still for a longer time than normal mammogram.

The air gap resulting from separation of breast from image receptor reduces scattered radiation.

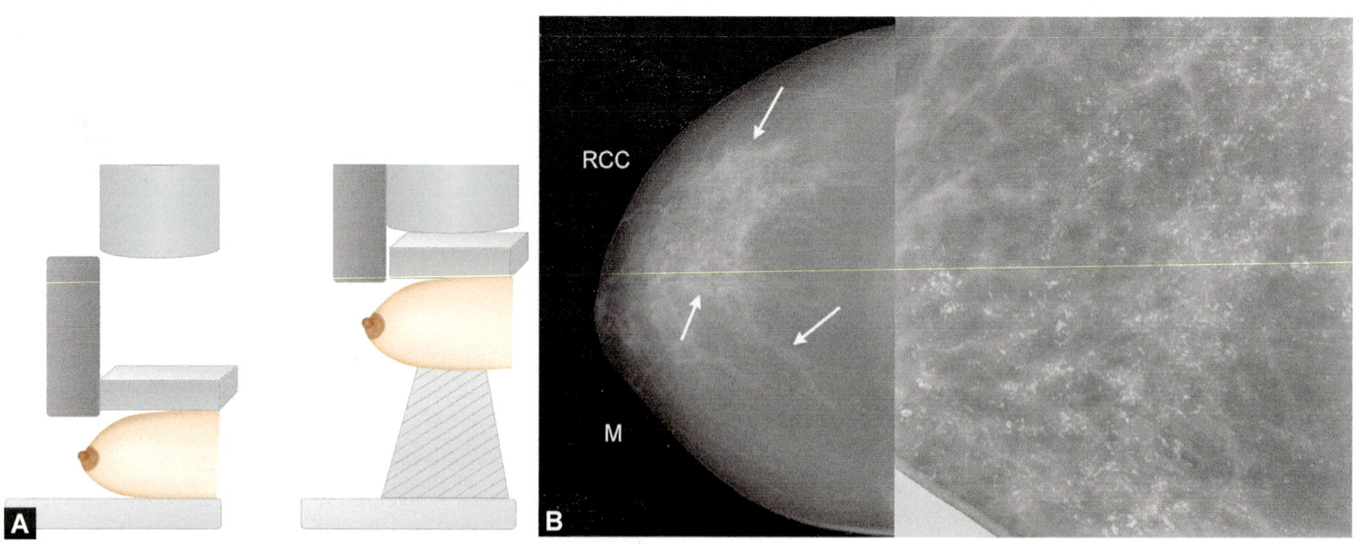

Figs. 9A and B: (A) Magnification view where the breast is positioned on top of the magnification stand, decreasing the focal spot and allowing for magnification; (B) Mammogram—magnification view showing location, morphology and the number of microcalcifications.

Rolled View

This view is done to separate superimposed structures, to confirm the presence of an abnormality, to determine the location of a finding seen on only one standard view (Fig.10).

Uses: To confirm the presence of an abnormality.

To determine the location of a finding seen on only one standard view.

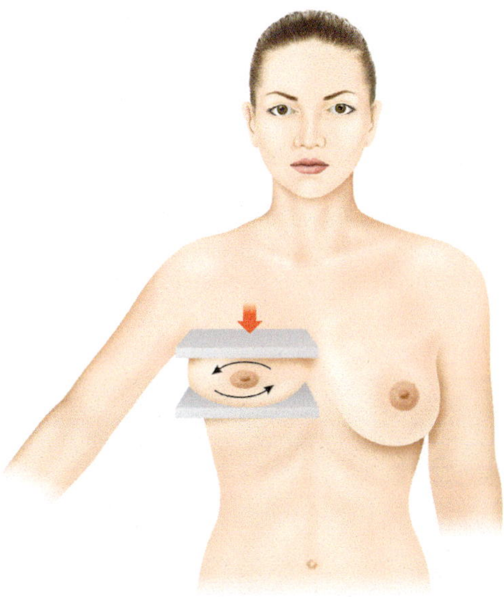

Fig. 10: Positioning for rolled view.

Technique

The patient should be repositioned in the same view in which abnormality was seen. The radiographer should put hands on either side of breast and roll the breast tissue in opposite direction applying compression at the same time. A marker should be positioned on the image receptor indicating the direction of roll.

Tangential View

This view is done mainly for lesion or calcifications which are in the skin or in superficial plane.

Technique

A lead marker is placed over the lump and X-ray beam is directed tangential to the lump so that it is seen properly (Figs. 11 and 12).

Caudocranial or from Below View

This view is performed in patients having kyphosis, patients with small breasts or male patients.

Since the compression comes from below, it does not exclude the posterior fixed tissue.

Eklund View for Implants

Imaging of breast with implants is challenging as the degree of compression is dependent upon the compressibility of

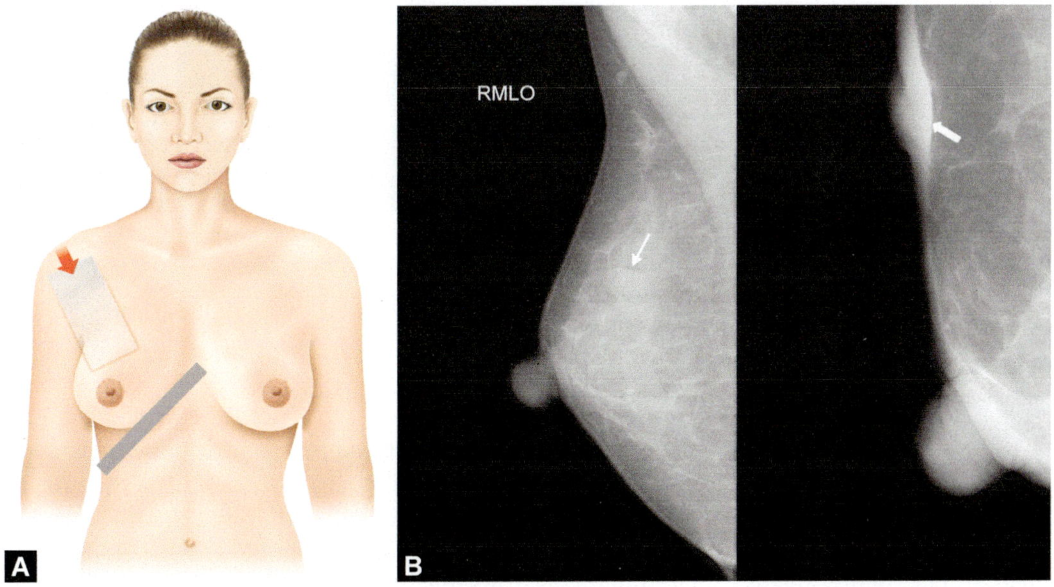

Figs. 11A and B: (A) Positioning for tangential view; (B) Mammogram MLO view showing an obscured density with a lucent halo superiorly which on tangential view was seen as arising from the skin. The patient had a skin nodule in that location. (MLO: mediolateral oblique).

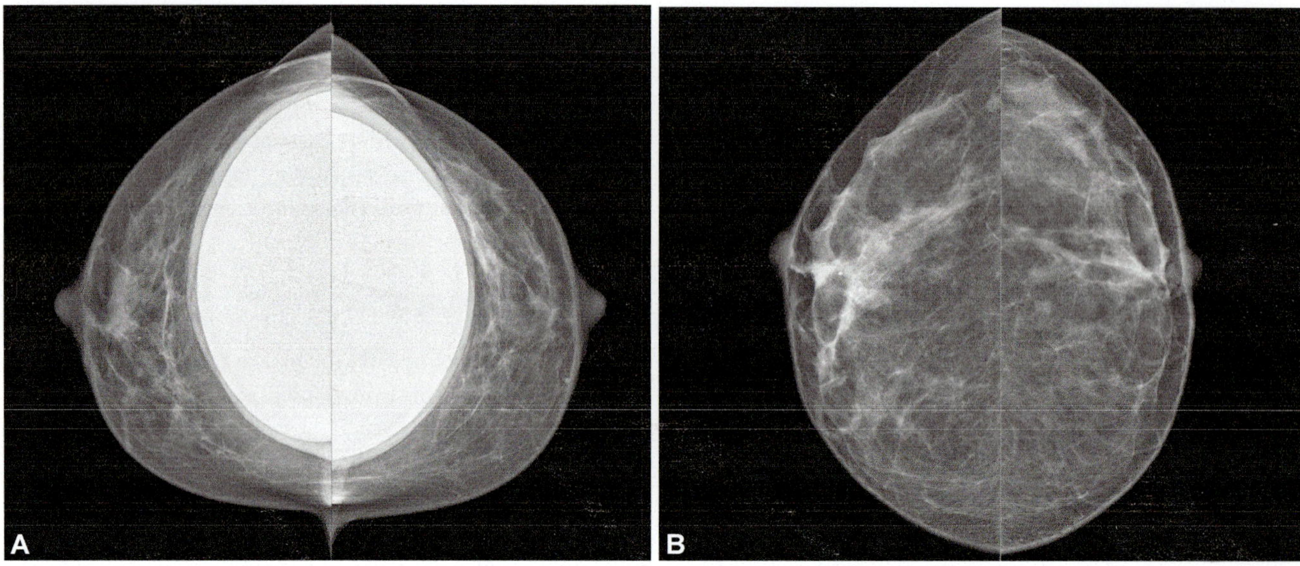

Figs. 12A and B: (A) Mammogram image showing submuscular breast implants on CC view; (B) Breast implants with Eklund view in which the breast tissue is pulled anteriorly and implant is pushed posterosuperiorly so that more of breast tissue is imaged. (CC: craniocaudal).

implants and exposure factors for CC and MLO view have to be set manually.

In this view, the implant is pushed posteriorly and superiorly against the chest wall while gently pulling the breast anterior to the prosthesis onto the image receptor and holding it in place with the compression device (Figs. 12A and B).

For a CC view with implant, the breast tissue superior and inferior to implant is pulled anteriorly.

For an MLO view with implant, the breast tissue that is superomedial and inferolateral will be pulled forward with the anterior tissue.

ARTIFACTS

Artifacts in mammography can create pseudolesions, mask abnormalities and degrade image quality leading to misinterpretation. A high-quality mammogram enhances the radiologist's skill to interpret mammograms. Familiarity with the numerous artifacts encountered while doing mammograms will enable radiologists to provide accurate diagnosis. Technologists should be able to recognize the artifacts and their causes to make corrections immediately and improve mammographic quality.

Artifacts in mammogram can be

- Patient related
- Technologist- and technique-related, including incorrect positioning
- Equipment related.

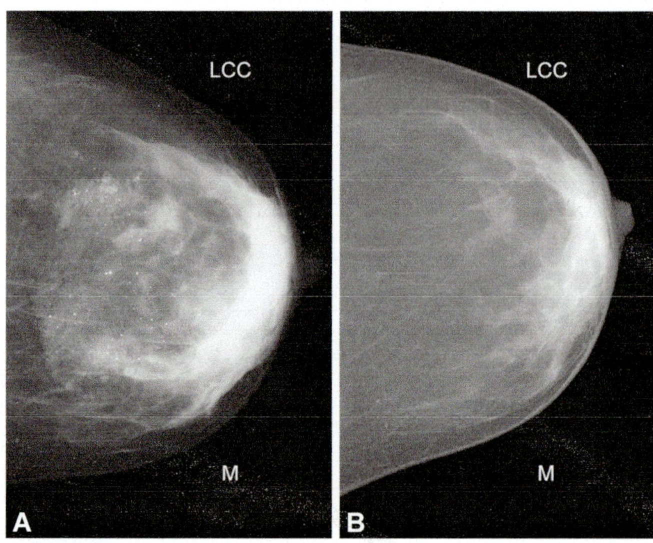

Figs. 13A and B: (A) Mammogram CC view with talcum powder which resembles microcalcifications; (B) Repeat view after cleaning the area appeared normal. (CC: craniocaudal).

Patient Related

The radiographer performing mammography should switch on the light beam during the time of positioning of patient so that overlapping shadows can be avoided.

The patient should be instructed not to apply deodorant or talcum powder before undergoing mammograms as these cause high-density foci resembling calcifications (Figs. 13A and B) because of presence of zinc or magnesium.

Medical devices, scars and nevus on the skin may create pseudomasses; hence, the patient's skin should be examined properly by the technologist. In the elderly patients, skin-fold artifact may be produced because of trapping of loose skin (Fig. 14) in compression paddle. Blurring is produced if the patient moves during compression (Fig. 15). Sometimes, artifacts are noted when the patient comes for a mammogram after an excision biopsy and has bits of adhesive plaster remaining on skin or the technologist does a mammogram without removing dressing from the skin surface (Figs. 16 and 17). The patient's hair should be properly tied as they can also produce artifacts (Figs. 18A and B).

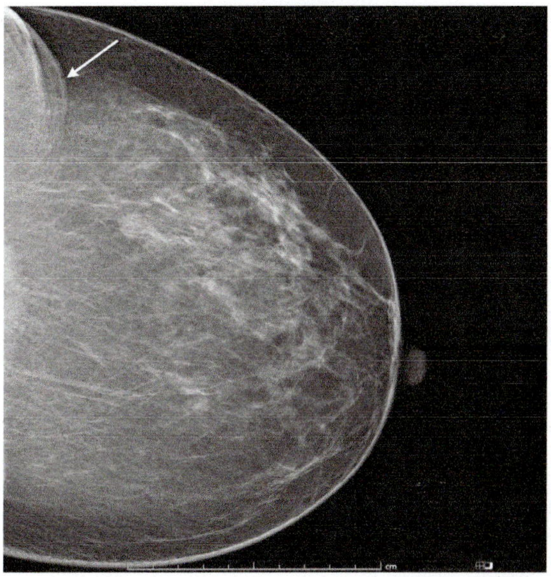

Fig. 14: Mammogram CC view of left breast showing skin fold (arrow). (CC: craniocaudal).

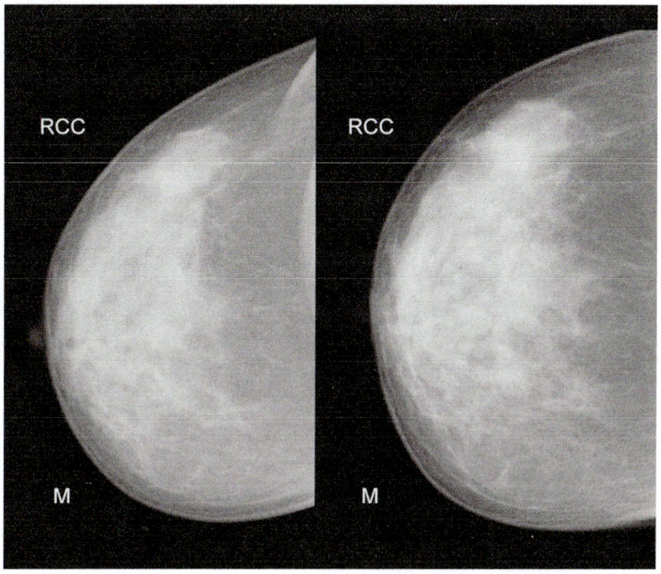

Fig. 15: Mammogram of right breast CC view—image with less compression causing unsharpness that was rectified on repeat view where the image appears sharp. (CC: craniocaudal).

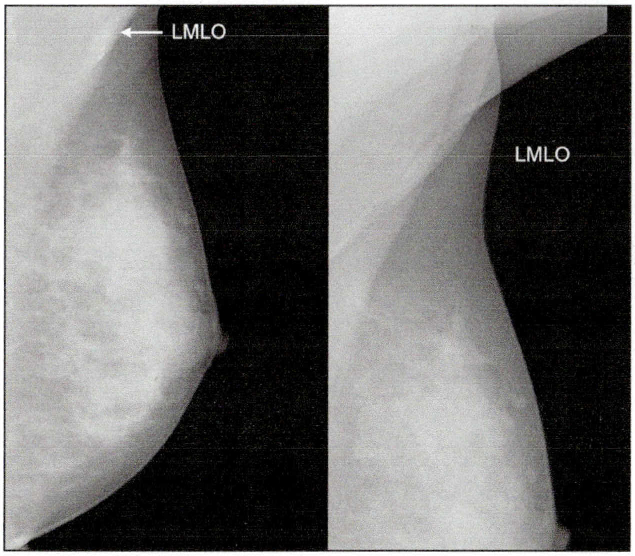

Fig. 16: Mammogram MLO view in a patient who had a lumpectomy for an axillary mass. Mammogram shows a few high-density foci arranged in a linear fashion. On examining the patient clinically, it was found that there were remnants of adhesive plaster. The view was repeated after thorough cleaning of the area. Repeat mammogram was normal. (MLO: mediolateral oblique).

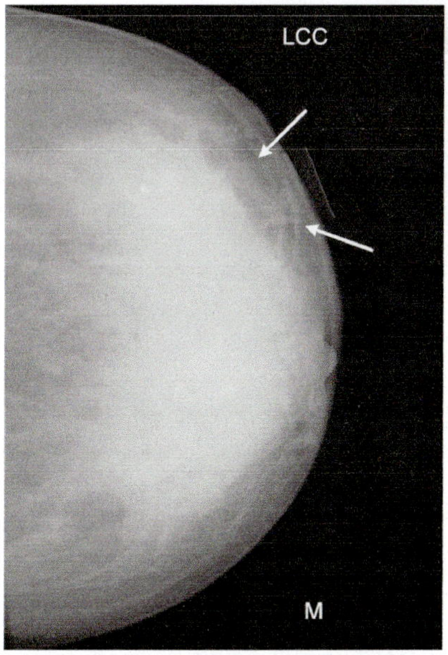

Fig. 17: Mammogram CC view shows a well-defined density (arrows) that was due to a dressing. Please note that the technologist had done the mammogram without removing the dressing. (CC: craniocaudal).

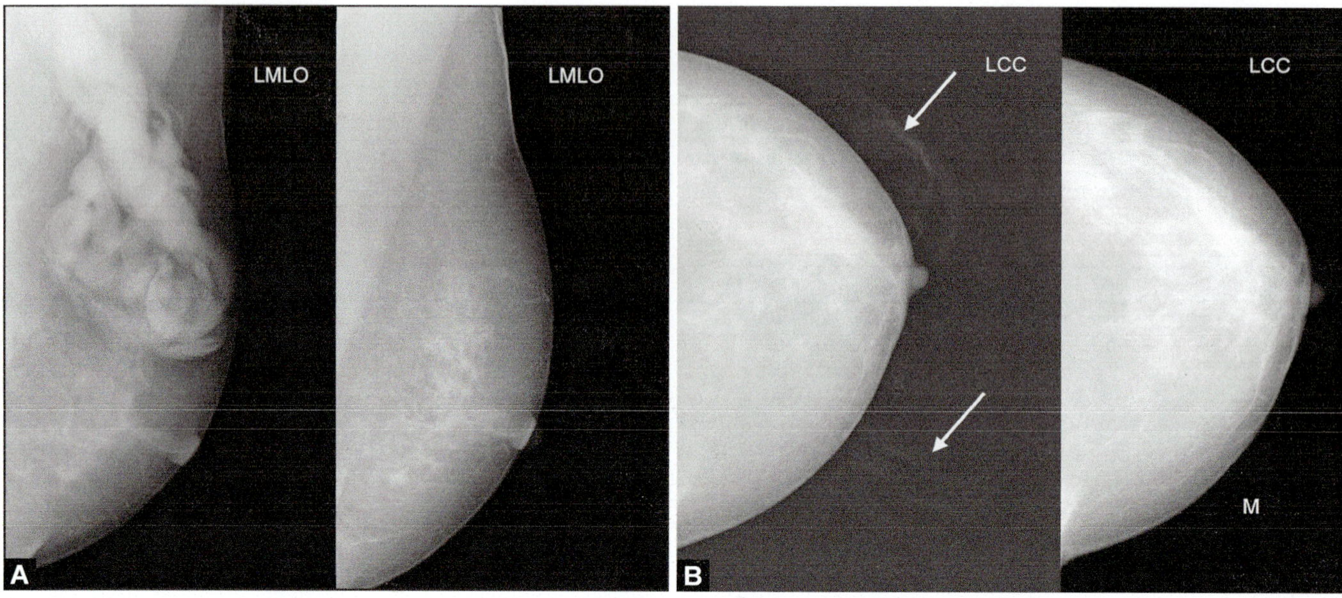

Figs. 18A and B: (A) Mammogram of left breast MLO view shows artifact due to hair (long braided plait) that was rectified on repeat view; (B) Similar artifact due to hair is seen in the CC view faint shadow (arrows). (CC: craniocaudal; MLO: mediolateral oblique).

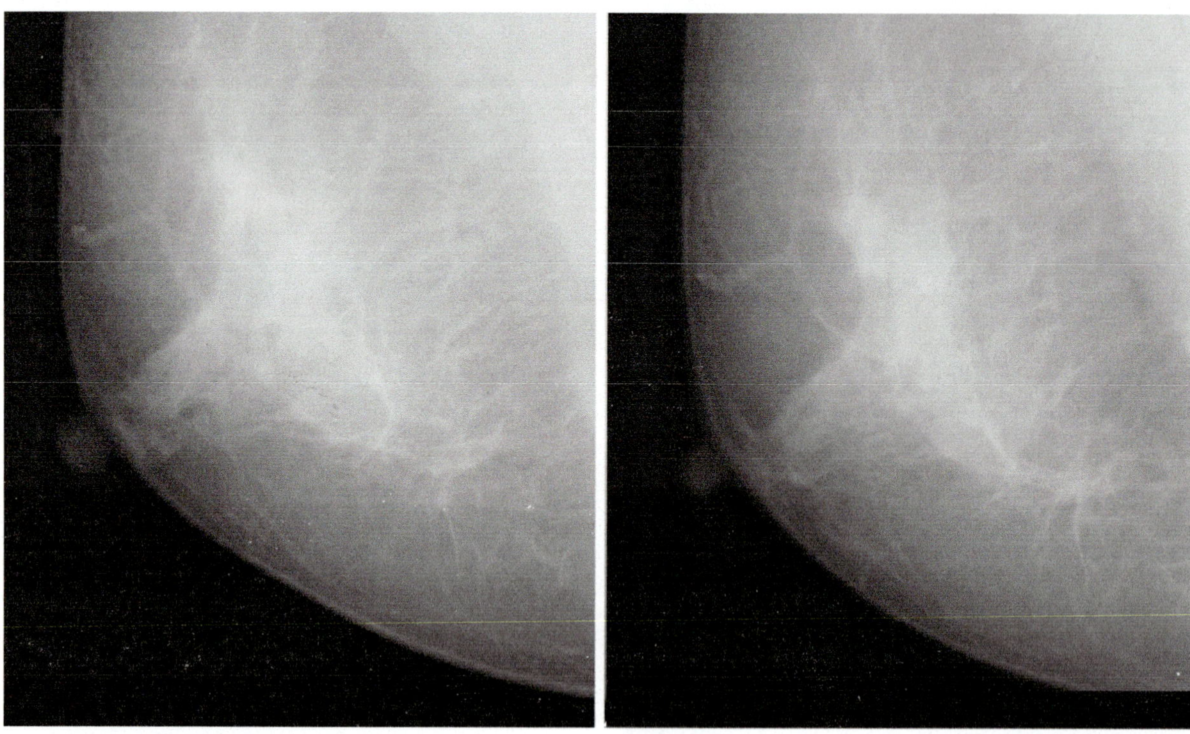

Figs. 19A and B: (A) Artifact due to dust particles on intensifying screen that disappeared on repeat view done after (B) cleaning the screen.

Technologist- and Technique-related

Proper care of the intensifying screens and cassettes should be taken and they must be cleaned at least weekly.

The most common artifacts are dust and dirt on the intensifying screen (Figs. 19A and B) that block the path of light during exposure so that there are white densities seen on the film which resemble calcifications.

Artifacts are also seen due to improper positioning by the technologist (Figs. 20 to 22) or because of sudden movement by the patient. The common artifacts noted are shoulder and chin artifact (Figs. 23 and 24).

Equipment Related

These artifacts may be due to incorrect collimation, incomplete grid motion, bucky failure, wear and tear and compression system failure (Figs. 25A and B; 26 to 30).

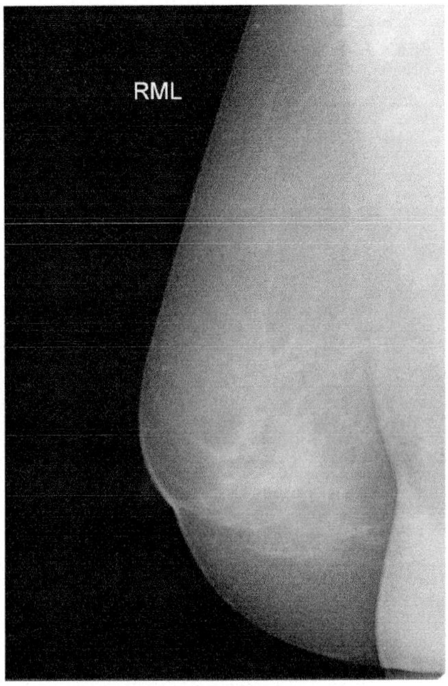

Fig. 20: Mammogram showing abdominal skin fold overlying the breast tissue.

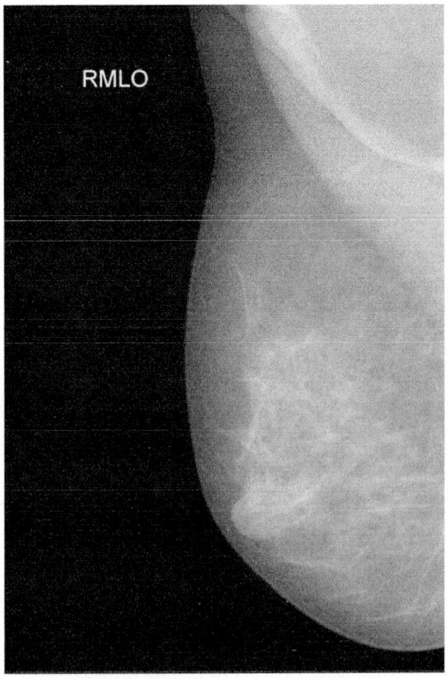

Fig. 21: Mammogram showing nipple en face on MLO. (Please note that nipple should be in profile). (MLO: mediolateral oblique).

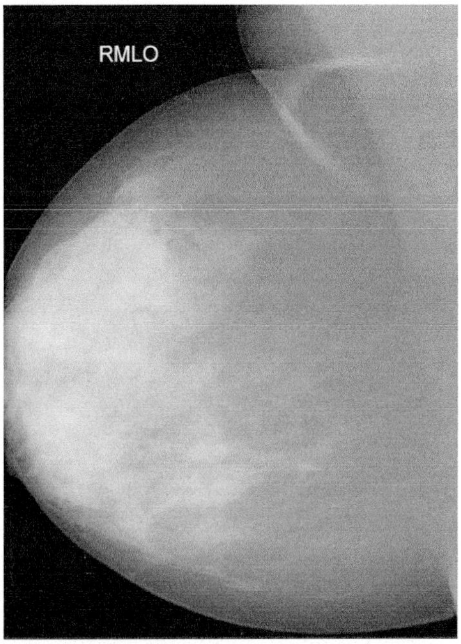

Fig. 22: The anterior portion of the breast is not included in MLO view. (MLO: mediolateral oblique).

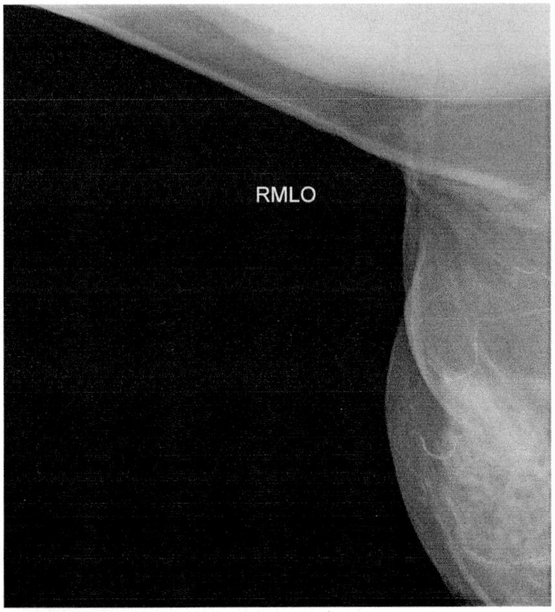

Fig. 23: Artifact due to shoulder on the MLO view due to improper positioning. (MLO: mediolateral oblique).

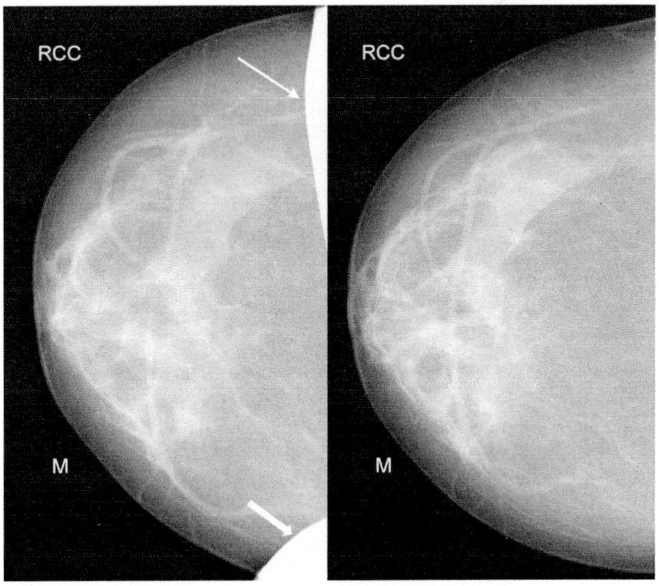

Fig. 24: Mammogram CC view showing chin (thick arrow) and shoulder (thin arrow) artifact due to improper positioning. Repeat view appears normal. (CC: craniocaudal).

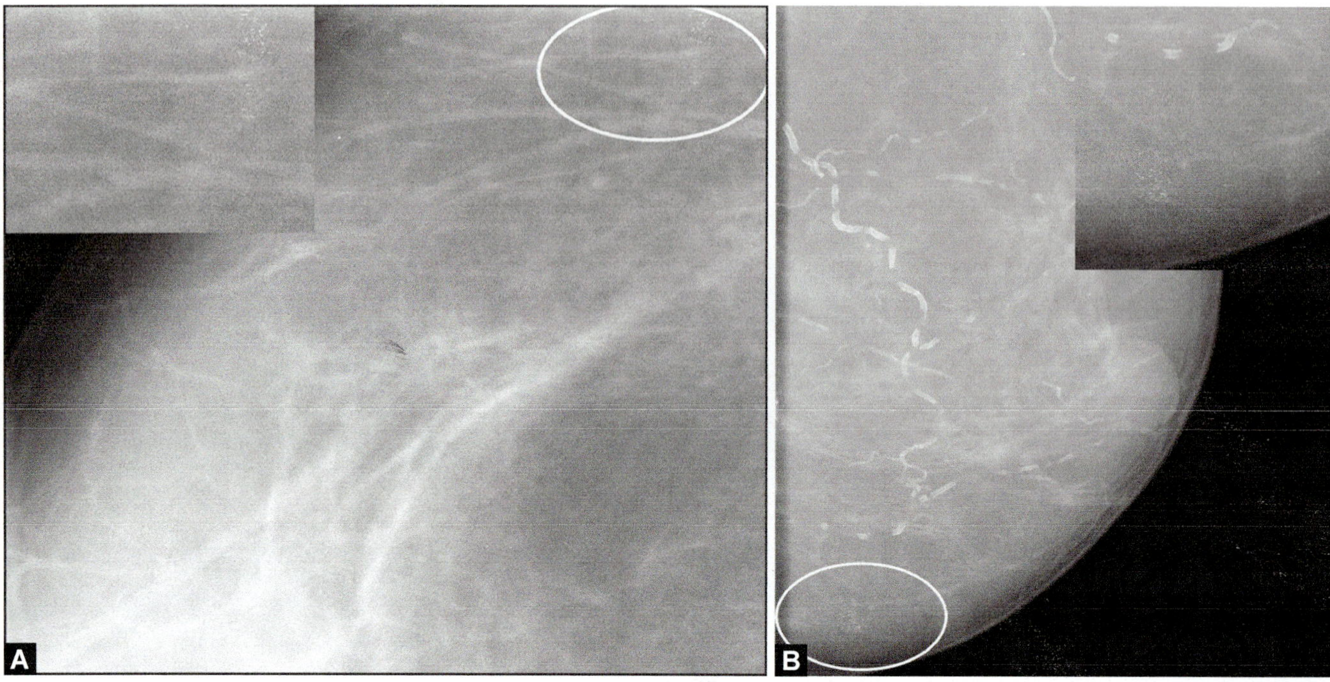

Figs. 25A and B: Artifact due to damaged intensifying screen (inset) which may simulate microcalcifications.

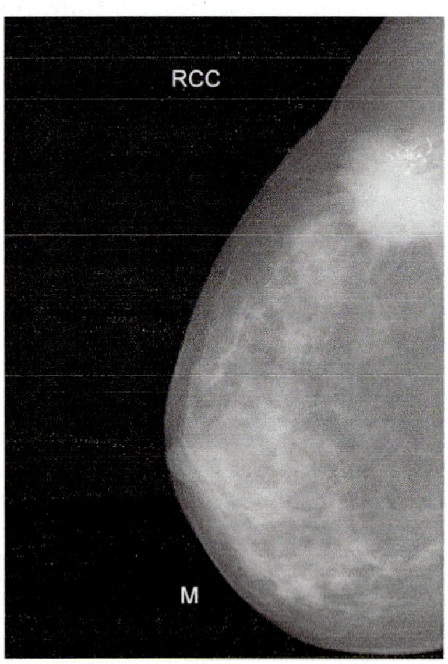

Fig. 26: Mammogram showing digitizer artifact.

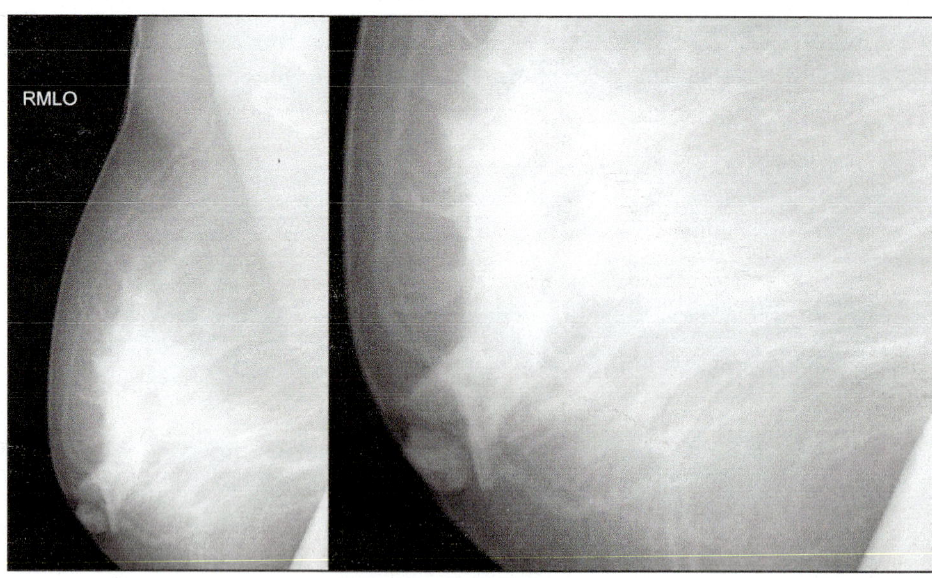

Fig. 27: Artifact due to grid lines is noted on mammogram MLO view.

The artifacts produced by equipment are similar in both analog and digital mammography. In addition laser printer artifact and image display monitor artifact are noted in digital mammography.

The most important factor to be considered in mammography is compression and positioning so that maximum amount of breast tissue is covered and imaged. If this is done properly most of the artifacts will be

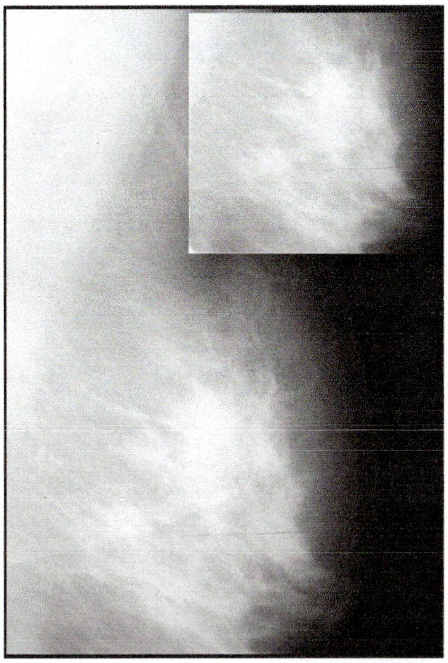

Fig. 28: Line artifact (inset) seen on this mammogram.

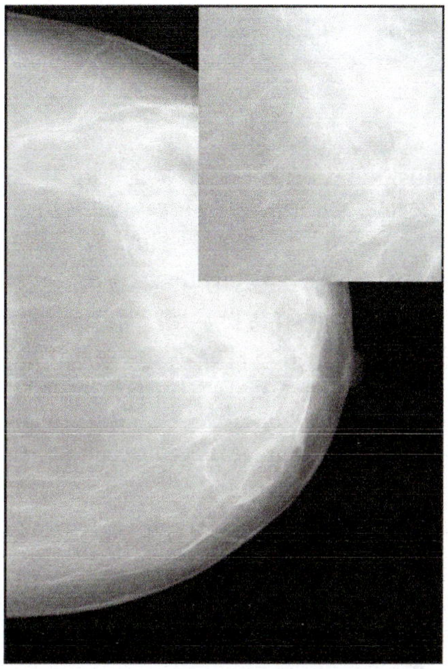

Fig. 29: Mammogram showing roller artifact.

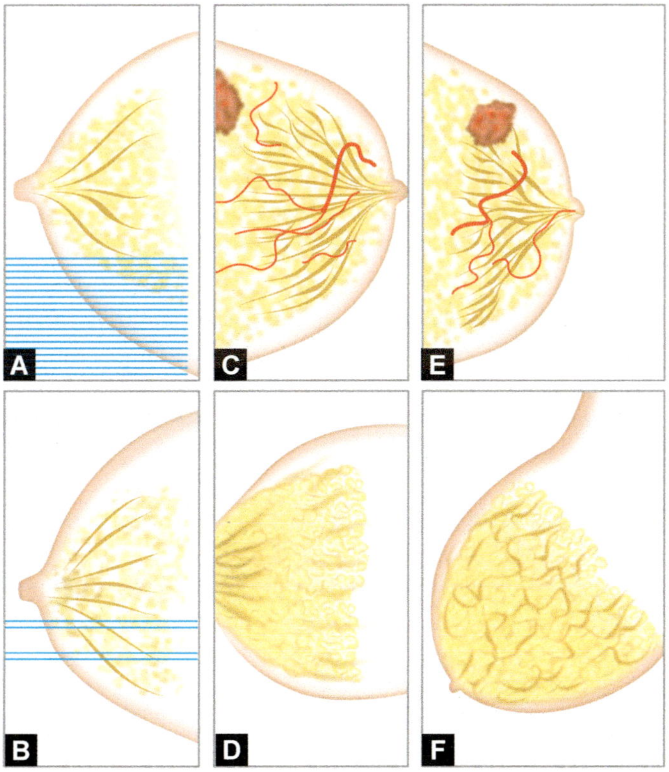

Figs. 30A to F: (A and B) Artifact due to digitizer and faulty rollers; (C to F) Inadequate coverage of breast tissue and breast mass.

removed. Therefore, it is absolutely important to train the radiographers who perform mammography.

REFERENCES

1. Lim GCC, Halimah Y, editors. Second report of the National Cancer Registry. Cancer incidence in Malaysia 2003. Kuala Lumpur: National Cancer Registry; 2004.
2. Faridah Y. Digital versus screen film mammography: a clinical comparison. Biomed Imaging Interv J. 2008; 4(4):e31.
3. Carney PA, Miglioretti DL, Yankaskas BC, et al. Individual and combined effects of age, breast density and hormone replacement therapy use on the accuracy of screening mammography. Ann Intern Med. 2003;138(3):168–75.
4. Pisano ED, Yaffe MJ, Kuzmiak CM, editors. Digital mammography. Philadelphia: Lippincott Williams & Wilkins; 2004.
5. Berns EA, Hendrick RE, Solari M, et al. Digital and screen-film mammography: comparison of image acquisition and interpretation times. AJR Am J Roentgenol. 2006;187(1):38-41.
6. Ranganathan S, Faridah Y, Ng KH. Moving into the digital era: a novel experience with the first full-field digital mammography system in Malaysia. Singapore Med J. 2007;48(9):804-7.
7. Pisano ED, Gatsonis C, Hendrick E, et al. Diagnostic performance of digital versus film mammography for breast-cancer screening. N Engl J Med. 2005;353(17):1773-83

2.2 Quality Assurance in Mammography

INTRODUCTION

Quality assurance (QA) is an integral part of mammography and there are guidance documents for maintaining quality that are available worldwide. These protocols and guidelines are mainly from American College of Radiology (ACR) and European Union Guidelines. They highlight the importance of dose assessment, testing the automatic exposure control (AEC) system[1] and also provide guidance on the frequency of these tests. It is important to remember that reference values and acceptability criteria vary for different protocols.

A lot of these tests are done at the time of installation of the equipment, whereas others are done periodically (yearly, 6 monthly, monthly, weekly or daily). There are reference values given for these as well as pass/fail criteria. As digital mammography is becoming widespread, revised versions of the present protocols will be produced for testing.

WHY IS QUALITY ASSURANCE REQUIRED?

Quality assurance (QA) is required so that subtle changes on mammogram can be seen and easily characterized in order to detect early breast cancers. An optimal QA program should be easy to implement in a clinical setting and adequate equipment for quality testing should be available. It should test various steps of image chain, namely, image acquisition, processing and display. The AEC system testing should be done regularly. The requirement of trained staff including radiographers, physicists and radiologists is mandatory as success of any QA program depends on team work and collaboration. The development of digital mammography in the last decade has led to development of QA tests[2] for digital mammography and has different parameters to be assessed. Mammography auditing plays a relevant role when discussing the quality of breast imaging, whether regarding the radiologist's interpretation or the quality of the images taken.

Stages of Image Chain

The following stages of image chain should be assessed regularly for QA:

Image Quality

Image acquisition: This is a very important component and includes:

- *Testing of X-ray generator and source, AEC system and breast compression system. The tests recommended are:*
  - Alignment of X-ray field and image receptor area
  - Repeatability and accuracy of tube output exposure
  - Half-value layer
  - Compression plate alignment
  - AEC response versus breast thickness and tube voltage compensation
- *Breast dose:* There are recommendations for testing breast dose and the parameter assessed is mean glandular dose. This can be done by different methods including using thermoluminescent dosimeter or phantoms, which varies depending upon protocols.
- *Image receptor:* There are different tests for digital mammography and computed radiography (CR) system.
- *Quality of acquired image:* This addresses the technical and clinical quality criteria using various test objects and phantoms.

For low-contrast image quality assessment, phantoms should be used, which differs between protocols used, for example, ACR phantom is used in USA and Canada.

The ACR phantom is used to test performance of a mammographic system by a quantitative evaluation of the system's ability to image small structures similar to those found clinically. The objects within the phantom simulate calcifications, fibrous calcifications in ducts and tumor masses. The phantom is designed to determine if a mammographic system can detect small structures that are important in the early detection of breast cancer. It helps in ensuring optimum image quality and peak performance of the mammographic system.

Image processing: This follows the recommendations of the manufacturer.

For screen film systems, performance of chemical processor should be assessed (time, temperature, base and fog levels) and artifacts resulting from chemical processing should be tested.

Image display:

Quality assurance for monitors: At least 5-Mega pixel monitors should be used for reading mammograms that provide the highest resolution resulting in better visibility of subtle masses and calcifications. There are recommendations regarding monitor luminance, contrast and lookup tables.

The monitor displays should have the ability to support zooming and panning and to view images in full resolution. QA of the monitors used for mammography should be regulated through each vendor's quality control program, as overseen by appropriate authority. A QA process ensures excellent quality, a good reputation and repeatable results.

Mammography-specific Training for Radiographers

The radiographer should have a basic knowledge of breast anatomy and physiology. In addition, they must be aware of the importance and role of compression while doing a mammogram. They should know the requisites for standard mammographic views and should have knowledge about additional views. A minimum number of examinations should be performed under the direct supervision of a qualified radiographer in order to work as a mammography radiographer.

Therefore, at the end of training, there should be a QA test by radiographer as mentioned above on a regular basis.

Optimal Environment for Reporting

Mammography reporting room: A proper workflow should be established so that a large number of mammograms can be read. The viewing room should have appropriate ambience, optimum lighting conditions and extraneous lights should be avoided as much as possible.

Viewing height: The chair–table combination should be such that the eye level of the radiologist should be at the level of top of the image.

Noise: The room's noise level can be controlled by several means; for example, acoustic tiles on the ceiling and carpets on the floor are used as traditional sound absorbers.

Ambient vicinity lighting: These are placed to illuminate the wall behind the displays to minimize the fatigue associated with looking back and forth between dark and bright.

Utility lighting for cleaning and service: If viewing films on a view box, a bright backlighting is needed in the view box that should be at least double of what is generally used in a standard view box. The edges of films should be masked for optimum visualization of image.

The mammogram images should be mounted in a standard and consistent manner on the view box. The films with mediolateral oblique (MLO) and craniocaudal (CC) view of each breast should be placed back to back as mirror images and the lateral portion in CC view should be placed at the top of the image. If there are two sets of images for comparison then new set of images should be placed on the bottom and older films above in the view box.

In digital mammography or a CR-based system, high-resolution (5 k) monitors are used, in which one can optimize the window width and window level settings. The images are placed and viewed in a similar fashion as when using a view box.

Role of Radiologist

The foremost role of radiologist is to maintain an optimum image quality, ensure proper positioning and take additional views when required which involves talking with the radiographer regarding the need on case to case basis. Substandard imaging should not be accepted and quality should be given utmost priority. The standard descriptors should be used for reporting as approved by ACR and proper recommendations should be advised.

Self-reflection and insights on our radiological practice is essential for improvements in breast cancer diagnosis and treatment. It may incentivize high-quality performance rates for mammography results, despite possible infrastructure and facilities limitations.

QUALITY CONTROL FOR DIGITAL MAMMOGRAPHY

The quality process for digital mammography emphasizes on assessing noise, contrast, spatial resolution and artifacts using a standardized phantom.[3] The phantom approved by the Mammography Quality Standard Act (MQSA) normally contains six fibers, five groups of calcifications and five masses. At least four fibers, three groups of calcification and three masses must be detected. At present, Food and Drug Administration (FDA) requires that specific steps for quality control testing must be those recommended by manufacture. Compression force should be sufficient and there should not be excessive compression.

Daily Quality Control

- *Warming up the machine*: The detector must be warmed for ≥10 min to ensure that detector reaches uniform temperature. Then only calibration should be done
- *Cleaning of workstation monitors*: Ensure that monitor is free of dust or finger prints.

Weekly Quality Control

- *Flat-field test*: This should be done to test detection function. There are five parameters that have to be tested in this—brightness non-uniformity, high-frequency modulation, SNR (signal-to-noise ratio) uniformity, bad region of interest (ROI) and bad pixel verification. If the detector does not pass these tests, then equipment recommendations should be followed to correct the abnormality
- *Phantom test*: This is done to check the performance of system by testing its ability to image small structures. This also helps in assessing artifacts
- *Contrast-to-noise (CNR) ratio*: This test is the ability of detector to distinguish between objects in image and image noise
- *Modulation transfer function (MTF)*: This measures the image sharpness and contrast delivered by detector
- *View box and viewing condition test*: This is to ensure good image viewing conditions.

Monthly Quality Control

- *Automatic optimization of parameter*: This tests the correct choice of parameters
- *SNR*: To test the correct level of SNR in image.

Semiannual Quality Control

Compression force: Compression should be adequate and not excessive. This is performed during installation and semiannually. Adequate compression ensures reduced motion artifacts, reduced scatter, improved X-ray penetration and reduced dose.

In conclusion, quality standards should be adopted to ensure that key goals of mammography are achieved. To implement a mammography/QA program, one has to select and prioritize the tests depending on available technology, expertise, resources and the relevance of the tests to local practices. A key factor to promote the success of a QA program for mammography is teamwork and the collaboration of all key staff (e.g. radiographers, radiologists, medical physicists and healthcare managers). There should be regular and continuous training and feedback mechanisms to improve the testing procedures and strengthen the outcomes of the program.[3]

REFERENCES

1. Reis C, Pascoal A, Sakellaris T, Koutalonis M. Quality assurance and quality control in mammography: a review of available guidance worldwide. Insights Imaging, 2013;4(5):539-53.
2. Marshall NW, Mackenzie AHI. Quality control measurements for digital X-ray detectors. Phys Med Biol. 2011;56:979-99.
3. Jayadevan R, Julie Armada M, Shaheen R, Mulcahy C, Slanetz P. Optimizing digital mammography image quality for full field digital detectors: artifacts encountered during QA process. Radiographics. 2015;35:2080-9.

2.3 Approach to Reading a Mammogram

INTRODUCTION

It is very important to adopt an organized and systematic approach while reading a mammogram as it influences the quality of reporting and final outcome. This involves a proper understanding of all aspects of breast imaging, a sharp observation, judicious use of additional views as and when required and use of appropriate descriptors. Finally the findings should be conveyed to the clinician in a comprehensive manner. The process starts right from quality control and image processing in the initial stages to recommendations and follow up in the later stage.

Screening mammogram done to detect cancer in asymptomatic women. The literal meaning of the word "screening" is sifting or filtering that requires a threshold. Mammography is used as a screening tool worldwide as it can detect small early stage cancers. Since detection must precede diagnosis hence, till such a time that preventive measures are discovered and improvement in therapies reach larger populations, mammography will continue to reduce mortality by early detection. For mammography to be effective, high-quality mammograms done by trained technologists and interpreted by experienced radiologists are needed to detect early cancers. Double reading is recommended in a screening setup to increase accuracy.

Diagnostic mammograms done in symptomatic patients, who present with positive clinical findings where mammogram can show features that may represent a benign or a malignant pathology. Sometimes even palpable abnormalities are not well visualized on standard mammographic views and specialized views have to be done to see the finding in question.

Clinical history: A detailed clinical history is required while reporting mammogram. The clinical details and relevant patient information can be recorded in a format in the request form for mammography as shown below:

- Age
- presenting complaints:
  - Pain/lump in breast/nipple discharge/skin puckering or thickening/axillary lump
  - Side: right/left
- Were any previous mammogram done? Yes/No. If yes, give details
- Personal history of breast cancer: Yes/No

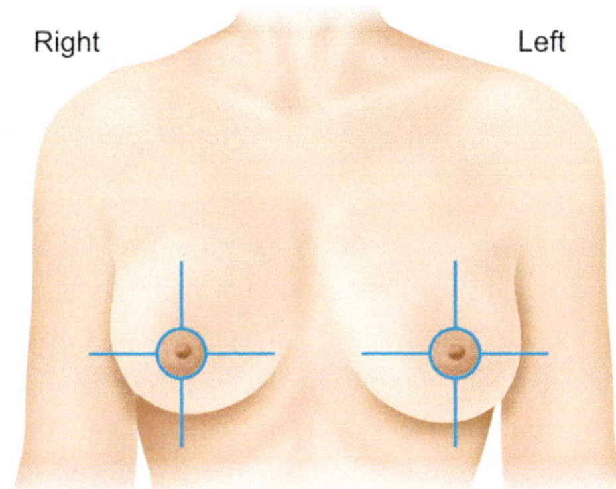

Fig. 1: Marking for presence of breast lump.

- Previous history of breast biopsy/breast surgery? Yes/No
  - If yes, Side: right/left
- History of radiation therapy to chest? Yes/No
- Hormone replacement therapy: Yes/No
- Family history of breast cancer in first degree relatives: Yes/No
  - If yes: Mother/sister/daughter/grandmother/aunt
- Breast implants: Yes/No
- If breast lump is present, please mark it in the diagram given in Figure 1.

SYSTEMATIC READING OF MAMMOGRAM

A standard viewing scheme should be followed step by step:

1. Check the identification of patient and labeling.
2. Mount the films on view box as mirror images with the chest wall side of breast against each other and labels on top of images. In the case of images displayed on PACS monitors, arrange them back to back so that mirror images can be seen properly.
3. Ensure that the positioning of the standard mammographic views is correct as per the criteria, breast compression is adequate, all the breast tissue is included and there are no artifacts.
4. There are five specific tasks to be done while reading a mammogram:
   a. Detection
   b. Verification
   c. Triangulation
   d. Identification
   e. Management.

DETECTION

- The images on both sides should be compared area by area to detect asymmetric densities, architectural distortion, mass and microcalcifications. Masking can be used in both horizontal and oblique directions to enhance perception of subtle findings. Asymmetry can be appreciated better when seen from a distance
- Whether the asymmetry is real or not, can be confirmed by (1) looking at two standard projections and (2) by comparing with previous study if available. If doubts persist, take a spot compression view to confirm that asymmetry is real or due to summation. Pay special attention if it is a developing asymmetry and do additional imaging to confirm it.
- *Skin and nipple areolar region*: Look at this region for skin thickening or nipple retraction. In a normal mammogram, skin is smooth and measures approximately 2–3 mm in thickness
- *Retroareolar region*: This area should be looked at carefully as it is often not compressed adequately and there is superimposition of ducts, vessels and fibrous tissue here. Since there is a rich network of lymphatics in this region, lymphatic spread is faster if mass is located here
- *Retroglandular tissue*: Always look at the gland-fat interface and the edge of the glandular tissue properly. It is important to remember that this edge should be concave. There should **not be any convex bulge or pulling in of tissue (tent sign)** (Fig. 2). If tenting is seen (Fig. 3), spot compression views should be done to look for underlying malignancy
- *Areas requiring special attention*: In breast imaging, forbidden, check or review areas are zones that according to Tabár, require special attention as shown below:[1]
  On craniocaudal view (Fig. 4):

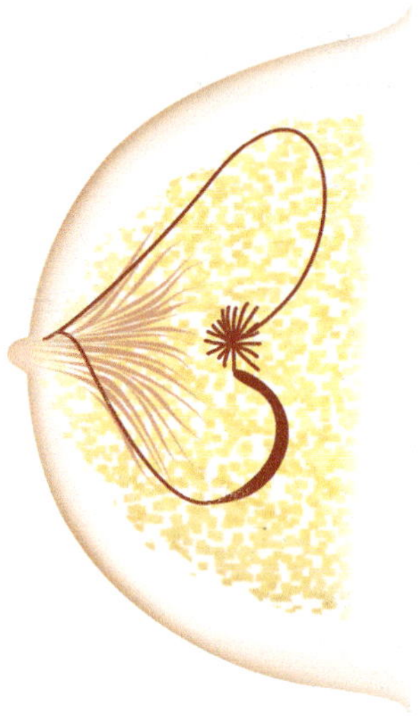

Fig. 3: If convex bulge or tent sign is seen, then additional views like spot compression views should be done to look for underlying malignancy.

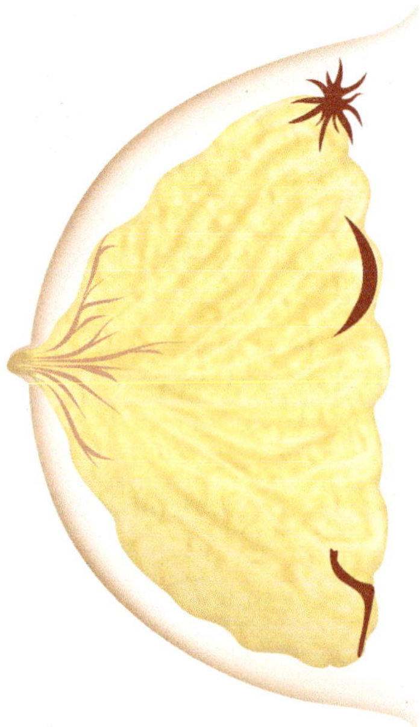

Fig. 2: Convex bulge and tent sign that are indirect signs of malignancy.

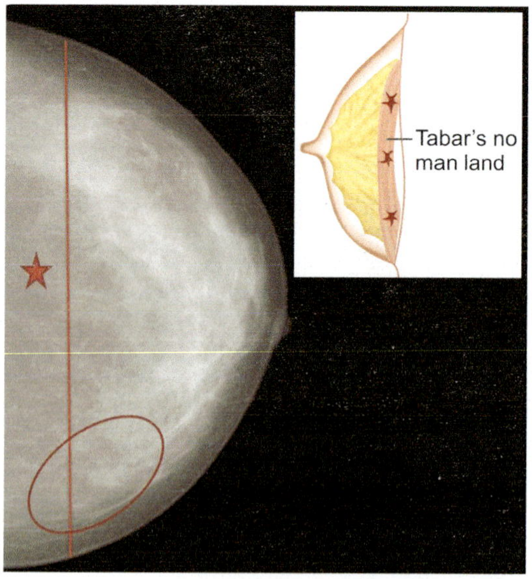

Fig. 4: Mammogram—CC view showing area requiring special attention, medial portion of breast (marked as red oval) and Tabár's no man land (inset) which is a strip of tissue in the retroglandular space (star). (CC: craniocaudal).

- The medial half of the breast
- "No man's land" (the retroglandular space) at the back of the breast behind the glandular tissue

On MLO view (Fig. 5):

- The "milky way" (retromammary fat): a 3-4 cm wide band parallel to edge of pectoral muscle
- Retroareolar region.

Asymmetric densities in these areas require special attention.

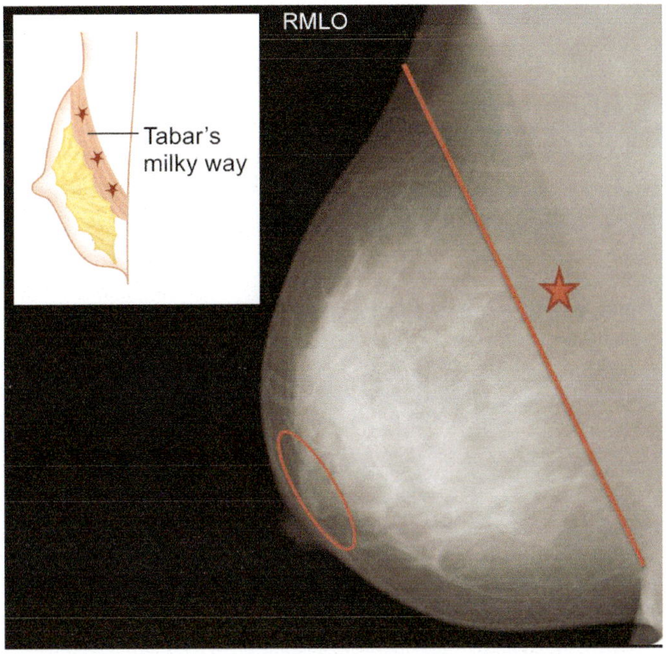

Fig. 5: Mammogram—MLO view showing retroareolar region (oval marked in red) and Tabár's milky way (inset) that is a wide 3–4 cm band parallel to pectoralis muscle (star). (MLO: mediolateral oblique).

VERIFICATION

The definition "forbidden areas" is based on the incidence and distribution of cancer or interval cancers identified in screening with clusters in the tail and inframammary fold on the MLO view and centrally and medial portions of the breast on CC view.

- *Calcifications*: Magnification views should be done if microcalcifications are present. They should be characterized according to their location, size, number, distribution and heterogeneity
- Comparison with previous mammogram films if available has to be done to check for developing new densities or to look for progressive changes
- If a mass is seen, it should be verified that it is a real three-dimensional structure by looking at the two views or by using triangulation method its location should be confirmed.

TRIANGULATION METHOD

Triangulation is a technique to determine if a questionable density is genuine or due to superimposition of structures.

For this, CC, MLO and lateral views should be taken for the side in question and should be put in the same order on viewing monitors (Figs. 6A and B).

Ensure that nipple on each view must be at the same level.

Using a measuring tool, one end of the scale should be put over the mass on the 90° lateral view, bringing it over the mass on the MLO view. Once kept in this way, one can find out the likely position of mass on CC view.

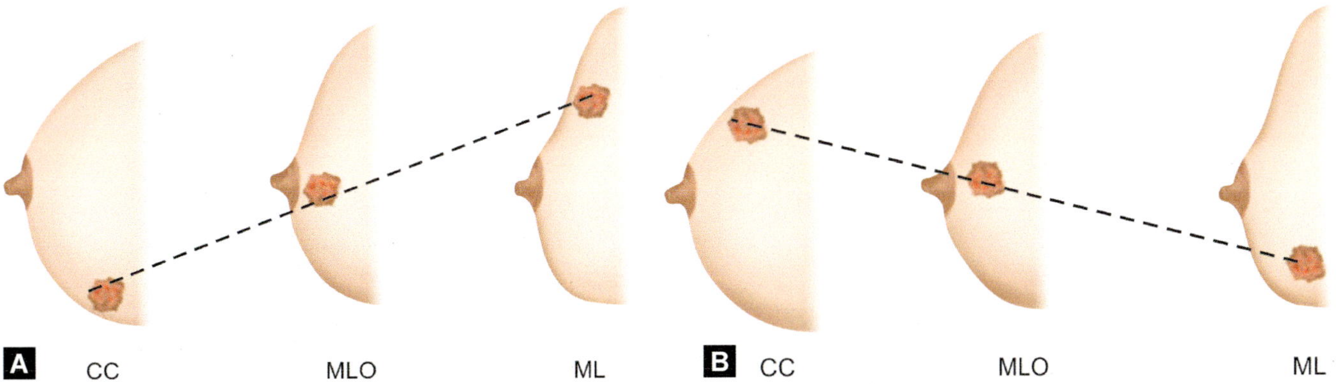

Figs. 6A and B: Triangulation method to localize position of mass on CC view based on movement of mass on MLO and lateral views. (CC: craniocaudal; MLO: mediolateral oblique; ML: mediolateral).

Interpretation

If the mass moves down on the lateral film or is located lower than it was on the MLO film, the lesion is in the lateral aspect of the breast.

If the mass moves up relative to the nipple or is located higher than it was on the MLO film, the lesion is in the medial aspect of the breast.

If no significant change in the location is noted, then the finding must be located in the central aspect of the breast.

Identification

Once a mass is localized, it should be assessed for its shape, margins, density using appropriate descriptors with mention of other associated features like architectural distortion, calcification, axillary lymph nodes etc. Using all these descriptors, it should be categorized into the assigned BI-RADS (Breast Imaging-Reporting and Data System) categories by ACR.

Management

Since most radiologists in India currently follow the BI-RADS reporting system by ACR, management recommendations are also according to BI-RADS.

In the next chapter, BI-RADS descriptors that are used for describing masses, asymmetry, architectural distortion and calcification are described in detail along with BI-RADS classification and recommendations for management.

REFERENCE

1. Kopans DB. A systematic approach to breast imaging. 3rd ed. Lippincott William and Wilkins; 2007. pp. 323-41 a Wolters Kluwer business.

2.4 The Breast imaging-reporting and Data System (BI-RADS) Classification

INTRODUCTION

The American College of Radiology (ACR) Breast Imaging Reporting and Data System (BI-RADS) lexicon was developed in 1993 with an aim to standardize breast imaging reports and improve communication with referring physicians. The fifth edition of the ACR BI-RADS lexicon was released in February 2014 and is currently followed by radiologists. During this revision, there were various additions and deletions and introduction of new terminologies to avoid ambiguity. Most importantly, these descriptors are helpful in speaking a common language in order to write a structured report and suggest further recommendations. As everyone reporting mammograms is aware, there is a steep learning curve for reporting and interpreting mammograms, one learns with experience and improves with regular follow up and audit of one's own cases.

BI-RADS lexicon: These are descriptors that are used to predict both benign and malignant lesions and eliminate ambiguity. In spite of using this lexicon, there is still interobserver variation depending upon the experience and expertise of the radiologist. With the use of patterned approach in reading mammograms, use of structured reporting and appropriate training this gap should get bridged slowly.

It is important to keep in mind that the most appropriate descriptors should be used while describing the findings so that its meaning is conveyed well to both fellow radiologists and treating clinicians.

Breast density: A varying amount of fatty and fibroglandular tissue is present in the breast and its proportion varies depending upon the age of patient. In the younger age group, there is increased breast density because of more fibroglandular tissue. As age advances, it is replaced by fatty tissue hence breast in an elderly woman appears entirely fatty.

According to ACR 2013, version 5, breast composition is characterized in Table 1 and Figures 1A to D.

Table 1: Categorization of breast density according to ACR.

Category	*Composition of breast*
A	The breasts are almost entirely fatty
B	Scattered areas of fibroglandular tissue
C	Heterogeneously dense tissue which may obscure small masses
D	Extremely dense breast which lowers the sensitivity of mammography

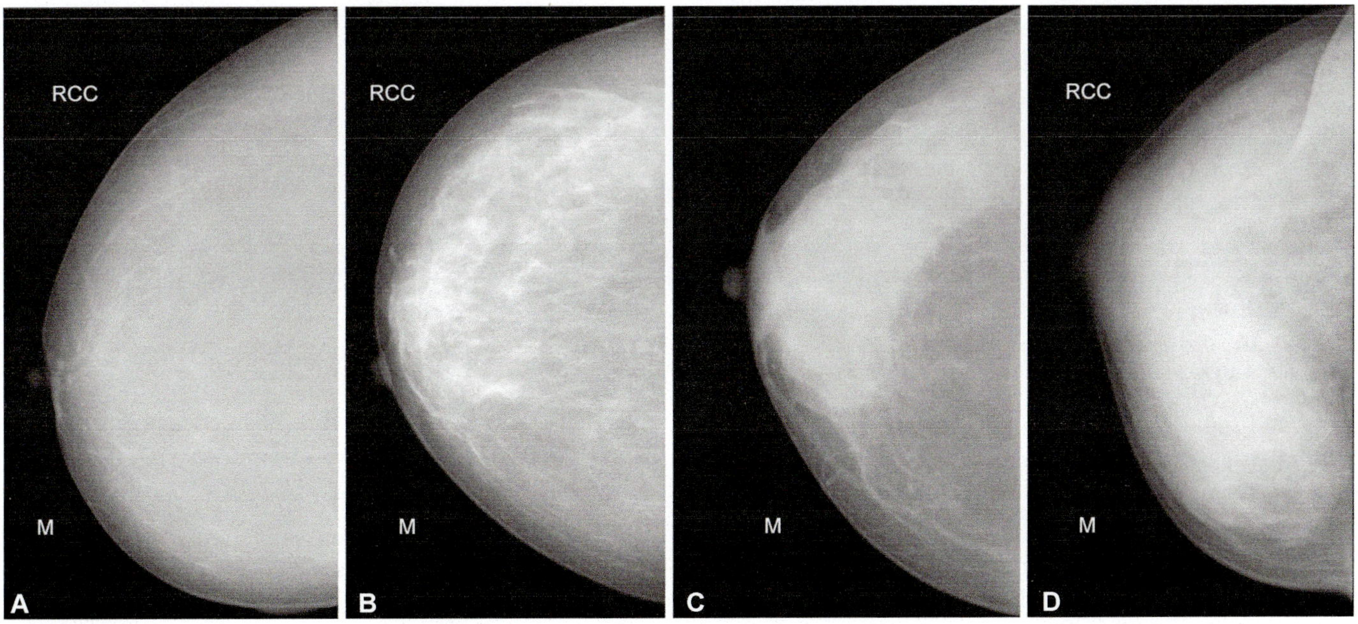

Figs. 1A to D: Mammogram images showing categorization of breast density as per ACR. (A) Almost entirely fatty breast; (B) Scattered areas of fibroglandular tissue; (C) Heterogeneously dense breast tissue that may obscure small masses; (D) Extremely dense breast that lowers the sensitivity of mammography.

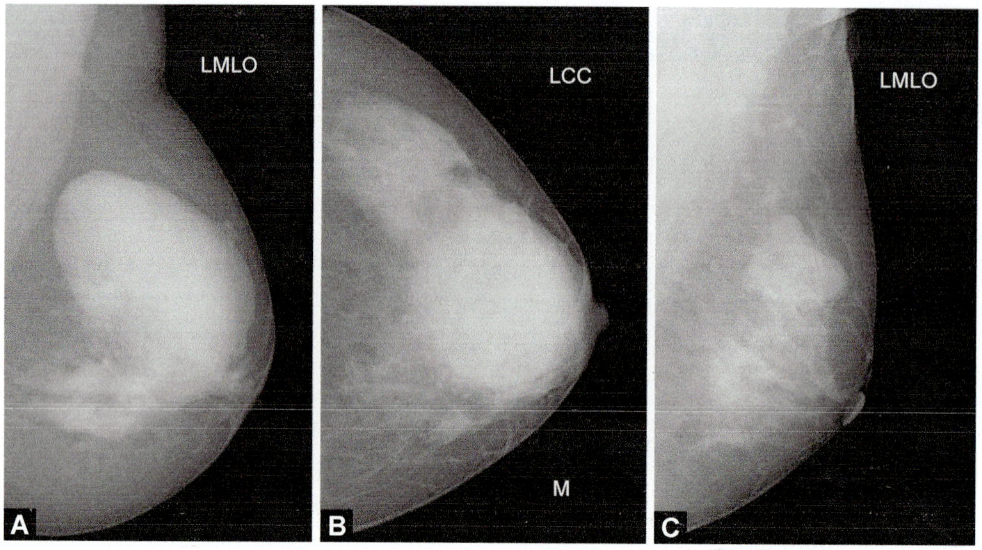

Figs. 2A to C: Mammogram showing shape of mass described as oval, round, or with two to three lobulations.

There is influence of hormones too and therefore a woman who has been started on hormone replacement therapy (HRT) shows an increase in breast density as compared to her previous mammograms prior to HRT.

BI-RADS lexicon uses the following descriptors:

1. **Mass:** It is a space occupying three-dimensional lesion that is seen in two different projections. If an abnormality/potential mass is seen in only a single projection it should be called an "asymmetry" until its three dimensionality is confirmed. Once it is determined that finding is a potentially concerning mass, its location should be established and categorization done based on level of suspicion
   a. ***Shape:*** The shape of mass is described as oval, round, lobulated (2 or 3 gentle lobulations) or irregular (Figs. 2A to C).
   b. ***Margins:*** The margins are described as circumscribed, obscured, microlobulated, indistinct and spiculated ranging from least suspicious to the most suspicious (Figs. 3 and 4).

Circumscribed margin: It can be seen in both benign and malignant masses though are more common in benign masses. The risk of malignancy for circumscribed lesions is categorized as probably benign (i.e. BI-RADS 3) is <2%.[1]

Circumscribed carcinomas are relatively less frequently seen than spiculated ones and these include medullary, papillary and mucinous carcinoma. It is important to look at the margins of the mass closely as sometimes, there may be a comet tail projection or a mild flattening in a small portion that can give a clue to the diagnosis. A compression view may be helpful in demonstrating it better, thereby increasing the confidence level.

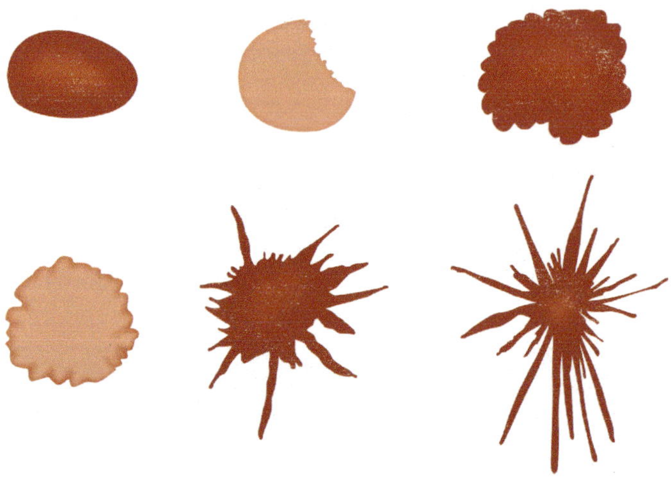

Fig. 3: Various margins commonly seen in breast masses.

Obscured margins: A portion of the margin is not seen clearly and may be silhouetted because of surrounding dense fibroglandular tissue or because of infiltration of malignancy into the normal parenchyma. Here again compression view can be helpful.

Microlobulated: These masses show closely placed undulations (1–2 mm) throughout the contour of the mass unlike the gentle undulations seen in benign masses. As mentioned earlier, it is possible that these are seen only in one portion and not the entire mass but **characterization should be done based on the most**

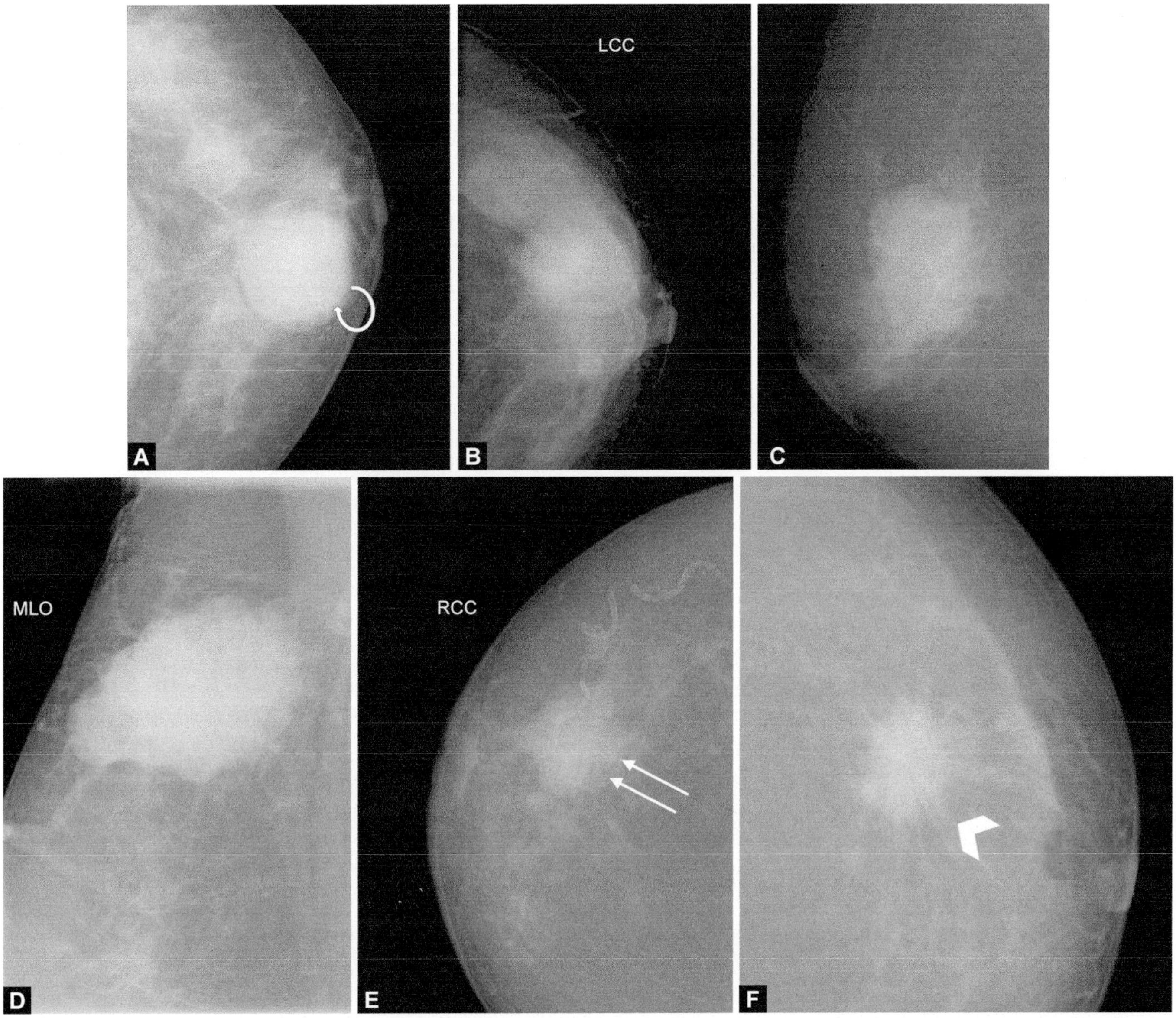

Figs. 4A to F: Mammogram showing margins of breast masses: (A) Circumscribed; (B) Obscured; (C) Indistinct; (D) Microlobulated; (E) Irregular; (F) Spiculated.

suspicious findings. Magnification view may be helpful to ascertain these as and when required in order to categorize the masses and suggest recommendations.

Indistinct: Indistinct margins are fairly suspicious because they indicate that there may be infiltration of the mass in the surrounding fibroglandular tissue.

Spiculated: Spiculated margins are seen as fine white lines radiating out from the borders of the mass and are due to dense fibrosis or desmoplastic reaction around the mass with growth and infiltration into the surrounding tissue.

A mass may have both circumscribed and obscured margins or a combination of the above-described margins. It is important to remember that in such cases, the decision has to be taken **based on the most suspicious findings**.

c. ***Density:*** The density of mass is divided into high, equal (Fig. 5), low or fat-containing (Fig 6A). In many cases, it cannot be reliably used to differentiate between benign and malignant masses. A malignant mass may have a high, equal, or low density though there are studies in literature where high-density mass is significantly

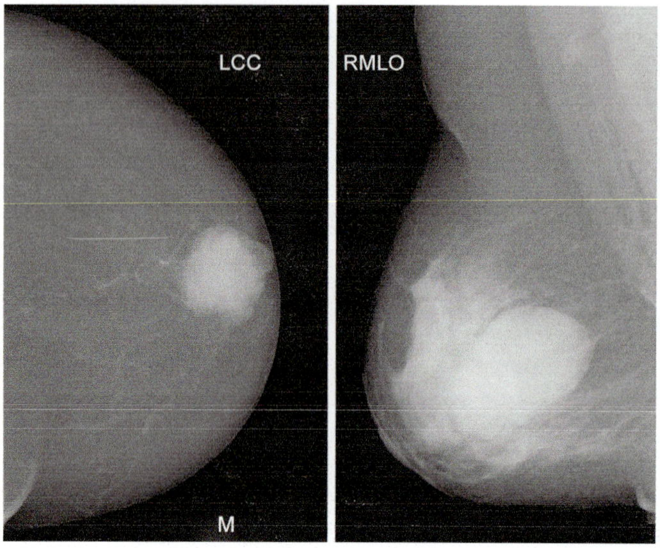

Fig. 5: Mammogram showing high and equal density masses in two different patients.

associated with malignancy in both retrospectively and prospectively assessed data sets, with moderate prospective-retrospective agreement.[2]

Benign masses like fibroadenoma commonly show equal density, while cysts may show an equal or low density with a partial or complete lucent halo around it. Amongst the malignancies, mucinous carcinomas show a low density.

Fat containing masses are definitely benign and do not require biopsy for confirmation. These include lipomas, hamartomas, fat necrosis (Fig 6 A) and galactoceles.

Lipomas are benign fat containing masses and are sometimes difficult to distinguish from normal fatty tissue especially if the breast is lumpy. They are slow growing masses and are more commonly seen in postmenopausal women. They have a thin fibrous pseudocapsule surrounding the mass that may require a spot compression magnification view to be demonstrated.

Fibroadenolipomas or hamartomas are due to benign proliferation of fibrous, glandular and fatty tissue in different proportions. They are also described as having a "Breast within a breast appearance." On mammogram, they are seen as well-circumscribed mixed density masses surrounded by a thin capsule though at times it is not well visualized.

Fat necrosis is commonly seen as small well-circumscribed lucent mass with a rim calcification in post-traumatic breast or in patients with history of breast conservative surgery.

Galactoceles (Fig. 6D) are fat-containing masses with a recent history of lactation. These are basically retention cysts resulting from lactiferous duct occlusion and on biochemical analysis show proteins, fat and lactose. The natural history of galactocele is spontaneous resolution. Its appearances on mammogram may be variable where it may be seen as multiple fat containing masses or cystic masses showing a fat-fluid level. In its acute phase, it is anechoic on ultrasound and water density mass may be seen on mammogram. When it appears hyperechoic or solid appearing on ultrasound, mixed fat and water

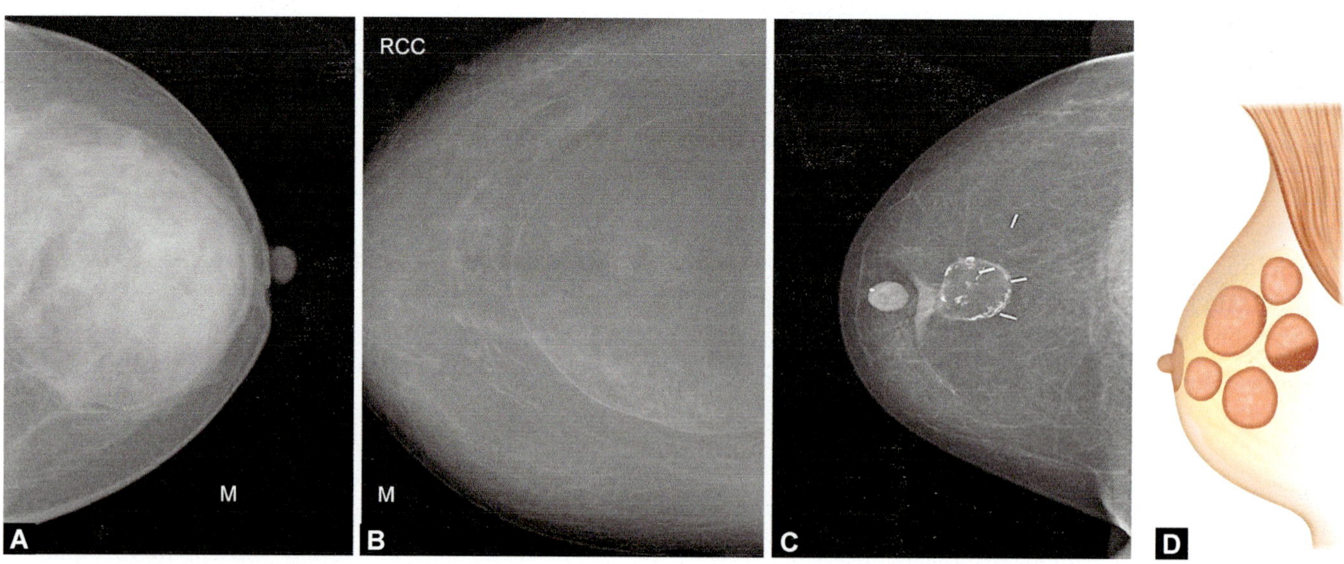

Figs. 6A-D: Masses with fat density: (A) hamartoma; (B) lipoma; and (C) fat necrosis on mammograms; (D) different appearances of galactocele on pictograph where they are seen as well circumscribed, round to oval fat density masses sometimes showing fat fluid levels.

density masses are seen on mammogram. As galactoceles become chronic, there is curdling of milk and formation of fat fluid level. Aspiration of galactocele reveals milky fluid.

2. **Calcifications:** These are classified based on their morphology (Table 2) and distribution. In the fifth version of BI-RADS, calcifications are consolidated into two categories: typically benign and suspicious morphology (Figs. 7 and 8). In the "typically benign" category, eggshell and lucent-centered calcifications have been combined into a new term " rim," while round and punctate calcifications are combined into the term "round."[3]

Amorphous, coarse heterogeneous, fine pleomorphic and fine linear or fine linear branching calcifications are now placed in the "suspicious morphology" category.

Table 2: Calcifications based on morphology.

Typically benign	*Suspicious*
Skin calcification	Amorphous
Vascular calcification	Coarse heterogeneous
Coarse or popcorn like	
Large rod like	Fine pleomorphic
Round (includes punctate and round)	Fine linear
Rim (includes lucent centered and egg shell)	
Dystrophic	
Milk of calcium	
Sutural	

According to distribution, the calcifications are categorized into diffuse, regional, grouped, linear and segmental.

(Calcification is dealt in detail in chapter on breast calcifications)

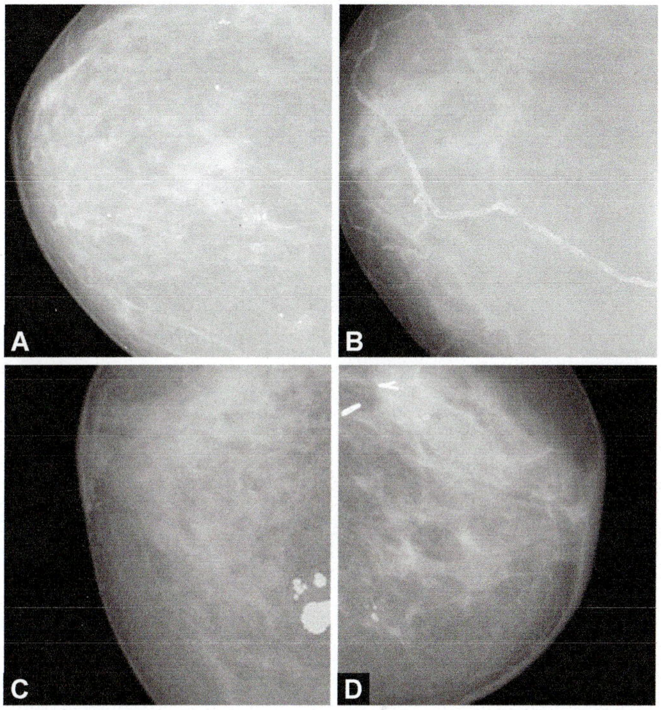

Figs. 7A to D: Benign calcifications seen on mammogram: (A) Secretory; (B) Vascular; (C) Involuting fibroadenoma; (D) Dystrophic. Calcifications are at the operative site in a conservatively treated breast.

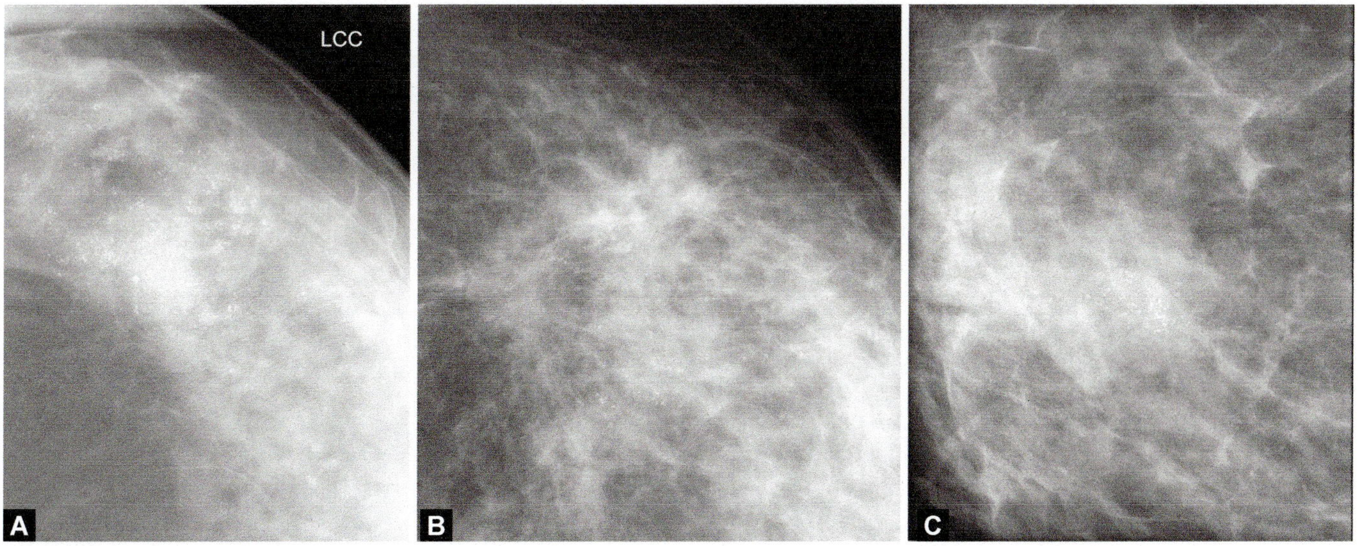

Figs. 8A to C: Coarse heterogeneous (A); Fine pleomorphic (B and C).

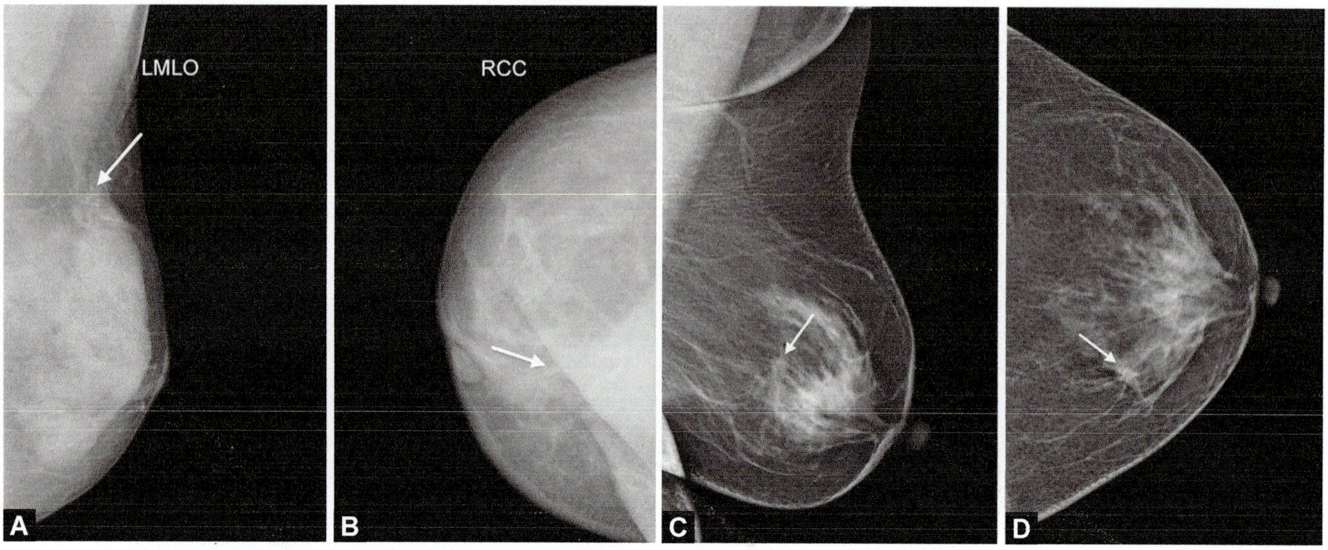

Figs. 9A to D: Mammogram showing (A) Architectural distortion in a patient who underwent breast conservative therapy; (B) Architectural distortion in a patient who underwent lumpectomy with wide local excision; (C and D) Mammogram CC and MLO view showing small spiculated mass with architectural distortion that was proved to be malignant on histopathology. (CC: craniocaudal; MLO: mediolateral oblique).

3. **Architectural distortion:** The term architectural distortion is used when the normal architecture is distorted but there is no definite mass. The causes of architectural distortion include malignancy, post-surgical or post-traumatic changes and radial scar. (Figs. 9A to D).

   On mammogram, it may be seen as thin straight lines or spiculations radiating from a point or as focal retraction/distortion or straightening at the edges of the parenchyma without any obvious mass. It is important to take additional views like compression views to confirm the findings.
4. **Asymmetries:** Asymmetry is different from a mass and should not be confused with it. The most common cause of asymmetry is superimposition of normal breast tissue because of summation. It is seen on one view only and normally disappears on repeat views (Fig. 10A).

A focal asymmetry (Fig. 10B) is visible on two projections and therefore is a real finding rather than superimposition and has to be differentiated from a mass. Spot compression on craniocaudal (CC) or mediolateral oblique (MLO) view helps in its delineation.

Global asymmetry consists of an asymmetry involving at least one quarter of the breast and is usually a normal variant.

Developing asymmetries are new and larger densities that are more conspicuous when compared to previous mammography examinations (Fig. 10C). These are important and have to be further assessed as they are suspicious for malignancy.

SPECIAL CASES

Intramammary lymph node: It is seen as a well circumscribed oval mass with lucent fatty hilum on the mammograms (Fig. 11).

Skin lesions: These can be demonstrated by a BB marker or by a tangential view (Fig. 12).

Solitary dilated duct: As a linear opacity in the subareolar region and may be due to an intraductal papilloma.

Associated features: These are skin retraction, nipple retraction, skin thickening, trabecular thickening, axillary lymphadenopathy, architectural distortion and calcifications (Figs. 13 to 15).

Location of lesion: The laterality, quadrant and clock face, depth and distance from nipple should be noted.

The nipple should be in profile. The location of the mass can be in anterior, middle and posterior one third of breast. Measure the distance from nipple in both views. It is important to remember that size, shape and margins of the mass should be similar in all views.

Correlating the Position of Mass in Mammogram and Ultrasound

Mammogram is divided into anterior third, middle third and posterior third on MLO view (Fig. 16 A). Once a mass

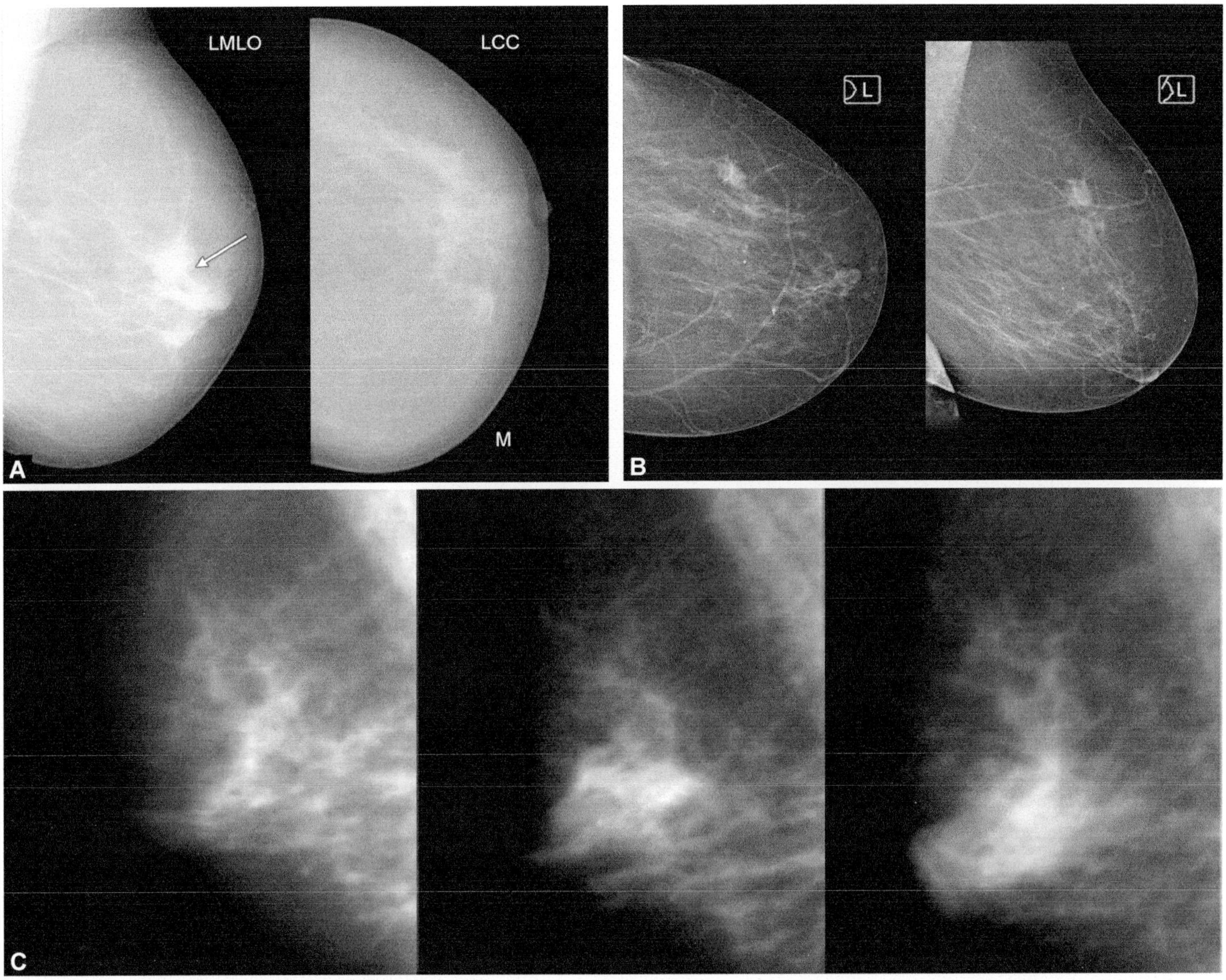

Figs. 10A to C: (A) Mammogram of left breast MLO and CC views showing asymmetric density due to summation in MLO view (arrow) which is not seen on the CC view; (B) Focal asymmetry seen in both MLO and CC views that showed a suspicious mass on ultrasound; (C) Serial mammogram showing developing asymmetry over a period of 3 years in a 52-year-old female which was seen as an irregular hypoechoic mass on ultrasound. Histopathology was s/o invasive ductal carcinoma. (CC: craniocaudal; MLO: mediolateral oblique).

is identified on mammogram on CC and MLO views, its clock position on ultrasound can be ascertained as shown (Figs. 16B and Figs. 17A to C). This is especially useful when there are multiple masses and one is looking for their imaging features on ultrasound.

Why is a Finding (Mass or Asymmetry) Seen in Only One View?

- Due to summation shadows
- Obscured in the other projection
- Far posterior location

What Should be Done Next?

This would depend upon the cause. Localization of the mass in these cases can be determined by using spot compression view in the most likely location visually and additional views may be done.

Due to Summation Shadows

Summation shadows due to overlapping normal structures are sometimes a cause of false concern and repeated views or spot compression views can help in taking care of these as these are not real and disappear.

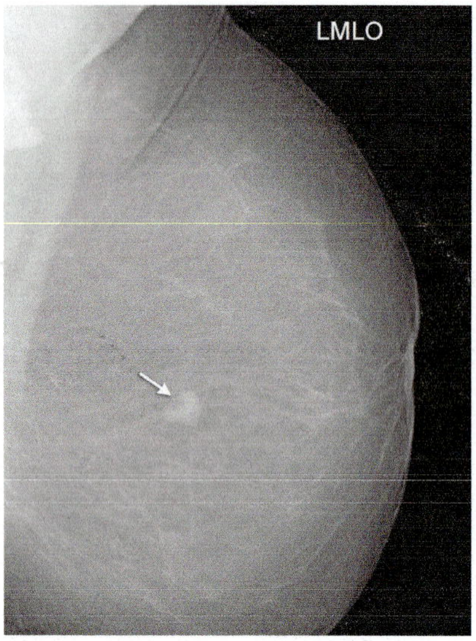

Fig. 11: Mammogram showing a circumscribed oval mass with a fatty hilum mass with radiolucency (arrow - fatty hilum) s/o intramammary lymph node.

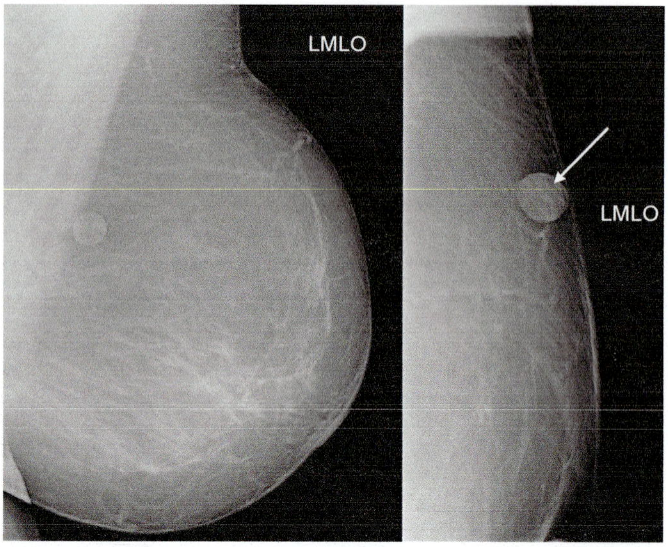

Fig. 12: Mammogram of left breast in a patient with dermal nodule showing a circumscribed mass (arrow) that correlated with the position of the nodule on clinical examination.

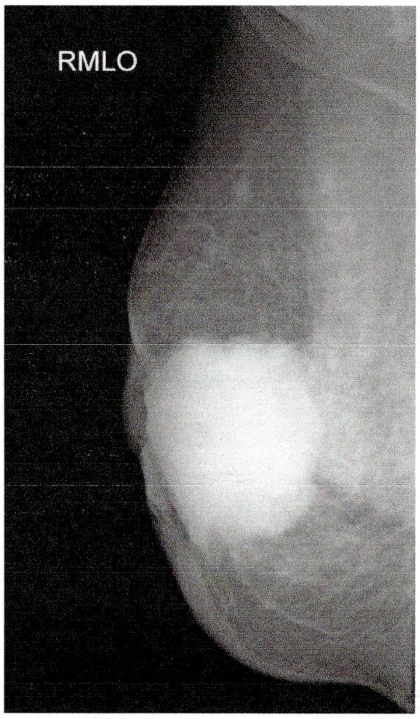

Fig. 13: Mammogram of right breast (MLO view) showing a high-density mass with irregular margins causing architectural distortion, overlying skin thickening and nipple retraction. Imaging features represent BI-RADS category 5 mass. (BI-RADS: breast imaging reporting and data system; MLO: mediolateral oblique).

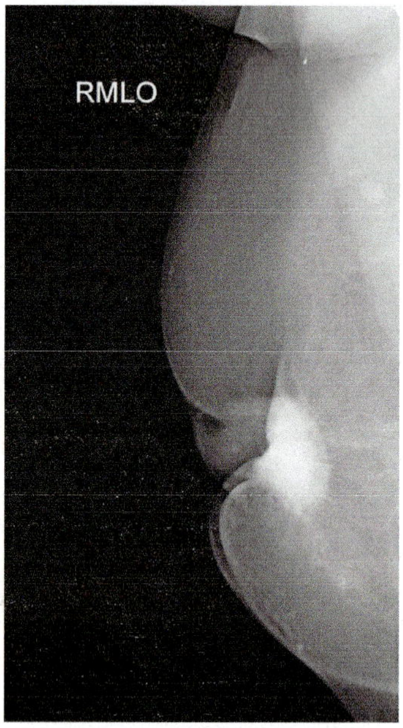

Fig. 14: Mammogram of right breast (MLO view) showing a circumscribed retroareolar mass with associated features as nipple inversion-BI-RADS category 5. Histopathology was s/o invasive ductal carcinoma. (BI-RADS: breast imaging reporting and data system; MLO: mediolateral oblique).

Obscured in the Other Projection

When a mass is obscured in the other projection or view, a spot compression view should be done, mediolateral view for an MLO finding and rolled CC view for a CC-only finding. While deciding upon lateral views (LM or ML), remember that tissue closest to the receptor is sharpest, hence for medial masses, LM view and for lateral mass or when one is not sure about location, a ML view should be taken.

Far Posterior Location of the Mass

Sometimes, the mass is very much posteriorly located and is not included on CC view. Check if the positioning is adequate and posterior most extent of breast is included in the view. A mediolateral view can be done in these cases.

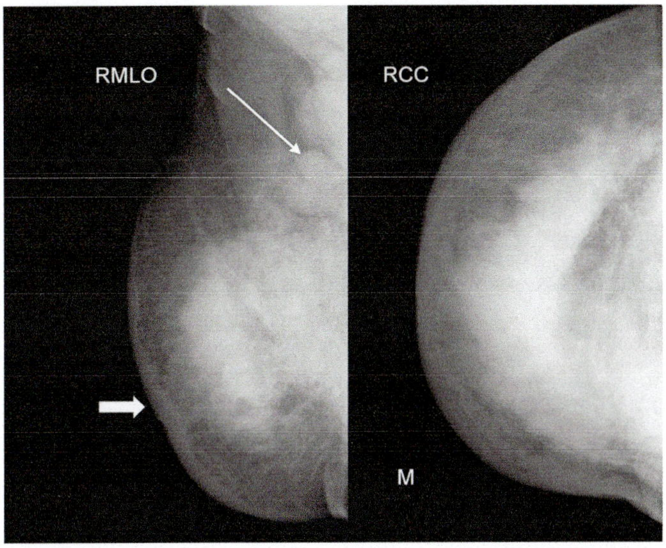

Fig. 15: Mammogram of right breast (MLO and CC view) showing an equal density mass with obscurred, indistinct margins and with associated features as architectural deformity, as skin thickening and axillary lymphadenopathy s/o BI-RADS category 5 mass. Histopathology was s/o invasive ductal carcinoma NOS. (BI-RADS: breast imaging reporting and data system; CC: craniocaudal; MLO: mediolateral oblique; NOS: not otherwise specified).

If mass is seen far posterior on MLO view, it usually means that the mass is lateral, so extended CC view should be done. If extended CC view does not show the mass then do not forget the upper inner quadrant and look for the mass there.

If the mass is seen far posterior on CC only, put a BB marker and do ultrasound.

If the mass is still not localized, then help of tomosynthesis, ultrasound, or MRI may be taken. It is important to remember that imaging features should be similar between various imaging modalities.

BI-RADS CLASSIFICATION (TABLE 3)

BI-RADS 0: This represents incomplete evaluation and signifies that further information or imaging is required, for example, special mammographic views like compression, magnification, or even ultrasound in some cases (Figs. 18 and 19A and B).

BI-RADS 0 is also used when previous images are not available for comparison at the time of reading of mammogram. It can be avoided by immediately doing additional imaging if patient is available. In the Indian setting, BI-RADS 0 is hardly ever used, since patient is available most of the times, and additional imaging can be done at the same sitting as and when required.

BI-RADS 1: *Negative examination:* The breasts are symmetric and there are no masses, architectural distortion or

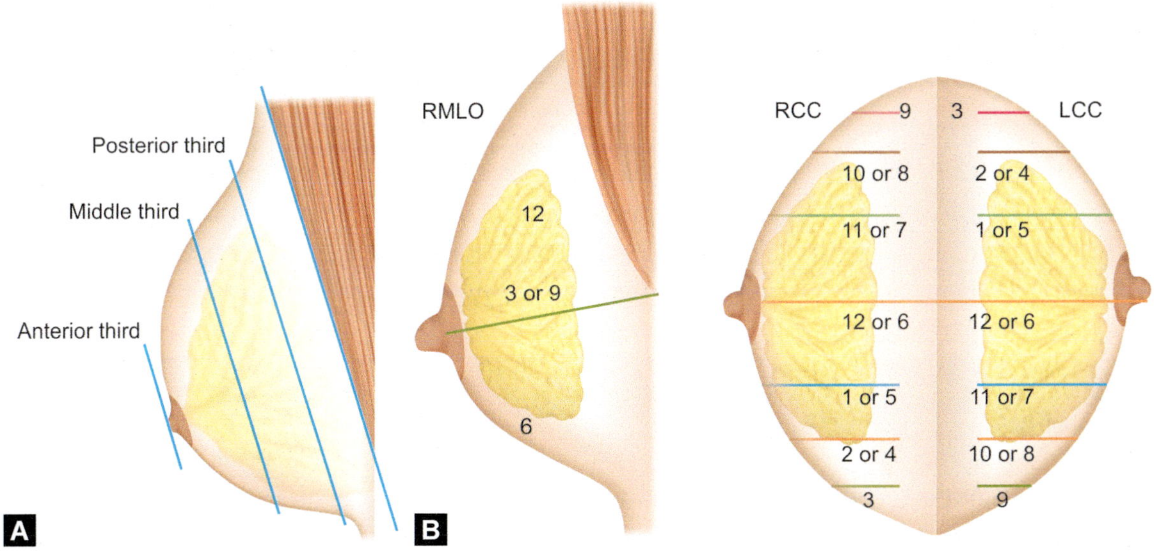

Figs. 16A and B: Mammogram: (A) MLO view showing division into anterior, middle and posterior third; (B) Mammogram (CC and MLO view) showing the corresponding position of mass on ultrasound. (MLO: mediolateral oblique; CC: craniocaudal).

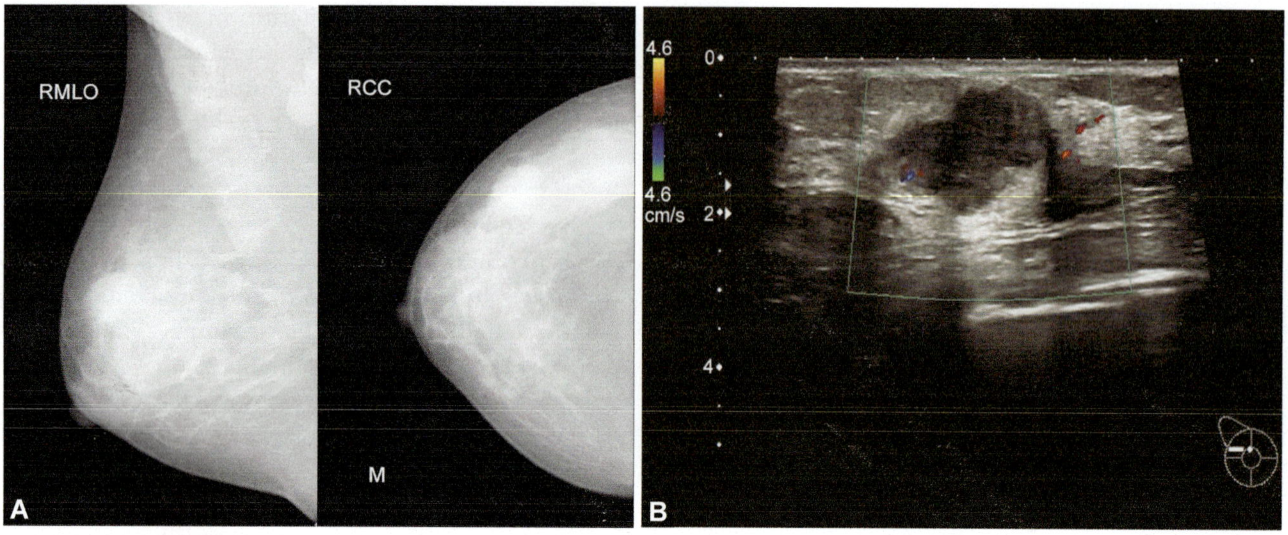

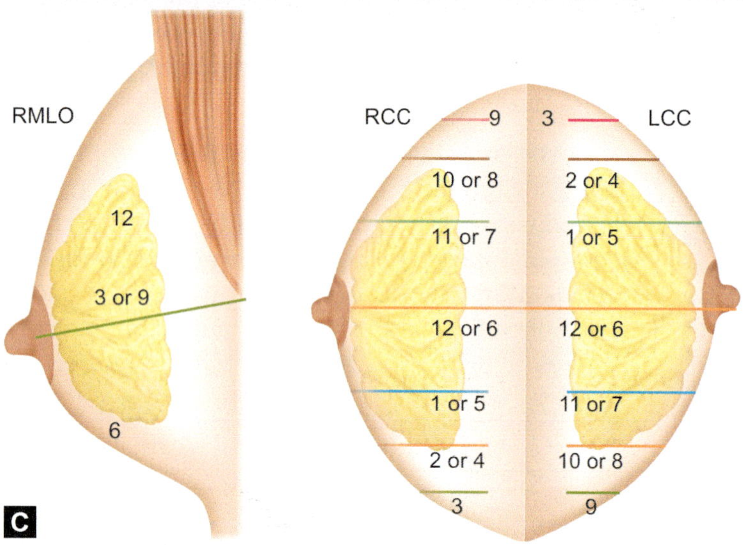

Figs. 17A to C: (A) Mammogram of right breast—MLO and CC views showing a mass with partially obscured margins in superolateral upper outer quadrant of right breast; (B) On ultrasound a hypoechoic mass with irregular margins was seen at 10 o'clock position; (C) Using the chart mentioned in Figure 16, one can see that the corresponding positions on ultrasound are correlating well with location of mass on mammogram. (CC: craniocaudal; MLO: mediolateral oblique).

Table 3: BI-RADS classification and recommendations.

BI-RADS category	*Management recommendations*	*Likelihood of cancer*
Category 0	Need additional imaging evaluation and/ or prior mammograms for comparison	NA
Category 1: Negative	Routine mammographic screening	0% Likelihood of malignancy
Category 2: Benign	Routine mammographic screening	0% Likelihood of malignancy
Category 3	Short interval follow-up (6 monthly) or continued surveillance	0% to ≤2% Likelihood of malignancy
Category 4: 4A low suspicion 4B moderate suspicion 4C high suspicion	Tissue diagnosis	2% But <95% likelihood of malignancy 2% to ≤10% 10%–50% >50% to <95%
Category 5: Highly suggestive of malignancy	Tissue diagnosis	≥95% Likelihood of malignancy
Category 6: Known biopsy proven malignancy	Surgical excision when clinically appropriate	NA

Source: Adapted from BI-RADS 5th edition.

suspicious calcifications (Fig. 20). This category denotes a normal or a negative examination that is very reassuring for the patient. However, if there is a palpable abnormality and a normal mammogram, a clinical evaluation and surgical consultation should be suggested.

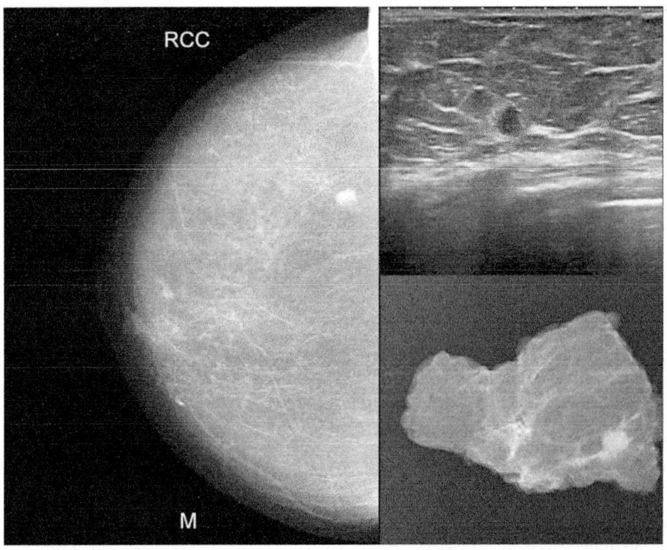

Fig. 18: Mammogram craniocaudal view shows a small mass in posterior one third of breast that was difficult to characterize. Targeted ultrasound showed a taller than wide mass s/o BI-RADS 5 which was resected. Histopathology was s/o invasive ductal carcinoma. (BI-RADS: breast imaging reporting and data system).

BI-RADS 2: This denotes a normal assessment that shows benign findings which should be described in the report. This category has a 0% likelihood of malignancy; hence, routine mammographic screening should be done as before.

The following are included in this category (Figs. 21A to K):

- Simple breast cysts
- Involuting calcified fibroadenomas
- Fat containing lesions such as oil cysts, lipomas, fibroadenolipoma/hamartomas
- Intramammary lymph nodes
- Architectural distortion related to breast conservative surgery
- Implants
- Benign calcifications like multiple secretory rod-like. calcifications, vascular calcifications and scattered macrocalcifications.

BI-RADS 3: This category includes probably benign masses that have a 0 to ≤2% likelihood of malignancy (Figs. 22 to 24). These include:

- Nonpalpable, circumscribed mass on a baseline mammogram (unless shown to be a cyst, an intramammary lymph node or another benign finding)
- Focal asymmetry due to fibroglandular tissue that becomes less dense on spot compression view
- Solitary group of punctate calcifications

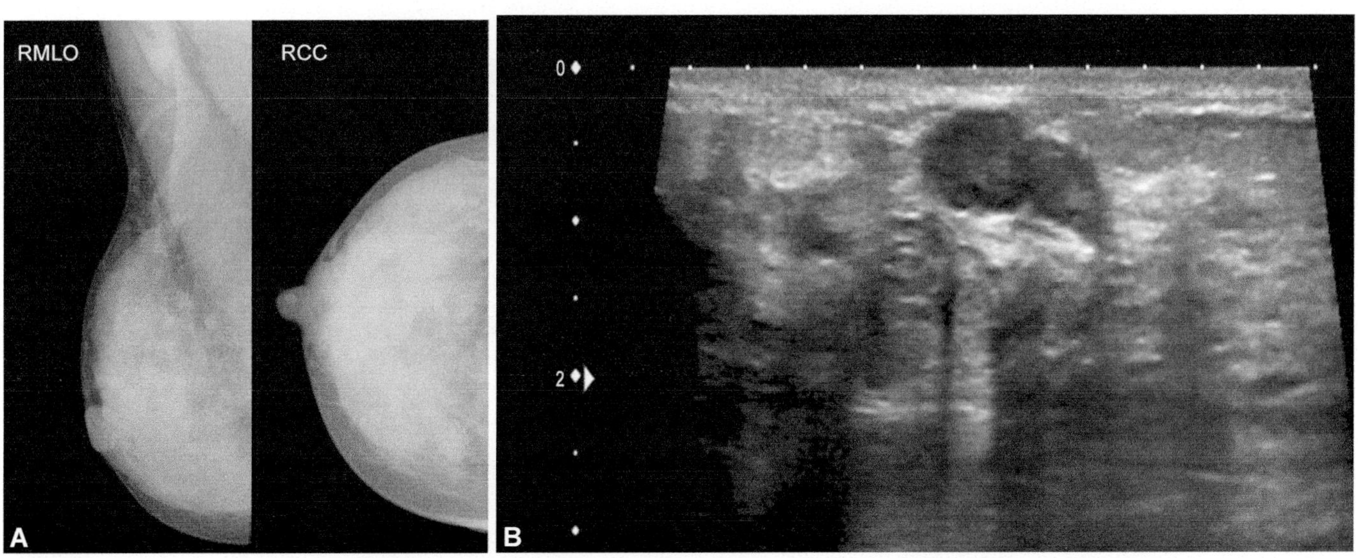

Figs. 19A and B: (A) Mammogram of right breast MLO and CC views views shows dense breast parenchyma with a circumscribed density on medial quadrant on CC view that was not seen well on MLO view, hence ultrasound was done; (B) Ultrasound shows a circumscribed, oval hypoechoic mass at 4 o'clock position s/o BI-RADS category 3. The patient was kept on short interval follow-up. (BI-RADS: breast imaging reporting and data system; MLO: mediolateral oblique; CC: craniocaudal).

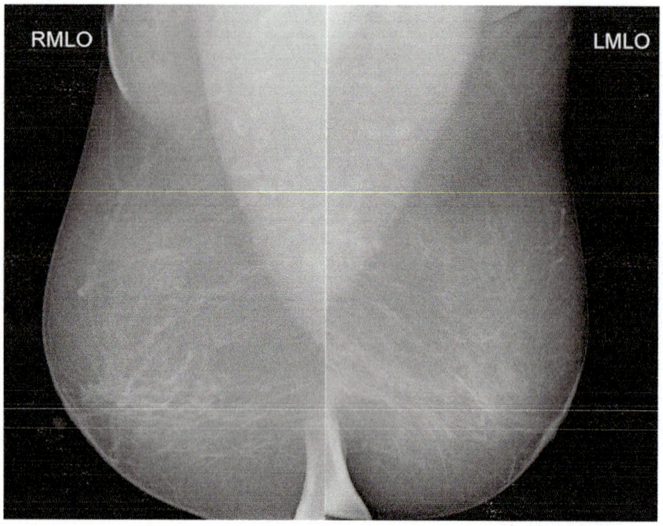

Fig. 20: Mammogram showing normal breast parenchyma on both sides s/o BI-RADS 1. (BI-RADS: breast imaging reporting and data system).

These are not expected to change over the 2-year follow-up interval but their stability should be established by doing regular follow-up imaging. A unilateral mammogram should be done at 6 months and bilateral follow-up mammogram at 12 months and 2 years.

If there is no significant change at 2 years, then final assessment is changed to BI-RADS 2 (benign), that is, mass is downgraded and no further follow-up is needed.

If any change in the mass is noted during follow-up period, then it is changed to BI-RADS 4 or 5, that is, mass is upgraded and biopsy should be performed.

BI-RADS 4: These do not have the classic appearance of malignancy but show sufficiently suspicious findings on imaging to justify a recommendation for biopsy. They have a suspicion of malignancy >2% but have a <95% likelihood of malignancy (Figs. 25 to 29).

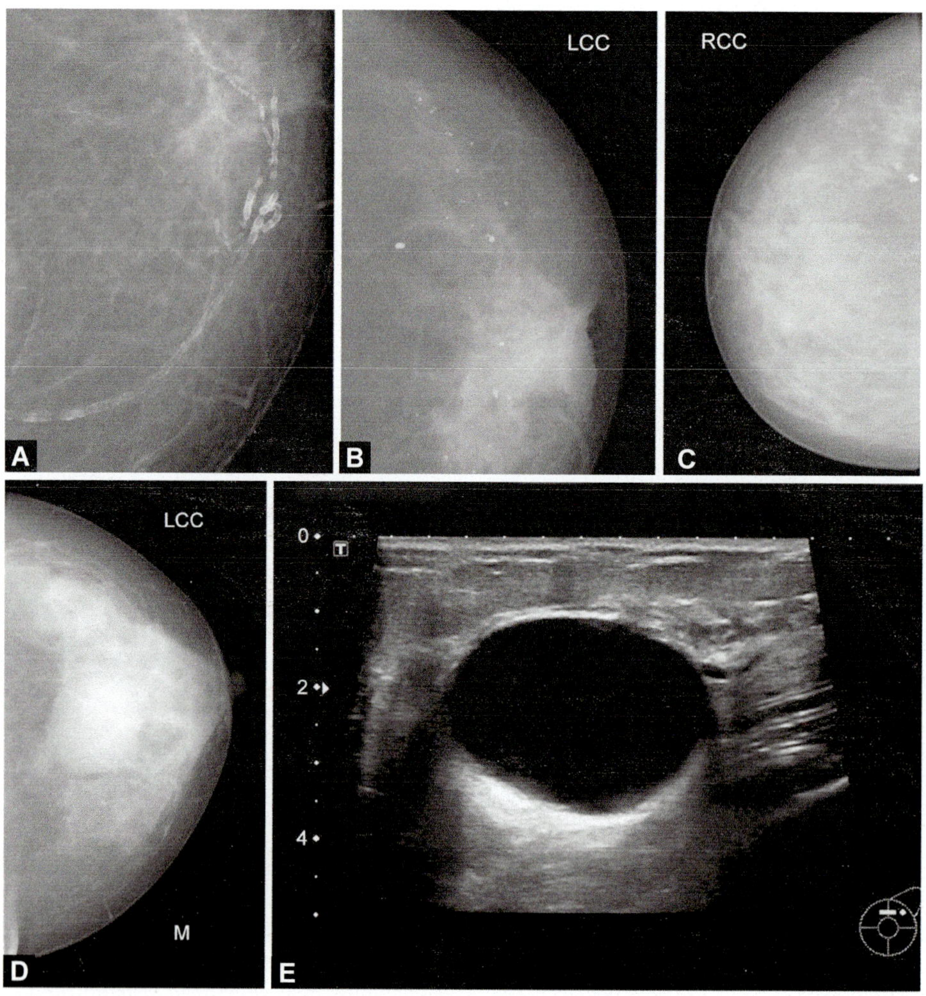

Figs. 21A to E: Mammogram showing findings which are included in BI-RADS 2 category: (A) Vascular calcification; (B and C) Secretory calcifications; (D and E) Simple cyst.

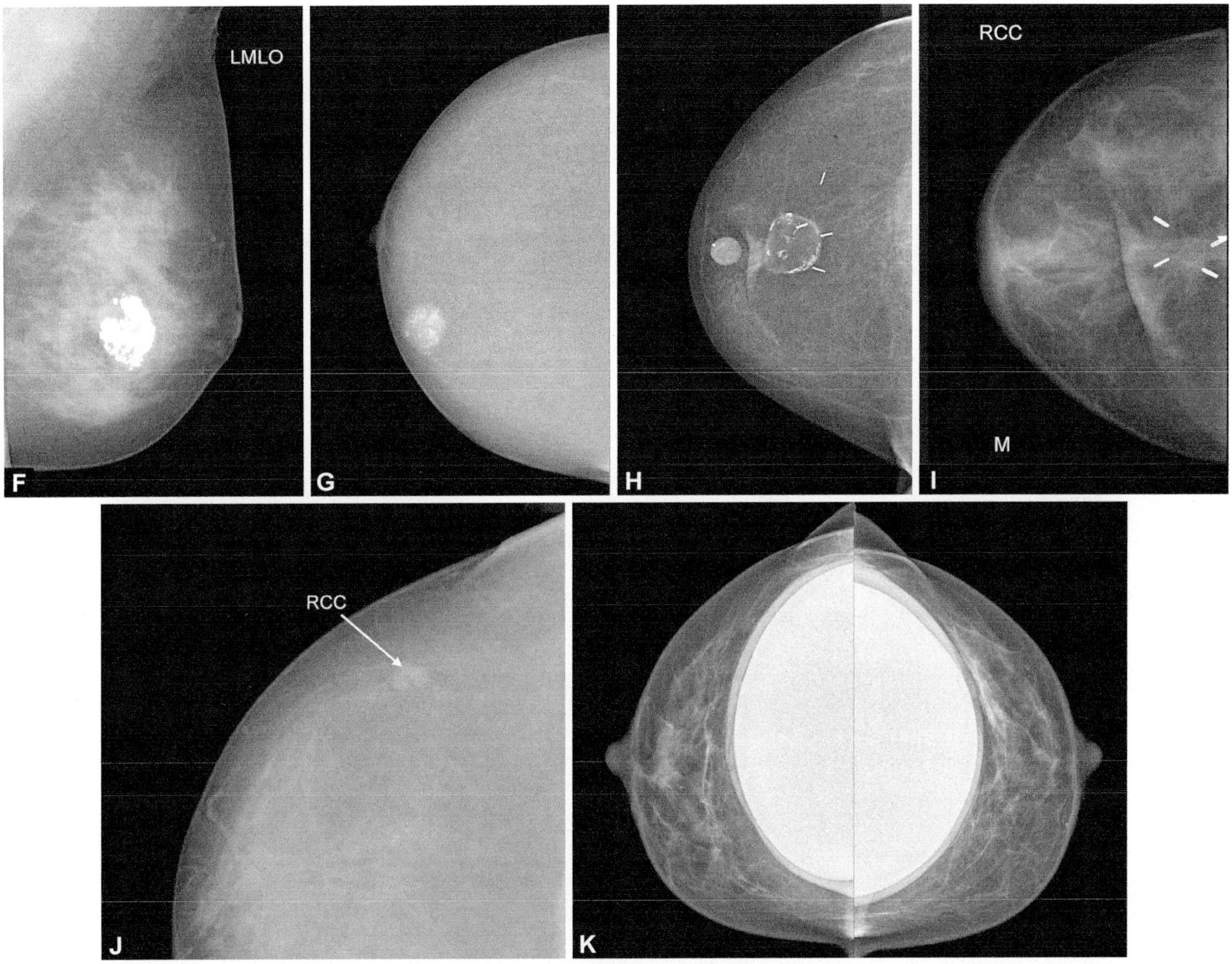

Figs. 21F to K: (F and G) Involuting calcified fibroadenoma; Mammogram showing findings which are included in BI-RADS 2 category: (H) Fat necrosis; (I) Postoperative changes in treated breast; (J) Intramammary lymph node; (K) Breast implants. (BI-RADS: breast imaging reporting and data system).

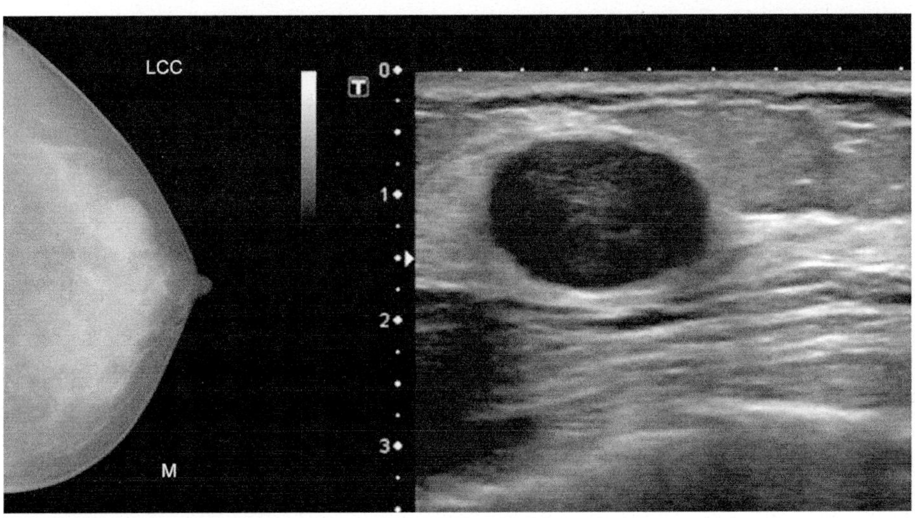

Fig. 22: Mammogram showing a circumscribed equal density mass that on ultrasound was hypoechoic and showed smooth margins. Features are s/o BI-RADS category 3. Histopathology was s/o fibroadenoma. (BI-RADS: breast imaging reporting and data system).

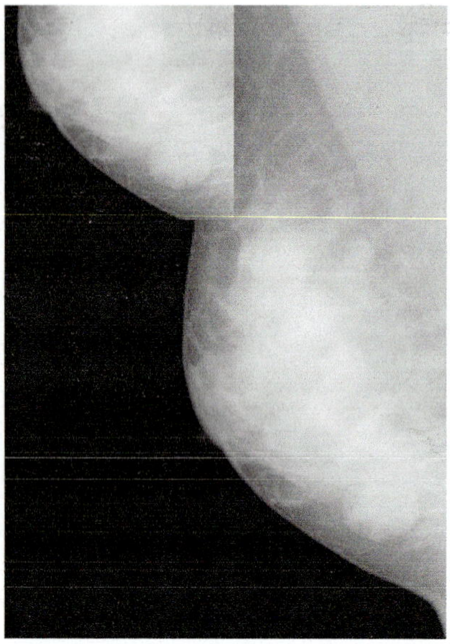

Fig. 23: Mammogram showing multiple well-circumscribed equal density masses in MLO view and in inset s/o BI-RADS category 3. (BI-RADS: breast imaging reporting and data system; MLO: mediolateral oblique).

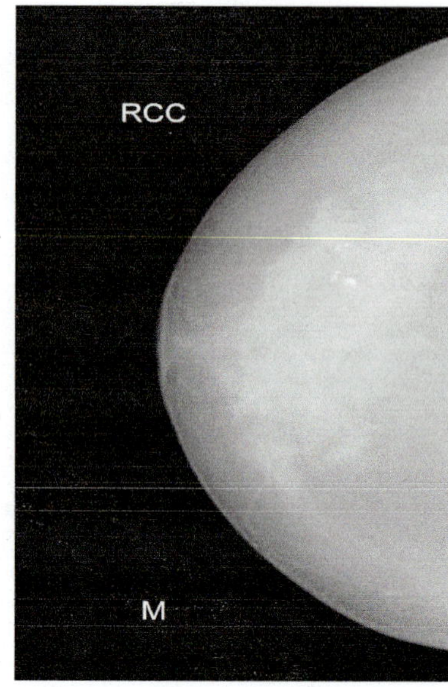

Fig. 24: Mammogram showing a group of secretory calcification s/o BI-RADS category 3. (BI-RADS: breast imaging reporting and data system).

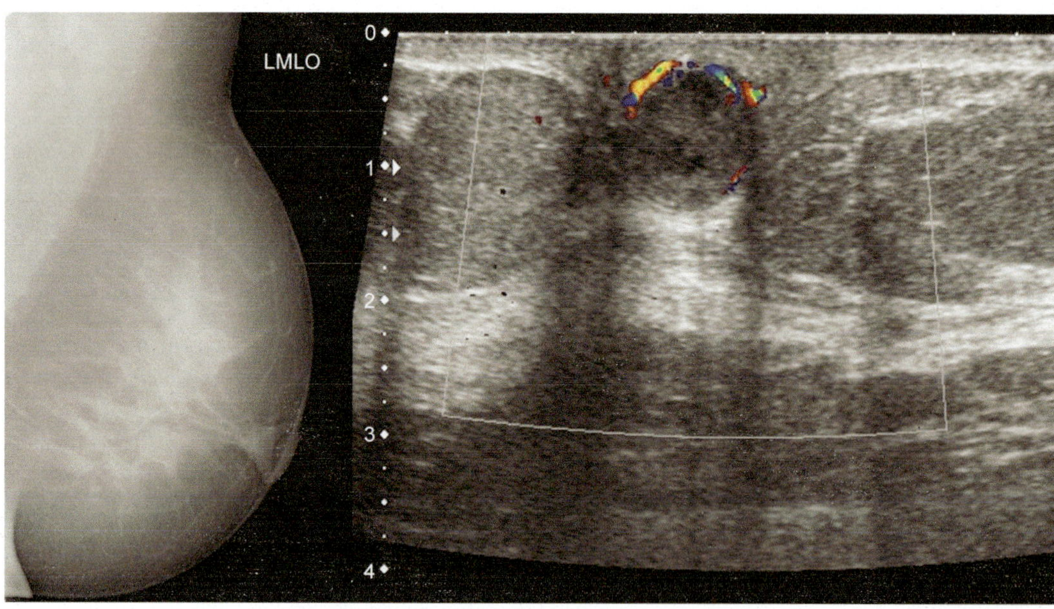

Fig. 25: Mammogram in a 49-year-old female showing a circumscribed mass in retroareolar region which on ultrasound is seen as a well-defined hypoechoic mass showing peripheral vascularity. Features are s/o BI-RADS category 4A. Histopathology was s/o chronic inflammatory pathology. (BI-RADS: breast imaging reporting and data system).

These are divided into three subcategories:

Category 4A: Low suspicion of malignancy 2% to ≤10%

Category 4B: Moderate suspicion of malignancy 10%–50%

Category 4C: High suspicion of malignancy >50% to <95%.

The positive predictive value of breast cancer for category 4C lesions is around 79%. The most important point to remember in this category is that whenever suspicious findings are seen, a biopsy should be recommended irrespective of subcategories as experience of radiologist forms an important component. So whenever there is suspicion of malignancy, biopsy is mandatory.

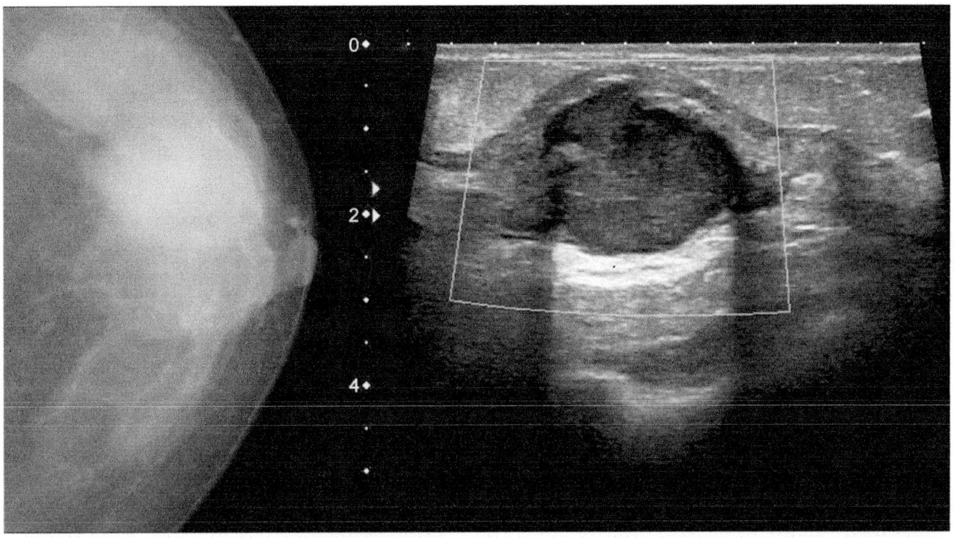

Fig. 26: Mammogram in a 54-year-old female showing a partially obscured mass that on ultrasound is hypoechoic and shows lobulation in one portion of the mass. Features are s/o BI-RADS category 4B. Histopathology was s/o invasive ductal carcinoma. (BI-RADS: breast imaging reporting and data system).

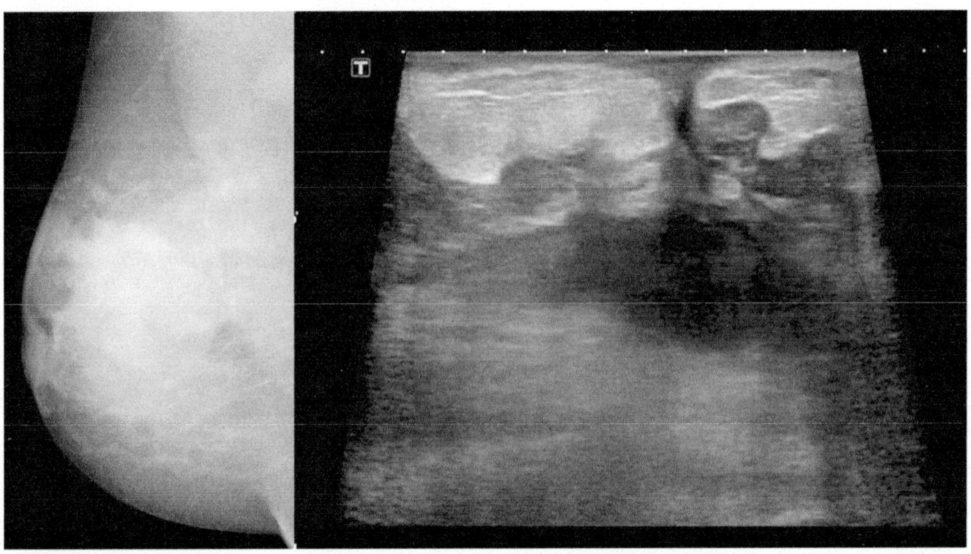

Fig. 27: Mammogram of right breast MLO view shows increased density in right breast in retroareolar region with thickening in nipple areolar complex. Ultrasound showed an ill-defined heterogeneously hypoechoic mass in retroareolar region with a track extending up to nipple areolar complex-BI-RADS 4B. Histopathology was s/o chronic granulomatous mastitis. (BI-RADS: breast imaging reporting and data system; MLO: mediolateral oblique).

This category should also be used in the presence of suspicious unilateral axillary lymphadenopathy without abnormalities/mass in breast.

BI-RADS 5: This category is used when findings are highly suggestive of malignancy with a ≥95% likelihood of malignancy (Figs. 30 to 34).
This includes
- Spiculated, irregular high-density mass
- Segmental or linear arrangement of fine linear calcifications
- Irregular spiculated mass with associated pleomorphic calcifications

BI-RADS 6: This is used when there is already a biopsy proven malignancy, for example, when the patient has undergone biopsy and is referred to a tertiary health center with a histopathological diagnosis of malignancy.

It should also be used for incomplete excise and to monitor response to neoadjuvant chemotherapy.

Writing a Structured Mammogram Report

Structured reports should be organized into several categories, including breast density, description of findings using appropriate descriptors and a final decision-oriented assessment and recommendation.

It is important to write a structured mammogram report because if a systematic reporting pattern is followed during reporting, there are less chances of missing any findings.
A structured report should include the following:

- Indication for the study. Screening, diagnostic or follow-up
- Relevant clinical history
- Composition of breast as per ACR into any of the four categories
- Description of any significant finding using standardized terminology or descriptors while describing mass, asymmetry, architectural distortion and calcifications
- Mention of associated features, like skin thickening, nipple retraction, calcifications, etc.
- If mammography and ultrasound, both are performed then a single report should be given integrating the ultrasound and mammogram findings
- Comparison with previous studies, if any, should be done and a final assessment category and management recommendations should be given
- BI-RADS categories from 0 to 6 should be used along with phrase associated with them while describing management recommendations
- The overall assessment however should be based on the most abnormal of the two breasts, based on the highest likelihood of malignancy.

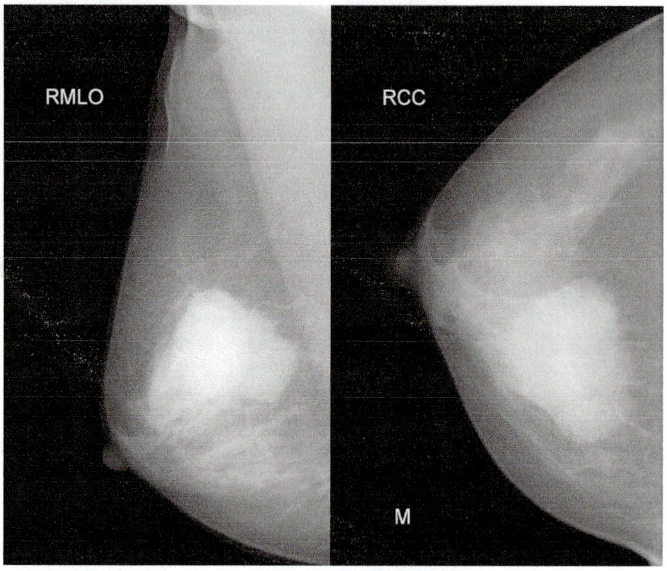

Fig. 28: Mammogram in a 48-year-old female shows a large high-density mass with partially obscured and indistinct margins s/o BI-RADS category 4C. Histopathology was s/o invasive ductal carcinoma. (BI-RADS: breast imaging reporting and data system).

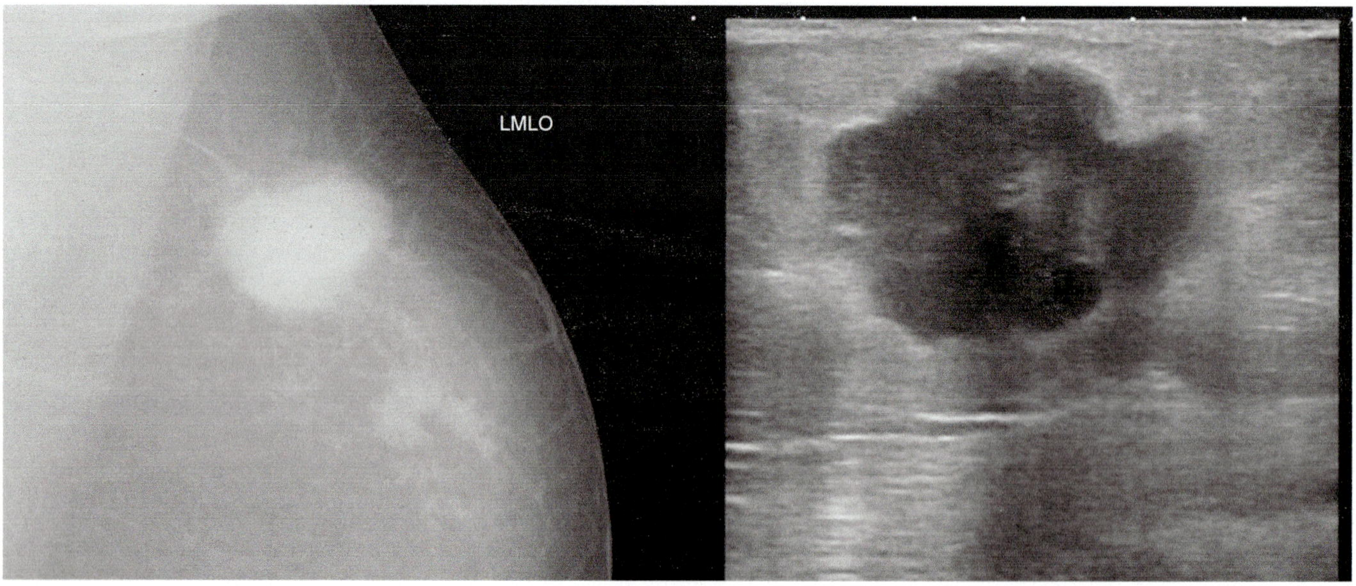

Fig. 29: Mammogram in a 50-year-old female shows an irregular round mass with indistinct margins at places. On ultrasound, the mass was hypoechoic and showed irregular margins with multiple lobulations. Features are s/o BI-RADS category 4C. Histopathology was s/o invasive ductal carcinoma. (BI-RADS: breast imaging reporting and data system).

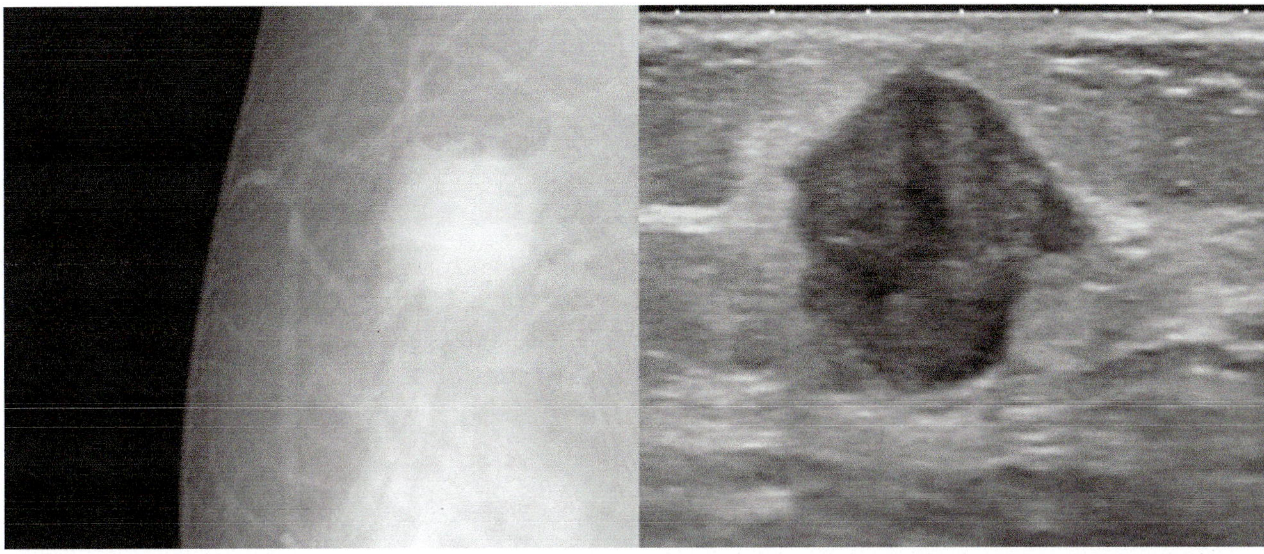

Fig. 30: Mammogram shows a irregular mass with surrounding architectoral distorsion. Ultrasound showed an irregular hypoechoic mass, taller than wide or antiparallel s/o BI-RADS 5. Histopathology was s/o invasive ductal carcinoma. (BI-RADS: breast imaging reporting and data system).

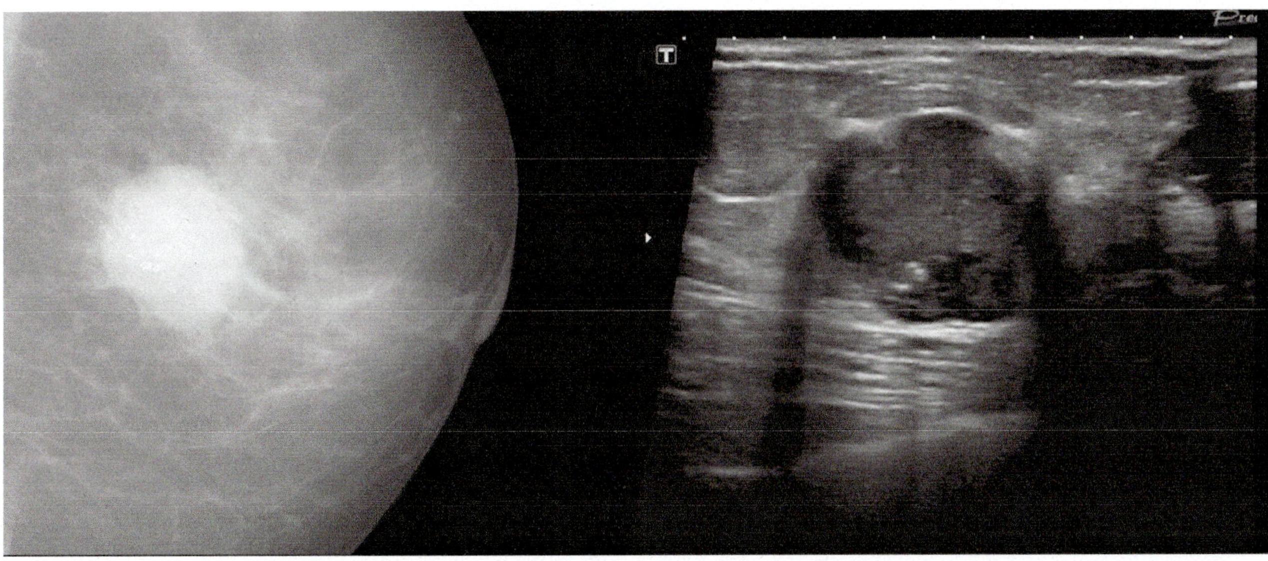

Fig. 31: Mammogram shows a high-density mass with irregular and indistinct margins. Linear pleomorphic calcification was seen in the mass. Features were s/o BI-RADS category 5. Histopathology was s/o invasive ductal carcinoma. (BI-RADS: breast imaging reporting and data system).

In conclusion, it is important to remember that one must not ignore any suspicious finding on mammogram however subtle they may appear. Many times the typical imaging findings of malignancy may not be seen in a mass for example "taller than wide" a term so commonly used for malignant masses may not be present in all malignant masses and it may instead be a "wider than tall" mass. Do not ignore that as it is important to be aware of the clinical context in which a patient is seen while reporting mammograms.

When a patient presents with a breast lump or symptoms suspicious of carcinoma, a triple assessment should be done and diagnosis should be established based on clinical assessment, radiological imaging and tissue sampling (cytological or histopathological).

BI-RADS 3 category is a category that causes anxiety for most patients. The recommendation for BI-RADS 3 mass is a short interval follow-up till 2 years following which a reassessment should be done to either upgrade or downgrade the mass.

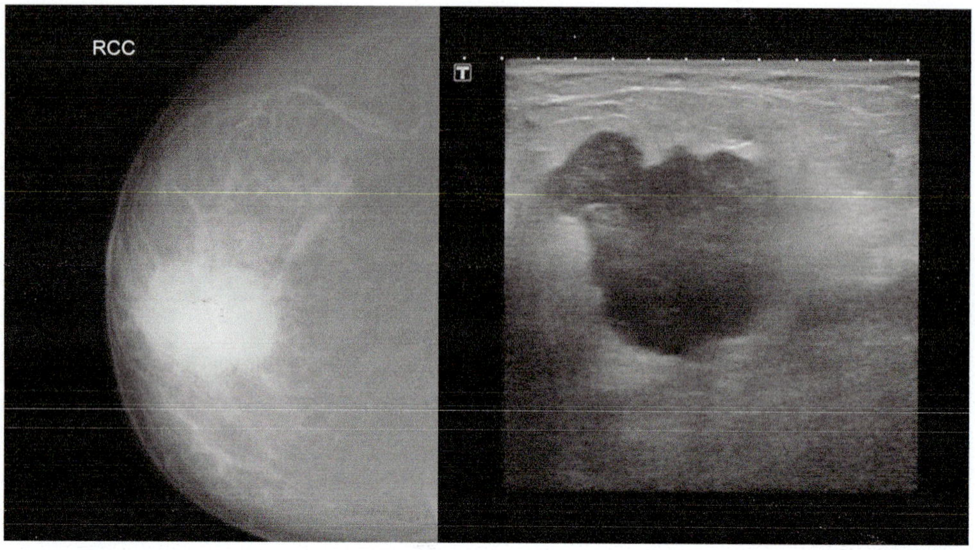

Fig. 32: Mammogram in a 54-year-old female showed a mass equal density mass with irregular margins and architectural distortion. Ultrasound showed an irregular hypoechoic mass with a few microlobulations. Features were s/o BI-RADS 5. Histopathology was s/o invasive ductal carcinoma. (BI-RADS: breast imaging reporting and data system).

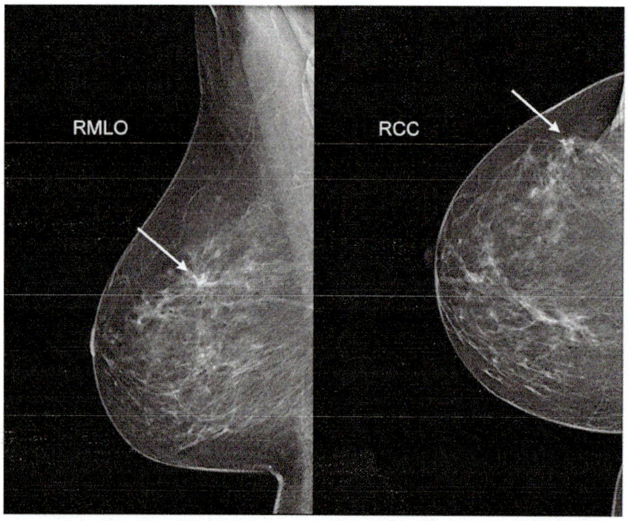

Fig. 33: Mammogram in a 57-year-old female showed a small spiculated mass in upper outer quadrant of right breast s/o BI-RADS category 5. Histopathology was s/o invasive ductal. (BI-RADS: breast imaging reporting and data system).

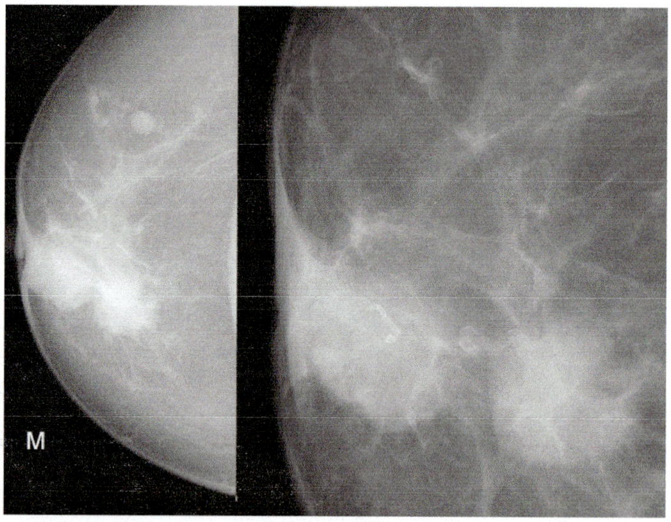

Fig. 34: Mammogram in a 48-year-old female showed two equal density masses with irregular margins in the retroareolar region s/o multifocal masses—BI-RADS category 5. Histopathology was s/o invasive ductal carcinoma. (BI-RADS: breast imaging reporting and data system).

In the Indian setting, it is not sometimes practical to assume that patients would come back for follow-up promptly and many times patients are lost to follow up. As far as possible, these patients should be convinced for a regular and sustained follow-up and in patients who are more apprehensive; a biopsy may be done after consulting the treating surgeon as per the local policy of the hospital.

REFERENCES

1. Sickles EA. Non-palpable, circumscribed, non-calcified solid breast masses: likelihood of malignancy based on lesion size and age of patient. Radiology. 1994;192:439-42.
2. Woods RW, Sisney GS, Salkowski LR, et al. The mammographic density of a mass is a significant predictor of breast cancer. Radiology. 2011;258(2):417-35.
3. Rao AA, Feneis J, Lalonde C, Ojeda-Fournier H. A pictorial review of changes in the BI-RADS fifth edition. RadioGraphics 2016;36:623-39.

2.5 Breast Calcifications

INTRODUCTION

Breast calcifications are commonly seen on mammograms and may represent benign or malignant pathology. However, it needs to be kept in mind that breast calcifications may be the only sign of cancer, they are best detected on mammography and best evaluated on magnification views.

Breast calcifications should be analyzed for their location, distribution, morphology and stability over time. Causes of calcification are infection, chronic inflammation, benign and malignant masses. Calcifications can form within the ducts or acini due to secretion from the epithelial cells or due to deposition of calcium in necrotic cells. These are usually calcium phosphate or calcium oxalate. The other sites of calcification include stroma, periductal area, arteries, skin and fat. It is important to identify dermal calcifications as these are benign and can be mistaken for calcification within the parenchyma leading to unnecessary biopsies. Artifacts due to talcum powder, dust particles and deodorant can simulate dermal calcification.

ANATOMY

Terminal ductal lobular unit (TDLU) is the basic functional unit of breast lobule, made up of 10–100 acini draining into the terminal duct which in turn drains into the larger duct and finally into main duct which drains into the nipple (Fig. 1).

Mechanism of Formation of Calcifications in Terminal Ductolobular Unit

Calcifications are described based on their morphology which, in turn, depends on the anatomical structure in which they form.

- *Round or punctate*: Calcifications in lobular acinus are round, regular, dense and sharply marginated. They are called **round** calcifications when of size >0.5 mm and **punctate** when they measure <0.5 mm. These generally form in fibrocystic changes and adenosis, where the secretions calcify over a period of time (Fig. 2)

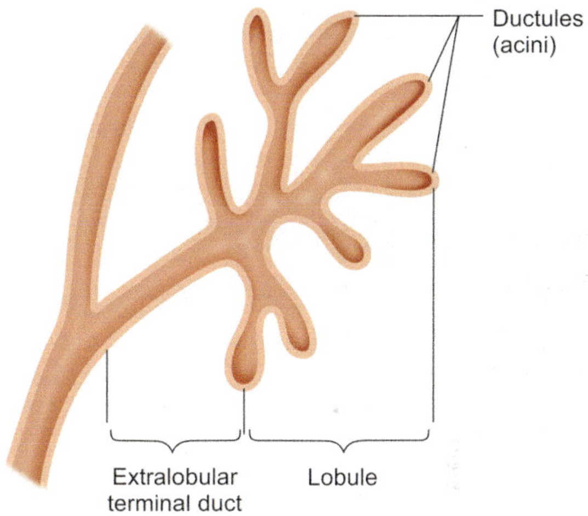

Fig. 1: Terminal ductolobular unit (TDLU).

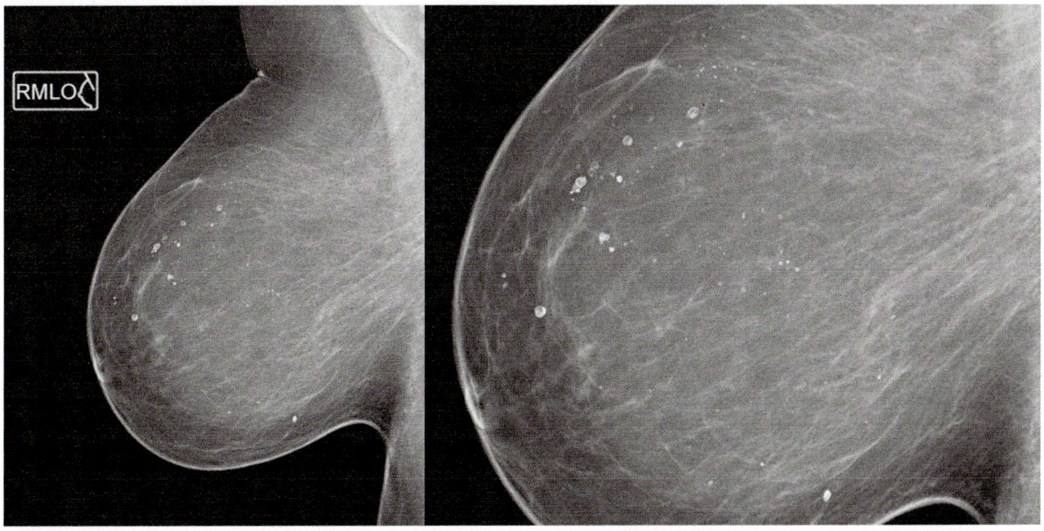

Fig. 2: Mammogram showing diffuse, round and punctate calcifications along with rim calcifications.

- *Coarse calcifications*: Large calcifications that form in the connective tissue of fibroadenomas (Figs. 3A and B) or in the stromal reaction of invasive cancer
- *Rod like calcifications*: Well-defined, linear and smooth calcifications formed due to accumulated secretions in larger ducts, such as in plasma cell mastitis. These are secretory calcifications (Fig. 4)
- *Amorphous calcifications*: Small roundish, hazy, flake-shaped particles that are too small and vague to characterize (200–300 μm). Amorphous calcifications (Fig. 5) can be seen in both benign and malignant pathologies:
  - Benign diseases like fibrocystic disease and sclerosing adenosis can sometimes have ductal extension with dilatation that result in indeterminate amorphous or indistinct calcifications
  - Low or intermediate grade Ductal Carcinoma in situ (DCIS) can cause obstruction leading to dilatation of ducts and acini with accumulation of secretions which calcify and form round or amorphous calcifications of different sizes[1]
- *Fine linear calcifications*: Comedocarcinoma completely fills and dilates the ducts with plugs of high grade tumor cells having central necrosis ("comedonecrosis"), thereby leading to linear microcalcifications (Fig. 6)

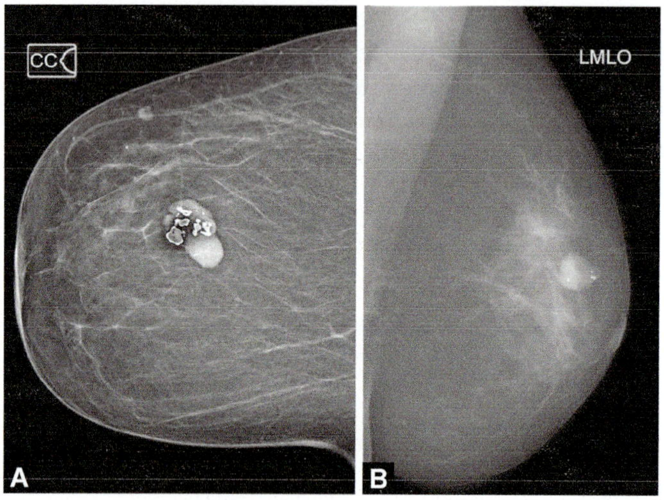

Figs. 3A and B: (A) Mammogram showing classic popcorn calcification in a circumscribed mass and (B) mammogram shows a lobulated mass that has started showing foci of calcifications. Features are s/o involuting fibroadenoma.

Evaluation of Microcalcifications

Calcifications which are <1 mm in diameter and can be characterized on mammography with a focal spot of 0.1 mm and magnification of 1.5 are called microcalcifications. These microcalcifications are seen in malignant masses (30%) and in ductal carcinoma in situ (85–90%).

Whenever there are suspicious microcalcifications on mammogram, magnification view should be done to see them clearly and further characterize them. This can be done by using a 0.1 mm focal spot and air gap magnification which leads to magnification by 1.8 times and further

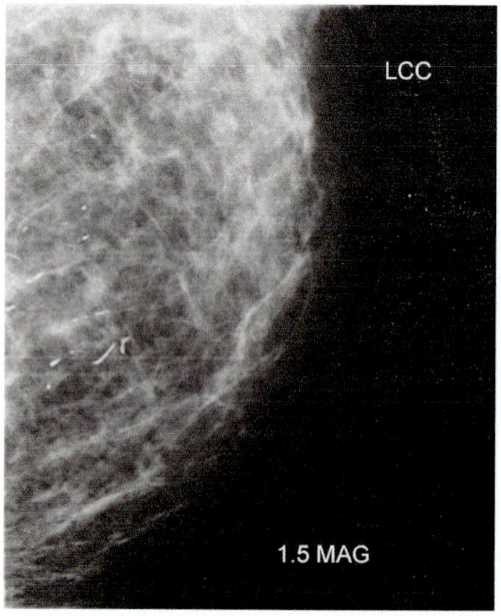

Fig. 4: Mammogram showing large, well-defined, smooth and linear calcifications in segmental distribution—due to secretions in large ducts as seen in chronic mastitis.

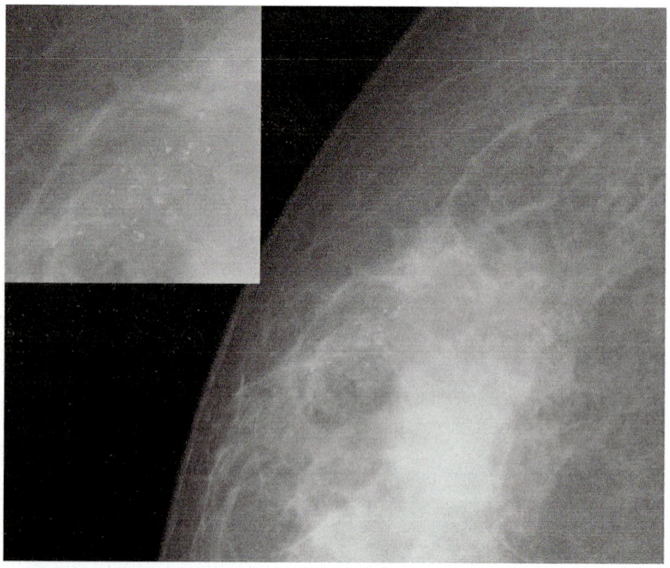

Fig. 5: Mammogram showing segmental amorphous calcifications. Histopathology was s/o DCIS.

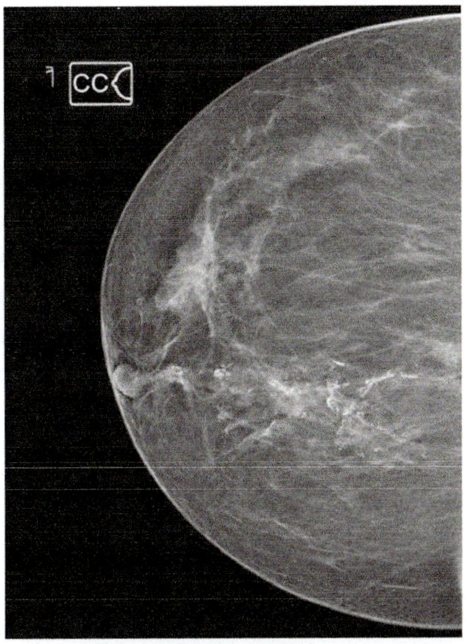

Fig. 6: Mammogram—CC view showing segmental fine linear calcifications. Histopathology was s/o DCIS. (CC: craniocaudal).

sharpens the image. Also, additional calcifications may be seen and grouped calcifications are seen more clearly, separately and distinctly.

In digital mammography, while the image can be magnified electronically to make microcalcifications appear bigger and more conspicuous, it is important to remember that electronic magnification on the workstation is not the same as performing air-gap magnification views, the former merely magnifies the calcifications without further characterizing them, often with degradation of clarity.

Number of calcifications: It is important to evaluate the number of calcifications in addition to their shapes. According to Sigfusson et al., if the number of calcification in a cluster or group is less than 5, the possibility of it being malignant is very low. Biopsy from such clusters should be performed only if the individual morphology of the calcifications is extremely suspicious or if the calcifications are present in a suspicious clinical scenario. A group of >10 microcalcifications in a volume of 1 cm^3 is more suspicious than a group of 5 microcalcifications of similar morphology in similar volume.

Stability of calcifications: One should not assume that if the calcifications are stable, they are always benign[2] and should confirm the findings by doing a biopsy. The decision to do a biopsy should be taken by looking at the **worst looking** individual calcification.

Significance of calcifications: Breast calcifications can be the only sign of malignancy hence all calcifications in a cluster should be analyzed individually and carefully. A group or cluster of suspicious calcifications should not be labeled benign simply because it also contains a few round benign-appearing calcifications. It is seen that even DCIS may have round and benign looking calcifications, when the malignant cells spread into the lobule and small, amorphous looking calcifications coexist with pleomorphic calcifications. It is the decision and responsibility of the radiologist to biopsy the worst looking calcification. It is important to note that sometimes magnification view may show more number and smaller calcifications than seen on the standard mammogram making it more significant.

Only the following groups of calcifications[3] should be followed up on mammogram:

- Few round or punctate clustered calcifications
- Few amorphous microcalcifications in a small cluster—beginning of calcification process in fibroadenoma
- Coarse heterogeneous microcalcifications grouped in a small volume representing a calcified or involuting fibroadenoma

BI-RADS CLASSIFICATION

Calcifications have an important place in the BI-RADS classification system. In **BI-RADS atlas version 5 (2013)**, the calcifications have been divided according to **morphology** into two major categories: (1) typically benign calcifications and (2) calcifications of suspicious morphology (Table 1).

Table 1: Benign and suspicious calcifications

Benign	*Suspicious morphology*
Skin	Amorphous: 4B
Vascular	
Coarse or popcorn like	Coarse heterogeneous: 4B
Large rod like	
Round/punctate	Fine pleomorphic: 4B
Rim calcification	
Dystrophic	Fine linear: 4C
Fat necrosis	
Milk of calcium	Fine linear branching:4C
Suture	

According to their location and distribution they are divided into following five groups:

1. *Diffuse*: Scattered or diffusely present and usually seen in benign pathology.
2. *Regional*: Arranged in a non-ductal distribution.
3. *Grouped*: A single group is more common in malignant pathology.
4. *Linear*: The entire duct and its branches are filled with calcifications.
5. *Segmental*: These are present in a ductal distribution.

MICROCALCIFICATIONS ACCORDING TO MORPHOLOGY

Typically Benign

- *Skin calcifications*: These are usually very small (about the size of the skin pores visible on the mammogram), formed by calcium deposition in sebaceous glands and often occur in skin folds like axilla, inframammary fold, areolar and parasternal region that are more rich in sebaceous glands.

On mammograms, they are classically seen as egg-shell, round or ring shaped calcifications with a lucent center (Figs. 7 and 8). Sometimes it may be difficult to distinguish them from intraparenchymal calcifications, but it should be remembered that configuration of skin calcifications remains the same on different projections. This is called the **tattoo** sign.[4] If the calcifications are located in breast parenchyma, their appearance on different views would change. A tangential view can also be used to confirm skin calcifications.

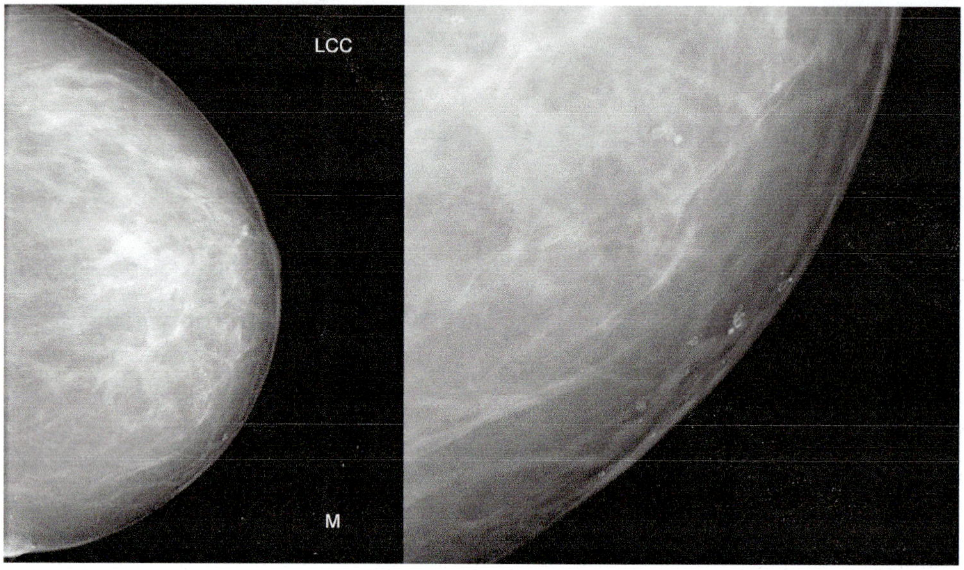

Fig. 7: Mammogram showing skin calcifications some of them having a lucent center.

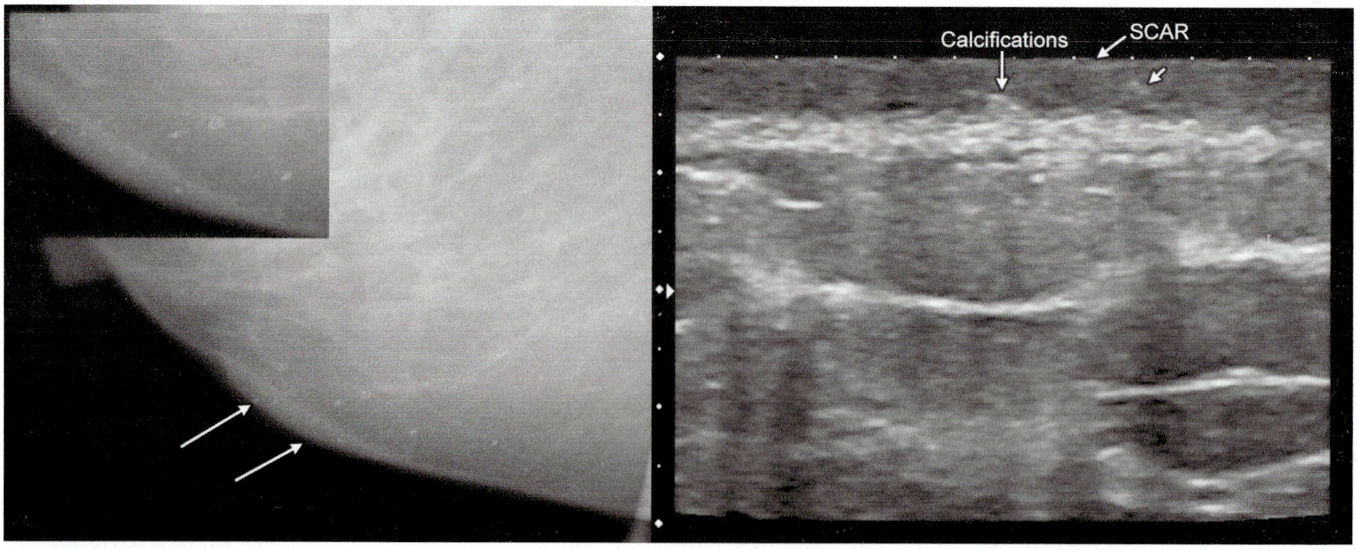

Fig. 8: Mammogram showing skin thickening with skin calcifications that are seen on ultrasound as echogenic foci with posterior acoustic shadowing.

- **Vascular calcifications:** These are because of athero-sclerotic changes and deposition of calcium in middle layer of arterial wall, also called Mönckeberg calcifications. These are thin calcifications involving the vessel wall circumference making it rigid and less distensible
  They are seen as parallel or tram track calcifications on mammogram (Figs. 9 and 10). In the initial stage when the vessel starts calcifying, only one wall may be involved that may look like intraductal calcification and may cause confusion.
- **Coarse or "popcorn-like" calcifications:** Large, chunky "popcorn-like calcifications" are classically seen in involuting fibroadenomas. (Figs. 11A and B). Sometimes small and numerous calcifications in the fibroadenoma may resemble malignant calcifications and may require to be biopsied for confirmation. Old hematomas can also calcify sometimes and show coarse calcifications (Fig. 12)

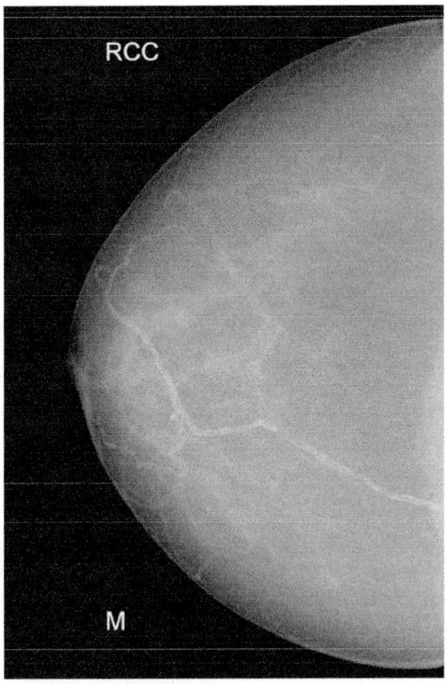

Fig. 9: Mammogram showing vascular calcifications having a parallel or tram track appearance.

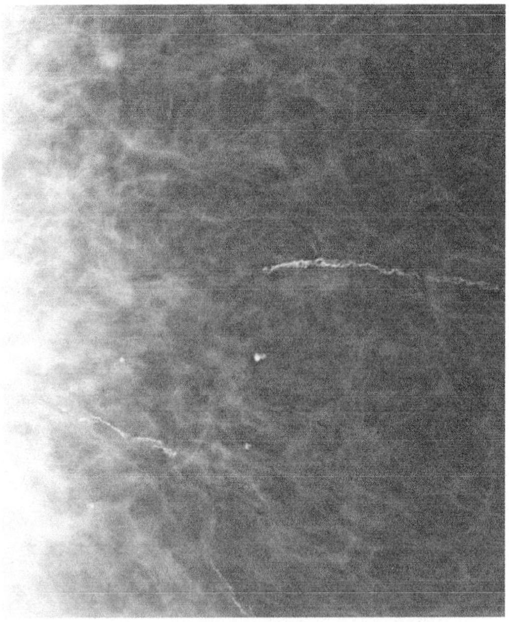

Fig. 10: Developing vascular calcifications on mammogram that appears partially calcified.

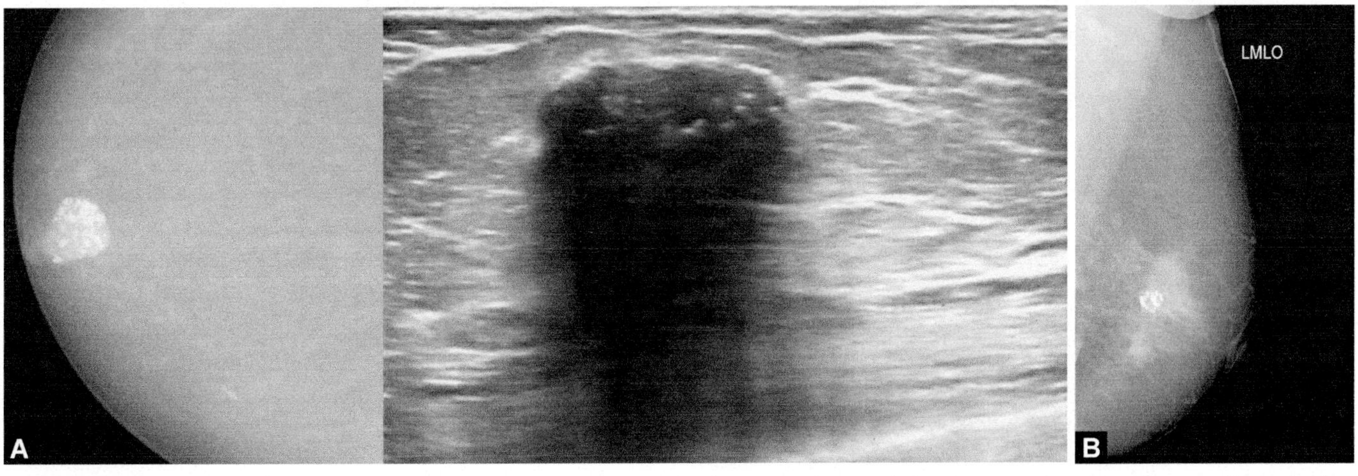

Figs. 11A and B: (A) Mammogram and ultrasound showing a circumscribed mass with large, calcifications showing posterior acoustic shadowing on ultrasound; (B) Mammogram in another patient shows a partially calcified circumscribed mass. Features represent involuting fibroadenoma.

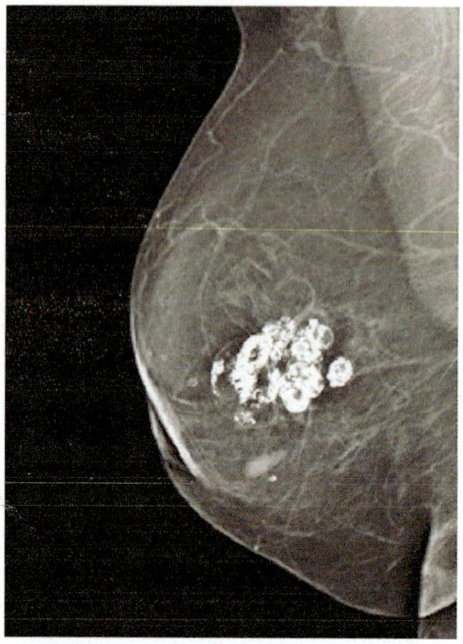

Fig. 12: Mammogram showing multiple well-defined calcifications in old hematoma.

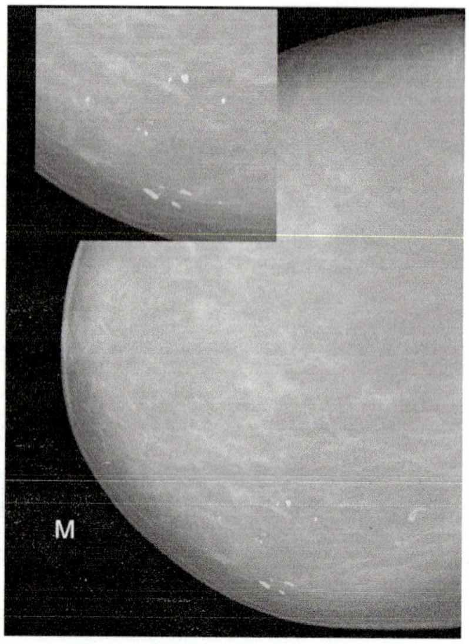

Fig. 14: Mammogram showing rod-like calcification.

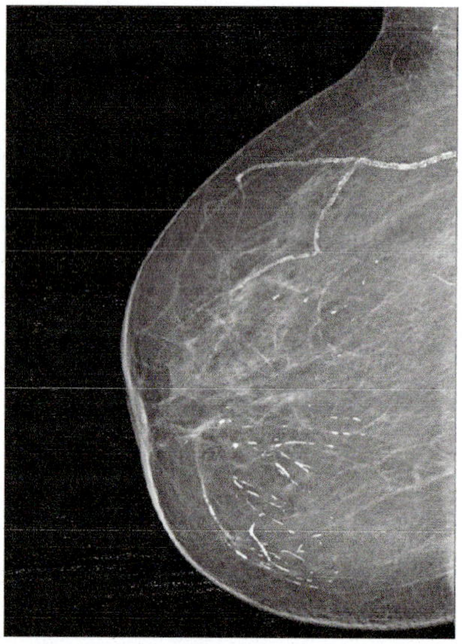

Fig. 13: Mammogram showing segmental large, rod-like calcifications in right breast. Vascular calcification is also noted.

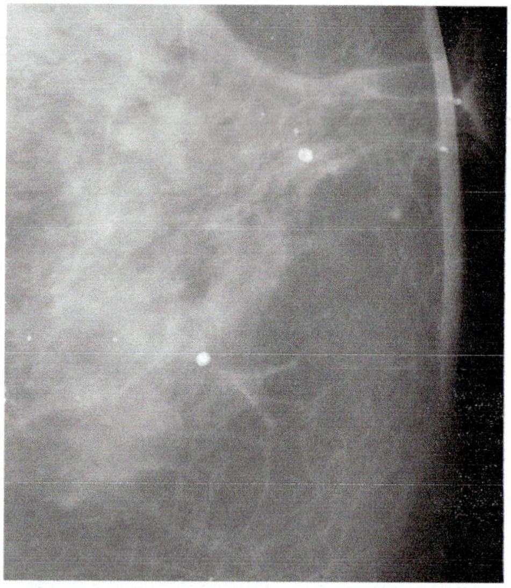

Fig. 15: Mammogram showing round calcification—benign.

- **Large and rod-like calcifications:** These are due to secretion produced within the ectatic ducts and appear as rod-like elongated calcifications (Figs. 13 and 14). These are generally larger (>1 mm) than fine calcifications seen in DCIS and is because of calcified walls and a lucent center. They are seen in a ductal distribution and are usually bilateral
- **Round calcifications:** These are small round calcifications which form within the acini and measure 0.5–1 mm in size (Fig. 15). Punctate calcifications are generally smaller than 0.5 mm in size.

The round calcifications are commonly seen in fibrocystic disease though similar appearance can be seen in artifacts due to talcum powder, skin calcification and rarely DCIS in which calcifications are much smaller and have a heterogeneous appearance in addition to distribution in cluster, linear or segmental location.

Round and punctate calcifications are classified as:

BI-RADS 2: When there are scattered round calcifications.

BI-RADS 3 or 4: When calcifications are in an isolated cluster (Fig. 16) or if they are new or ipsilateral to a cancer.

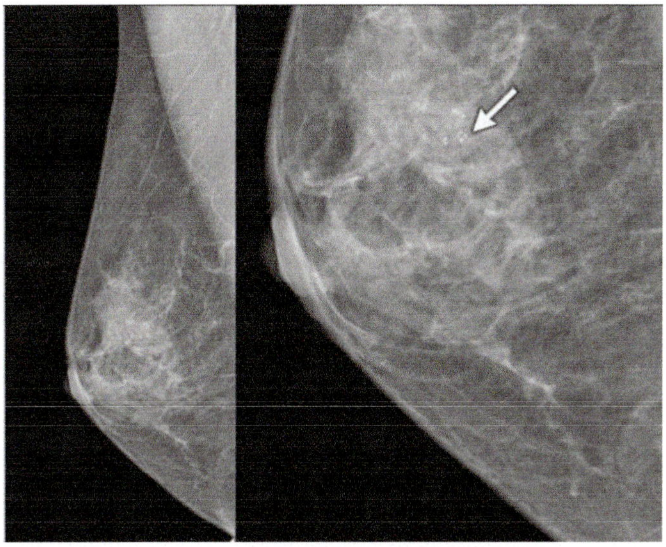

Fig. 16: Mammogram showing a group of round and punctate calcifications. Histopathology was s/o low grade DCIS.

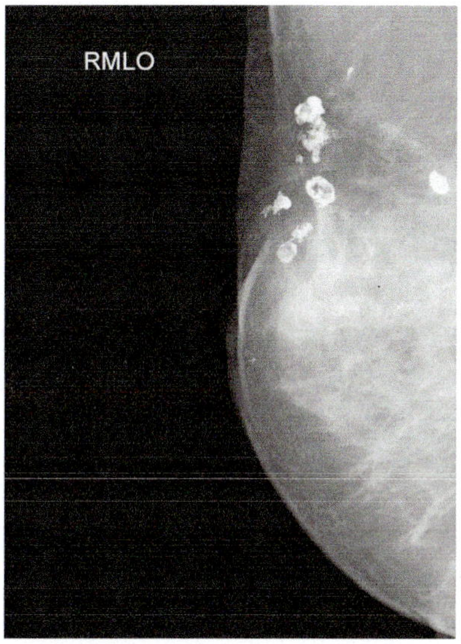

Fig. 17: Dystrophic calcifications seen in a woman who has undergone breast conservative therapy.

- *Rim calcifications*: These are thin (<1 mm) calcifications and include calcifications in cyst wall or fat necrosis.
- *Dystrophic calcifications*: These are coarse calcifications that are larger than 0.5 mm in size and show central lucency. These are generally seen in postoperative breast or irradiated breast a few years after treatment (Fig. 17)
- *Milk of calcium*: They are benign sedimented calcifications in macro- or microcysts that appear fuzzy, round or amorphous on craniocaudal views.[5] An apparent change in shape is noted when comparing them on MLO view (where there is layering of calcium) and on 90° mediolateral view (where they appear semilunar or crescent shaped "tea cups").
  However, many calcifications representing milk of calcium within microcysts do not layer on horizontal beam radiographs.
- *Suture calcifications*: These are due to calcium deposition on suture material and are typically linear or tubular in appearance. Sometimes knots may be visible.

Calcifications of Suspicious Morphology

1. **Amorphous:** More than 60% of these calcifications are benign with common conditions being fibrocystic disease and sclerosing adenosis. Still there may be approximately 20% of these that may be malignant which includes low grade DCIS (Figs. 18 to 20).
   The amorphous calcifications can be classified as:
   BI-RADS 2: When diffuse and bilateral
   BI-RADS 3: When multiple bilateral clustered
   BI-RADS 4: When unilateral clustered or appearing on follow-up or in a patient with a cancer in the contralateral breast.

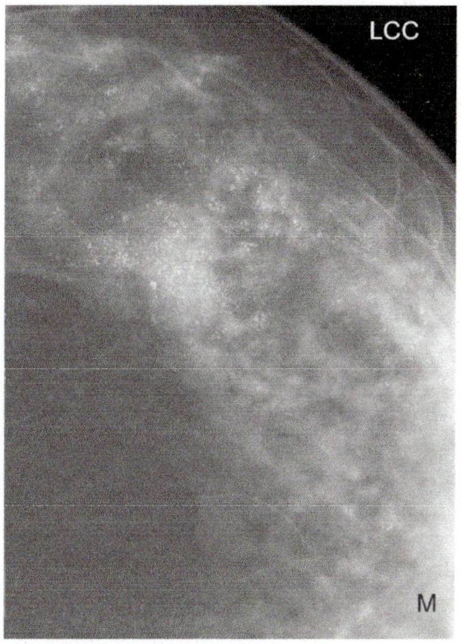

Fig. 18: Amorphous and coarse heterogeneous calcification seen in a woman on a routine mammogram. Histopathology was s/o low grade DCIS.

2. **Coarse heterogeneous microcalcifications:** These are large calcifications that are >0.5 mm in size (Figs. 21 and 22). Their distribution in a segmental or linear distribution points toward DCIS. It is important to distinguish them from fine pleomorphic calcification seen in malignancy.[1]

The differential diagnosis of **coarse heterogeneous calcifications** includes

- Fibroadenoma
- Fibrosis
- Post-traumatic, representing evolving dystrophic calcifications (fat necrosis)
- DCIS.

3. **Fine pleomorphic calcifications:** These are more conspicuous (Fig. 23) and prominent and are linear in distribution as compared to amorphous calcification and have a 25%–40% risk of malignancy.
4. **Fine linear or fine linear branching (casting) calcifications:** They are seen in **DCIS** or invasive ductal cancer, formed within the DCIS (Figs. 24 to 26) as it grows within in branching ducts, making tiny irregular casts of the duct and its branches forming X, Y, or Z-shaped forms.

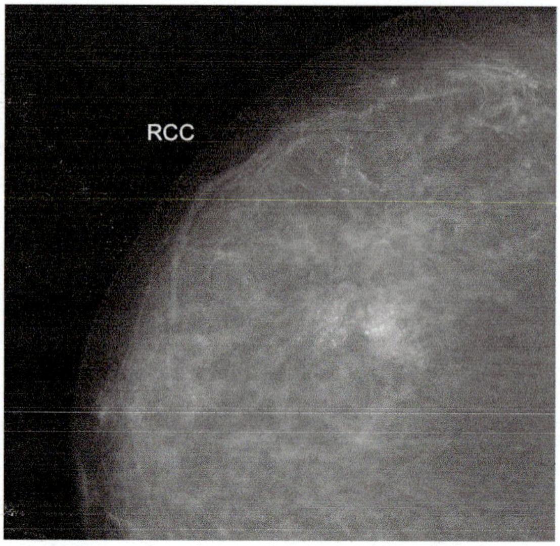

Fig. 19: Amorphous and fine linear segmental calcification seen on mammogram. Histopathology was s/o DCIS with invasive cancer.

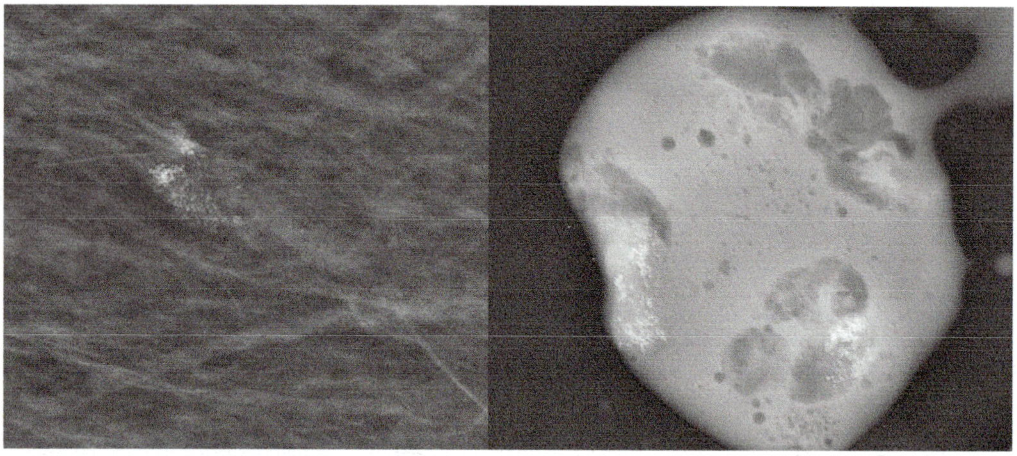

Fig. 20: Amorphous grouped calcification seen on mammogram and on specimen. Histopathology was s/o intermediate grade DCIS.

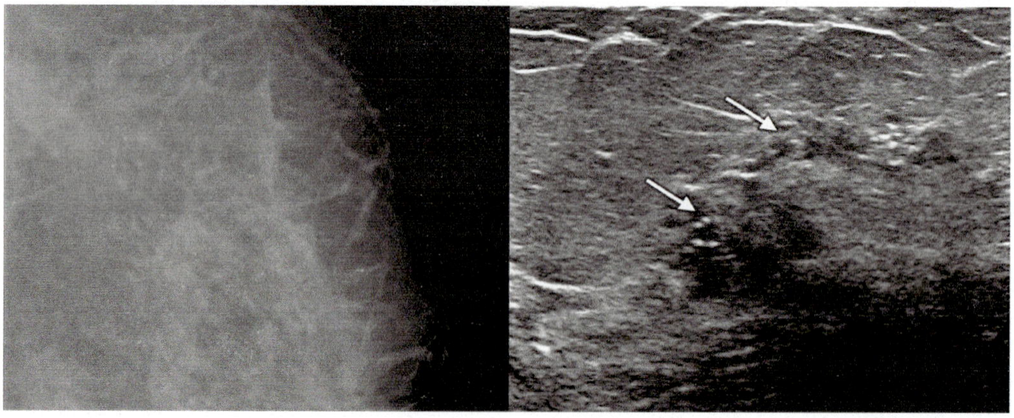

Fig. 21: Segmental coarse heterogeneous calcification on mammogram which were seen as multiple small echogenic foci (arrows) with posterior acoustic shadowing on ultrasound. Histopathology was s/o DCIS.

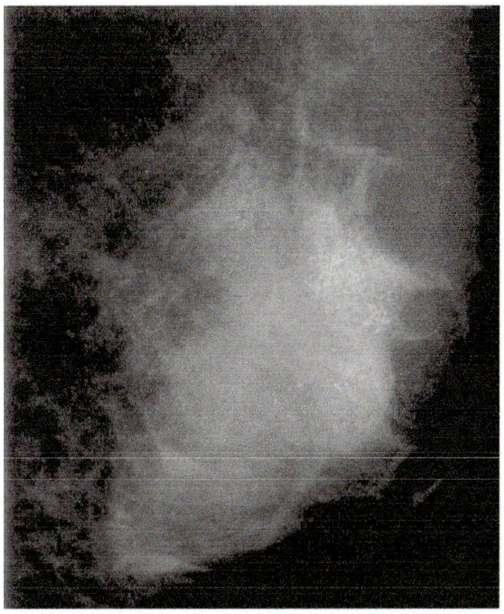

Fig. 22: Coarse heterogeneous segmental calcification seen on mammogram.

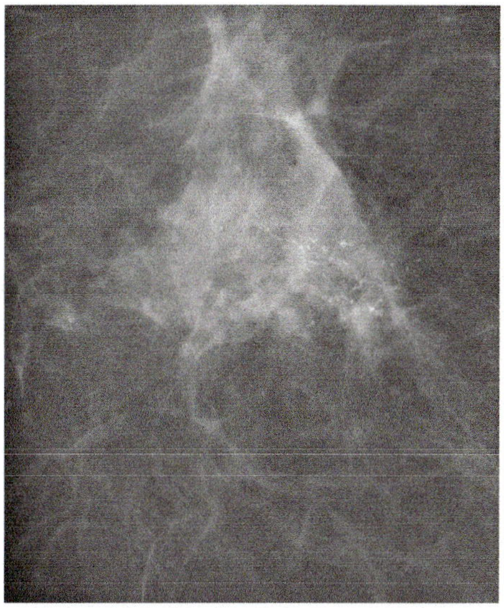

Fig. 24: Mammogram showing fine, linear calcifications. Histopathology was s/o DCIS.

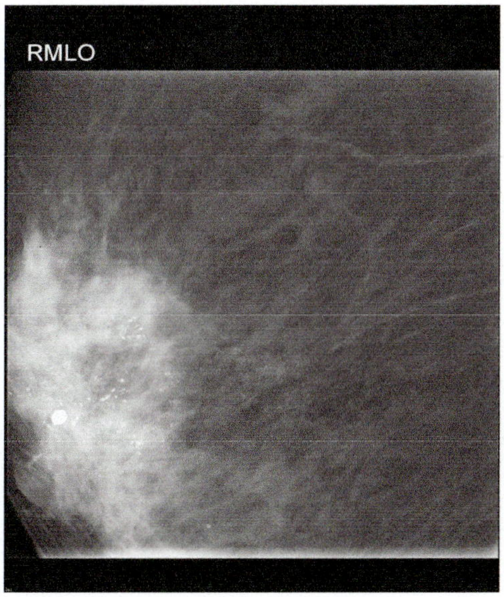

Fig. 23: Fine, pleomorphic calcification seen on mammogram. Histopathology was s/o DCIS.

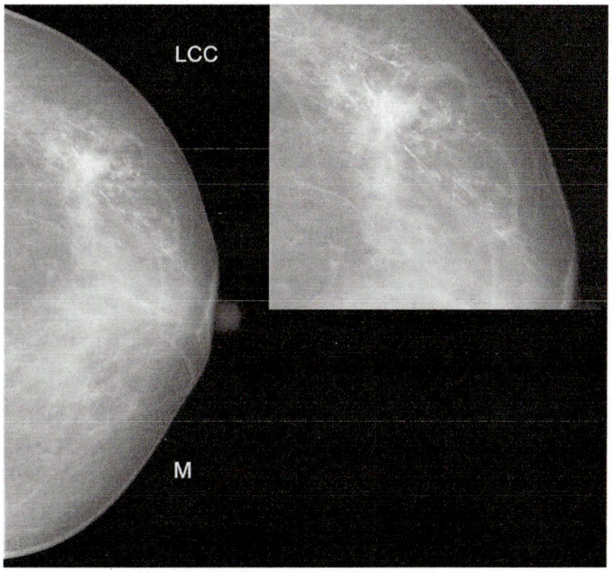

Fig. 25: Fine, linear and branching calcification in a segmental distribution is seen on mammogram. Histopathology is s/o DCIS.

Based on histopathology, DCIS is classified as high, intermediate and low grade. In comedocarcinoma, there is secretion of a thick tenacious material that calcifies in the central portion and is seen on mammogram.

The other types are micropapillary, solid and cribriform type. In micropapillary type, there is secretion of mucin and necrotic material that breaks off and gets calcified leading to loosely placed calcifications giving rise to a dotted, fragmented and casting type of calcification on mammogram.

Sometimes there are isolated cluster of calcifications restricted to a small volume. These can be due to various causes like fibrocystic disease, DCIS, sclerosing adenosis, etc. In such cases, one has to analyze both the individual calcification structure as well as shape and structure of cluster to know the cause.

Calcifications are also seen within a mass sometimes which can be appreciated both on mammogram and ultrasound (Figs. 27 and 28).

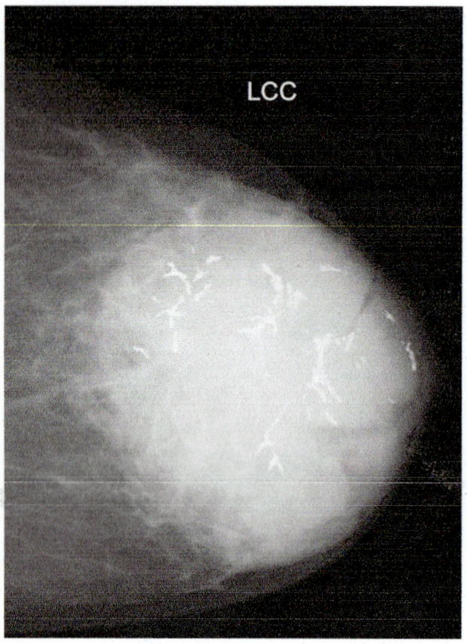

Fig. 26: Fine, linear and branching calcification in a mass is seen on mammogram. Histopathology is s/o invasive cancer with DCIS.

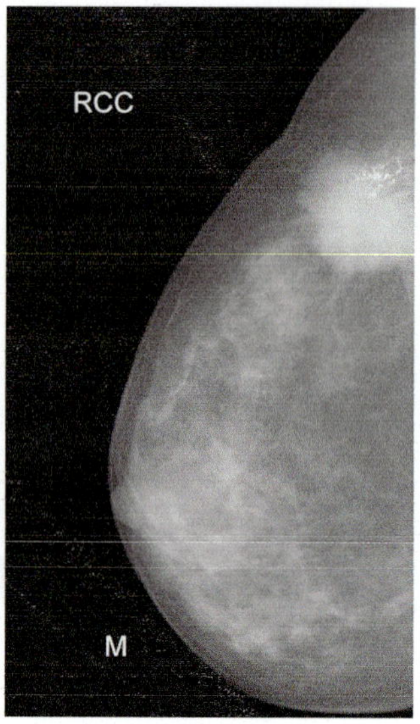

Fig. 27: Mammogram showing a irregular mass with spiculated margins showing fine linear calcifications within s/o BI-RADS category 5. (BI-RADS: breast imaging reporting and data system).

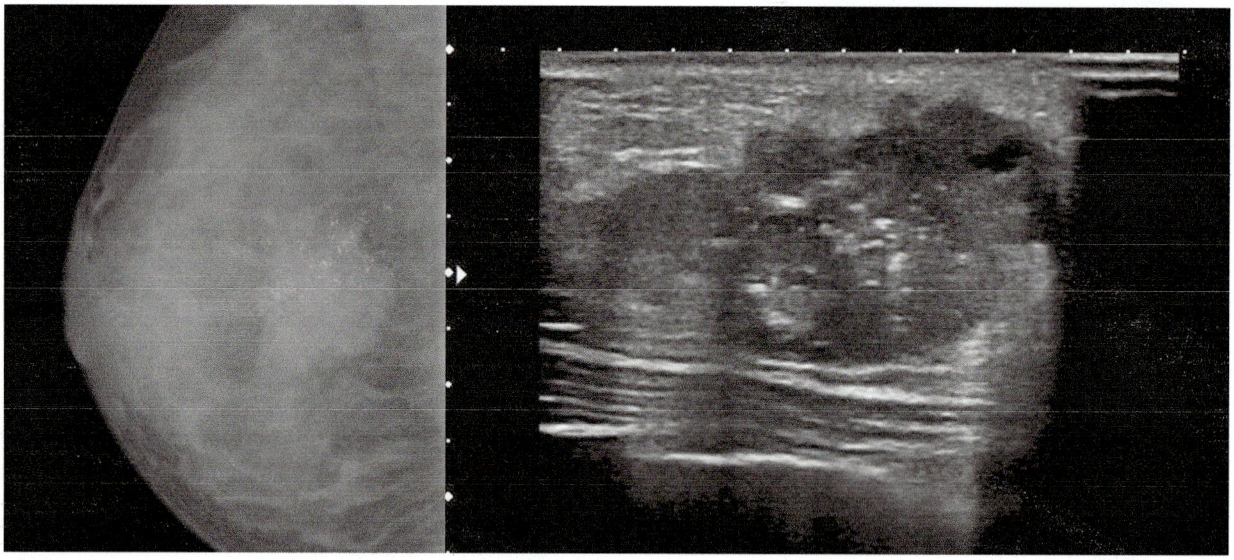

Fig. 28: A mass with irregular margins and coarse heterogeneous calcification on mammogram which are seen as echogenic foci on ultrasound—BI-RADS category 5. (BI-RADS: breast imaging reporting and data system). Histopathology was s/o invasive cancer with DCIS

DISTRIBUTION

Diffuse calcifications: These are scattered throughout the breast and favor a benign process like fibrocystic changes. **Regional** calcifications are seen in a large area covering more than one ductal distribution. If the distribution is non-ductal, it goes more in favor of a benign pathology. Sometimes it is difficult to distinguish between "segmental" and "ductal" distribution on a mammogram and the distribution and worst appearing imaging findings decide the decision to biopsy.

Segmental: These are calcium deposits in ducts and branches of a segment or lobe. Segmental calcifications cover slightly less than a quadrant and form in a triangle with its apex pointing at the nipple. A segmental distribution is suspicious for cancer because it suggests a process within a branch and its ducts (ductal distribution).

Linear pleomorphic, linear branching and segmental: Also suggest a process within a duct and its branches. The term linear describes calcifications in a line and can represent tumor in a duct or a focal benign process.

Grouped or Clustered

In grouped calcifications, ≥5 microcalcifications are present in a group. When they are scattered in breast they point toward a benign cause while a single group is more in favor of a malignant cause.

How to Distinguish Clustered Calcifications from Scattered Calcifications?

Sometimes it becomes difficult to distinguish grouped and scattered calcification on CC view because of superimposition. On MLO view, the scattered calcifications are seen distributed diffusely without any superimposition while grouped calcifications remain superimposed on both the views.

Fibroadenoma

The calcifications in fibroadenoma can be amorphous, grouped or coarse heterogeneous.

Adenosis

Adenosis is hyperplasia and hypertrophy of the glandular elements. In this condition, the number of acini is considerably increased and lobules are correspondingly enlarged.

Sclerosing Adenosis

Sclerosing adenosis may show suspicious calcifications. It is one of the histopathological types of adenosis, others being blunt duct and microglandular types. Unless there is calcification, sclerosing adenosis cannot be detected on mammogram. The calcifications seen are tiny cotton ball or powdery calcifications which are not resolved individually.

In conclusion, microcalcifications indicate a pathological process that can be identified by the location, morphology and distribution of calcification. A proper approach should be followed to ascertain the cause. At times, there may be an overlap in findings but the distinction between benign and suspicious calcification should be made so that cancer is not missed.

In addition, it is also important to evaluate stability of calcification over time as stable calcifications may not always indicate a benign pathology.

REFERENCES

1. Holland R, Hendriks J, Verbeek A, Mravunac M, Schuurmans SJ. Extent, distribution and mammographic/histological correlations of breast ductal carcinoma in situ. Lancet. 1990;335:519-22.
2. Lev Toaff AS, Feig SA, Saitas VL, Finkel GC, Schwartz GF. Stability of malignant breast microcalcifications. Radiology. 1994;192:153-6.
3. Henrot P, Leroux A, Genin P. Breast microcalcifications: the lesions in anatomical pathology. Diagn Interv Imaging. 2014;95:141-52.
4. Loffman Felman RL. Signs in imaging. Radiology. 2002;223: 481-2.
5. Linden SS, Sickles EA. Sedimented calcium in benign breast cysts: the full spectrum of mammographic presentations. Am J Roentgenol. 1989;152:967-71.

2.6 Digital Breast Tomosynthesis

INTRODUCTION

Breast tomosynthesis is also called 3D mammography or digital breast tomosynthesis. In this technique, three-dimensional volumetric image of breast is obtained by capturing multiple images of breast using different angles. To put it simply, it is a modified digital mammography.

Equipment and technique: A full-field flat panel digital detector is used, which can perform a rapid read out without distorting the image. The detector is made up of cesium iodide crystals or amorphous silicon or selenium. The positioning of patient and breast compression are as in digital mammography. Multiple projections are taken after positioning the patient and giving instructions to hold breath. During this, the X-ray tube source moves through a 15° arc to acquire 15 low-dose projections images with a movement of 1° between each projection. This process is repeated four times to get two craniocaudal and two mediolateral oblique (MLO) views. The raw data from the tomosynthesis projection images obtained in each projection are reconstructed into a stack of tomosynthesis slices separated by 1 mm and then displayed on the work station for interpretation.

Advantages and disadvantages of breast tomosynthesis: In spite of the fact that radiation dose is higher as compared to standard mammography, it is still within the limit approved by FDA. The advantage of tomosynthesis is that lesion in the selected cross section of breast tissue is seen clearly. Apart from that, there is increased visibility of overlying objects helping in delineating the border of the lesion (Figs. 1A to C). It improves the accuracy of screening and diagnostic mammography as breast can be seen in three dimensional format with multiple slices which remove the confounding factors due to overlapping structures. This helps in proper and definitive interpretation of the mass and increases confidence level of the interpreting radiologist.

Breast tomosynthesis helps by:

- Increasing lesion conspicuity: There is a subjective improvement in assessing conspicuity of both benign and malignant lesions.
- Three dimensional localization of lesions: With 3D reconstruction, this is possible without the need of additional views.
- Slice by slice evaluation is possible so that false positive due to overlapping structures leading to asymmetric densities can be avoided. At the same time false negative due to normal structures hiding underlying mass can be avoided.

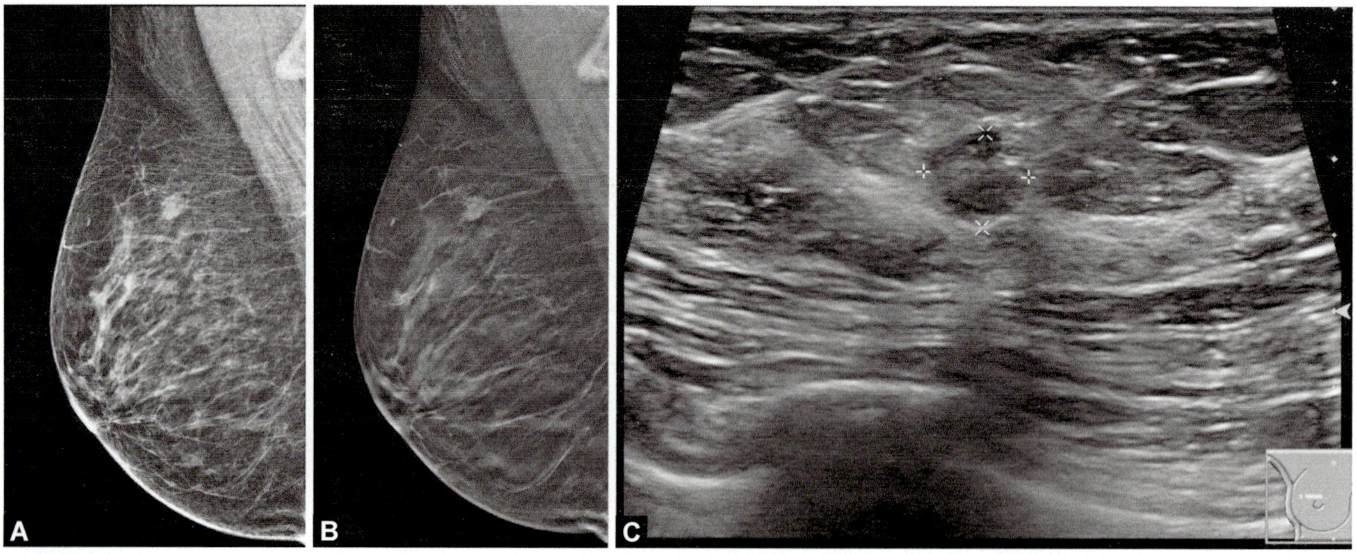

Figs. 1A to C: A 58-year-old female who underwent hysterectomy Ca endometrium. She came for a routine mammogram. Mammogram MLO view shows (A) an irregular mass whose margins appear spiculated on (B) Tomosynthesis s/o BI-RADS 5; (C) Ultrasound images show the same findings. (BI-RADS: breast imaging reporting and data system; MLO: mediolateral oblique).

Courtesy: Dr Sabita Desai, Hinduja Hospital, Mumbai, Maharashtra, India, for the contribution of this case.

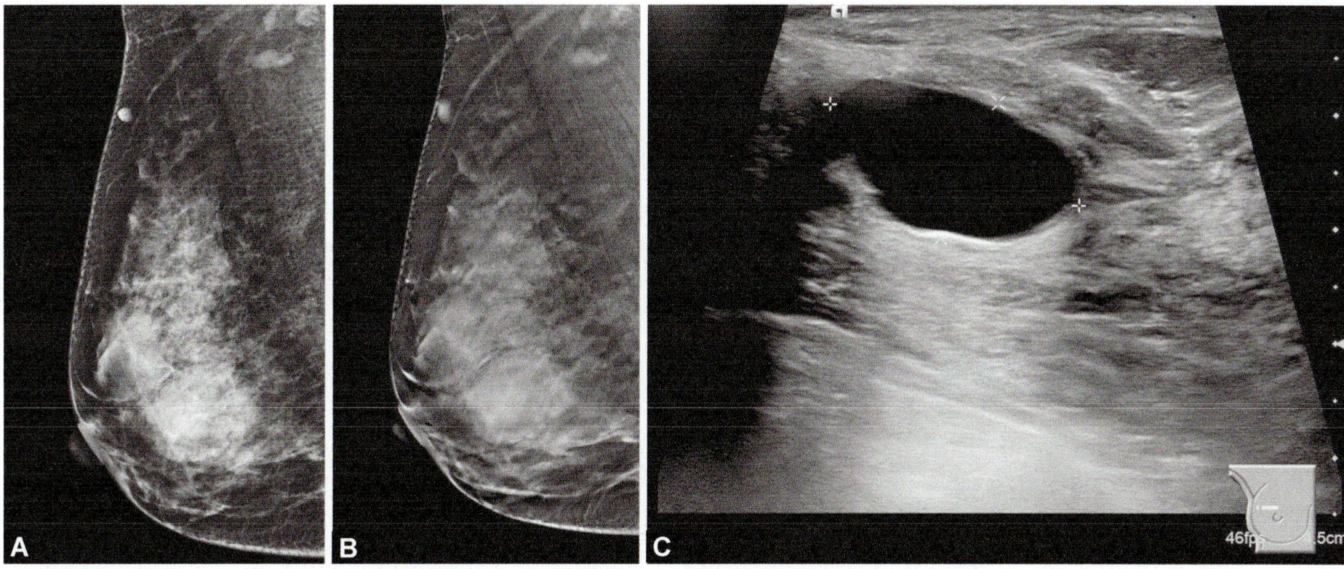

Figs. 2A to C: Mammogram MLO view in a 45-year-old female showed circumscribed (A) equal density masses whose margins were appreciated well on (B) Tomosynthesis. Ultrasound confirms circumscribed; (C) simple cysts. (MLO: mediolateral oblique).
Source: This case is contributed by Dr. Sabita Desai, Hinduja Hospital, Mumbai, India.

Breast tomosynthesis is especially useful in women with dense breasts as it is often difficult to visualize masses with certainty in these cases. It is observed that the number of masses, their margins and other findings like involvement of ducts or any associated microcalcifications are seen clearly by tomosynthesis. This helps in categorizing the mass into benign or malignant mass (Figs. 2A to C).

It has been shown in various studies that "call back or recall" rates are lesser when breast tomosynthesis is used for screening. It also helps in early detection of breast cancer. The time taken to interpret tomosynthesis images is definitely longer than that to evaluate digital mammography images. Breast tomosynthesis has accuracy comparable to spot compression views. When suspicious asymmetric density is seen, the use of tomosynthesis increases sensitivity of the lesion to characterize. There have been studies that have shown that if digital mammography is combined with digital tomosynthesis; it increases the concordance between the readers for BI-RADS classification. The image quality and diagnostic value of tomosynthesis is better than full-field digital mammography (FFDM) and is almost similar to FFDM + MAG Magnification when microcalcifications have to be evaluated. Advantages of breast tomosynthesis:

- Breast cancers that are hidden or are not clearly visible due to their small size are detected at an early stage
- The morphological features of mass like size, shape and location are seen more accurately. This avoids unnecessary biopsies
- Multiple breast masses are seen clearly

Ultrasound

CHAPTER 3

3.1 Equipment and Technique

INTRODUCTION

Breast ultrasound was first introduced in the 1950s when its role was primarily to distinguish cystic from solid masses. It was in 1995 that Stavros published his landmark study which demonstrated that benign and malignant breast masses could be characterized confidently using grayscale imaging features.[1]

Ever since, ultrasound has been a mainstay of breast imaging as a diagnostic tool and is evolving continuously. It has become an indispensable adjunct to mammography, especially in women with dense breasts where can detect early stage mammographically occult breast cancers. It is also recommended as the initial imaging modality in younger women with palpable breast lesions and in acute inflammatory lesions of the breast. With the use of high-frequency transducers, it is possible to see malignancy associated with clustered microcalcifications as an irregular mass, dilated duct or multiple echogenic foci. Its role as a screening tool is limited at the moment; however, there are several studies evaluating its role as an adjunct to screening mammography, especially in women with dense breasts.

Since ultrasound examination is operator dependent, the knowledge and understanding of technical parameters for producing an optimum imaging quality is a must. In some countries, ultrasound is performed by sonographer and the static images thus saved are later interpreted by the radiologist. In this regard, it is important to remember that real-time scanning can never be replaced by interpreting static images as subtle, but important findings like irregular or indistinct margins and architectural distortion cannot be captured adequately on static images. The mobility of lesion and its relationship with surrounding structures can be assessed only on real-time scanning. Therefore real-time scanning is a must for complete and proper evaluation of ultrasound images.

GOALS OF ULTRASOUND

The most important goal of ultrasound is to evaluate the consistency of mass followed by its characterization based on the imaging features. At the same time, it also helps in correlating or synthesizing the findings seen on other modalities and assimilating the clinical information to make a diagnosis that helps provide best patient care. While targeted ultrasound is used for evaluation of a palpable abnormality or a mammographic abnormality, non-targeted ultrasound is mainly used for evaluation of mastalgia or nipple discharge. Ultrasound is also used for breast interventions for guiding biopsies, cyst aspirations and fine needle aspiration cytology. Sometimes a second look ultrasound is useful after MRI in arriving at a diagnosis. There have been various advances in ultrasound technology over the last few years which include higher resolution transducers, compound imaging, harmonic imaging, power Doppler and more recently, elastography and 3-D ultrasound. Harmonic imaging selects higher frequencies thereby removing lower frequency reverberation echoes allowing better characterization of simple cysts.[2]

INDICATIONS OF BREAST ULTRASOUND

- Symptomatic breast lumps in women <35 years of age
- Confirmation and further characterization of a palpable mass or mammographic or MRI abnormality
- Nipple discharge
- Infection or mastitis
- Lump during pregnancy or lactation
- Cancer detection in asymptomatic women with mammographically dense breasts
- Mastalgia
- *Occult primary*: Lymph node metastases from breast primary in dense breasts with no mammographic abnormality

- Palpable axillary lumps
- Augmented breast/breast implants
- Guidance modality for interventional procedures
- Follow-up of patients treated with neoadjuvant chemotherapy
- Second look ultrasound following MRI.

EQUIPMENT AND SETTINGS

Ultrasound should be performed with a high-resolution scanner and proper gain settings, focal zone selections and fields of view should be optimized to obtain high-quality images. Breast ultrasound requires a high-frequency transducer of 8–15 MHz with a wide footprint probe. A lower frequency transducer may be used for larger breasts or large inflammatory masses. The use of a standoff may be required for evaluating nipple, superficial lesions or skin lesions.

The use of high-frequency transducers provides better lateral resolution, short axis focal zone of 1.5 cm, continuous electronic focusing on transmit and receive, broad band width and short pulse lengths and give the best combination of spatial and contrast resolutions for breast ultrasound. Low pulse repetition frequency (PRF) color and spectral Doppler capabilities are required for assessing vascularity of lesions.

Recent advancement in ultrasound equipment like coded harmonics and spatial compounding improve contrast resolution while maintaining or improving spatial resolution helping in making more specific diagnosis. Harmonic imaging leads to improved resolution and reduced reverberation and near-field artifacts and is especially useful in distinguishing a purely cystic mass from a hypoechoic mass. Extended or panoramic views provide a better perspective of the lesion in relation to the rest of the breast especially in larger lesions, and also help in accurate assessment of size and in measurement of distance of multifocal lesions.

Transducer: High-frequency linear transducers are used for breast imaging (Fig. 1). For women with breast thickness of >3 cm, a 12–5 MHz transducer must be used and for women with smaller breast and thickness <3 cm, a 17–5 MHz transducer is good. The use of 17–5-MHz probe provides good spatial and soft-tissue resolution for examining superficial structures; however, visualization of deeper and posterior structures will be compromised.

Before one starts ultrasound of the breast, it is important to set parameters like gain and time gain compensation (TGC) at an optimal level. Almost all the latest ultrasound machines are user friendly and knobs can be easily located on the control panel (Fig. 2). The depth and focus can be adjusted depending upon the lesion location. Without having a knowledge of technical parameters, optimum quality images are not produced compromising on the overall diagnosis.

Gain: The gain settings must be adjusted in a way that fat at all the levels is seen as midlevel gray. In comparison to fat, most of the masses are hypoechoic while structure like skin, coopers ligaments and fibrous tissue are hyperechoic (echogenic).

TGC: This is used to adjust the image brightness at various depths from the skin in order to compensate for the attenuation of ultrasound as it penetrates deeper tissues. This can be done manually or automatically depending upon the equipment used.

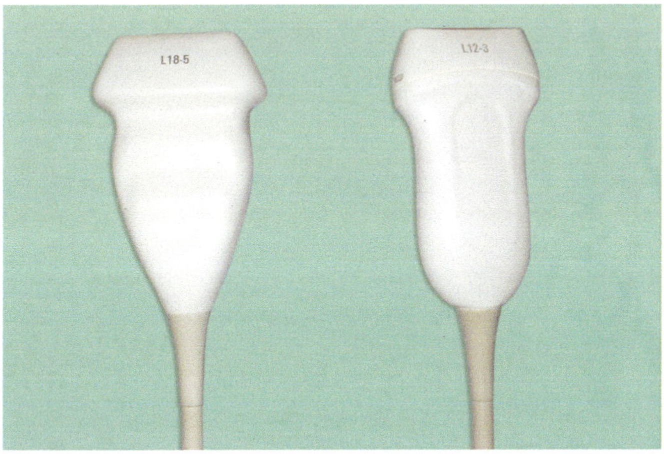

Fig. 1: High-frequency linear probes used for doing ultrasound of breast having a frequency of 18–5 and 12–3 MHz.

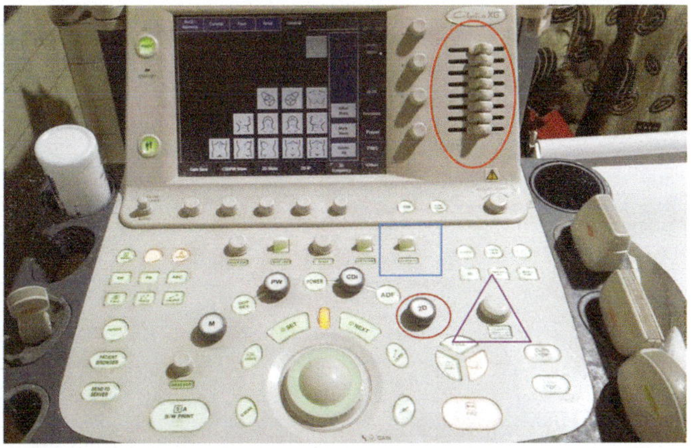

Fig. 2: Control panel of ultrasound machine showing the various knobs to optimize the parameters: Red: TGC, Blue: 2-D focus, Purple: depth and Maroon: gain. (TGC: time gain compensation).

Depth: When scanning is begun the depth is set in such a way that the pectoral muscle is seen just along the posterior margin of field of view. This depth can be adjusted and changed during real-time scanning, for example, decrease in depth will show more superficial structures while increased depth will show deeper or posterior structures clearly. Beginners often make a mistake in depth adjustment, thereby compromising on the quality of image and features of the lesion under examination (Figs. 3A and B).

Focal zone: If a single focal zone is chosen, then focus should be placed at the area of interest or just posterior to it for optimum image quality (Figs. 4A and B). Multiple focal zones are also available as an option and it increases the resolution at multiple levels with a slight decrease in frame rates.

TECHNIQUE OF PERFORMING ULTRASOUND

Optimization of ergonomics setup: The person performing ultrasound should sit or stand in a neutral and comfortable position to reduce stress and strain. Newer ultrasound machines have adjustable worktops (monitor and control panels) according to the requirement of the person doing ultrasound.

Position of patient: The patient should be positioned supine with ipsilateral arm relaxed and flexed behind the head to minimize the thickness of the portion of the breast being evaluated. Adequate amount of coupling gel should be applied on the breast to get an optimum image. While evaluating lesions in, on, or just beneath the skin,

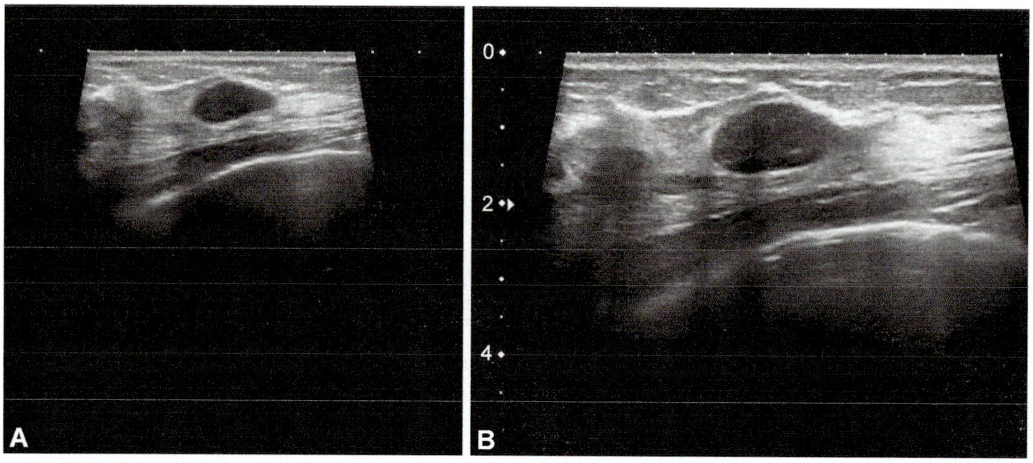

Figs. 3A and B: Ultrasound of a breast lesion showing: (A) Incorrect depth; (B) Correct depth. If the lesion is placed superficially depth is decreased and for deeper lesions, depth is increased.

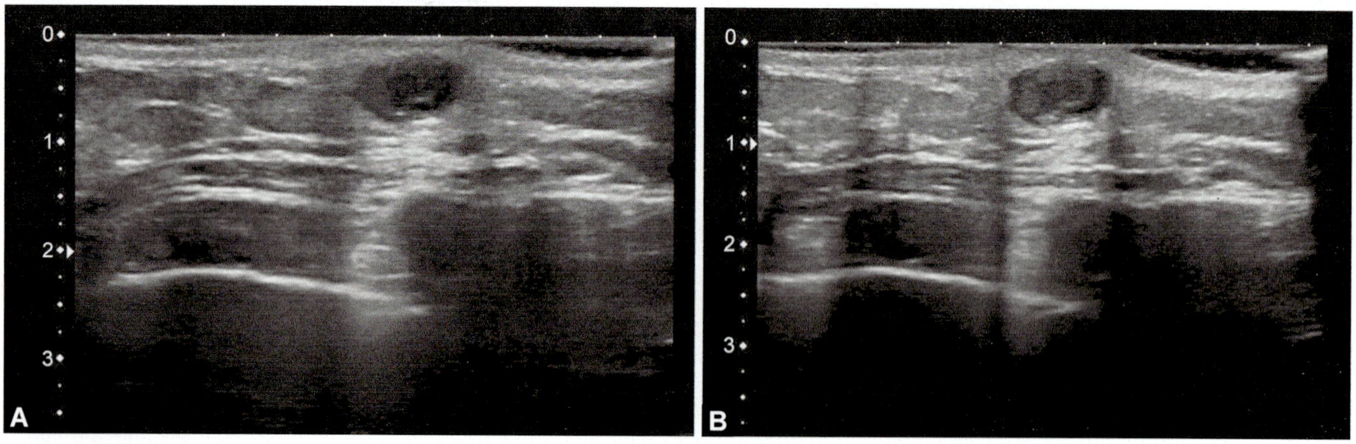

Figs. 4A and B: Ultrasound of a superficially placed mass showing: (A) Incorrect focus placed too posterior to lesion; (B) Optimum focus placed just posterior to lesion.

a stand-off device or thick layer of gel should be put. For medial masses in breast, supine position is better, while for evaluation of lateral lesions and axilla, a lateral decubitus position or contralateral oblique position is used. If the patient feels a thickening in sitting position, then ultrasound examination should be done in the sitting position also.

Planes and scanning technique: There should be a planned approach while performing an ultrasound examination so as not to miss any findings. The breast should be scanned in radial and antiradial planes (Fig. 5) and, if required, transverse and longitudinal planes. Radial and antiradial planes are better because they are along the normal axis of ducts and lobar tissues making it easier for lesion detection and ductal extension.[3] One can adapt his or her own scanning technique according to convenience, but it's always better to scan in a systematic manner. One can start from 12 o'clock position and scan in a clockwise direction in radial plane till one finishes the entire extent of breast and return to 12 o'clock position again. While doing ultrasound for a palpable mass, it should be ensured that the area under question has been scanned properly which can be ascertained by placing a finger on the palpable abnormality before placing the transducer on the region. If no mass is seen in the region of palpable abnormality and only normal breast tissue is seen, it is useful to palpate the lump and do simultaneous scanning to be sure and this should be mentioned clearly in the report.

Role of compression: Strong compression should be avoided as it may push the lesion out and may deform normal tissue structures. Light compression on the other hand can cause prominent shadowing from Cooper ligaments especially in dense breasts.[4] This shadowing from Cooper ligaments disappears when the scanning plane is changed and shows continuity with surrounding tissues without any shadowing. This is a commonly observed finding and therefore it is important to remember that shadowing in only one plane is not a real finding. Optimal compression on the other hand is useful for identification of fat lobule and sometimes in cystic masses to identify the cystic component. For a beginner, it is often difficult to differentiate normal from abnormal tissue and many times pseudolesions which are due to interspersed fat within glandular tissue are described as fibroadenomas. Scanning in different planes would solve this dilemma.

Split screen imaging: This can very useful to compare mirror image locations in left and right breast (Figs. 6A and B) especially while correlating mammographic findings like asymmetric density in one breast which can be due to fibroglandular tissue. Split screen imaging can also be used to document dynamic events, for example, effect on a lesion with or without compression. This can be done by storing image with compression on one side of the screen and without compression on the other side. While documenting images without compression, a light scanning is required, barely touching the skin.

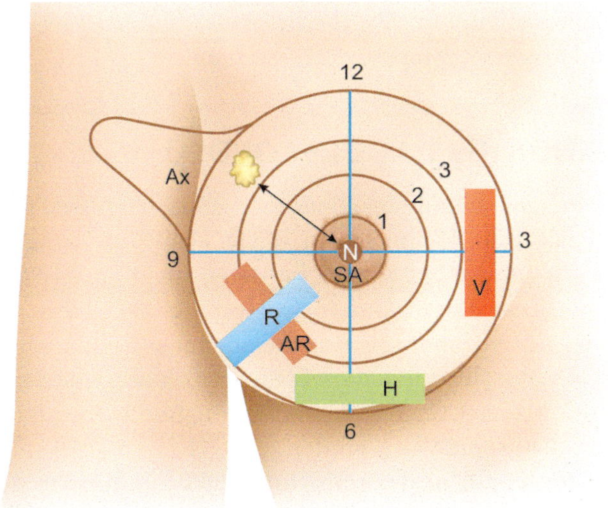

Fig. 5: Clock position and various planes for doing ultrasound of breast. (V: vertical, H: horizontal, R: radial, AR: antiradial).

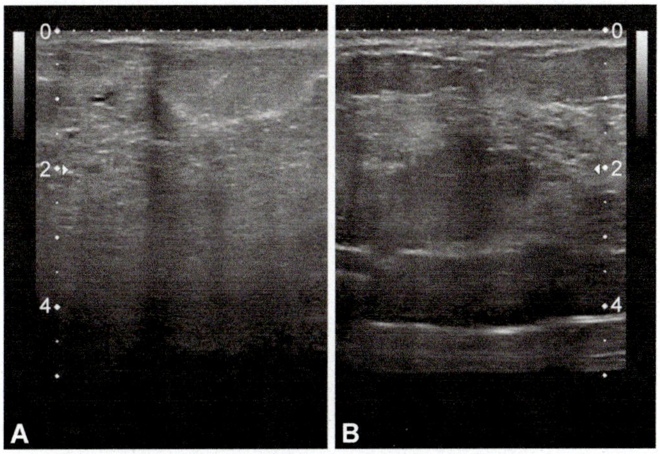

Figs. 6A and B: Split screen imaging showing mirror image location in both breasts for comparison: (A) Increased echogenicity of the fat lobules and parenchyma s/o inflammation; (B) Same location on the opposite breast shows normal parenchyma.

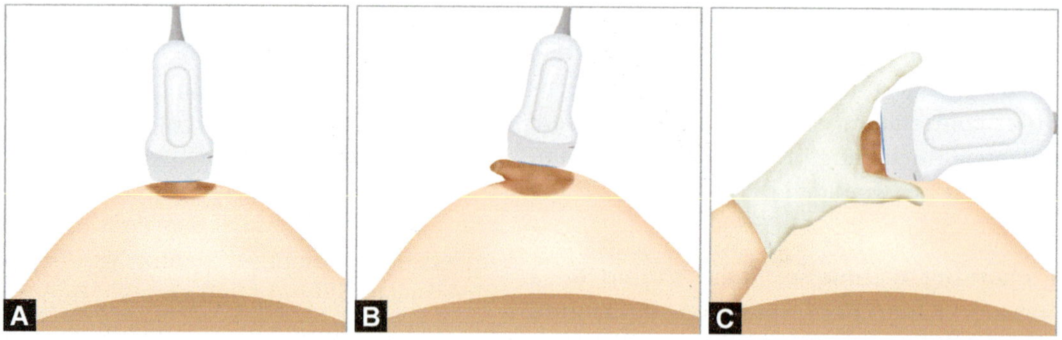

Figs. 7A to C: Evaluation of nipple: (A) Transducer kept on nipple with shadowing behind the nipple causing it difficult to evaluate this area; (B) Rolled nipple technique to depict the portion of the mammary duct within the nipple; (C) The two-handed compression technique for better visibility of the duct where it enters the base of the nipple.

Split imaging with and without compression is also used to:

- Assess mobility of echoes within an enlarged echogenic duct
- Evaluate compressibility of an enlarged duct
- Look for movement of debris in abscess.

While evaluating ducts, dynamic maneuvers like ballottement of duct can be done with transducer to demonstrate movement of thick echoes and differentiate inspissated secretions from papilloma.

One must remember that specific lesions should be correlated with both clinical and mammographic findings (if available) and documented properly so that they are clearly identified on stored images. The easiest and most consistent way to correlate mammographic and sonographic findings is to compare the transverse sonographic plane with craniocaudal view on mammogram.

The axilla should also be examined in the same sitting especially if one finds a suspicious malignant mass as lymph nodal involvement should be assessed and commented upon in the report. *(Please note: Axillary lymph node assessment is dealt within chapter on "Evaluation of Axilla.")*.

NIPPLE–AREOLAR REGION

Evaluation of the nipple and subareolar portions of the mammary ducts requires angulation of the transducer so that the ultrasound beam is perpendicular to the long axis of the duct during peripheral compression. When the transducer is held at an appropriate angle against the periphery of the nipple, it is easier to maintain steady contact and pressure needed to achieve optimal depiction of the duct. If one puts the transducer directly upon the nipple, the nipple is pushed into the breast, producing intense shadowing behind it making it difficult to visualize the subareolar region. In this position, the ducts run parallel to the ultrasound beam.

The use of a standoff pad or copious amount of gel helps in removing shadowing caused by air trapped in the crevices within the raised nipple. The application of maneuvers including the rolled-nipple technique and two-handed compression technique (Figs. 7A to C) described by Stavros may help in improving the detection of clinically significant lesions located near or in the nipple.

The **rolled-nipple technique** is used to depict the portion of the mammary duct within the nipple. In this position, ultrasound beam is perpendicular to the long axis of duct and there is no acoustic shadowing from the duct. The **two-handed compression technique** is used to achieve better visibility of the duct where it enters the base of the nipple and to assess intraductal lesions and ductal compressibility. In this, the breast is supported by other hand to optimize nipple probe contact.

FINDINGS TO BE RECORDED

The images should be labeled as right or left breast along with location of the lesion using clock face notation. The size of a mass should be determined by recording its maximal dimensions in two orthogonal planes. The measurements should be taken from outer to outer margin of the mass. The orientation of the transducer with respect to the breast (e.g. transverse or longitudinal, radial or antiradial) should be recorded.

The length of the transducer face (footprint), usually between 3.5 and 5 cm, can be used to estimate the distance of the lesion from the nipple. Remember that measurements should not be made from the edge of the areola, as areolar width is widely variable.) The depth of the lesion from skin surface should also be recorded.

Extended or panoramic views can be done especially in larger lesions to show its entire extent in relation to the rest of the breast and multiple lesions. This is an advanced technology where imaging is done beyond the foot print of transducer using free-hand technique in which the operator slides the transducer along the region of interest in a particular direction without lifting the transducer. This finally gives rise to a single large field of view image[4] and can be used especially in measuring distances between multifocal (same quadrant, within 4–5 cm of index cancer along the same ducts) and multicentric lesions (lesions in different quadrant or >4–5 cm along different ducts). If the probe slips during sliding of transducer, then image becomes distorted and the process has to be repeated.

Ultrasound reporting: The ultrasound report should be concise and structured. Correlation of any clinical, mammographic and MRI findings with the sonographic findings should be specifically stated in the report.

If the lump is palpable, concomitant palpation and scanning is useful and if there is no lump in the region of palpable abnormality, it should be mentioned clearly in the report. Multiple simple cysts or a combination of multiple simple and complicated cysts need not be reported individually. If any masses have been biopsied previously, they should be noted in the report together with the prior biopsy results, if known.

The annotation should be as follows:

- Side of breast
- Clock face
- Size of mass in two orthogonal planes-maximal dimensions (images should be captured with and without calipers to assess the margins adequately on static images).
- Distance of the lesion from the nipple
- Depth of the lesion from the skin surface
- Axillary assessment

There are five descriptors to know the **location** of the lesion (Fig. 8):

1. The first is the side-right or left written as R or L.
2. The second descriptor tells the clock position.
3. The third defines distance of the lesion from the nipple. The distance descriptor has five locations: 1, 2, 3 SA and axillary (Ax). The numbers 1, 2, 3 are equal width rings from the areolar margin to the periphery of breast. Alternatively, distance of the lesion from the nipple can be measured in centimeter.
4. The fourth descriptor is depth of the lesion and A, B, C is used where A is the most superficial and C is the deepest. Alternatively depth of the lesion from skin surface can be used.
5. The fifth descriptor is for scan plane-transverse (tr), longitudinal (lo), radial (rad) and antiradial (ar).

If there are multiple lesions, then the findings can be recorded in tabular form as shown bottom of page.

STRUCTURED ULTRASOUND REPORT

Indication: The indication for the examination, relevant clinical history and relevant risk factor information should be clearly stated. If it is a follow-up for a specific mass or area of concern then the dates of comparison should be clearly mentioned in the report.

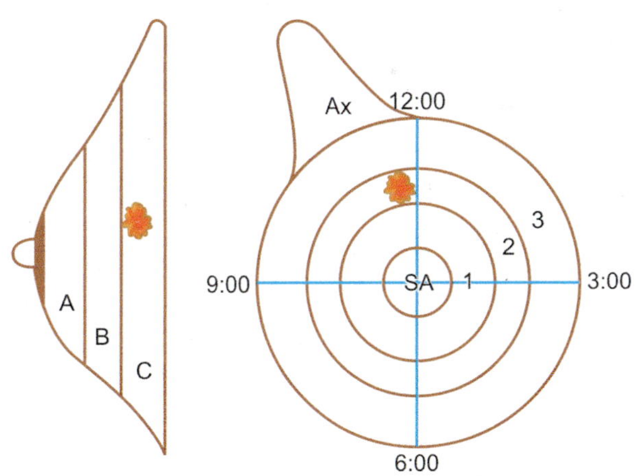

Fig. 8: Descriptors for knowing location of mass: the distance descriptor has five locations: 1–3, SA and A. Depth of the lesion is marked as A, B, C where A is the most superficial and C is the deepest. (Ax: axillary; SA: subareolar).

S. No	*Side*	*Ultrasound features*	*Size*	*Clock position*	*Distance from nipple (cm)*	*Depth (cm)*

Whether the examination was directed or targeted to a specific location, or whether it was performed for supplementary screening should be clearly mentioned.

REPORTING FORMAT

- *Breast composition*: It should be mentioned as follows:
  - Homogeneous background echotexture—fat
  - Homogeneous background echotexture—fibroglandular
  - Heterogeneous background echotexture—both fat and fibroglandular tissue
- *Mass*: If a mass is seen, its location in terms of clock position and distance from nipple along with morphological descriptors of shape, margin and orientation (parallel versus not parallel) should be mentioned. Findings like posterior features, echogenicity and size in at least two dimensions should be clearly written. The associated findings like architectural distortion should also be mentioned. If Doppler is done and there is any positive finding, it should be recorded
- When more than one lesion or abnormality is located in the same scan frame, then its distance from the skin to the center or anterior aspect of the mass should be measured to differentiate one lesion from another
- For bilateral findings, all the findings in each breast should be described in a separate paragraph
- When more than one type of examination for a mass or abnormality (e.g., mammography and ultrasound is performed on the same day), the findings for each examination should be described in separate paragraphs with an overall assessment and management recommendations for the combined examinations
- The combined final assessment should reflect the highest likelihood of malignancy assessed at the two examinations and categorized in breast imaging reporting and data system (BI-RADS) category
- Clear recommendations should be made as to the next course of action as per the BI-RADS assessment category and further management suggested. If an image guided interventional procedure is recommended, then the type of imaging should also be suggested.

Conclusion: Ultrasound is operator dependent, has a learning curve and one must get used to the normal appearance of breast tissue which varies in density depending upon the age of the patient. It is important to optimize and standardize the ultrasound technique at any given institution. The knowledge of correct patient position, technical parameters, amount of transducer pressure, various planes and maneuvers to get an optimal image is essential to make an accurate diagnosis.

REFERENCES

1. Stavros AT, Thickman D, Rapp CI, et al. Solid breast nodule: use of sonography to distinguish between benign and malignant lesions. Radiology. 1995;196:123-34.
2. Weinstein SP, Conant EF, Sehgal C. Technical advancement in breast ultrasound imaging. Semin Ultrasound CT MR. 2006;27:273-83.
3. Stavros AT. Breast ultrasound. Philadelphia, PA: Lippincott, Williams and Wilkins; 2004. pp. 46.
4. Park JM, Yang L, LaraoiaA, Franken Jr EA, Fajardo L. Missed and/or misinterpreted lesions in breast ultrasound: reasons and solutions. Can Assoc Radiol J. 2011;62:41-9.
5. Stafford RJ, Whitman GJ. Ultrasound physics and technology in breast imaging. Ultrasound Clin. 2011;6:299-312.

3.2 Breast Imaging-reporting and Data System (BI-RADS) Classification

INTRODUCTION

Ultrasound is a widely used modality for evaluating breast masses and though it is available in every nook and corner of the country, there exists considerable variability in the quality of assessment of breast masses on ultrasound depending on the technique, experience and expertise of the observer. This leads to disparity and confusion in lesion interpretation, assigning final assessment categories and in suggesting recommendations.

In order to speak a common language and use a terminology that is understood by everyone, we are currently following the breast imaging reporting and data system (BI-RADS) reporting system by American College of Radiology (ACR). The ultrasound BI-RADS lexicon is based on the already established BI-RADS Mammography lexicon. There are some descriptors which are unique to ultrasound, for example orientation, echo pattern and posterior features with a few descriptors showing interobserver variability. **It is important to remember that categorization and recommendation must be based on the most suspicious finding.**

Composition of breast: The breast parenchyma can have varied appearances on ultrasound depending upon the age of patient. It can appear thin and membrane like as in elderly patients or thick and almost isoechoic during lactation. The breast in a young nulliparous woman demonstrates great variation in echogenicity and pattern that ranges from a homogenously echogenic tissue to a diffusely heterogeneous almost striped appearance due to ducts and periductal hypoechoic tissue. The parenchyma may also show focal thickening, which may occasionally cause a palpable abnormality. In a middle-aged woman, parenchyma is usually heterogenous with both fatty and fibroglandular tissue.

Other age-related changes include ductal ectasia often seen in older women which can be completely asymptomatic or associated with nipple discharge.

Ultrasound descriptors used for breast composition: The breast tissue composition on ultrasound is primarily determined by echogenicity which is compared with that of subcutaneous fat. The subcutaneous fat is medium gray and darker than fibroglandular tissue which is light gray in color. When the term heterogeneous breast is used, it means that there is an admixture of hypoechoic and more echogenic areas.

According to BI-RADS Atlas 5th edition, breast composition is described and categorized as follows (Figs. 1A to C):

- Homogeneous background echotexture—fat
- Homogeneous background echotexture—fibroglandular
- Heterogeneous background echotexture.

The **other descriptors** which are discussed in BI-RADS 5th edition are shown below.

Mass: A mass should be described using the morphological descriptors of shape, margin, orientation, echo pattern and posterior features.

1. **Shape:**
   a. Oval shape (wider than tall) indicates that the sagittal and transverse dimensions are greater than the anteroposterior dimension and there are 2–3 undulations (Fig. 2).
   b. Round
   c. Irregular (Fig. 3).

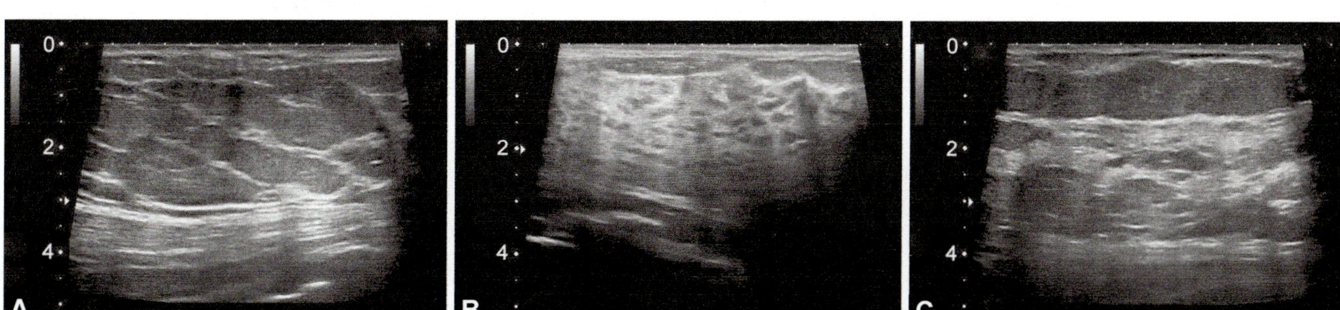

Figs. 1A to C: Ultrasound showing different types of breast density: (A) Fatty breast; (B) Fibroglandular and (C) Heterogeneous background echotexture.

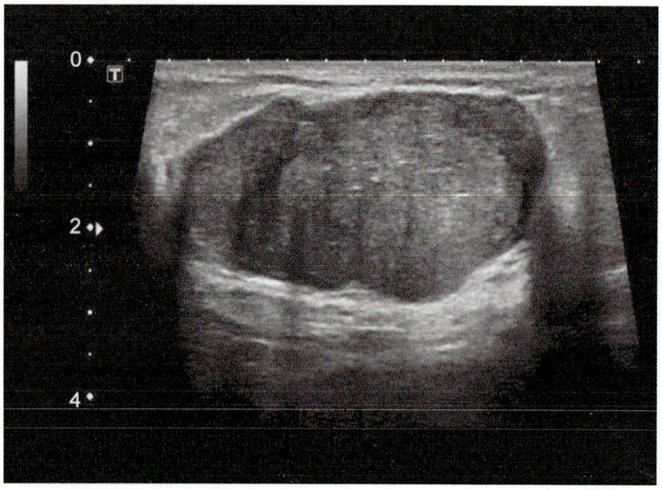

Fig. 2: A circumscribed oval mass with 2–3 undulations and parallel orientation. Histopathology was s/o fibroadenoma.

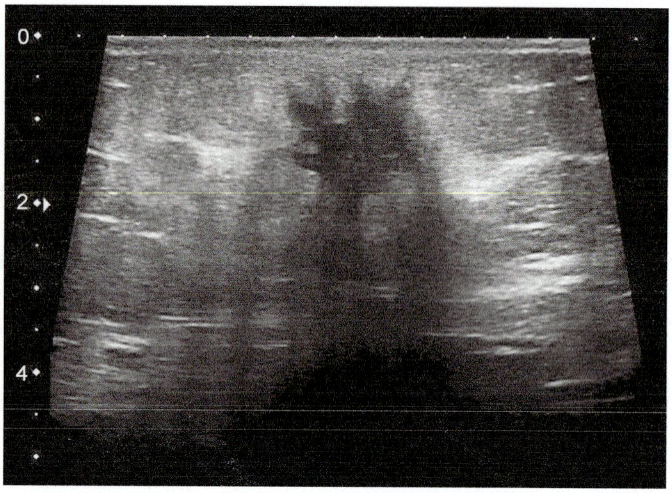

Fig. 4: A 62-year-old female presented with a palpable lump in left breast. Ultrasound showed a hypoechoic mass with angular margins. Histopathology was s/o infiltrating ductal carcinoma.

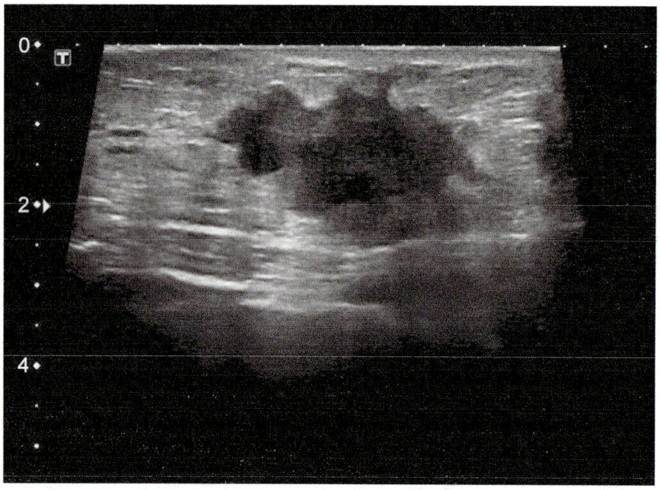

Fig. 3: A hypoechoic mass with irregular shape in a 55-year-old woman. Histopathology was s/o infiltrating ductal carcinoma.

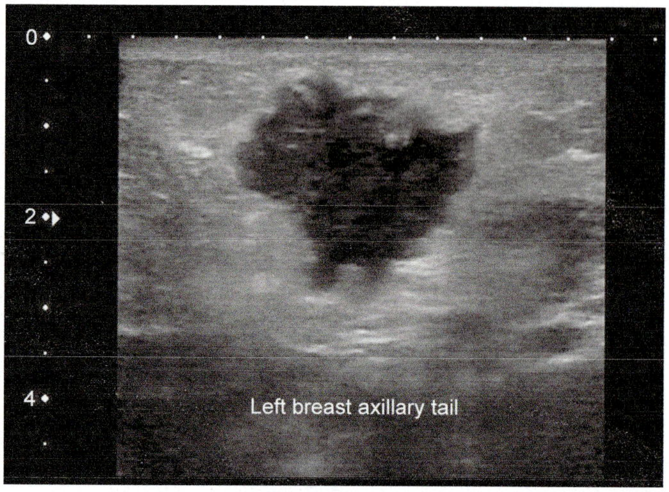

Fig. 5: A mass with microlobulations in a 64-year-old female presenting with a palpable lump. Histopathology was s/o infiltrating ductal carcinoma.

2. **Orientation:** It is defined as parallel (benign) or not parallel (suspicious finding) to the skin surface.
3. **Margins:**
   a. **Circumscribed margins**: Sharp and well defined.
   b. **Not circumscribed margins**:
      - *Indistinct margins:* These are not demarcated clearly
      - *Angular margins:* These refer to the junction between the relatively hypoechoic or isoechoic central part of the solid nodule and the surrounding tissue and has sharp corners to make acute angles (Fig. 4).
      - *Microlobulated:* Microlobulation is analogous to the mammographic finding and is recognized by the presence of many small (1–2 mm) lobulations on the surface of the solid breast nodule (Figs. 5 and 6).
      - *Spiculated:* These appear like sharp and thin lines projecting from the mass and are similar to mammographic spiculation. It consists of alternating hyperechoic and hypoechoic straight lines that radiate perpendicularly from the surface of the solid nodule. A thick echogenic "halo,"

best seen around the lateral edges of a malignant nodule, also represents hypoechoic spiculations.

4. **Echo pattern:** The echo pattern is categorized as:
   a. Anechoic
   b. Hyperechoic
   c. Complex cystic and solid
   d. Isoechoic
   e. Hypoechoic
   f. Heterogeneous.

   The echo pattern is always described using the subcutaneous fat in breast as a reference. Generally, the masses which are hyperechoic in comparison with fat are benign. The majority of breast masses are hypoechoic irrespective of being benign or malignant.

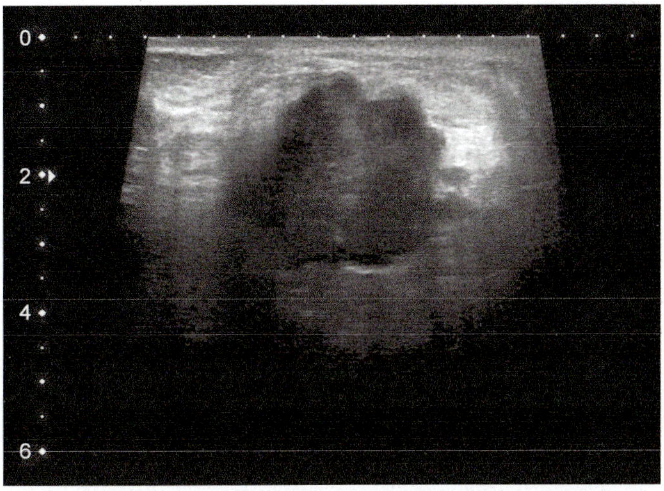

Fig. 6: Microlobulated margins in a mass in another patient with palpable lump which turned out to be a malignant mass.

5. **Posterior features:** Posterior features like enhancement or shadowing (Fig. 7) represent the attenuation characteristics of a mass with respect to its acoustic transmission and is of additional value though alone it has little specificity.

The posterior features are categorized as:

a. *No posterior features*
b. *Enhancement:* This is a benign feature and is seen in simple cyst, complicated cyst and papilloma (Fig. 8)
c. *Shadowing:* Shadowing exists when an area has relatively less through-transmission of sound than is present in surrounding tissues. This is a suspicious finding and may be seen in infiltrative ductal carcinoma (Fig. 9), postoperative scar and patients with dense breast tissue.
d. *Combined pattern*

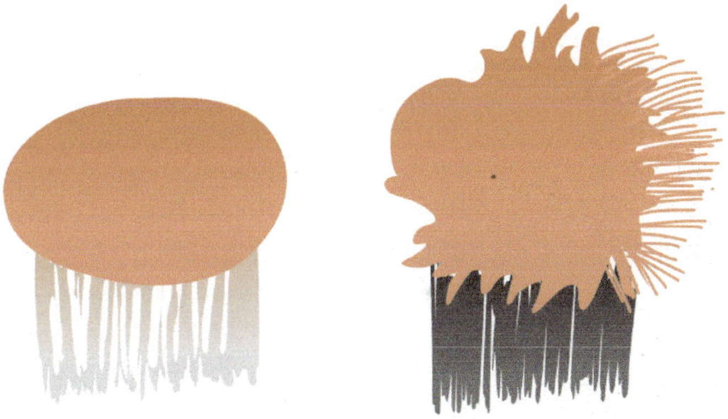

Fig. 7: Posterior features of a mass—enhancement and shadowing.

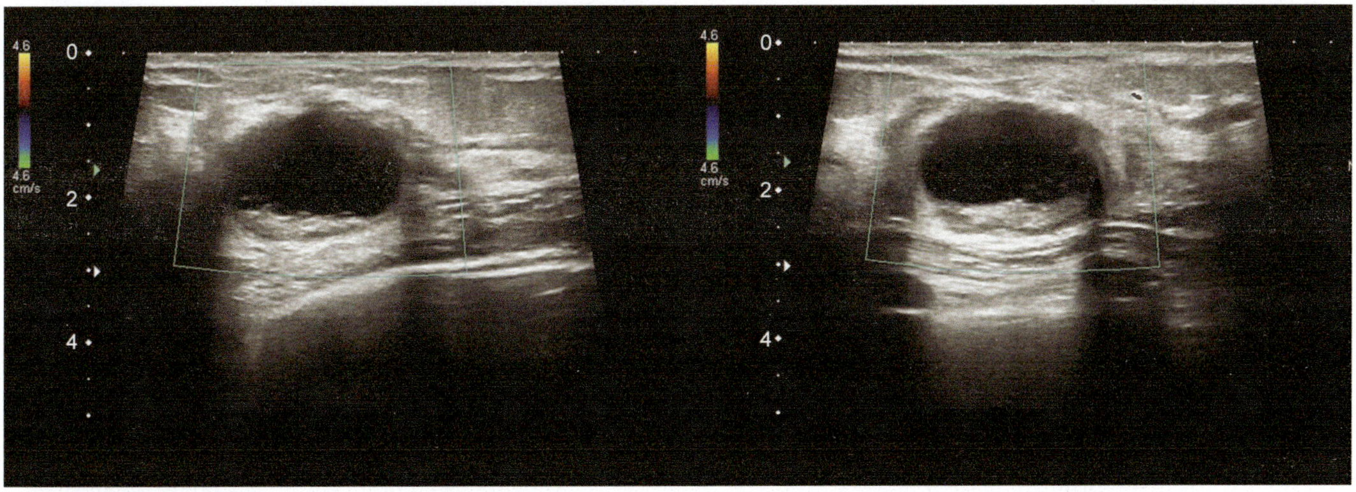

Fig. 8: Complicated cyst showing dependent debris and posterior acoustic enhancement.

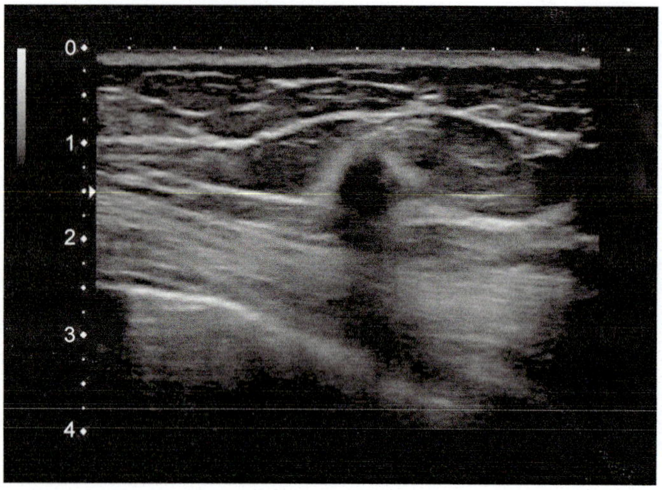

Fig. 9: Mass showing posterior acoustic shadowing which was proved to be infiltrating ductal carcinoma on histopathology.

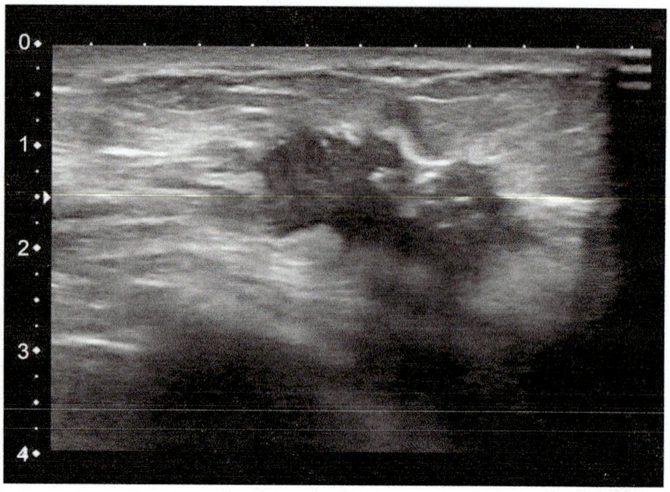

Fig. 10: Malignant mass showing small echogenic foci s/o punctate calcifications.

The ultrasound descriptors used to differentiate between benign and malignant masses are as shown in Table 1.

Table 1: Benign and maligant features of a mass.

Ultrasound descriptor	*Benign features*	*Malignant features*
Shape	Oval	Round, irregular
Orientation	Parallel	Not parallel
Margin	Circumscribed	Indistinct Microlobulated Angular Spiculated
Echo pattern	Anechoic, hyperechoic	Complex cystic and solid, hypoechoic
Posterior features	Enhancement	Shadowing, combined

Calcifications: These are poorly characterized on ultrasound as compared to mammography, but can be recognized as tiny echogenic foci, particularly well seen when present within a mass.

Calcification is categorized as follows:

- *Calcification in a mass*: Punctate calcifications that are sonographically visible within solid nodules are more likely to be associated with malignant than benign lesions (Fig. 10)
- Calcification outside a mass
- Intraductal calcification.

The following **Associated features** (should also be looked for):

- Architectural distortion
- Duct changes
- Skin changes in the form of skin thickening/skin retraction
- Edema
- *Vascularity*: The vascularity may be absent, central, peripheral or mixed.

Elasticity assessment: A lesion can be categorized as soft, intermediate or hard based on elasticity

EVALUATION OF CYSTIC MASSES

- *Simple cysts*: These are anechoic, circumscribed lesions with thin, echogenic outer wall, enhanced through transmission and thin edge shadows (Fig. 11).
- *Complicated cyst*: These are cystic lesions with homogeneous low-level echoes that otherwise meet the criteria of a simple cyst. Circumscribed cystic lesions with imperceptible wall and fluid-debris level (Fig. 12) are included as complicated cystic lesions.
- *Clustered microcysts*: These are lesions which are composed entirely of clusters of tiny (2–5 mm) anechoic foci with no discrete solid component (Fig. 13). Clustered cysts or cysts with thin septations (<0.5 mm) arise in the terminal ductolobular unit (TDLU) (Fig. 14) and each represents a cystically dilated intralobular tubule.
- *Complex cystic mass*: These are cystic masses with solid or intracystic component within.

Complicated cysts: Complicated cysts are one of the commonest cystic lesions seen in the breast and can have multiple features as described below:

- *Uniform isoechoic thickening of cyst wall*: The normal thin echogenic wall becomes edematous and appears isoechoic with fat and is suggestive of inflammation.

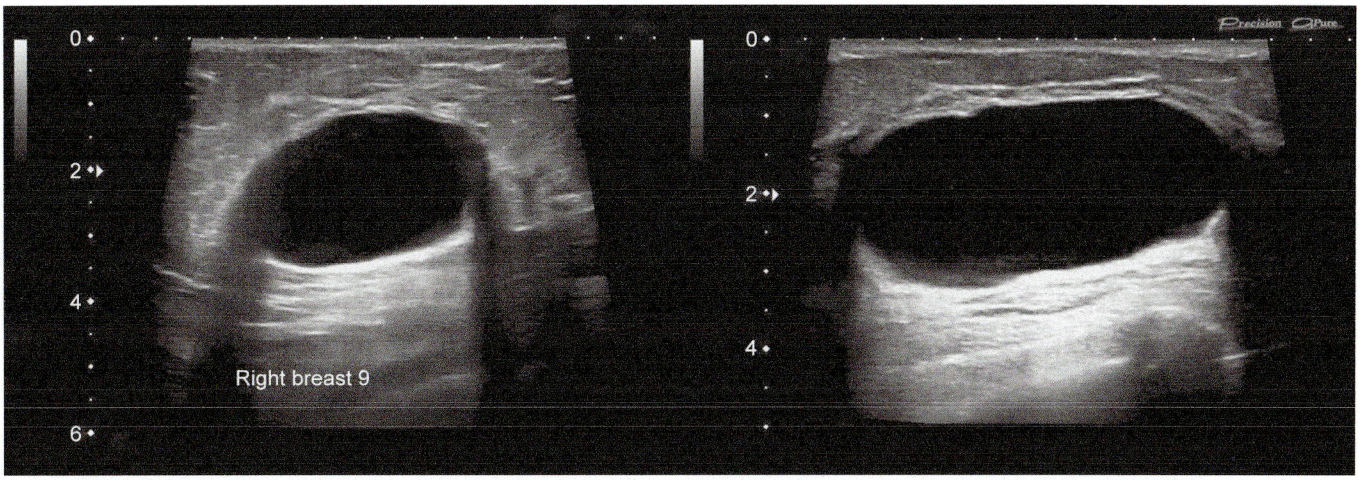

Fig. 11: Ultrasound showing an anechoic, well circumscribed mass with thin, echogenic outer wall, enhanced through transmission and thin edge shadows s/o simple cyst.

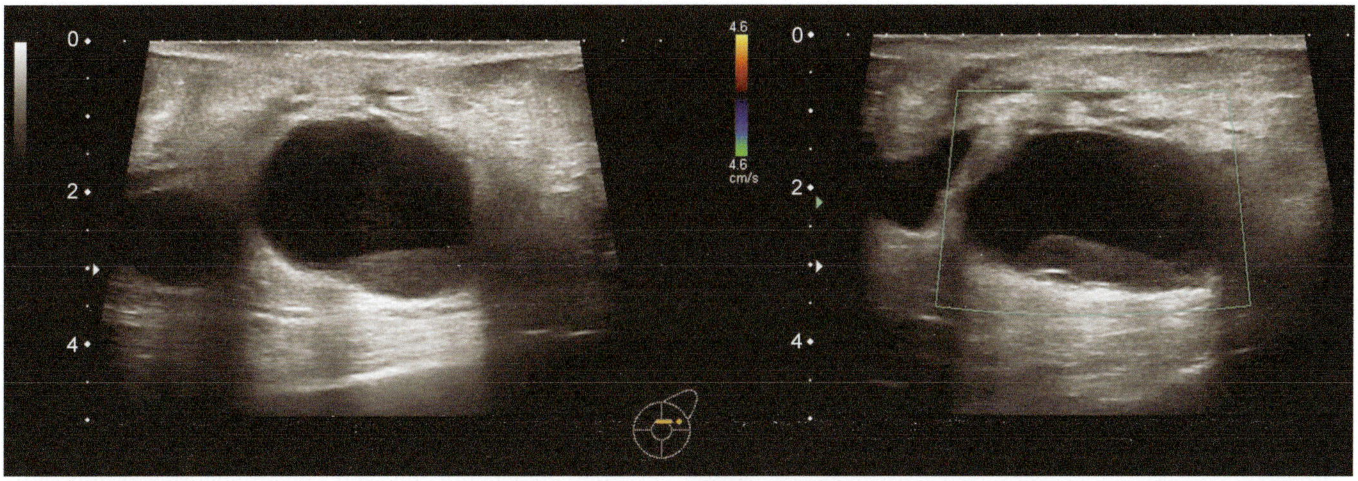

Fig. 12: Complicated cyst showing fluid debris level and posterior acoustic enhancement.

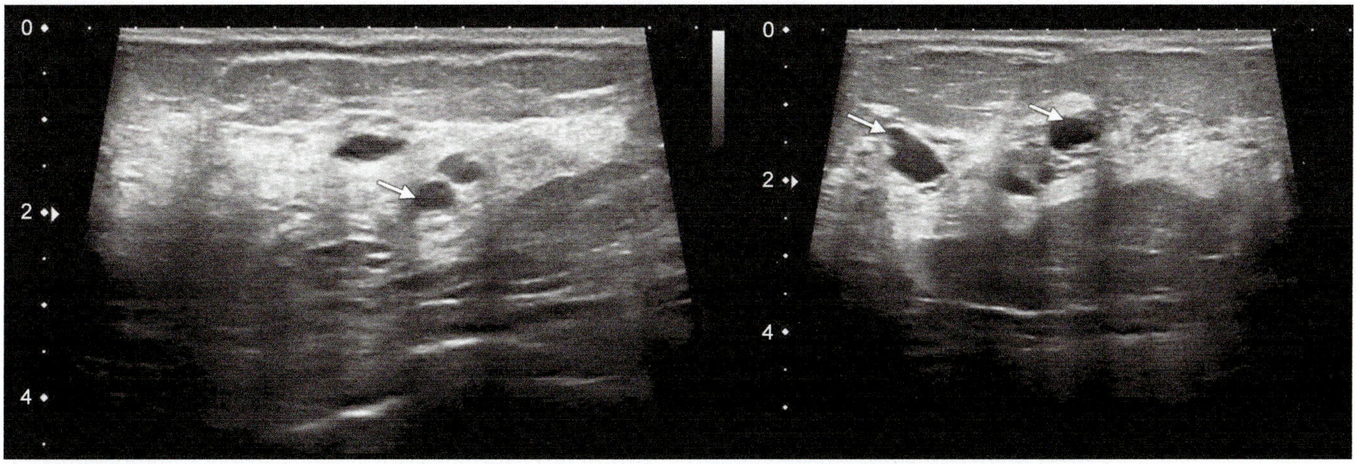

Fig. 13: Ultrasound showing clustered microcysts which are small cysts (2–5 mm) without any solid component.

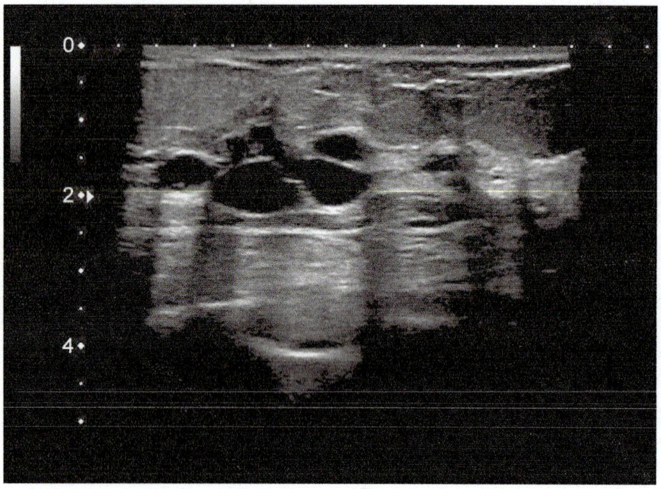

Fig. 14: Ultrasound showing cyst with thin septations (<0.5 mm) where each represents a cystically dilated intralobular tubule.

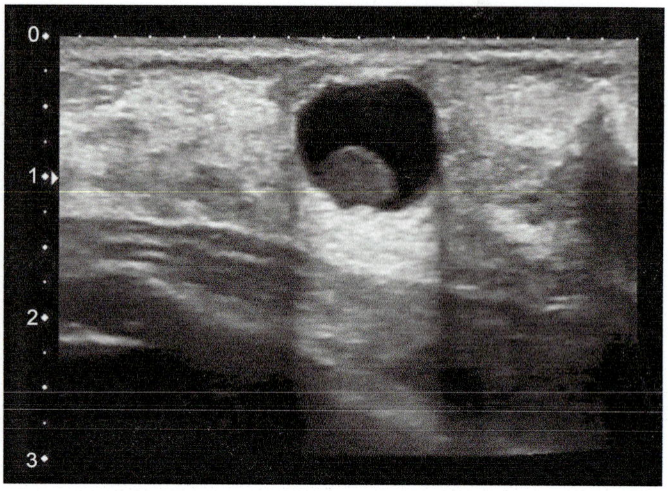

Fig. 16: A complicated cyst showing a mural nodule kind of appearance due to thick inspissated sludge.

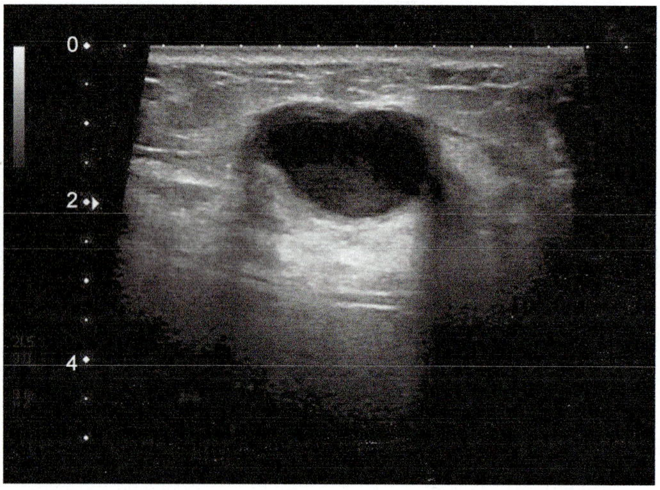

Fig. 15: Ultrasound showing infected cyst with thickened wall and low-level echoes.

- *Hyperemia of wall*: Acute inflammation leads to increase in vascularity of cyst wall.
- *Fluid-debris level*: This is due to large dependent particles that are cellular, white blood cells or red blood cells and settle down into layers that change with change in patient's position. Once the acutely inflamed cyst is aspirated, the residual thickened wall (Fig. 15) may remain and the fluid should be sent for gram stain and culture rather than cytology as there can be inflammation in the spectrum of fibrocystic disease. Sometimes, a mural nodule kind of appearance is seen because of tumefactive sludge (Fig. 16).
- *Lipid cysts or fat fluid level in cyst*: These are seen commonly in spectrum of fibrocystic disease and shape and orientation of fat fluid interface may vary from straight, concave, or convex (Fig. 17). Sometimes, the lipid layer appears immobile and may be mistaken for mural nodule.
- *Milk of calcium*: These occur as echogenic foci in dependent portion of cyst which change with change in patient's position. Because of their small size, they do not generally cause posterior acoustic shadowing.
- There may also be small **punctate calcification** seen in the cyst wall. At other times, there are arc like or circumferential calcifications which represent egg shell calcifications as a consequence of lipid cyst. Initially, the cyst is filled with lipid which appears echogenic, later the wall becomes echogenic and causes shadowing and in the last stage only the anterior wall is visible and deeper portions are obscured by intense shadowing.

Internal echoes within cysts: There are various other causes of internal echoes within a cyst apart from papilloma or carcinoma. These are seen as spectrum of findings in fibrocystic disease and include:

- Cell debris
- Protein globules
- RBCs
- Inflammatory cells and macrophages
- Epithelial cells: floating, papillary
- Apocrine cells: floating, papillary.

Artifactual echoes: It is important to remember that there can be artifactual internal echoes within the cysts due to reverberation, ring down, speckle and side lobe artifact. This happens when transducer frequency, band width and dynamic range are pushed beyond their limits.

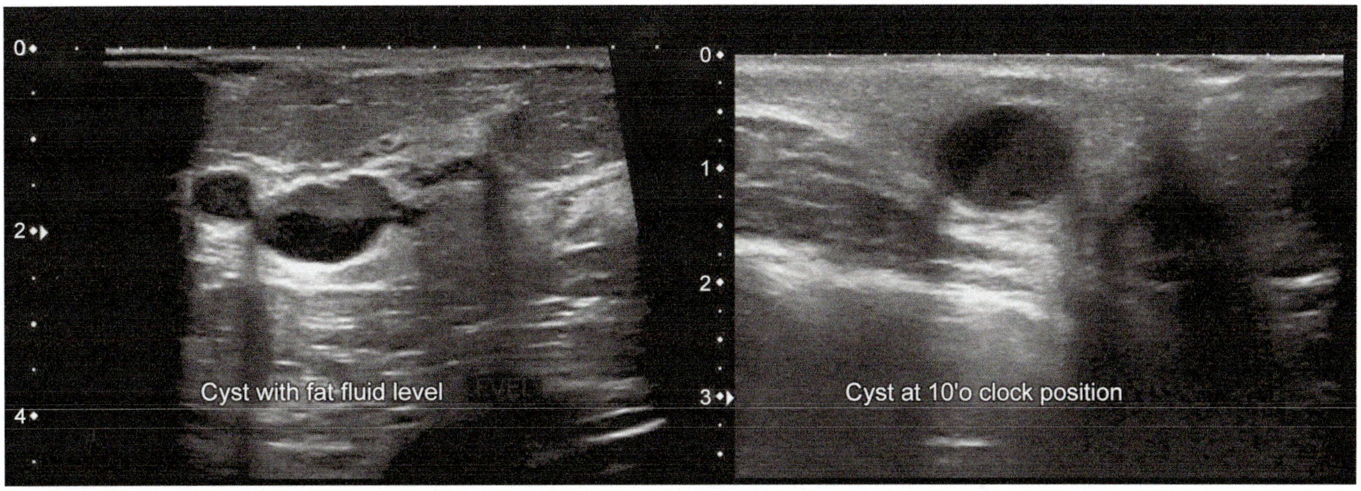

Fig. 17: Ultrasound showing a lipid cyst with fat fluid level forming layering.

If gain is excessive, artifactual internal echoes can appear. Reverberation echoes have a characteristic appearance and are parallel to the anterior wall of the cyst and can be reduced by angulating the transducer slightly so that the ultrasound beam does not intersect the anterior cyst wall. High-frequency coded harmonics show reduced clutter, reverberation and speckle artifacts within cyst.

COMPLEX CYSTIC MASS

The ultrasound findings of a complex cystic mass are:

- *Thick isoechoic septations*: These are worrisome for malignancy.
- *Mural nodule*: Majority of mural nodules are caused by benign proliferative disorders that are part of fibrocystic spectrum which include papillary apocrine metaplasia (PAM). These generally have a smooth attachment to cyst wall and thin echogenic capsule is preserved. The nodule due to intracystic papilloma has an irregular and angular point of attachment to cyst wall. Tumefactive sludge, clot and pus can simulate mural nodule and should be seen in different positions of patient.
- *Presence of fibrovascular stalk*: There are differences in blood supply to mural nodules caused by papillomas, carcinomas and PAM. Papillomas are the most vascular lesions with even a tiny lesion having blood flow (Fig. 18) within fibrovascular stalk - this is not seen in PAM. Since papillomas are very soft and sensitive to pressure, a copious amount of gel should be applied and scanning done with minimal transducer pressure.

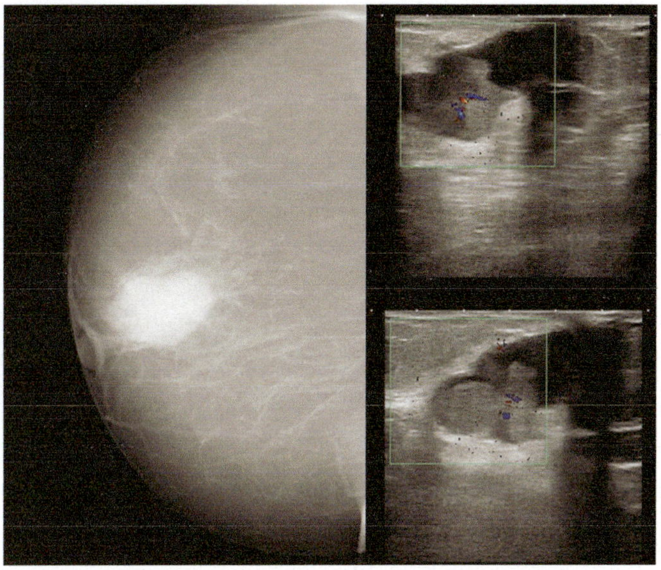

Fig. 18: A 49-year-old female presented with nipple discharge on and off from right breast. A circumscribed mass was seen in the retroareolar region on mammogram. Ultrasound showed a complex cystic mass with vascularity within the solid component. Excision biopsy was done and histopathology was s/o infarcted ductal papilloma with atypical ductal hyperplasia.

- *Microcystic microlobulated appearance*: This appearance is also seen in multiple enlarged ductules filled with high nuclear grade ductal carcinoma in situ (DCIS) which resemble a clustered microcyst.

When fluid is aspirated from a complex cystic mass, risk of false negative cyst fluid cytology is high; therefore, vacuum assisted biopsy should be done under ultrasound guidance followed by deployment of marker clip for identification later.

BREAST MASSES HAVING COMPLEX CYSTIC APPEARANCE DURING COURSE OF DEVELOPMENT

There are several conditions in breast which have a cystic phase while at other time they may appear solid. These include:

- Galactocele
- Mastitis and abscess
- Seroma
- Hematoma
- Fat necrosis
- Hemangioma and venous malformations.

Galactocele: These are cystically dilated terminal ducts and ductules filled with milk and are seen during third trimester of pregnancy or lactation. The ultrasound appearance varies with the stage of development and location. In acute phase it is anechoic and seen as unilocular cyst or thinly septated multiloculated cyst (Fig. 19). There may be low-level echoes due to multiple interfaces formed by interspersed lipid globules and fluid. Peripheral galactoceles are multilocular and central are generally unilocular involving the lactiferous sinus portion.

With time, the galactoceles become echogenic and have diffuse low-level echoes because of uniform admixture of lipid and water component. Some galactoceles in which curdling of milk has occurred may even appear solid but are still soft and compressible. In chronic galactoceles, water content is totally absorbed and they become pure lipid cysts.

Mastitis and abscess: These are common breast lesions showing cystic phase (Figs 20, Fig 21A and B) and are

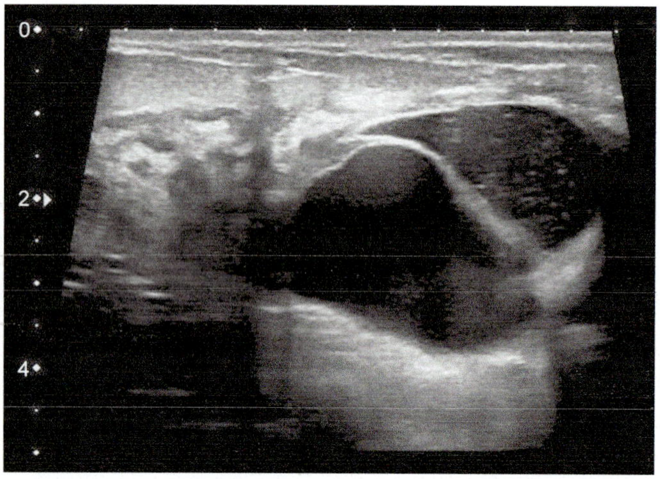

Fig. 19: Galactocele showing septations and echoes within.

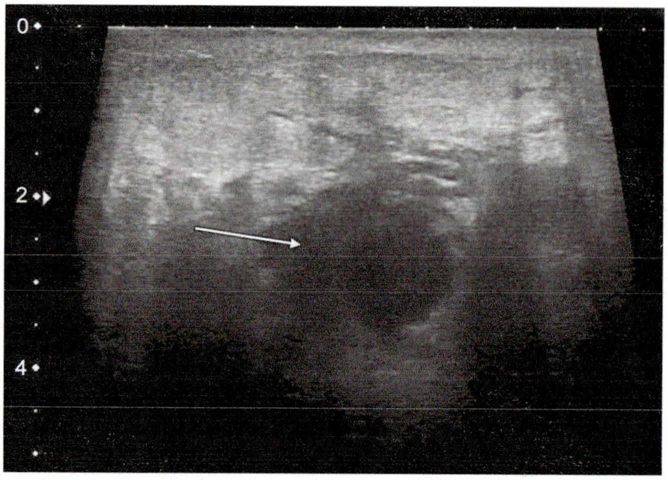

Fig. 20: Mastitis noted in the form of inflamed echogenic fat along with abscess formation (arrow).

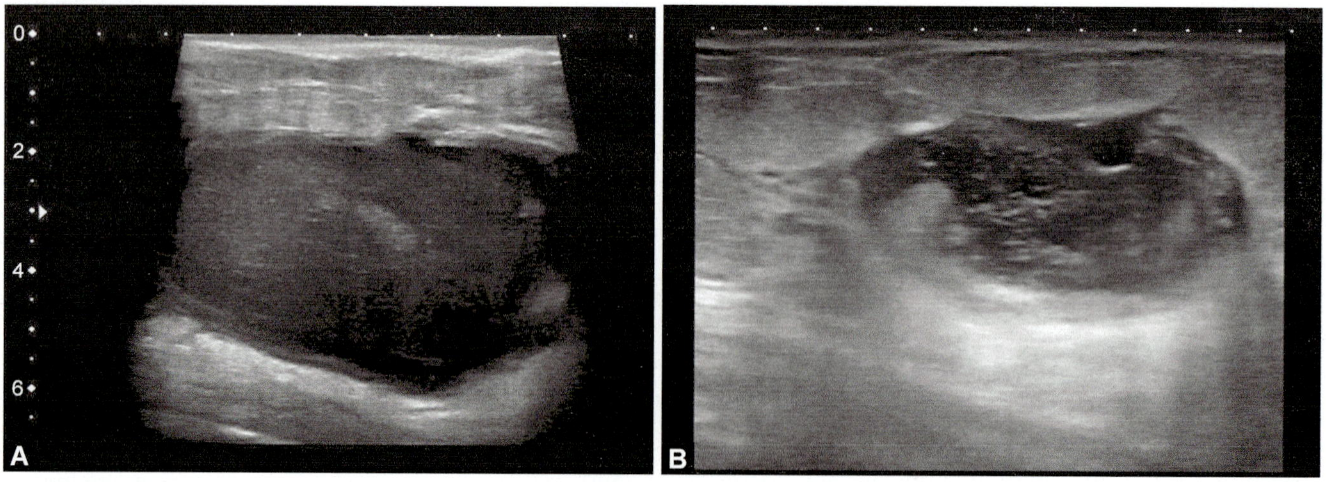

Figs. 21A and B: Ultrasound showing (A) Abscess with closely packed echoes and (B) Abscess with thick wall and echoes.

discussed in detail in the chapter on inflammatory diseases of breast.

Seroma: This is a due to localized serous fluid collection within a lumpectomy cavity. Most of these appear as simple cysts or complex cysts with low-level echoes (Fig. 22). There may be thin or thick echogenic avascular septations coursing through the fluid due to fibrinous adhesions.

Hematomas: These appear completely anechoic in hyperacute stage while in acute stage they are usually seen as hypoechoic masses with heterogenous echotexture (Fig. 23). Subacute hematomas appear as irregularly marginated complex cystic masses with thickened hyperechoic wall, mural nodule and thick avascular septations. Chronic hematomas are hypoechoic with septations and irregular wall and show posterior acoustic enhancement. There may be a fluid debris layer simulating a mural nodule.

Fat necrosis: The ultrasound findings vary greatly depending upon the stage of development.

Initially, there is edema of fat lobules which is seen as increased echogenicity compared to adjacent area of breast parenchyma. As the fat necrosis extends beyond the edema stage, a complex cystic lesion forms which represents fibrous encased lipid cysts. Gradually, an echogenic wall develops around the hypoechoic area (Fig. 24).

When fat necrosis evolves from a hematoma, the complex lipid cyst has a thick echogenic wall, mural nodule or thick septations simulating a chronic hematoma.

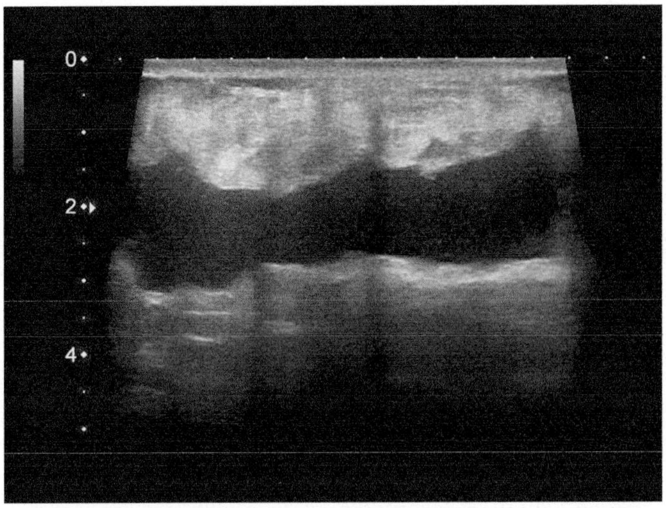

Fig. 22: An encysted collection at the lumpectomy site in a postoperative breast s/o seroma.

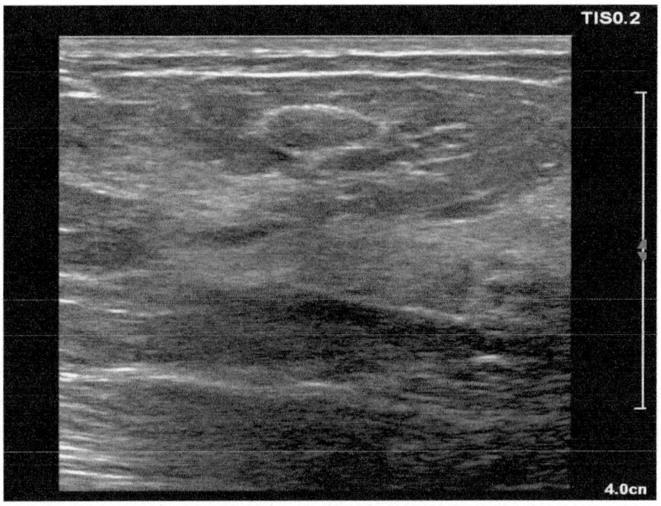

Fig. 24: Fat necrosis seen with an echogenic rim.

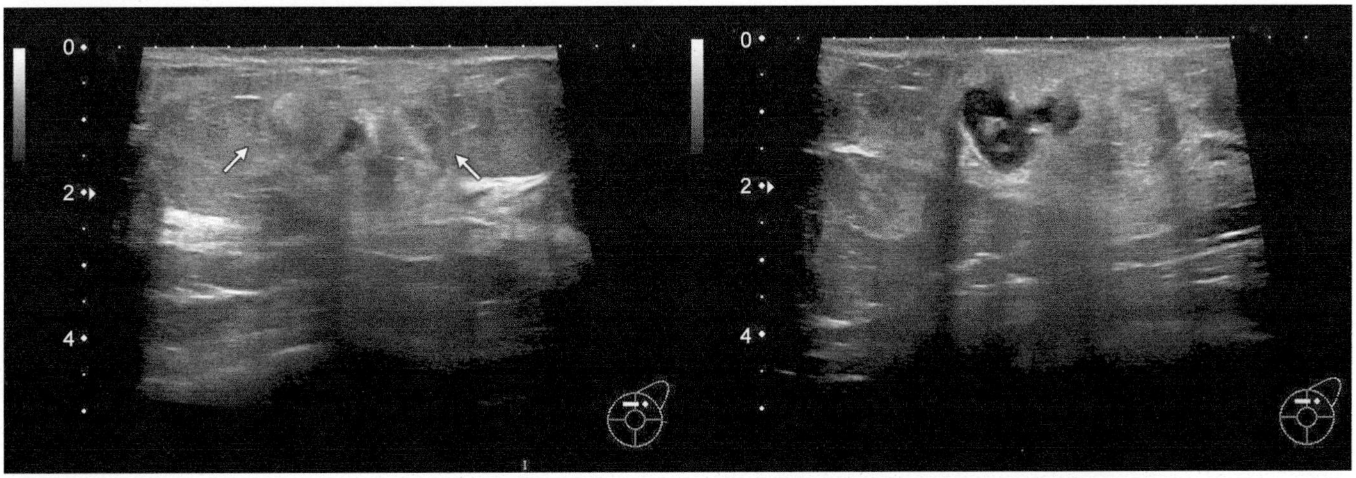

Fig. 23: A young woman presented with history of fall with bruising of skin over the breast. Ultrasound shows focal increase in echogenicity of fat s/o edema with heterogenously hypoechoic area s/o hematoma.

When fat necrosis evolves from a seroma, the complex cyst has an isoechoic wall with thin septations and anechoic fluid. Late in the process of fat necrosis, there is development of severe fibrosis which may show irregular margins.

Hemangiomas and venous malformations: Cavernous hemangiomas and venous malformations may be mistaken for cystic lesions of breast. Venous malformation can undergo spontaneous thrombosis resembling Mondors disease.

CYSTS ARISING FROM SKIN

These include sebaceous cyst, Montgomery gland cyst and epidermal inclusion cyst. The findings seen are (Figs. 25A to C):

- Lesion lies entirely within the skin: These can be scanned with acoustic stand-off pad.
- Most of the lesion lies within subcutaneous tissue, has a 'claw' of hyperechoic skin around edge of the lesion.
- The lesion lies entirely within subcutaneous fat but the gland neck/hair follicle from which the lesion took origin is seen coursing through the skin.
  - *Sebaceous cyst*: These are quite common and have a variable appearance based on internal echogenecity ranging from anechoic to hyperechoic depending on the relative amount of fluid and keratin (Fig. 26 A and B). If it is chronic with long standing obstruction, the keratinized material within the cyst becomes hyperechoic. They get frequently inflamed and may appear hypoechoic.
  - *Epidermal inclusion cyst*: These are similar in appearance to sebaceous cyst (Fig. 27). Epidermal inclusion cyst is caused by penetrating trauma, needle biopsy or surgery. There is formation of continuous adherent layers of keratin giving rise to a multilaminar appearance called onion skin appearance in a typical case of epidermal inclusion cyst.

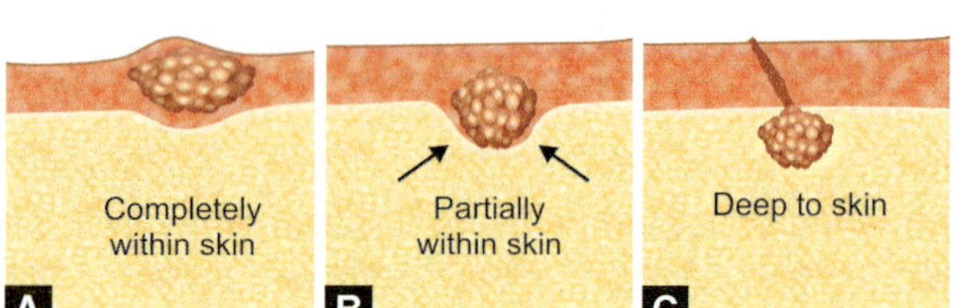

Figs. 25A to C: Cysts arising from skin: (A) Lesion is entirely within skin; (B) Most of the lesion is within subcutaneous tissue but shows a claw sign; (C) Lesion is within subcutaneous fat but the gland neck /hair follicle is coursing through the skin.

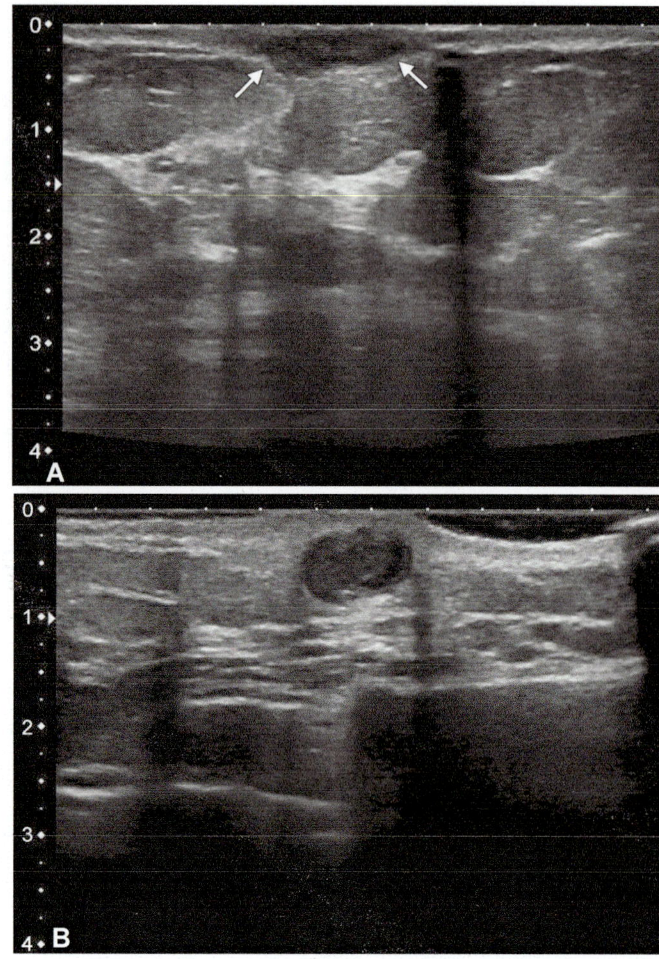

Figs. 26A and B: Ultrasound showing a circumscribed hypoechoic mass in two different patients: (A) Within the skin and (B) Partially within the subcutaneous tissue. Histopathology was s/o sebaceous cyst.

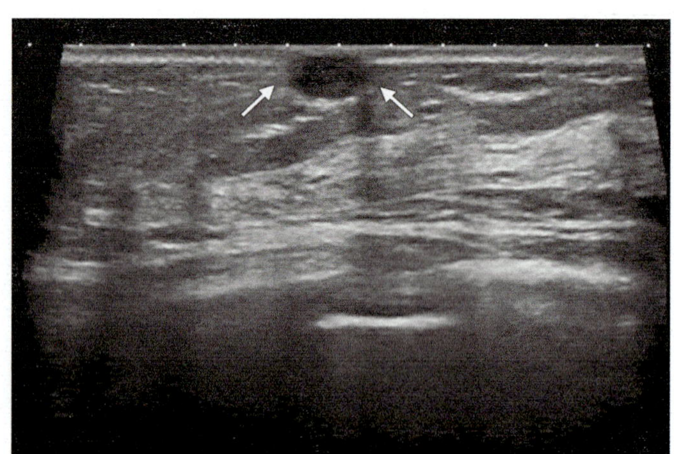

Fig. 27: Histopathologically proven case of epidermal inclusion cyst showing a circumscribed hypoechoic mass in skin and subcutaneous tissue.

SOLID LESIONS ON ULTRASOUND

Ultrasound reflects the gross morphology of solid lesions and, based on imaging features, it indirectly indicates the invasive histology of a mass.

It is important to remember that breast cancer is heterogeneous and this heterogeneity is not only from one lesion to another but also within the same mass. This means that **some parts of a mass may show benign features and other parts may show malignant features.**

The spectrum of solid masses can range from circumscribed to spiculated masses with the middle peak having both circumscribed and spiculated lesions.

Stavros had categorized solid breast masses into benign and malignant based on imaging findings.[1] The histological and morphologic features like desmoplasia, cellularity and vascularity affect the sonographic appearances of masses.[2]

Desmoplasia and inflammation: These features are because of host response to a tumor. To put in simple words, desmoplasia is host's response to a tumor to wall it off from normal tissue and prevent its spread. This is a slow response and is seen in a slow growing tumor. Therefore, spiculated masses showing desmoplastic reaction (Fig. 28) usually are low to intermediate grade malignancies which have taken time to grow.

In contrast, fast growing tumors like high grade ductal carcinoma are generally well circumscribed (Fig. 29) allowing no time for desmoplastic reaction to develop. Instead, these tumors incite an inflammatory response.

Both spiculated and circumscribed masses can develop both kinds of response albeit in a different proportion, for example, spiculated lesion have more desmoplastic reaction than inflammatory response, while circumscribed lesion have more inflammatory response than desmoplastic reaction.

Tumor cellularity: Circumscribed lesions are more cellular compared to spiculated lesion.

How does desmoplasia and cellularity affect ultrasound appearance of a solid mass?

The acoustic shadowing posterior to a mass is because of desmoplastic reaction; therefore, low-grade tumor with desmoplastic response has partial or complete posterior shadowing. High-grade circumscribed tumors with increased cellularity generally show enhanced through transmission.

Therefore, it is important to remember that those are two ends of a spectrum and one can find mixed features in the intermediate range. While assessing a mass, always try to look for the most suspicious features and let it guide your decision regarding biopsy and further management.

It is important to remember that assessing a single parameter is not enough to make a diagnosis as many malignant lesions may be missed. One has to look at a complete set of parameters before arriving at the final diagnosis.

Vascularity: Circumscribed lesions are more vascular because increased cellularity generates more angiogenesis factors. Moreover, the inflammation per se also incites a hyperemic response.

Spiculated lesions are paucicellular and have lesser vascularity.

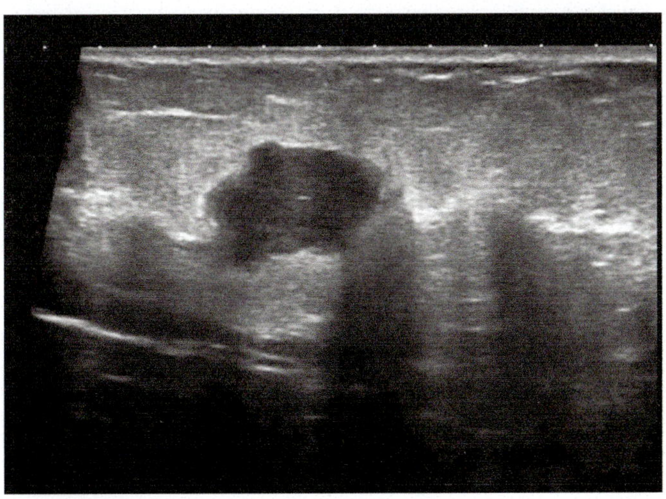

Fig. 28: Malignant mass showing microlobulations and posterior acoustic shadowing.

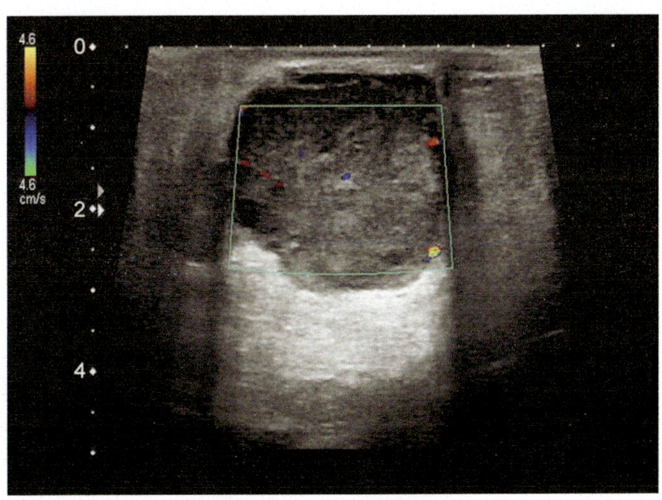

Fig. 29: A circumscribed mass showing posterior acoustic enhancement. Biopsy was s/o metaplastic carcinoma.

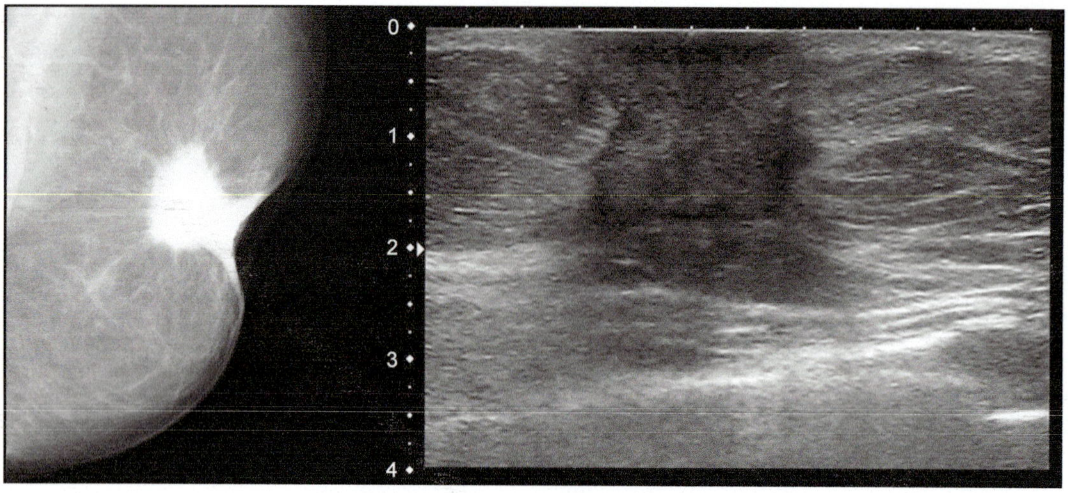

Fig. 30: A malignant mass with spiculations in retroareolar region with nipple retraction. Ultrasound showed a hypoechoic mass with spiculations which are seen as alternating hypoechoic and relatively hyperechoic straight lines.

Spiculations: It reflects invasion of mass into surrounding tissue and is seen as alternating hypoechoic and relatively hyperechoic straight lines radiating out perpendicularly from the surface of mass (Fig. 30).

Hypoechoic lines are seen better in a background of thick echogenic fibrous tissue. Please remember that these may be seen in only one portion of lesion and not the entire lesion.

Spicules are better appreciated on the lateral aspect of lesion because they are perpendicular to ultrasound beam and make bright specular reflections.

Thick echogenic halo: These most likely represent hyperechoic spicules that are too small to resolve sonographically (Fig 31). Real-time spatial compounding can show spicules better.

Sometimes a thick, irregular echogenic halo is seen because of peritumoral edema caused by intense peritumoral inflammation or from lymphatic obstruction due to lymphatic invasion.

Benign entities with spiculated margins are:

- Radial scar
- Sclerosing adenosis
- Fat necrosis
- Biopsy scar.

Angular margins: Angles on the surface of mass may be very acute, 90° or even obtuse. They may be seen in only a small portion of mass; therefore, the entire surface should be scanned in two orthogonal planes. Even if most of the mass is smooth and rounded and angular margin is seen along just one surface then mass should still be categorized as BI-RADS 4 rather than BI-RADS 3.

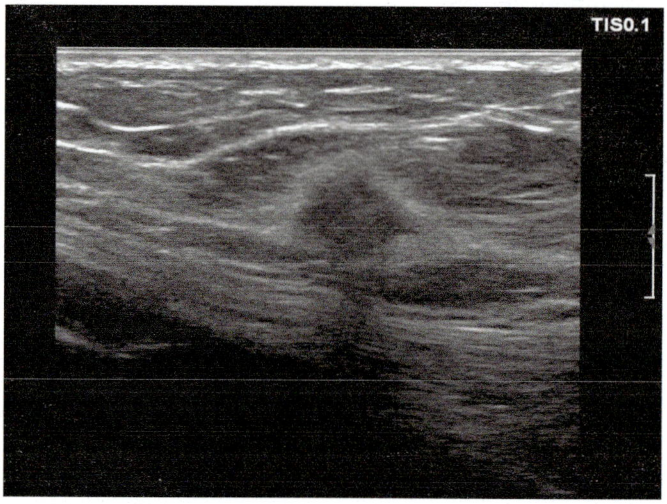

Fig. 31: A malignant mass with thick echogenic halo which represent hyperechoic spicules that are too small to resolve sonographically.

It is important to remember that invasion into surrounding tissue occurs along path of least resistance. Masses that are surrounded by fat invade easily and have randomly distributed angles along all surfaces. Masses close to anterior mammary fascia and fibrous tissue offer high resistance. The anterior mammary fascia acts as a barrier to the spread of tumor (Fig. 32). Therefore, the tumor grows horizontally along the under surface of fascia till point of low resistance is encountered at the intersection of Cooper ligament. The angular shape occurs when the tumor grows into the base of Cooper ligaments.

Microlobulation: These are small (1–2 mm) in size, numerous and placed close together. Even if part of mass

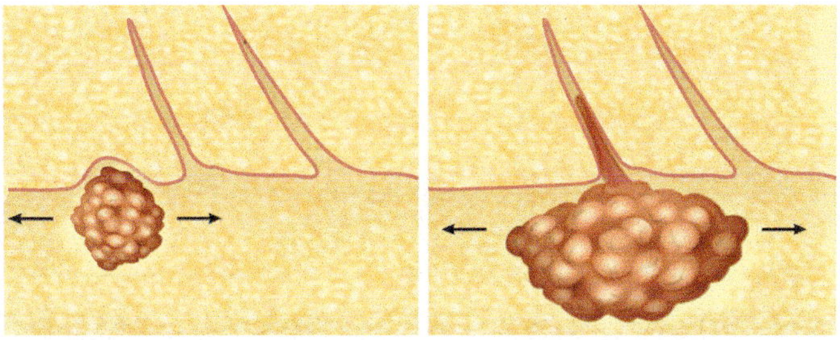

Fig. 32: Anterior mammary fascia and the high resistance offered by it to spread of malignant tumor. The tumor grows horizontally on undersurface of the fascia till it reaches the point of low resistance at intersection of Cooper ligament with fascia. Here it grows into the base of Cooper ligament where it is seen as angular shape.
Source: Adapted from Stavros.

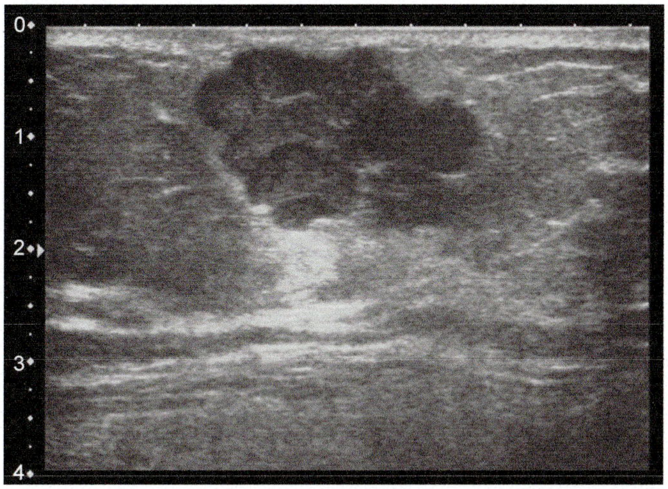

Fig. 33: Ultrasound showing a microlobulated hypoechoic mass which was confirmed to be malignant on histopathology.

is smooth and another part shows microlobulation, the entire nodule is assigned a higher risk category (Figs. 33 and 34).

There can be three possible reasons for microlobulation:

1. Invasive tumor: These have angular configuration.
2. DCIS: These microlobulations are round and thinly encapsulated.
3. DCIS with invasive cancer. The microlobulations coexist with spiculations, thick halo and angular margins. Larger the microlobulations, the more likely it is for the lesions to be high grade.

Other entities in which microlobulations are seen are:

- Fibrocystic disease
- Sclerosis adenosis
- Intraductal papilloma
- Complex fibroadenoma.

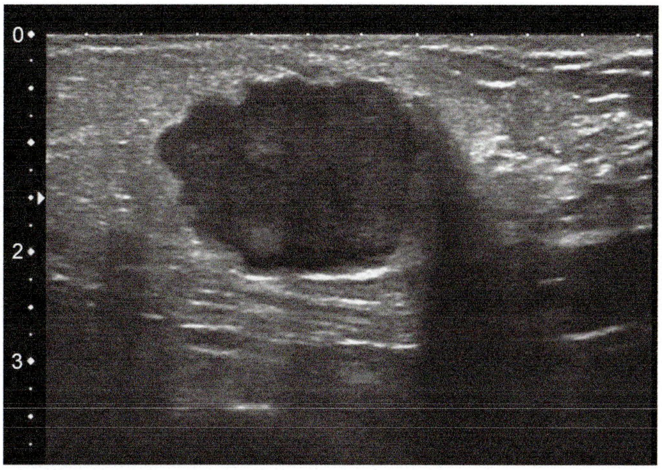

Fig. 34: A hypoechoic malignant mass with closely placed microlobulations.

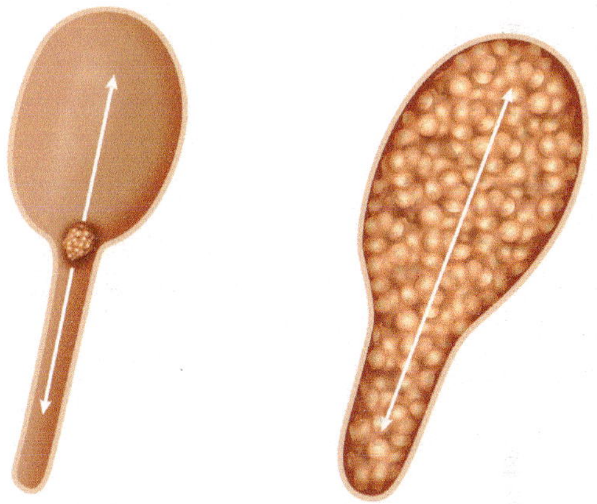

Fig. 35: Growth pattern of carcinoma. Carcinomas arise at TDLU at junction of extralobar terminal duct with lobule and proximally into terminal duct and large duct. (TDLU: terminal ductolobular unit).
Source: Adapted from Stavros.

Taller than wide configuration: Most carcinomas arise at TDLU at junction of extralobar terminal duct with lobule (Fig. 35). DCIS grows proximally into terminal duct and large duct. It grows peripherally into lobule and intralobular ductule.

Fibroadenoma arise at lobule but cannot grow into terminal duct or main duct. They grow perpendicular to long axis of lobule (Fig. 36).

Duct extension and branch pattern: These findings are often appreciated only when specifically looked for. Duct extension is usually a single large projection of tumor into a centrally located duct away from tumor. This involves the lactiferous sinus portion of the duct. Branch pattern involves smaller peripheral ducts away from nipple.

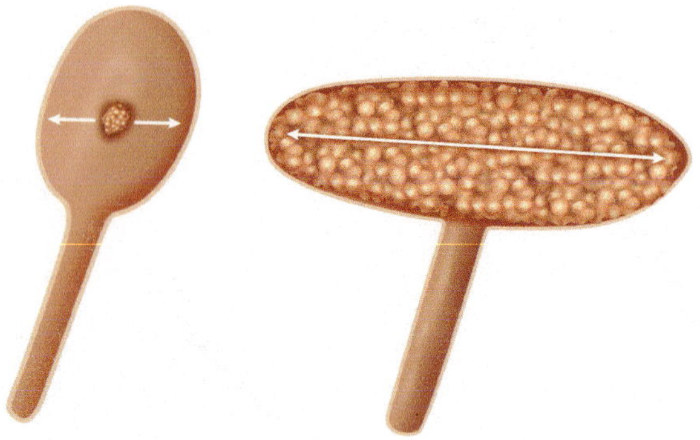

Fig. 36: Growth pattern of fibroadenoma. These arise from lobules and grow perpendicular to long axis of terminal ductolobular unit.

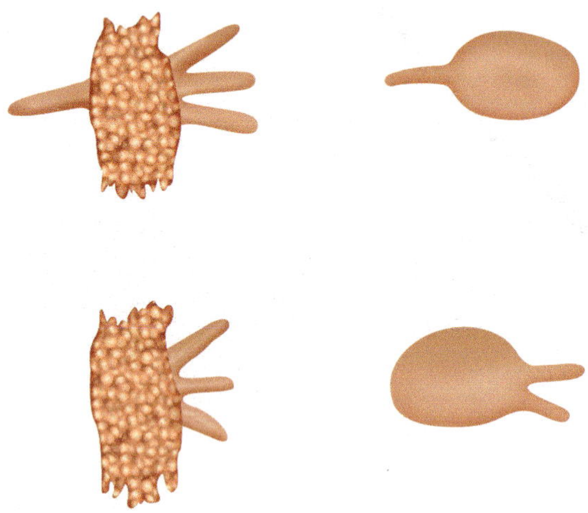

Fig. 37: Ductal extension and branch extension from a mass.

Duct extension and branch pattern (Fig. 37) without mass or other suspicious findings may represent benign papillomas, DCIS or atypical ductal hyperplasia (ADH).

Hypoechoic mass: Markedly hypoechoic masses are seen in both DCIS and invasive cancer. The echogenicity of solid nodule should be compared to echogenicity of fat (which should be at a midgray level) and not with hyperechoic fibrous tissue. Medullary carcinomas are extremely hypoechoic so much so that they almost look cystic and have a pseudo cystic appearance.

Individual benign nodule findings:

- Hyperechoic
- Elliptical or oval
- Gentle lobulations (<3)
- Thin capsule

Findings suspicious for malignancy:

- Spiculations
- Thick echogenic halo
- Angular margins.

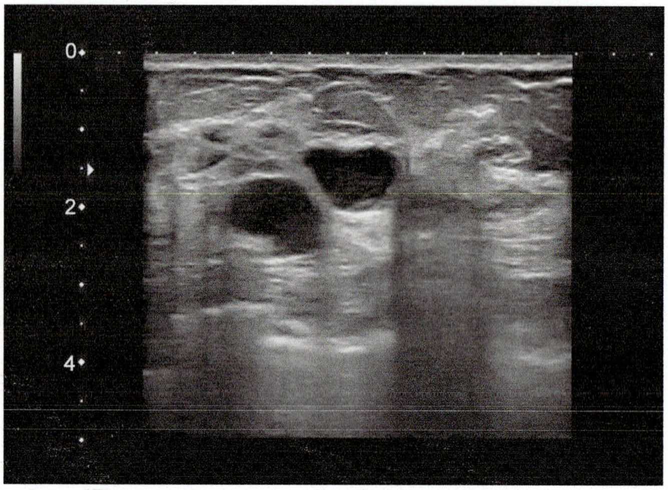

Fig. 38: Circumscribed anechoic lesions are seen s/o cysts—BI-RADS category 2. (BI-RADS: breast imaging reporting and data system).

Stavros had given a classification of solid breast masses in 1995 with a 99.5% negative predictive value.

In a study by Hong et al, descriptors having high predictive value for benignity and malignancy were described. The descriptors and predictive values for benign masses were circumscribed margins (90%), parallel orientation (78%) and oval shape (78%).

The common features of malignant masses are irregular shape (62%), spiculated margins (86%) and non-parallel orientation (69%).

BI-RADS CATEGORIZATION OF BREAST MASSES

After having discussed the BI-RADS lexicon and the salient features of benign and malignant masses, let us describe the BI-RADS classification.

BI-RADS 0: Incomplete assessment. This needs additional imaging evaluation and/or comparison with prior images. This category indicates that there is a finding for which additional imaging evaluation is needed.

BI-RADS 1: This category is used when ultrasound examination is normal and there is no abnormality. Sometimes, there is a clinically palpable abnormality but mammogram and ultrasound are normal. The management would depend upon the clinical level of concern.

BI-RADS 2: This category is used when definitely benign findings are seen on ultrasound and include simple cyst, breast implant, stable postsurgical changes, lipoma (Fig. 39), hamartoma and involuting fibroadenomas (Figs. 40A and B) or those fibroadenomas which have remained stable in successive studies for ≥2 years. Therefore, category 2 should be used when describing one or more specific benign sonographic findings in the report.

BI-RADS 3: This includes masses which have <2% chance of being malignant (Figs. 41 and 42). A follow-up is extremely important which should be done 6 monthly till 2 years, still classifying the lesion as BI-RADS 3 during this interval imaging. After 2 years, there may be possibility of the mass remaining stable or increasing in size and depending on it, a properly worded report should be given changing the assessment category which seems appropriate to the current reader. If the mass is stable, downgrade it to BI-RADS 2 and if it increases in size, upgrade to BI-RADS 4 and recommend a biopsy.

BI-RADS 4: This category is reserved for findings that do not have the classic appearance of malignancy but are sufficiently suspicious to justify a recommendation for biopsy. It has a possibility of malignancy ranging from 2% to 95%. It is further divided into 4A (Fig. 43 and Fig 44), 4B (Figs. 45) and 4C (Fig. 46) as follows:

- Category 4A: Low suspicion for malignancy, >2% to <10% likelihood for malignancy

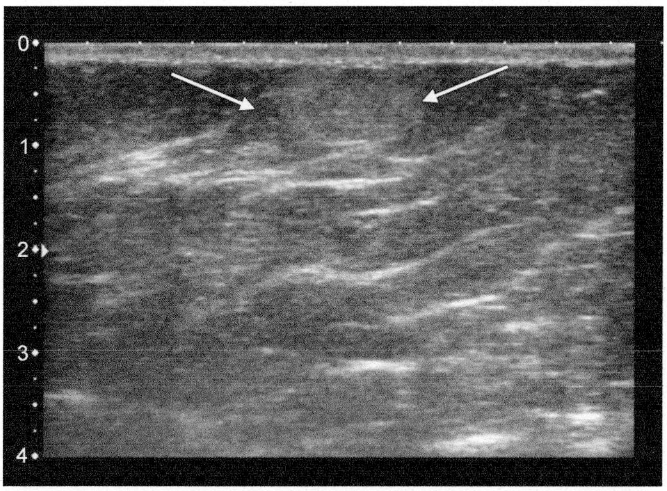

Fig. 39: A circumscribed hyperechoic mass is seen s/o lipoma—BI-RADS category 2. (BI-RADS: breast imaging reporting and data system).

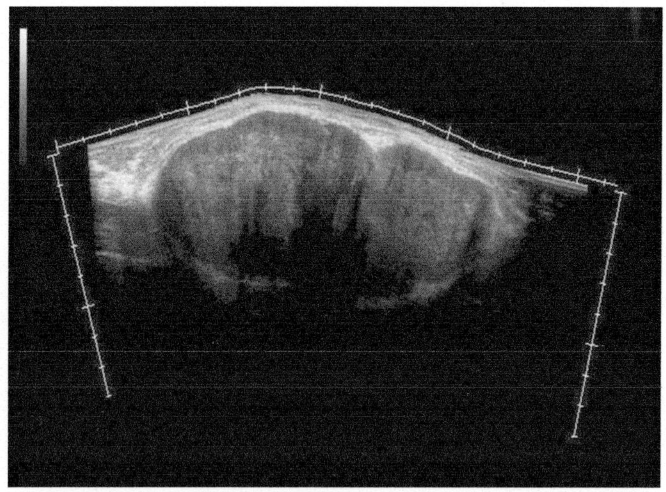

Fig. 41: A circumscribed mass with gentle lobulations in a 16-year-old girl—BI-RADS category 3. Histopathology was s/o fibroadenoma. (BI-RADS: breast imaging reporting and data system).

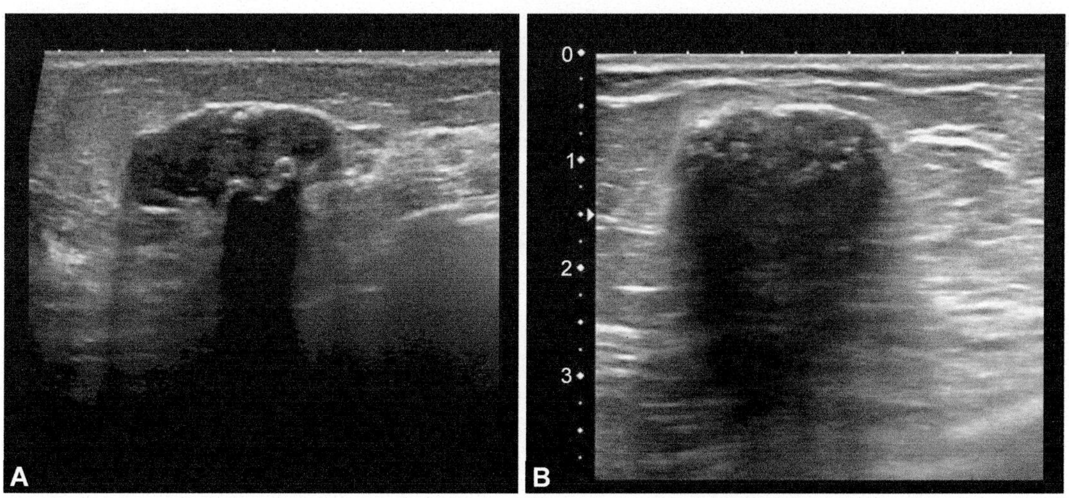

Figs. 40A and B: Ultrasound (A and B) showing circumscribed hypoechoic mass having echogenic foci with posterior acoustic shadowing s/o involuting fibroadenoma—BI-RADS category 2. (BI-RADS: breast imaging reporting and data system).

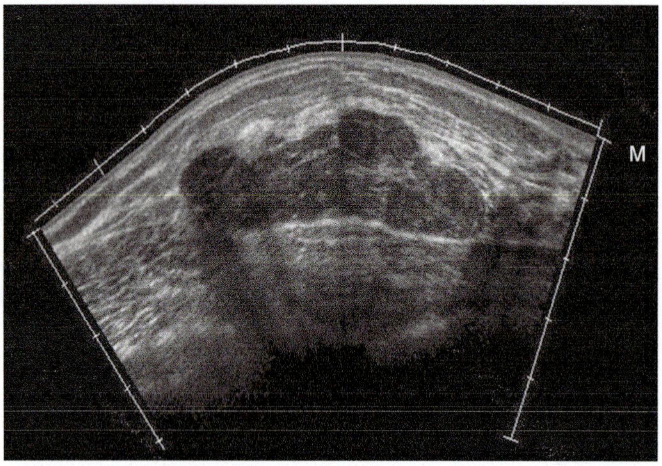

Fig. 42: A circumscribed, horizontally placed heterogeneously hypoechoic mass with smooth undulations in young girl—BI-RADS category 3. Histopathology was s/o fibroadenoma. (BI-RADS: breast imaging reporting and data system).

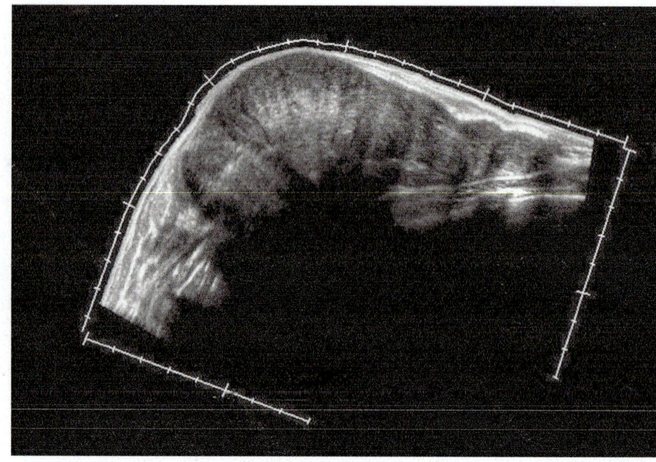

Fig. 44: A circumscribed horizontally placed lobulated mass in a 50-year-old female—BI-RADS 4A. Histopathology was s/o benign phyllodes tumor. (BI-RADS: breast imaging reporting and data system).

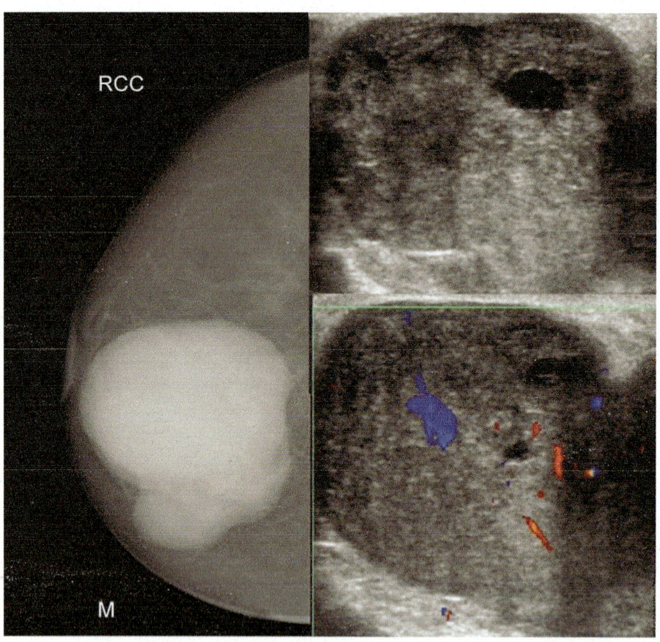

Fig. 43: A large circumscribed round mass with cystic area and vascularity in 35-year-old woman—BI-RADS 4 A. Histopathology was s/o benign phyllodes tumor. (BI-RADS: breast imaging reporting and data system).

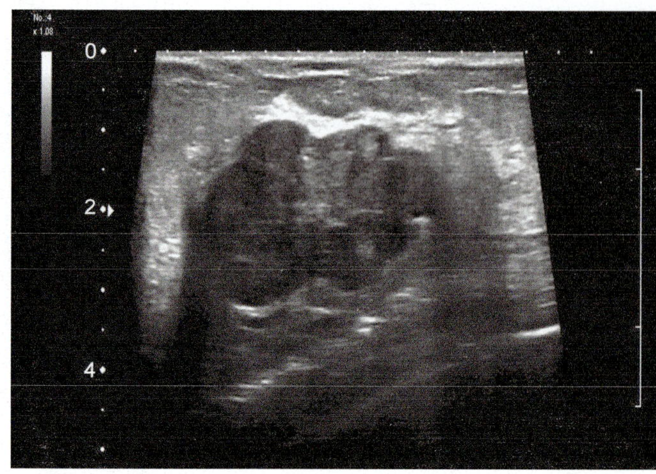

Fig. 45: A circumscribed hypoechoic mass with multiple lobulations—BI-RADS 4B. Histopathology was s/o infiltrating ductal carcinoma. (BI-RADS: breast imaging reporting and data system).

- Category 4B: Moderate suspicion for malignancy, >10% to <50% likelihood for malignancy
- Category 4C: High suspicion for malignancy, >50% to <95% likelihood for malignancy
- This is final comment to the whole BI-RADS 4, it does not need dot here

BI-RADS 5: These masses have typical features of malignant masses and have >95% likelihood of malignancy (Figs. 47 and 48). The fifth edition provides more directed management recommendation, "biopsy should be performed in the absence of clinical contraindication."

BI-RADS 6: This category includes biopsy proven cases of malignancy (imaging performed after percutaneous biopsy but prior to surgical excision), in which there are no abnormalities other than the known cancer that might need additional evaluation.

Importance of follow-up of masses on ultrasound: The purpose of follow-up on ultrasound is to look for stability or for any change in size of mass. The BI-RADS category 3 masses are the ones which have to be followed up meticulously but in our set up, we sometimes find that patients do not return for follow-up.

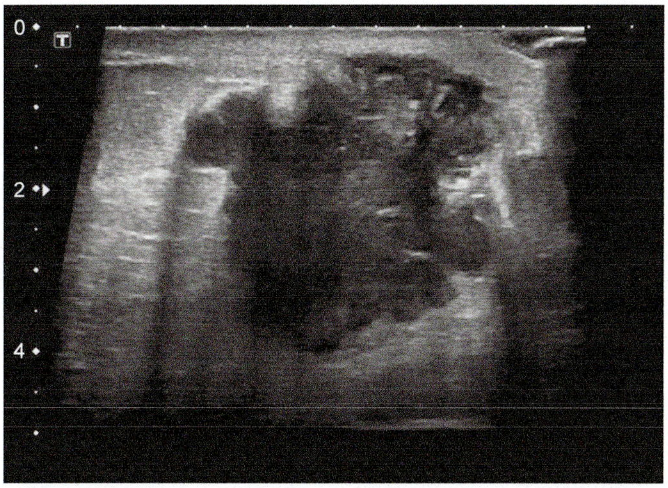

Fig. 46: An irregular multilobulated hypoechoic mass in an elderly woman with a portion of mass showing obscured margins—BI-RADS 4C. Histopathology was s/o invasive ductal carcinoma. (BI-RADS: breast imaging reporting and data system).

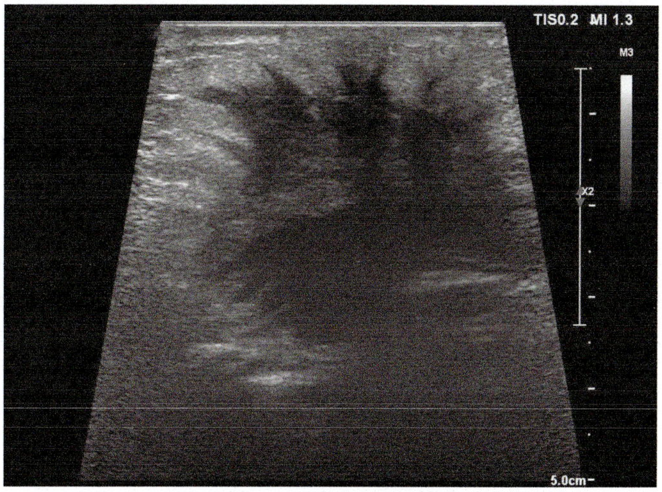

Fig. 48: An irregular hypoechoic mass with spiculated and angular margins—BI-RADS category 5. Histopathology was s/o invasive ductal carcinoma. (BI-RADS: breast imaging reporting and data system).

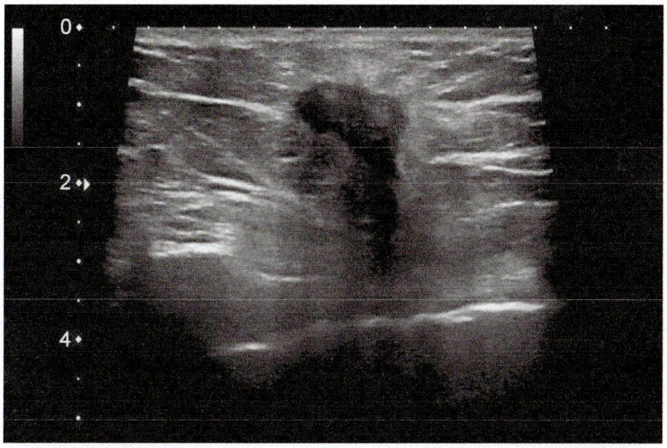

Fig. 47: A hypoechoic mass in a 55-year-old female showing partially obscured margins, echogenic halo and posterior shadowing—BI-RADS category 5. Histopathology was s/o invasive ductal carcinoma. (BI-RADS: breast imaging reporting and data system).

In a study by Goodman, there was only 54% compliance rate for follow-up after a benign result at biopsy while Raza et al. found that 82.6% patients returned for imaging follow-up in BI-RADS category 3 masses. The patients returning for follow-up after a benign biopsy result are lower as compared to imaging follow-up till 2 years.

It is important to note that while making a recommendation for biopsy in BI-RADS category 3 mass, the final category need not be changed, for example, in an elderly patient, biopsy can be done in the setting of benign imaging finding.

There are situations where **clinical factors** play more crucial role than imaging.

For example, an abscess may resemble a malignancy but in an appropriate clinical scenario of tender mass with fever in a young female, an aspiration should be done after assigning a category 4A.

In a post-traumatic scenario, a hematoma or fat necrosis is the most likely possibility even though the imaging findings may resemble malignancy. Hence, a follow-up is advised to look for resolution of hematoma or findings of fat necrosis. Fat necrosis may have various forms including solid mass, complex cystic mass, mural nodule or necrotic mass.

Conclusion: Breast cancer is a heterogeneous disease with heterogeneity seen even in an individual nodule. Ultrasound is useful in characterization of breast masses into benign and malignant. The categorization of masses in BI-RADS categories helps in characterizing the masses thereby helping to decide as to which masses should undergo biopsy and which should be kept on a follow-up. **The follow-up of BI-RADS 3 masses should be done at 6 months rather than 1 year as high grade invasive ductal carcinomas grow rapidly so that a change can be detected within 6 months.**

REFERENCES

1. Stavros TA, Thickman D, Rapp CL, et al. Solid breast nodules: use of sonography to distinguish between benign and malignant lesions. Radiology 1995;196:123-34.
2. Thomas Stavros A. Ultrasound of solid breast nodule: distinguishing benign from malignant. In: Breast ultrasound. Philadelphia, PA: Lippincott Williams & Wilkins; 2004;. pp. 445-527.

3.3 Ultrasound Features of Breast Masses

INTRODUCTION

Benign Masses

Fibroadenomas: These are benign tumors arising from terminal ductolobular unit (TDLU) which have variable amounts of stromal and epithelial elements. The stroma can be paucicellular or highly cellular and may undergo myxoid change, hyalinization and calcification. Giant and juvenile fibroadenomas have a highly cellular stroma.

CLINICAL FEATURES

These are more common in young adults <30 years of age with a peak incidence in third decade. They present as palpable masses which are firm, rubbery, mobile and painless. Estrogen stimulation is important in formation and growth of these masses. They appear softer with cellular and myxomatous stroma and hard with sclerotic or hyalinized stroma.

IMAGING FEATURES

Shape: These are generally oval or elliptical in shape with two or three gentle lobulations (Figs. 1 and 2). As they grow in size, the number of lobulations may increase and microlobulations may be seen. If microlobulations are seen, these should be put as BI-RADS 4A and biopsy should be done. Sometimes, smaller fibroadenomas <1 cm appear round and are difficult to distinguish from complex cysts seen in fibrocystic disease.

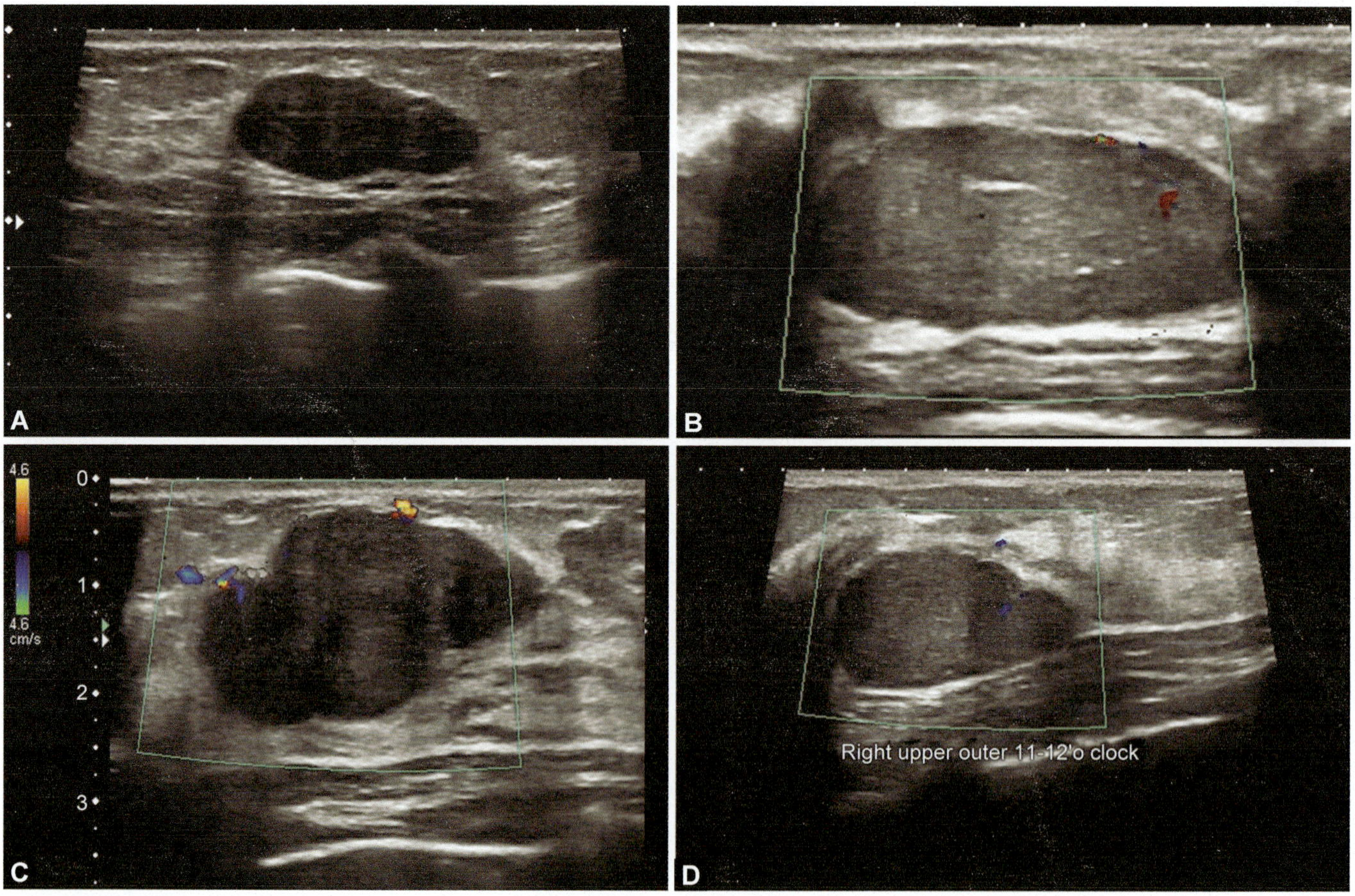

Figs. 1A to D: Ultrasound showing various appearances of fibroadenoma on ultrasound. Fibroadenomas are circumscribed, oval, hypoechoic masses placed horizontally and may show gentle lobulations (2–3).

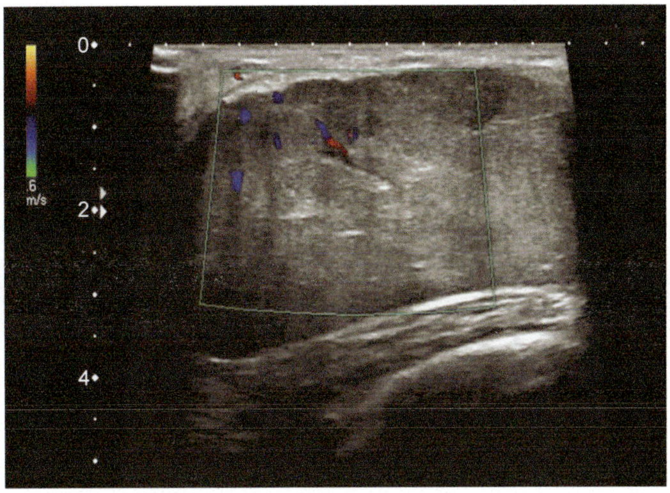

Fig. 2: A circumscribed hypoechoic mass with vascularity within. Histopathology was s/o fibroadenoma.

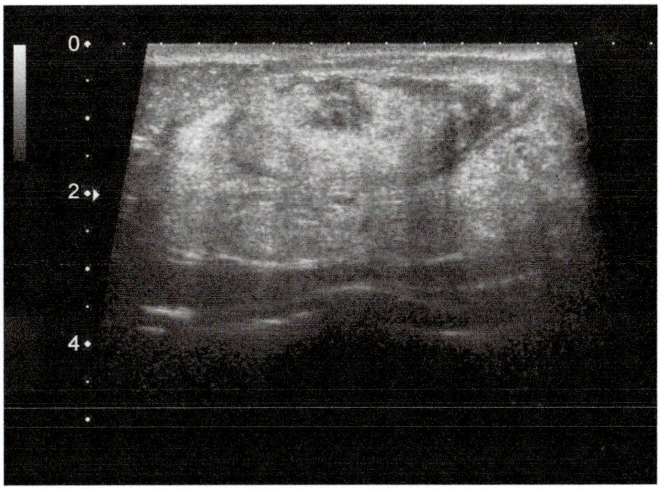

Fig. 3: A circumscribed heterogeneous mass showing a "breast within breast appearance" s/o hamartoma.

Orientation: These are generally aligned parallel to skin surface.

Echotexture: They are isoechoic or mildly hypoechoic with respect to fat and their appearance depends upon the amount of epithelial and stromal elements. Nodules which are hypoechoic are perceived better than isoechoic nodules.

Most fibroadenomas are homogenous in echotexture. A typical finding seen in fibroadenoma is a thin echogenic traversing line or septa that is non-enhancing on MRI.

Capsule: A thin echogenic capsule is generally seen which indicates that the leading edge of mass pushes rather than infiltrates the surrounding tissues.

Acoustic enhancement: The classic fibroadenoma with more cellular stroma shows acoustic enhancement with respect to surrounding tissue. Those with hyalinized or sclerotic stroma can show acoustic shadowing. A thin edge shadowing may also be seen.

Mobility: These masses are generally mobile relative to parenchyma, the only exception being those with infarction. Cellular fibroadenomas are softer in comparison with those with sparse cellularity.

Complex fibroadenoma: These fibroadenomas contain epithelial proliferative changes like cyst formation, apocrine metaplasia, epithelial hyperplasia with calcifications and sclerosing adenosis and have a marginally increased risk of malignancy. The ultrasound features to be looked for complex fibroadenoma are punctate calcifications, small cysts and heterogeneous echotexture.

VARIANTS OF FIBROADENOMA: TUBULAR ADENOMA AND LACTATING ADENOMA

Both these occur during the reproductive years with lactating adenoma commonly seen during third trimester of pregnancy or lactation, when it enlarges rapidly and may get infarcted which is associated with pain.

On ultrasound, tubular adenomas appear as fibroadenoma and have tendency to appear fusiform in shape. Lactating adenomas are elliptical, have increased through transmission and may show small cystic spaces which is due to lactational lobules. They are generally soft and compressible and may show increased vascularity on Doppler because of stimulation by hormones.

Hamartoma: These are composed of normal lobules, fibrous tissue and fat in various proportions. They are frequently seen in asymptomatic patients but may present as palpable lumps.

On ultrasound, the findings are variable depending upon histology. In general they are heterogenous and composed of a variable mixture of fat, fibrous tissue and lobular elements (Fig. 3). An echogenic pseudocapsule may be present whose thickness depends upon the amount of compressed breast tissue. Lesions with more fat are isoechoic and more compressible than those with increased fibrous content and are difficult to distinguish from lipoma.

Lipoma: These are benign overgrowth of fatty tissue and present as soft, mobile, palpable lumps (Figs. 4 and 5).

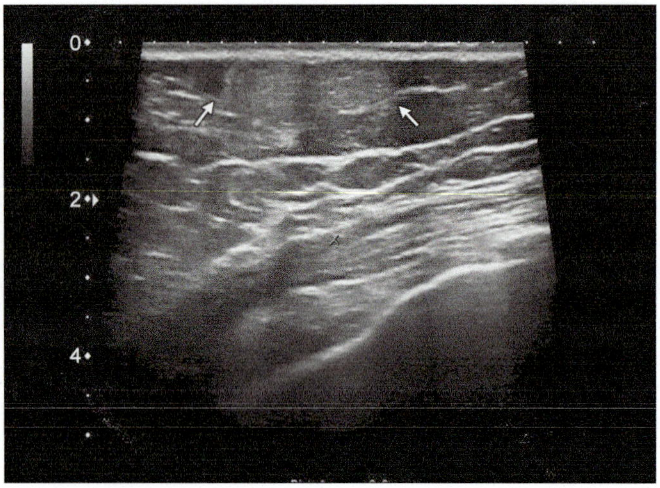

Fig. 4: A circumscribed oval hyperechoic mass s/o lipoma.

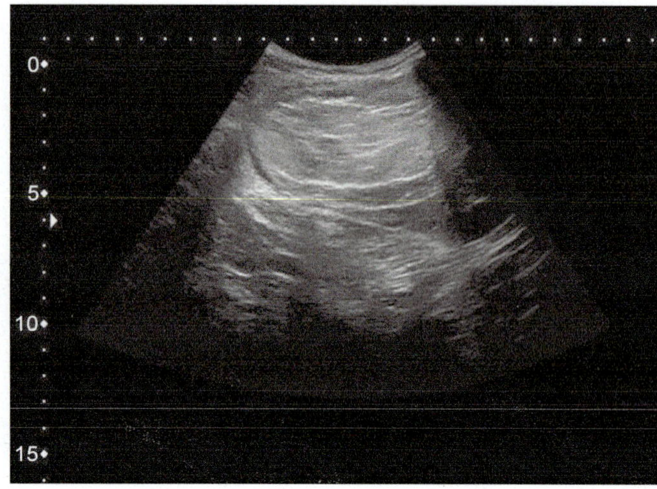

Fig. 5: A heterogeneously hyperechoic mass with an echogenic capsule s/o lipoma.

They may have the following appearances:

- Isoechoic with surrounding fat lobules
- Mildly hyperechoic with surrounding fat lobules
- Isoechoic with surrounding fat lobules showing thin internal echogenic septa

Sclerosing Adenosis: The enlargement of lobules due to adenosis is a variant of ANDI (aberration of normal development and involution) where there is increase in number and size of the TDLU.

On ultrasound, it can be seen as a solid nodule with central echogenic focus or a nodule with irregular margins. Punctate foci of calcifications may be seen.

MALIGNANT MASSES

Medullary Carcinoma

These present as well-defined palpable, mobile lumps or may be asymptomatic.

On ultrasound they are seen as circumscribed masses with enhanced through transmission because of increased cellularity. They are hypoechoic to fat giving rise to pseudocystic appearance. They have a thin echogenic capsule and show increased vascularity. These features appear like benign lesion hence they are often placed in BI-RADS category 3; however, its shape and presence of a thick halo should also be taken into account before considering it as a benign lesion.

Their differential diagnosis includes phyllodes, lymphoma and large fibroadenomas.

Mucinous Carcinoma

These tumors are more common in elderly women above 75 years of age with average age of 63 years. They present clinically as a palpable lump.

They occur in pure and mixed forms. On ultrasound, they are seen as circumscribed isoechoic to heterogeneously hyperechoic masses with a thin echogenic capsule. They are wide than tall and may show microlobulations. Masses >1.5 cm in diameter generally show enhanced through transmission.

The differential diagnosis includes: normal fat lobules, lipoma and fibroadenomas with a myxoid stroma.

3.4 Evaluation of Nipple: Areolar Region

INTRODUCTION

Nipple discharge is a common complaint at presentation, that causes distress and anxiety to the patient. Ultrasound is a widely available modality to evaluate the nipple-areolar region which requires a different technique as positioning of the transducer is of utmost importance.

Approximately 2%–5% of the women visiting the health providers present with nipple discharge.[1]

Anatomy of nipple-areolar region and ductal system of breast: Embryologically, milk line or paired mammary ridges develop on ventral surface of embryo from axilla to midthigh during the 6th week of gestation. They involute everywhere except in pectoral region where the breasts develop. Incomplete involution of milk line can lead to accessory nipple or nipples (polythelia) and accessory true mammary gland (polymastia) which is relatively rare. The common sites for accessory nipples is axilla or inframammary fold.

The nipple-areolar complex (Fig. 1) has large sebaceous glands called Montgomery glands opening at Montgomery tubercles which are 1-2 mm raised papules at areola. It also has sensory nerve endings and abundant lymphatics—subareolar or Sappey plexus.

Each lobe of breast parenchyma consists of a number of lobules which contains approximately 10–100 acini or blind ending sacs. These lobules and lobes are drained by interlobular, intralobar and interlobar ducts uniting to form a lactiferous duct which converges toward the nipple and dilates into an ampulla before terminating at the nipple (Fig. 2A). The terminal ductolobular unit (TDLU) is the functional unit and basic building block of lobule and consists of extralobular duct, intralobular duct and acini or ductules (Fig. 2B).

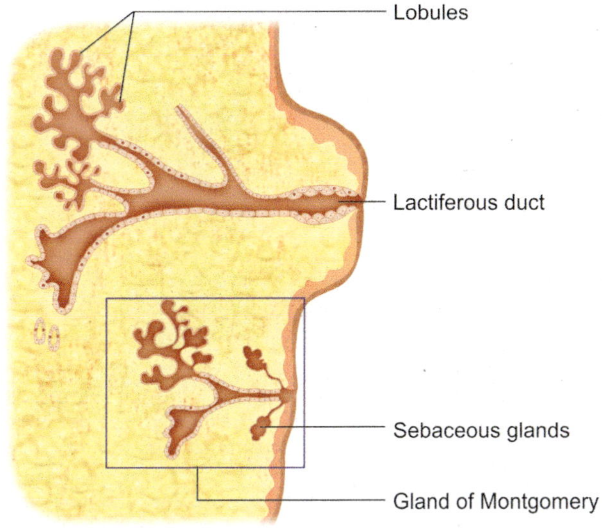

Fig. 1: Anatomy of nipple–areolar region.

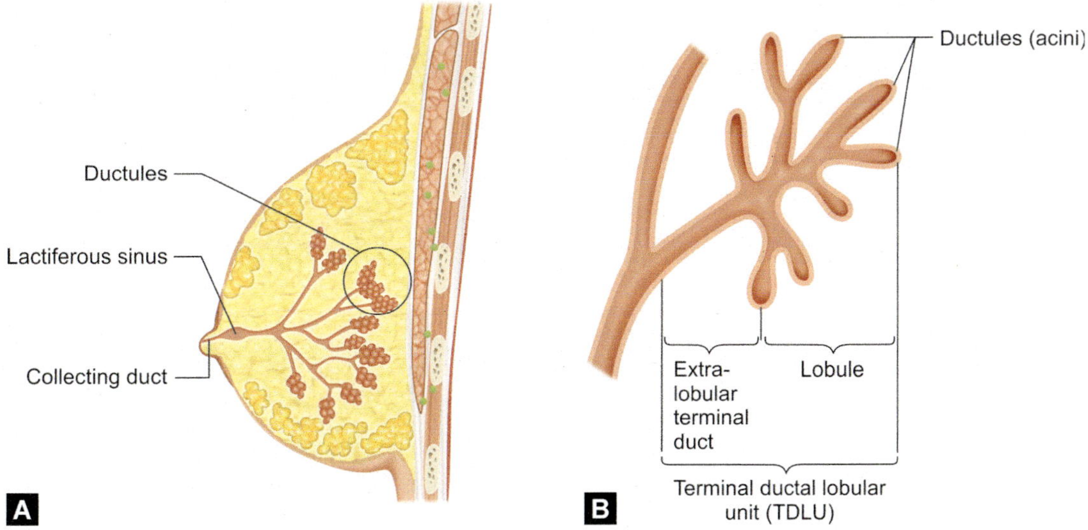

Figs. 2A and B: (A) Ductal anatomy of breast; (B) Anatomy of the terminal ductolobular unit.

Clinical presentation: The patients with involvement of nipple-areolar region may present with nipple inversion, skin changes/cracks around nipple, nipple enlargement, ulceration (Fig. 3), polypoidal mass or polyps (Fig. 4) and prominent or enlarged Montgomery's tubercles (Fig. 5). It is important to **distinguish nipple retraction from** inversion, both of them may be congenital or acquired. In retraction, a slit like area is pulled in centrally while in inversion the entire nipple is pulled inward.

Bilateral, slowly progressive, long-standing nipple inversion is generally benign. A unilateral inversion can be due to chronic inflammatory pathology, periductal mastitis or malignancy (Fig. 6) and should be evaluated further.

Paget's disease of the nipple presents with a bloody discharge from the nipple, itching, erythema, scaly or flaky skin, nipple erosion or ulceration, nipple retraction or a palpable mass.

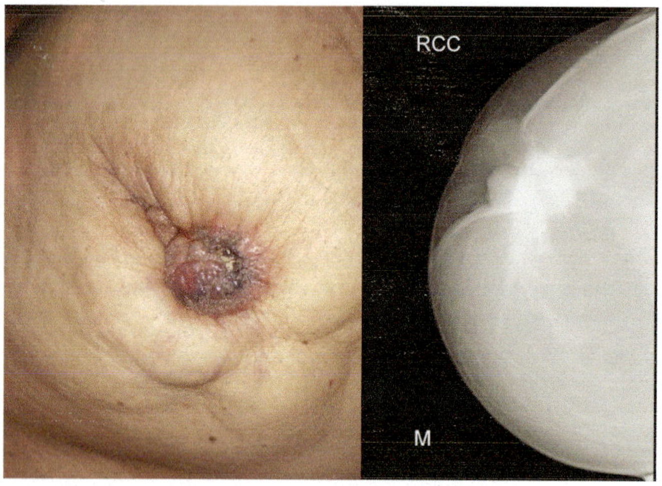

Fig. 3: A 55-year-old female presented with ulceration in nipple–areolar region with nipple retraction. Mammogram showed a irregular retroareolar mass with spiculated margins causing nipple retraction—BI-RADS category 5. Histopathology was s/o invasive ductal carcinoma. (BI-RADS: breast imaging reporting and data system).

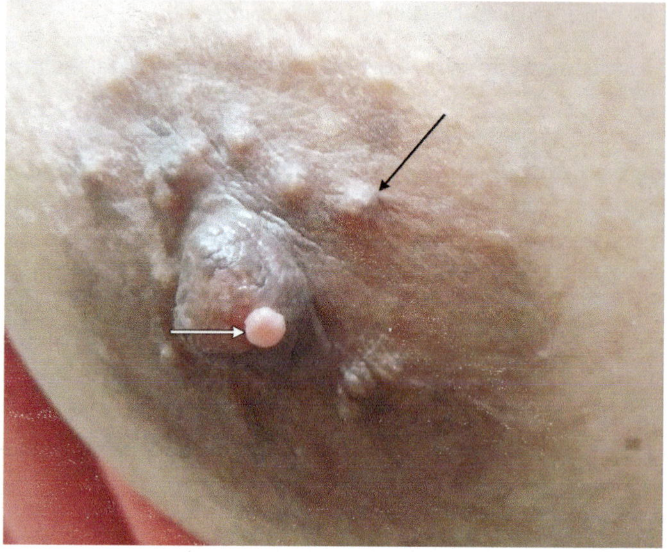

Fig. 5: A 35-year-old female presented with a small polypoidal growth on nipple (white arrow) with prominent Montgomery tubercles (black arrow). Histopathology was s/o benign papillary adenoma of nipple.

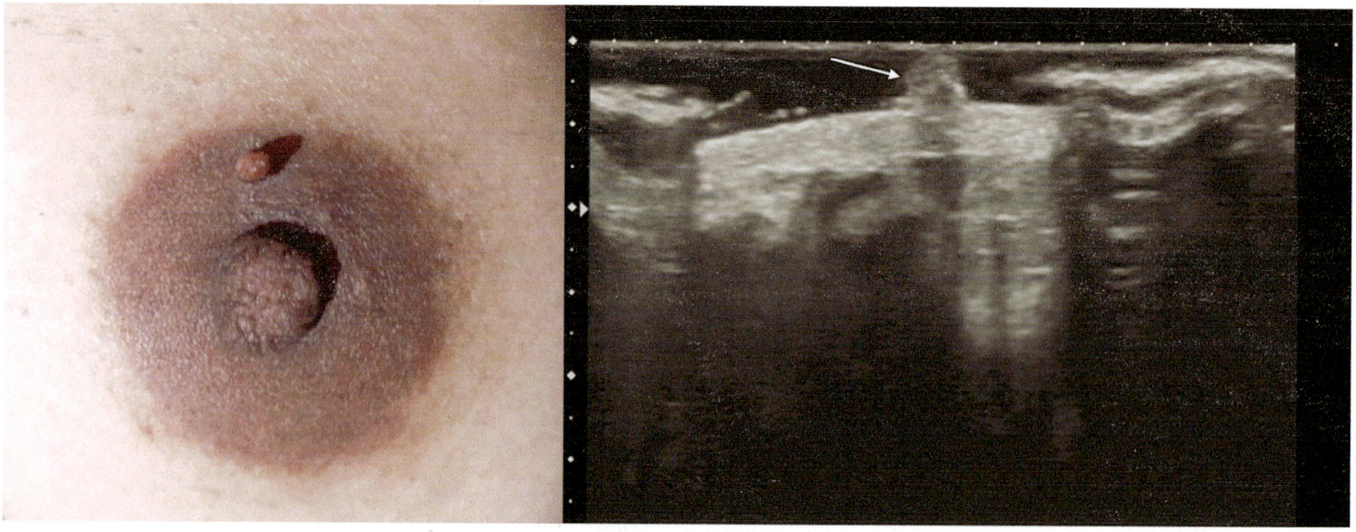

Fig. 4: A 25-year-old female presented with a small polypoidal growth in the nipple–areolar region. Ultrasound showed small well-defined echogenic nodule arising from the skin. Histopathology was s/o ulcerated fibroepithelial polyp.

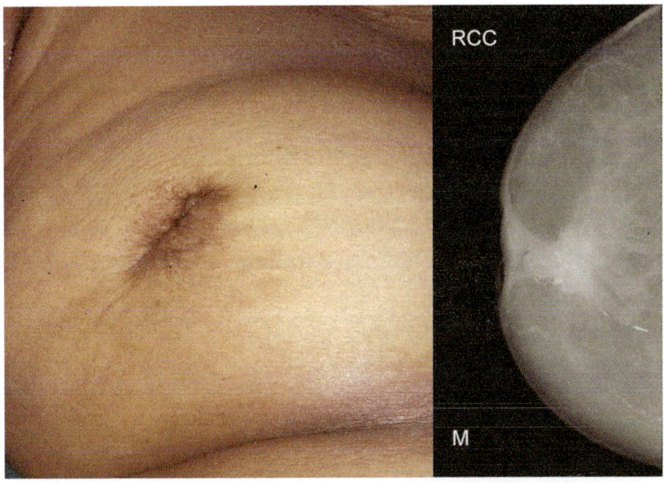

Fig. 6: A 65-year-old female presented with nipple inversion. Her mammogram showed a retroareolar mass with nipple retraction and overlying skin thickening. Histopathology was s/o invasive ductal carcinoma.

The patient with ductal disease may have a myriad of presentations like serous, serosanguineous or bloody nipple discharge, lump in retroareolar region, papillomas or inverted nipple.

TYPES OF NIPPLE DISCHARGE

There are two kinds of nipple discharge: physiological and pathological and in order to differentiate between the two, it is important to take a proper clinical history along with a careful clinical examination.

Spontaneous nipple discharge must be regarded as abnormal unless a proper evaluation rules out underlying pathology.

The most frequent and **physiological** cause of ductal distention and nipple discharge is lactation, when the lobules and ducts become dilated due to hormonal changes. It is usually bilateral, involves multiple ducts and may be white or clear, straw colored, gray, yellow or brown in color.

The lobules are responsible for production of a proteinaceous fluid which peaks during the secretory phase of the menstrual cycle. This fluid is turbid in appearance and is resorbed normally. When it is not resorbed fully, it collects within the ducts thereby causing obstruction and dilatation of ducts. Since there is an alkaline environment within the ducts, calcifications are produced which are detected on mammogram.

There are certain medications which cause nipple discharge physiologically. These include hormonal preparations; psychotropic, antihypertensive and antiemetic drugs, H2 receptor antagonist group and dopamine which causes galactorrhea.[2]

Pathological nipple discharge is spontaneous, unilateral, bloody, serous or clear and may be associated with an intraductal mass. The common benign causes of pathological discharge are duct ectasia, blocked ducts due to debris leading to ductal obstruction, inflammatory infiltrates, periductal mastitis, apocrine metaplasia, intraductal papillomas and papillomatosis. Normally cytology is not advised in these cases because it has a low sensitivity (~27%) for detection of carcinoma.[3] The nipple discharge obtained may be tested for blood with a Hemoccult test. Ductal carcinoma in situ (DCIS), invasive ductal carcinoma and Paget disease are some of the malignant causes of nipple discharge.

IMAGING OF DUCTAL DISEASE

Ductal disease commonly presents as nipple discharge and is evaluated mainly by ultrasound, though a combination of modalities like mammography, ductography and MRI are also used for evaluation of ductal disease. One has to look for dilatation of duct which may be diffuse or focal and any intraductal pathology like intraductal mass or thick secretions which appear as low-level echoes

With the availability of high resolution transducers, the ducts are very well seen and intraductal pathology can be diagnosed easily on ultrasound.

MAMMOGRAPHY

When nipple-areolar region is involved, the nipple may appear inverted on mammography, as seen on a properly taken profile view. A proper history and careful clinical examination is an essential part of workup.

One of the common cause of nipple inversion is a chronic inflammatory process which may be unilateral or bilateral. Sometimes, nipple inversion develops rapidly and in these cases a fast growing malignancy should be ruled out.

The additional views on Mammogram include spot compression view with the nipple in profile (to determine whether there is a retroareolar mass) as well as craniocaudal and lateral spot magnification views to assess microcalcifications. If the mammographic views are normal, ultrasound should be performed.

Duct ectasia is seen as an area of increased density or presence of a dilated duct in retroareolar region, which can be confirmed on a targeted ultrasound.

Mammography is indicated in a patient with spontaneous nipple discharge but according to some studies, it has a low sensitivity (59%) and positive predictive value (16.7%) in diagnosing a malignant pathology.[4] The mammogram findings seen (Fig. 7) in a patient with spontaneous nipple discharge depends upon underlying pathology and may be normal or show a retroareolar density or mass, developing asymmetry, architectural distortion, nipple retraction, microcalcification in nipple-areolar region, periductal microcalcifications or suspicious microcalcifications distributed in a linear or branching manner.[5] Sometimes, a developing asymmetry may be associated with a new onset nipple discharge which is suspicious for an underlying carcinoma and biopsy should be performed.

Benign appearing calcifications may be seen in 25% cases.[6] Secretory calcifications are well defined and rod like in appearance (Fig. 8). Sometimes, microcalcifications are seen in nipple-areolar region in chronic inflammatory conditions (Fig. 9) of the nipple. Indeterminate calcifications may be seen in a variety of causes like hemorrhage, fibrosis or DCIS.

DCIS is typically seen as microcalcifications on mammography, though in approximately 14% cases, it may present as a solid mass with (Fig. 10) or without microcalcifications. Microcalcifications are more common in high-grade than non-high-grade DCIS (Fig. 11).

Small papillomas may be occult on mammogram if present in the retroareolar region, while larger lesions with round or oval shape and circumscribed margins are easily seen. Papillomas may be solitary or multiple with the solitary one located just below the nipple-areolar region. Multiple papillomas are seen in approximately 10% of intraductal papillomas especially in younger women. Papillary carcinomas may be seen as round, oval or lobulated masses with circumscribed, indistinct or spiculated margins in areas of invasion.[7] Spiculated margins are generally not seen in papillomas as fibrotic reaction is less. Nipple adenoma, also known as florid papillomatosis, erosive adenomatosis and superficial papillary adenomatosis, is an

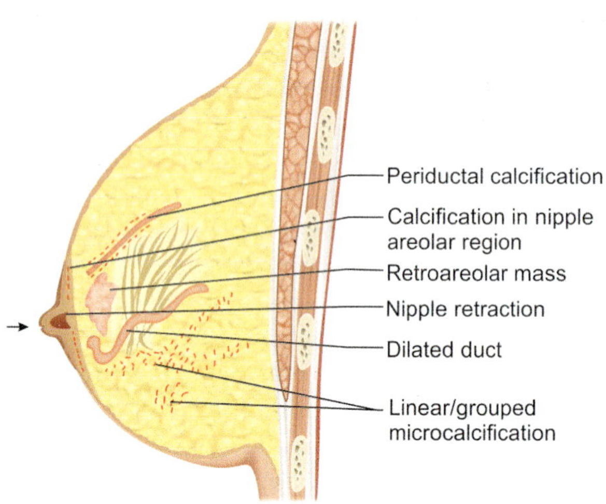

Fig. 7: Line diagram showing common mammographic findings in a patient presenting with spontaneous nipple discharge.

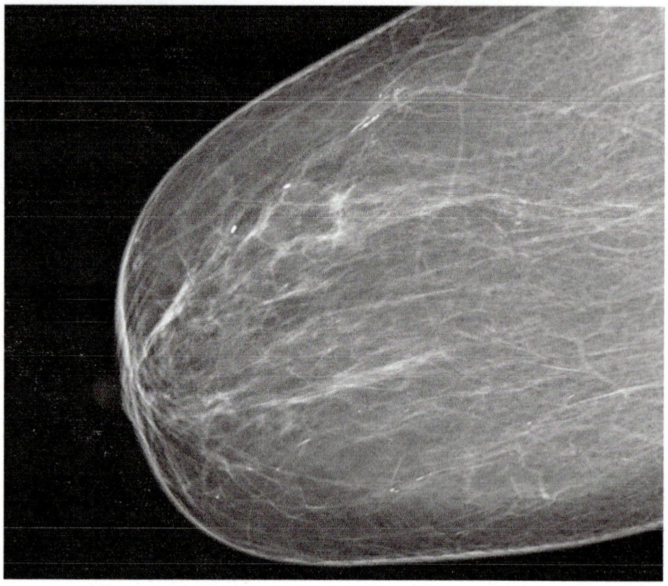

Fig. 8: Mammogram of right breast in a 49-year-old female with colorless watery nipple discharge. Shows rod like elongated benign calcifications.

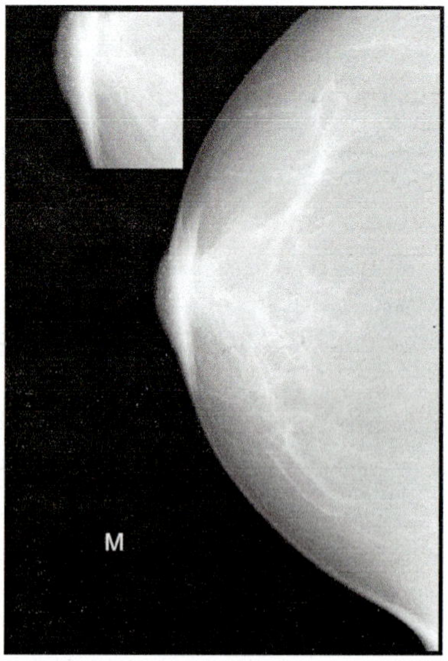

Fig. 9: A 45-year-old female presented with thickening in nipple-areolar region in right breast. Mammogram shows thickening and microcalcification confined to nipple–areolar region. Histopathology was s/o chronic inflammatory pathology.

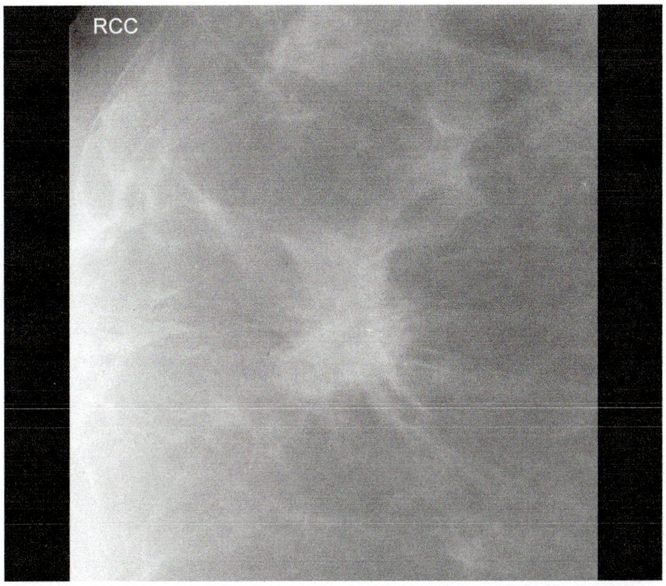

Fig. 10: Mammogram in 52-year-old female shows a spiculated mass with linear and pleomorphic calcifications. Histopathology was s/o DCIS with invasive ductal carcinoma. (DCIS: ductal carcinoma in situ).

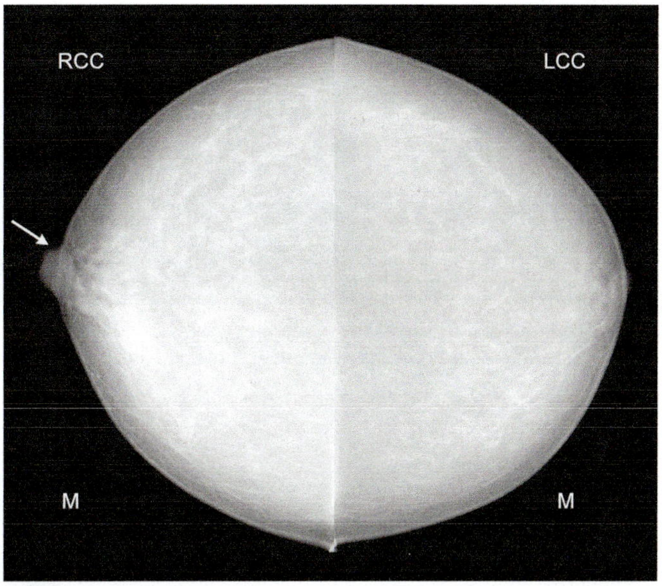

Fig. 12: A 40-year-old female presented with enlarged nipple on right side with ulceration. Mammogram shows enlarged nipple on right side. No mass or suspicious microcalcifications seen in both breasts.

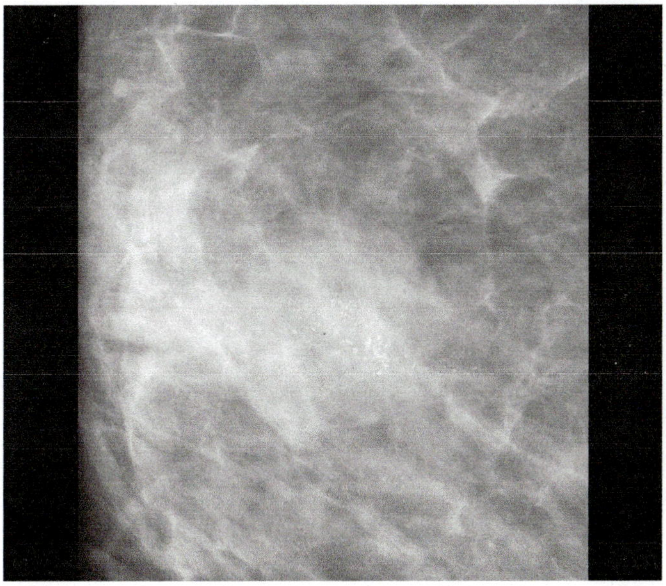

Fig. 11: A 55-year-old female presented with a blackish red nipple discharge on and off for 6 months. Mammogram of right breast magnification view shows segmental pleomorphic calcifications. Histopathology was s/o DCIS with microinvasion. (DCIS: ductal carcinoma in situ).

uncommon variant of intraductal papilloma that involves the nipple (Figs. 12 and 13).

Ultrasound: It is very useful in evaluation of nipple discharge as it is non-invasive, cost effective, widely available and is more accurate because of higher resolution providing greater details of the ductal anatomy. Involvement of a single duct or multiple ducts can be ascertained with ease and morphology of intraductal masses can be seen clearly. ***It has been observed that in a patient with pathological nipple discharge, ultrasound has a sensitivity of 97%, specificity of 60% and positive predictive value of 95%.***[8]

SONOGRAPHIC TECHNIQUE FOR EVALUATING NIPPLE DISCHARGE

While evaluating the nipple–areolar region, the technique is very important. The transducer has to be angulated in such a way that ultrasound beam is at 90° to the long axis of duct when peripheral compression is applied.

The nipple does not transmit sound well and shadowing behind the nipple interferes with visualization of ducts within and deep to nipple (Fig. 14A).

When the position of the transducer is correct, then it is easier to maintain a steady contact thereby showing the ductal anatomy well.

There are two maneuvers described by Stavros[9] which are commonly used: rolled-nipple technique and two-handed compression technique which can tip the nipple to one side. In the rolled nipple technique the entire duct is seen within the nipple (Fig. 14B) and any echogenic inspissated secretions, intraductal papilloma, etc. can also be seen. In the two-handed compression technique (Fig. 14C), scanning direction is changed and nipple in its

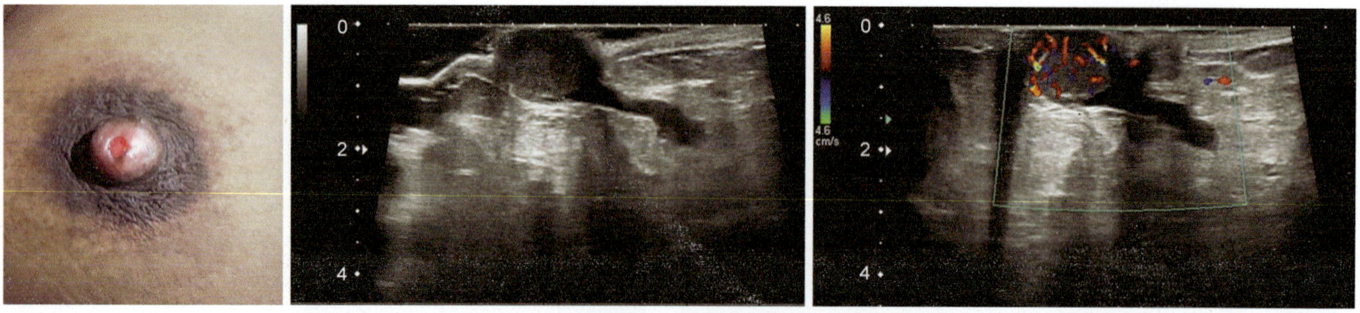

Fig. 13: Clinical picture and Ultrasound of the same patient as in Figure 12 shows a well-defined hypoechoic mass showing increased vascularity in the retroareolar region just behind the nipple with intraductal extension and duct dilatation. Histopathology was s/o nipple adenoma.

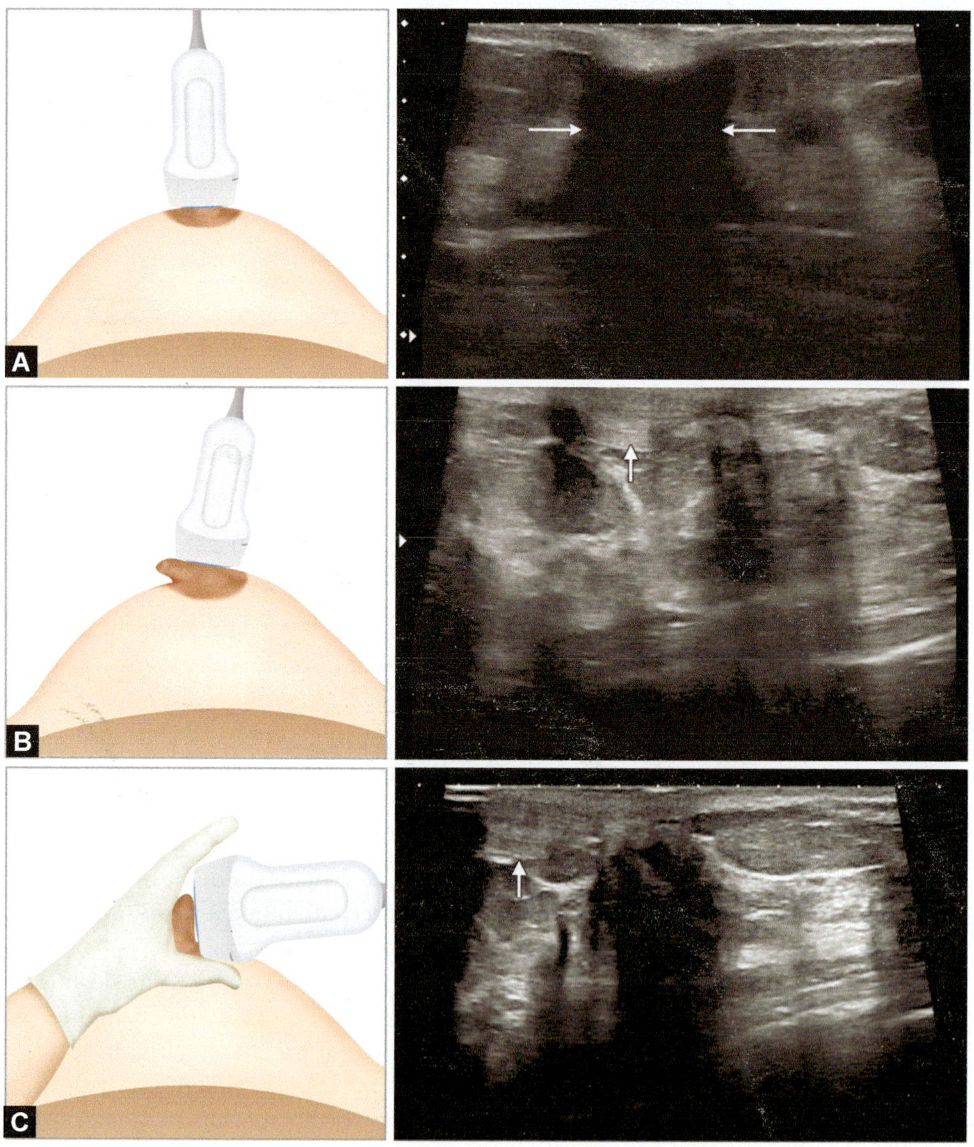

Figs. 14A to C: (A) Transducer kept on nipple with ultrasound image showing shadowing behind nipple; (B) Rolled nipple technique with ultrasound showing duct within the nipple; (C) Two-hand compression technique showing proper angulation of transducer with nipple and ultrasound showing normal nipple.

entirely is pressed against the transducer while the other hand supports the nipple. With this maneuver, the entire duct is seen from the base of nipple and duct compressibility can be assessed.

Sometimes in ductectasia, the secretions become thick, cheesy and viscous and are difficult to differentiate from a papilloma. In these cases, a dynamic maneuver like ballottement of the duct with transducer can help as it may show movement of inspissated secretions back and forth with alternating compression.

The location of discharging duct orifice on nipple surface can be helpful in targeting the scan area of greatest interest. If the discharging orifice is in the center of nipple, scanning is begun at 12 o'clock and when it is in the periphery of nipple its clock face position usually indicates the quadrant from where secretions are coming.

BENIGN PATHOLOGIES

The benign ductal pathologies are ductal inflammation, periductal mastitis, blocked ducts in lactating women, inflammatory infiltrates and papillomas.

A normal duct is usually collapsed and may not be seen. If it is visible, it is seen as a tubular hypoechoic structure (1–2 mm), wider at the nipple and tapering peripherally and distally.

Ductectasia: It is seen as dilated duct (>2 mm) in the retroareolar region (Figs. 15A to D) and is associated with periductal inflammation. It may be asymptomatic or may present with a palpable mass. There may be fluid or low-level echoes and inspissated secretions within the duct. The echogenicity of the secretions depends upon the viscosity and sometimes the secretions appear so echogenic that they appear like a mass. When several ducts are ectatic, some may show anechoic fluid while others may show echogenic secretions. Use of color Doppler or dynamic maneuver like ballottement with transducer can help create movement of echoes.

Ductectasia often has an inflammatory component involving its walls which can spread into the periductal tissues causing periductal mastitis. Periductal mastitis is commonly seen in premenopausal women where ducts below the nipple become inflamed and infected. The patient may present with a serous or serosanguineous discharge and sometimes an inverted nipple (Fig. 16) or abscess formation in retroareolar region.

Sonologically, there may be ductectasia , ductal wall thickening, edema of periductal tissue and increase

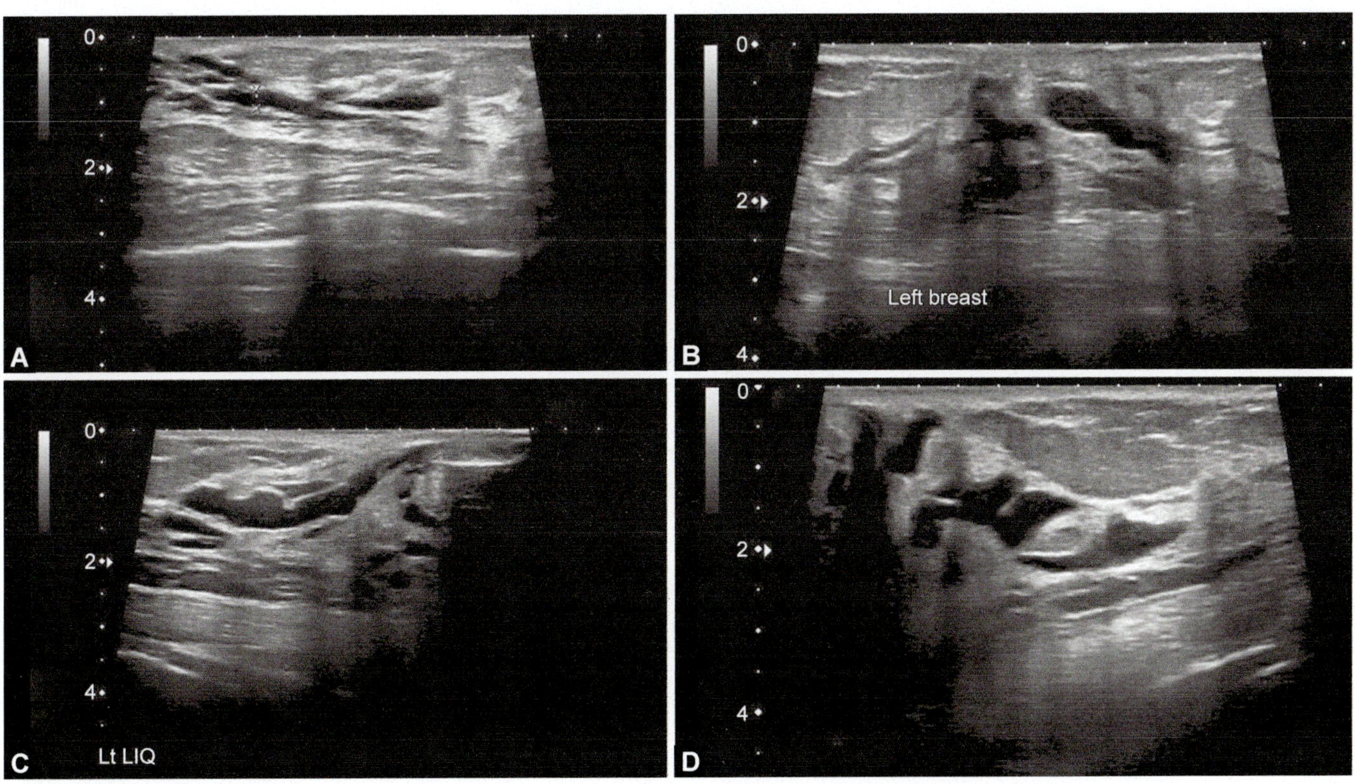

Fig. 15A to D: Ultrasound showing ductectasia (caliber >2 mm) in different patients.

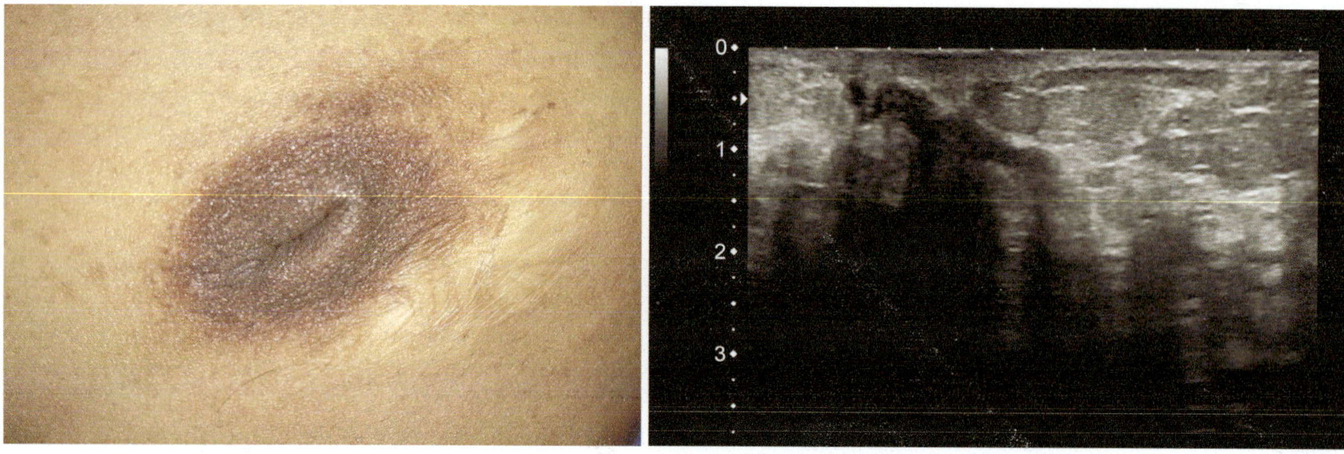

Fig. 16: A 48-year-old female presented with nipple inversion and a long-term history of nipple discharge. Ultrasound of nipple–areolar region shows a dilated duct in retroareolar region with echogenic debris. Features are s/o ductectasia with periductal inflammation.

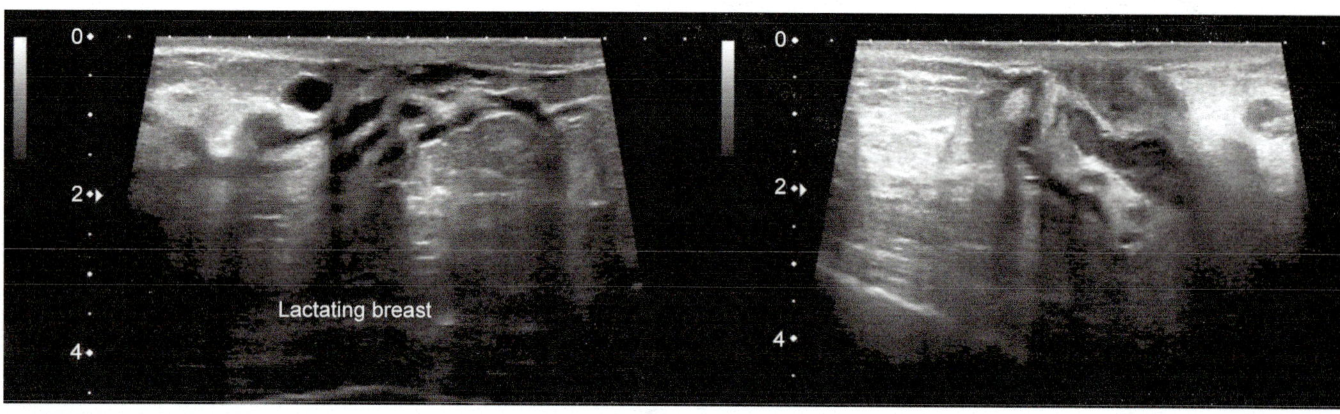

Fig. 17: Ultrasound showing ductectasia in a lactating breast where some of the ducts are seen filled with echogenic debris.

vascularity in periductal tissue on color Doppler. Periductal location of calcification is typically seen in chronic ductectasia and can be appreciated both on ultrasound and mammogram.

On aspiration of fluid from ducts, there may be inflammatory infiltrates and cellular debris which are usually sterile, but sometimes, there is anaerobic infection and antibiotics may have to be started. One must differentiate ductectasia due to a benign cause from that due to a malignant cause.

Ductectasia is also noted during lactation where the ducts may become blocked due to incomplete drainage of milk leading to ductal dilatation which is seen as dilated tubular structures filled with echogenic material with surrounding inflammation (Fig. 17).

Hyperprolactinemia can also cause ductectasia and nipple discharge and is usually bilateral.

Patients with fibrocystic changes can also present with nipple discharge when there is a communication of cyst with a duct. When its drainage to the duct is obstructed the discharge stops. Therefore, a typical alternating history of discharge and lump is seen in these patients.

Papillomas: They are the most common benign intraductal epithelial tumors and have a characteristic frond like structure with a central fibrovascular core. They may be asymptomatic or present with serosanguineous discharge. The bloody nipple discharge may be attributed to twisting of the papilloma on its fibrovascular pedicle, leading to necrosis, ischemia and intraductal bleeding. Papillomas occur in major ducts 2–3 cm away from nipple and cause duct obstruction. They may be solitary or multiple. Central or large duct papillomas are seen in the subareolar region near the lactiferous sinuses.

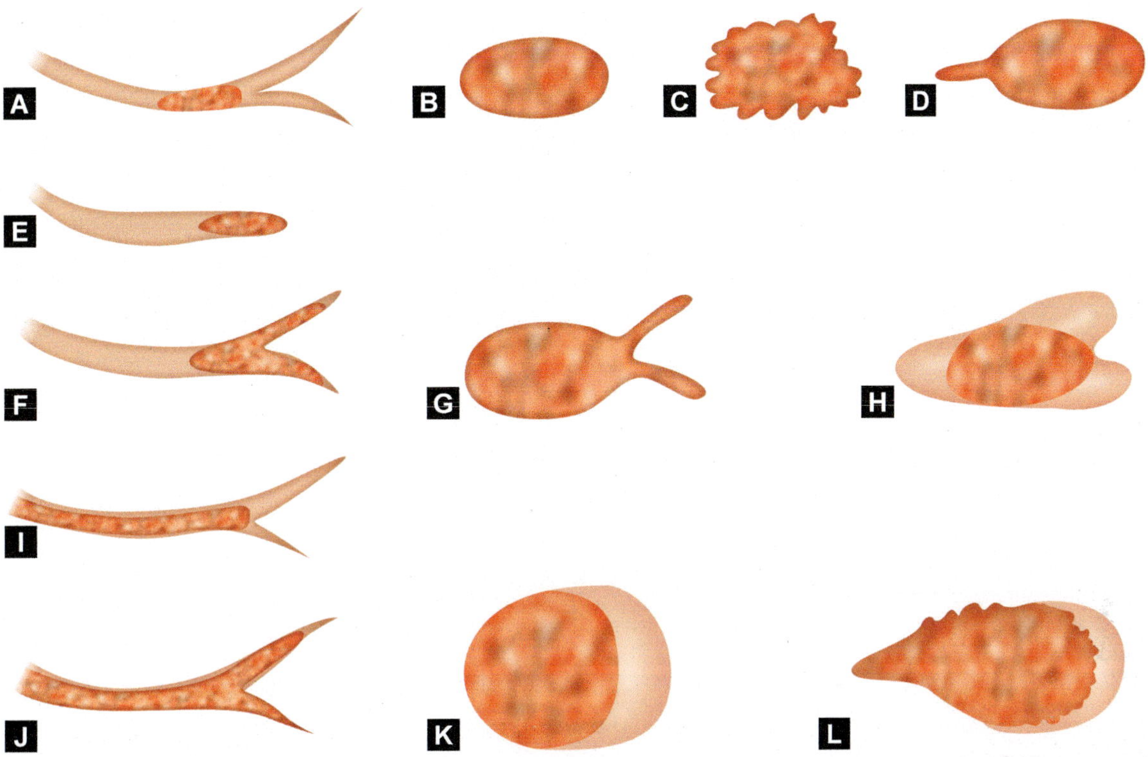

Figs. 18A to L: Ultrasound appearances in papilloma: (A) Small ovoid nodule with ductectasia proximally and distally; (E) Small nodule with ductectasia only distally; (F) Long papilloma extending into two branch ducts; (I) Long papilloma filling entire central duct; (J) Long arborizing papilloma extending into branch ducts. Papilloma without duct ectasia are seen as (D) Round or ovoid nodule; (C) Microlobulated nodule; (D) Nodule with duct extension; (G) Nodule with branch pattern; (H) Small nodule and isolated minimal duct ectasia; (K) Intracystic papilloma; (L) Intracystic papilloma with duct extension.
Source: Adapted form Stavros.

Papillomas have various appearance on ultrasound, (Figs. 18A to L) depending on the location,[9] (centrally or peripherally located), length and width of papilloma, presence of fluid within duct, duct dilatation due to papilloma and extension of papilloma in branches. Papillomas which are not associated with dilated ducts or cyst are generally seen as solid masses which are difficult to distinguish from other solid masses like fibroadenomas. These appear as heterogeneously hypoechoic nodules and may show a thin echogenic capsule which represents the wall of duct from where they arise. They may also show multiple microlobulations and extend into the duct toward the nipple. When papillomas obstruct a duct and secrete fluid, the duct becomes grossly distended and loses its shape to become spherical or elliptical cyst, hence the name intracystic papilloma.

The other appearances of papillomas are dilated duct with circumscribed intraductal solid or mural based nodules (Figs. 19A and B). Vascularity (Fig. 20) may be seen in the vascular pedicle of a papilloma.[10]

It is difficult to determine on ultrasound if intraductal lesion represents a benign papilloma, atypical ductal hyperplasia (ADH) or DCIS as there is a 6%–13% risk for atypia or malignancy, hence a biopsy should be done. Once a diagnosis of papilloma is confirmed by core biopsy, surgical excision is done because some of the papillomas may show atypia that is, atypical ductal hyperplasia or atypical lobular hyperplasia. There is increased risk of malignancy when this lesion is diagnosed; hence, compliance with screening recommendations for such patients is strongly advisable. The features which are suspicious for malignancy include size >1 cm, location of lesion >3 cm from nipple and age of patient >50 years.[11]

Sometimes, the secretions within ductal ectasia may show a fluid-debris level which simulates a papillary lesion. In these cases, changing the patient's position may help or balloting with the transducer can show movement of echoes or secretions within the duct.

Multiple papillomas or papillomatosis occurs in distal ducts in TDLU and is less common than solitary papillomas.

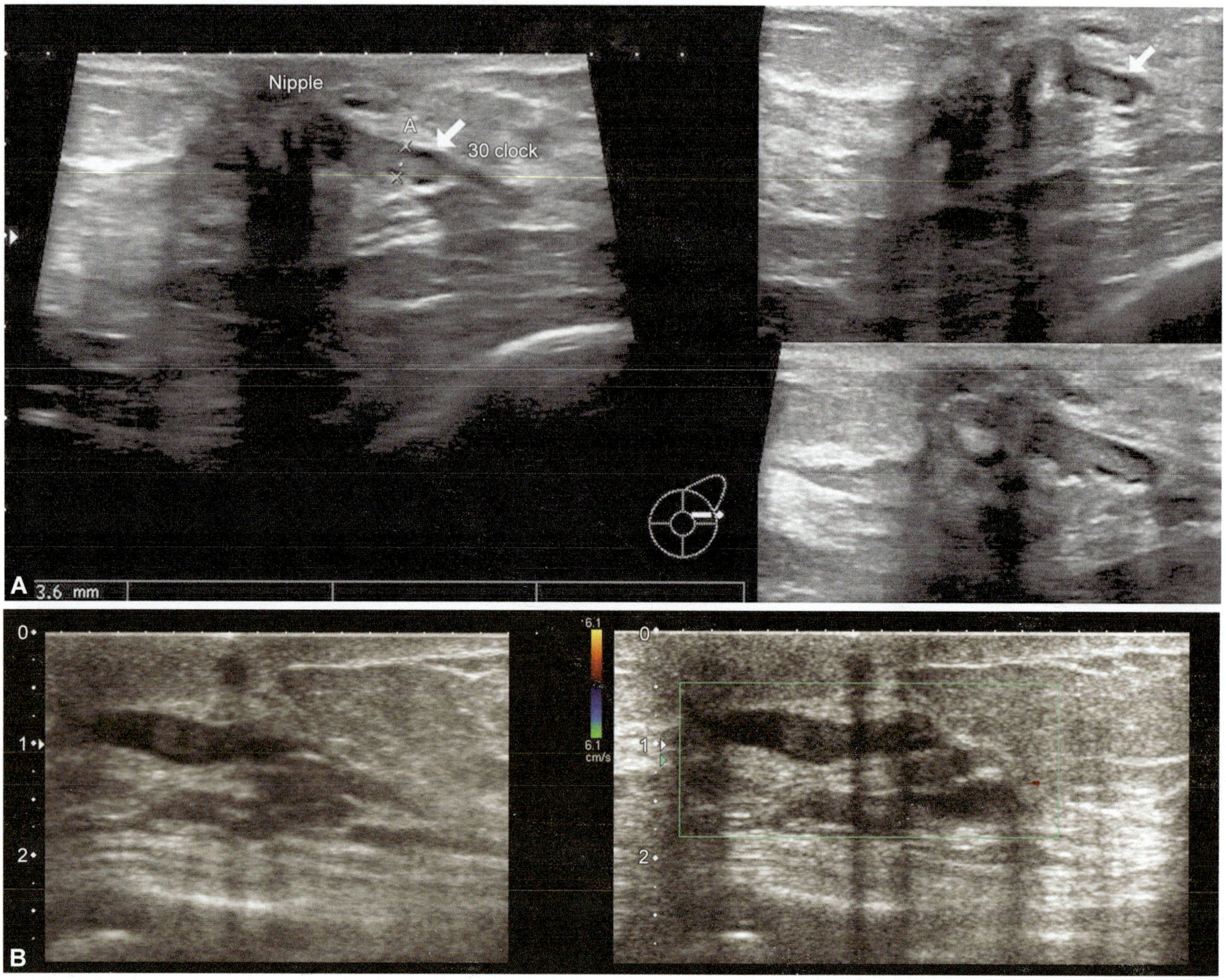

Figs. 19A and B: (A) A 35-year-old female presented with bloody nipple discharge of 6 months duration. Ultrasound shows dilated duct with a focal echogenic mass within. Histopathology was s/o papilloma; (B) A 45-year-old female presented with reddish black discharge from right breast for 6 months. Ultrasound showed a dilated duct with focal area of echogenic material which did not show vascularity on color Doppler. Histopathology was s/o papilloma.

They have an association with atypia or DCIS. They typically present as a palpable mass and are rarely associated with nipple discharge. On ultrasound, these are seen as multiple lobulated and irregular solid hypoechoic, subcentimeter masses with vascularity.

MALIGNANT PATHOLOGY

Papillary carcinomas are rare tumors which represent in <2% of breast cancers. They are common in postmenopausal women and their common location is retroareolar region.[12]

These are seen as hypoechoic solid mass or as complex cysts with septations or mural-based nodules. Duct ectasia due to malignancy is generally peripheral, has irregular duct margin, focal wall thickening and adjacent hypoechoic tissue.[13]

DCIS can show subtle findings on ultrasound and if there is calcification on mammogram, then ultrasound is done to look for an invasive component.

Microcalcifications are seen as echogenic foci if there is good spatial and contrast resolution, but sometimes, these are subtle and difficult to see due to volume averaging in a background of echogenic breast tissue and only an increase in number of ducts is seen (Fig. 21).

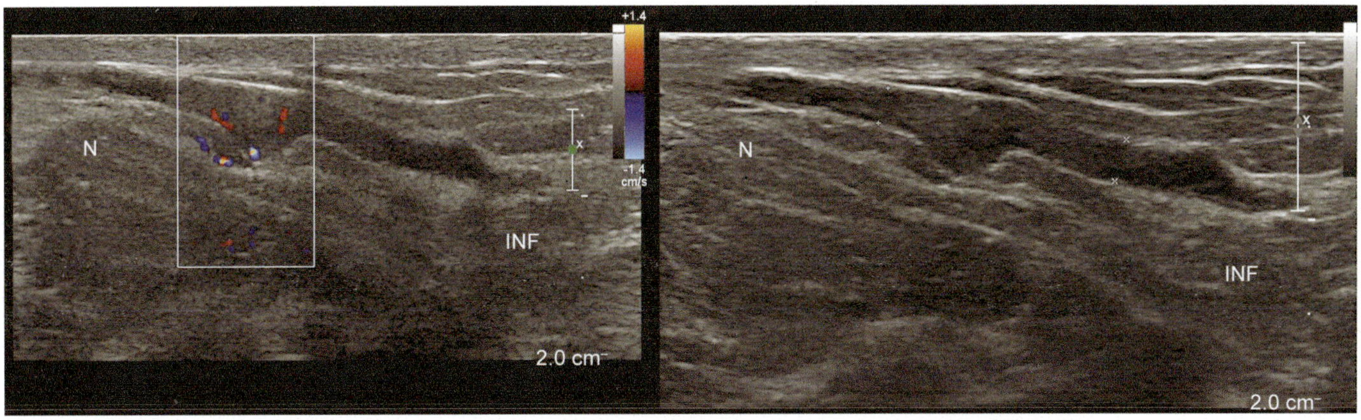

Fig. 20: A 42-year-old women present with blood stained nipple discharge on and off from right breast since 3 months. Ultrasound of the right breast showed a single dilated duct with a focally dilated portion having an intraductal hypoechoic mass with vascularity within. Histopathology was s/o papilloma.

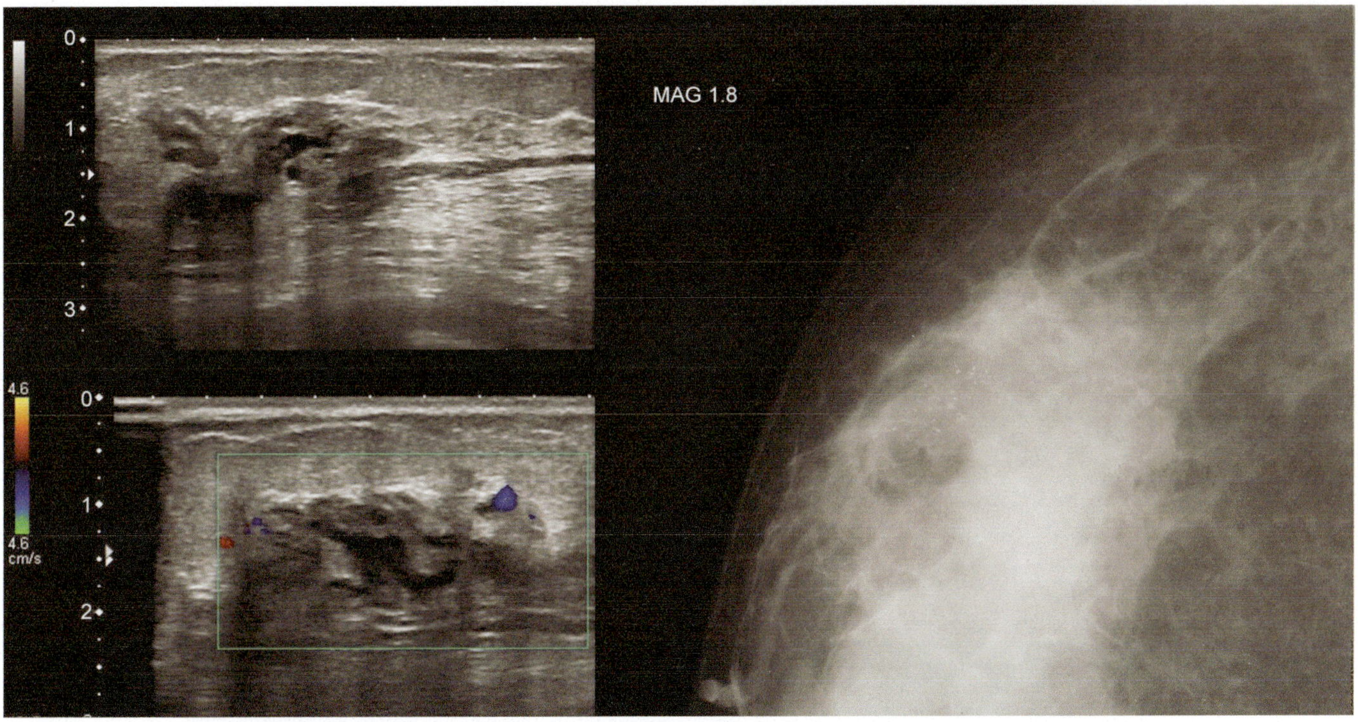

Fig. 21: A 56-year-old female presenting with vague discomfort and pain in right breast. Ultrasound showed ducts increased in number with hypoechoic area surrounding it which on Mammography correlated with a focal area of fine and pleomorphic calcifications. Histopathology was s/o DCIS with microinvasion. (DCIS: ductal carcinoma in situ).

In noncalcified DCIS, a wide variety of findings may be seen on ultrasound (Figs. 22A to I). These range from[14] hypoechoic mass with irregular or microlobulated margins with (Figs. 23 to 25) or without ductal extension, pseudomicrocystic appearance, area of altered echotexture, tubular mass, complex cystic mass, an increase in the number of ducts with ductal distention, architectural distortion, heterogeneous mass with microlobulation, hypoechoic mass with cystic area and intraductal mass (Fig 26) with vascularity, which increases the positive predictive value of ultrasound. Some of these findings may overlap with benign entities like fibrocystic changes, microcyst, apocrine metaplasia and adenosis.

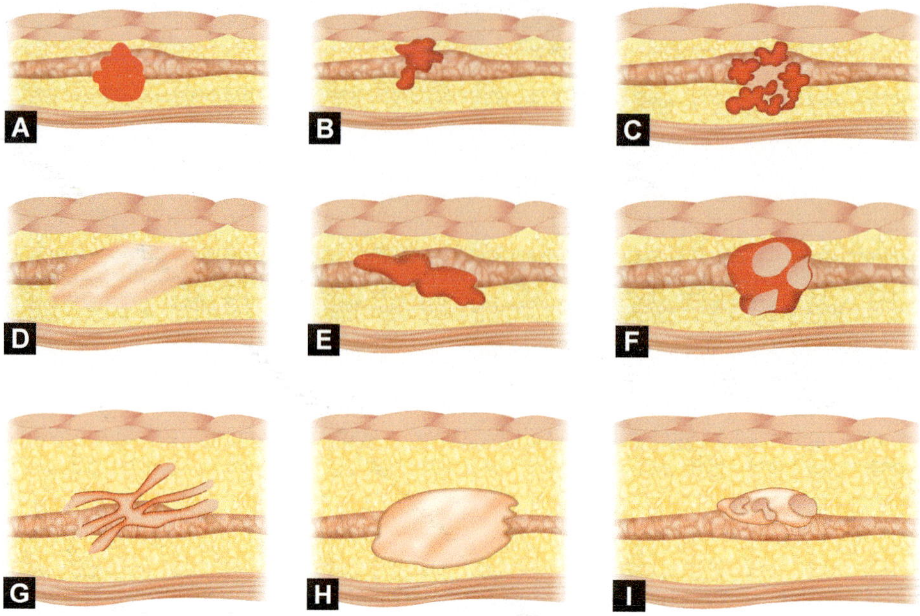

Figs. 22A to I: Ultrasound findings in noncalcified DCIS: (A) Hypoechoic mass with microlobulation in one portion; (B) Mass with irregular margins; (C) Pseudomicrocystic appearance; (D) Area of altered echotexture; (E) Hypoechoic tubular mass; (F) Complex cystic mass; (G) Increase in number of ducts; (H) Heterogeneous mass with microlobulations; (I) Hypoechoic mass with cystic area and vascularity.

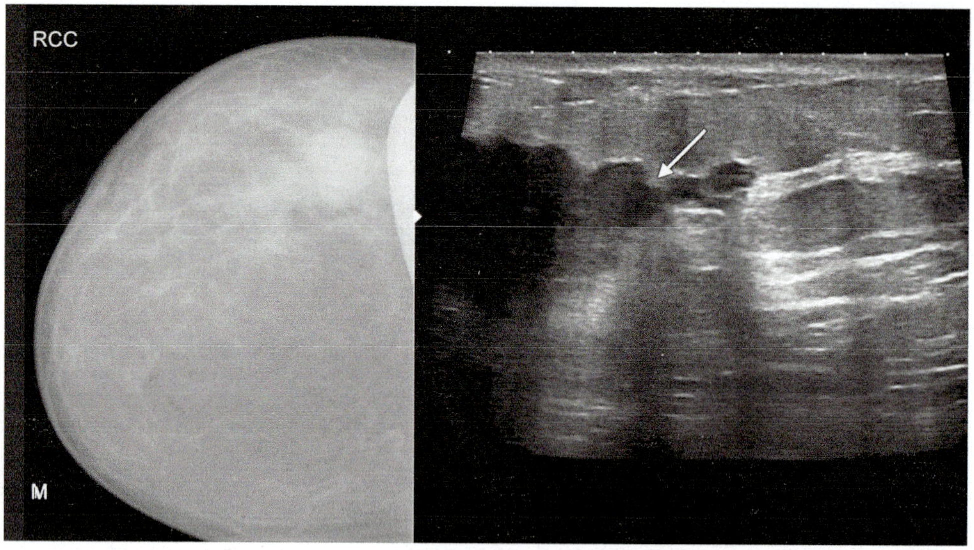

Fig. 23: Mammogram in 48-year-old female who presented with a palpable lump shows a mass with partially obscured margins on CC view which on ultrasound is seen as a hypoechoic mass having irregular margins and ductal extension (arrow).

CONVENTIONAL DUCTOGRAPHY

Ductography is a mammographic examination performed after retrograde filling of the lactiferous ducts with contrast material. It is still a valuable tool with the breast radiologist if mammogram and ultrasound are negative in a patient with unilateral, spontaneous nipple discharge which is bloody, serous or clear and involving a single duct.

The relative contraindications of ductography are:

- Discharge which is not spontaneous and has to be expressed.
- Bilateral nipple discharge
- Nipple discharge involving multiple ducts
- Green, gray, black or milky color discharge (note: It is significant if it is from a single duct and/or is bloody).
- Acute inflammation or abscess in the involved breast.

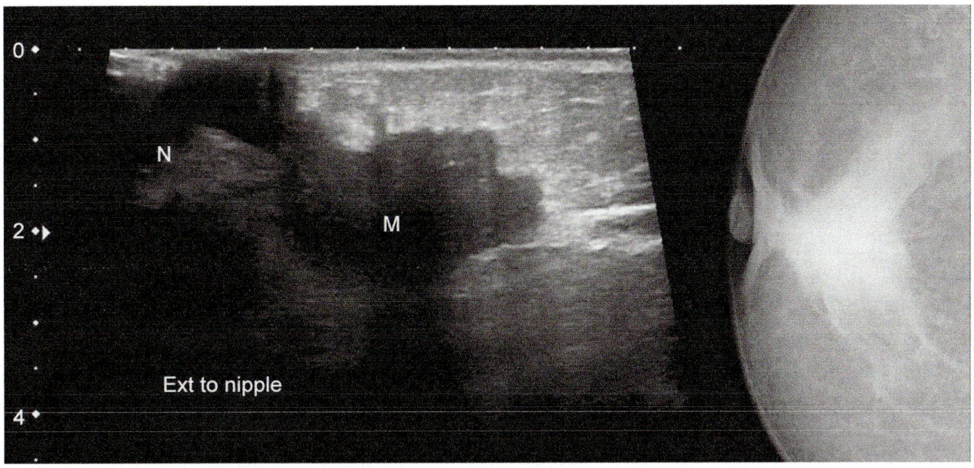

Fig. 24: Ultrasound in a 55-year-old female presenting with lump showed a mass in nipple–areolar region with ductal extension reaching up to nipple with nipple retraction. Histopathology was s/o invasive ductal carcinoma.

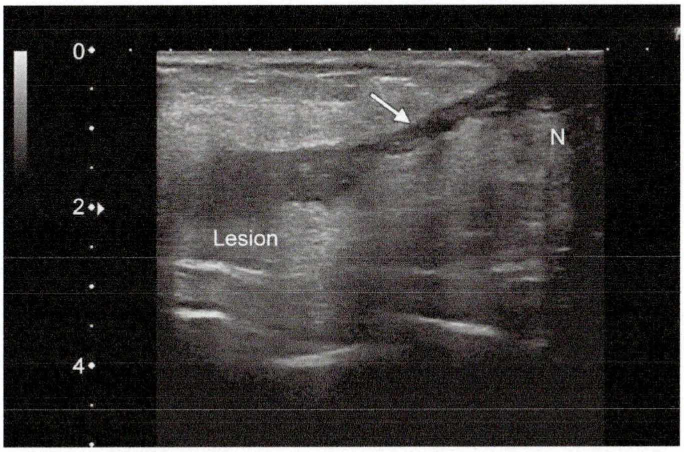

Fig. 25: Ultrasound in 42-year-old female with serosan guineous nipple discharge showing a mass in retroareolar region with ductal extension (arrow) reaching up to nipple (N). Histopathology was so DCIS with invasive ductal carcinoma. (DCIS: ductal carcinoma in situ.)

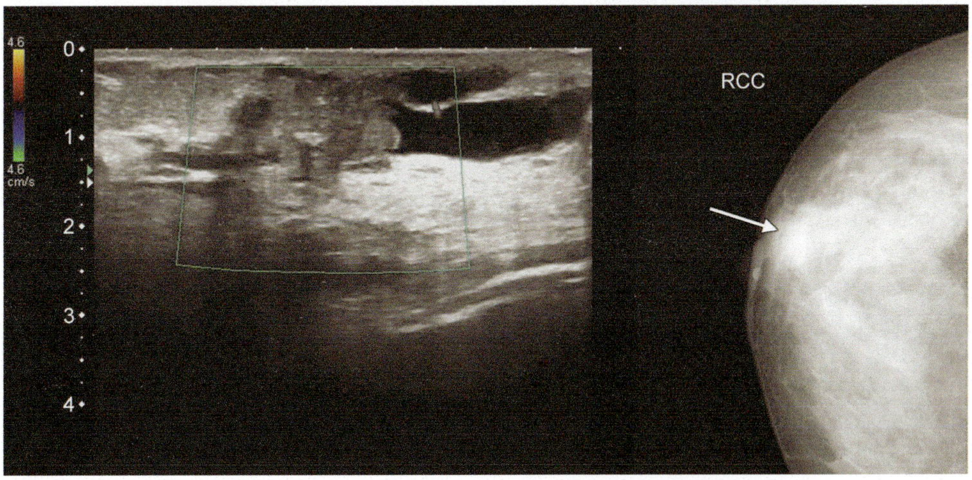

Fig. 26: A 58-year-old female presented with spontaneous serosanguineous discharge on and off since 7 months. Ultrasound showed a dilated duct in retroareolar region with intraductal hypoechoic mass also seen on mammogram. Histopathology was s/o papillary carcinoma.

Materials required: A 30-gauge straight or right-angled sialography cannula, 2-mL syringe, water soluble iodinated contrast, sterile gauze, sterile anesthetic gel, magnification lens.

Technique: A craniocaudal magnification view is done to look for suspicious calcifications or masses.

The patient is made to lie in supine position and using aseptic precautions, the nipple-areolar region is cleaned thoroughly and a gentle pressure is applied to elicit discharge. A trigger point is a focal area in breast which when compressed reliably produces discharge. A sialography cannula is then used to cannulate the duct by identifying the pore from which droplet of discharge is elicited. A magnifying lens may be useful in identifying the pore. Once the pore is identified, the tip of cannula is placed on the pore and gently manipulated till it descends or enters into the duct. Approximately 0.2–0.3 cm^3 of water soluble contrast is injected. Mammogram is taken in Cranio-caudal CC (magnification view) and mediolateral view (90°). After the examination, excess fluid should be expressed out and area covered with sterile gauze piece. If cannulation is unsuccessful, sterile anesthetic gel or warm compresses are applied to the nipple-areolar region and procedure attempted again.

The cannula may pierce through small masses and outline the duct with immediate reflux.

Precautions: Do not apply force or inject if it is painful. Remove air from the cannula before injecting contrast. Artifacts can be seen due to air bubbles which are well defined and round in shape and rise in upright position.

Complications: If too much pressure is applied and excess amount of contrast is injected, there may be perforation of duct and extravasation of contrast (Fig. 27).[15,16] If there is extravasation, the examination should be repeated after 1–2 weeks. There may also be infection and inflammation leading to mastitis in some cases.

DUCTOGRAPHY FINDINGS

The findings on ductography can be classified as:[17]

- Technically inadequate investigation
- Normal findings
- Ductal ectasia (i.e., duct over 2 mm)
- Filling stops
- Filling defects
- Ductal distortions.

Normal ducts have smooth walls and a branching appearance extending toward the chest wall (Fig. 28).

An ectatic duct is defined as a dilated duct >2 mm in diameter (Fig. 29) with an ampullary portion measuring approximately 3 mm.

Intraductal papillomas have a variety of appearances. They may be seen as circumscribed filling defects which can be lobulated and mural based. There can be large irregular filling defects sometimes with dilated ducts or

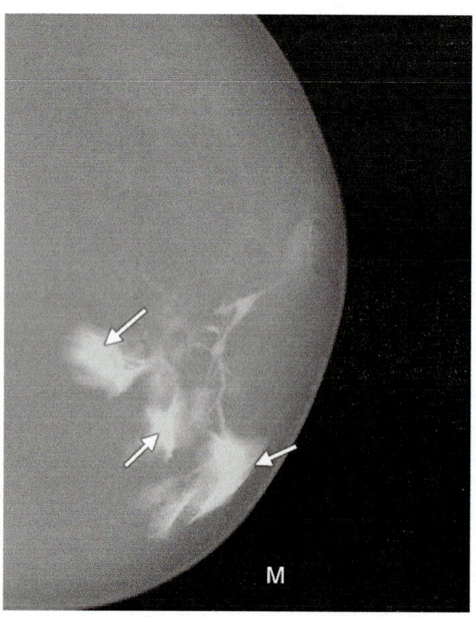

Fig. 27: Technically inadequate ductogram shows extravasation of contrast (arrows) obscuring the ductal anatomy.

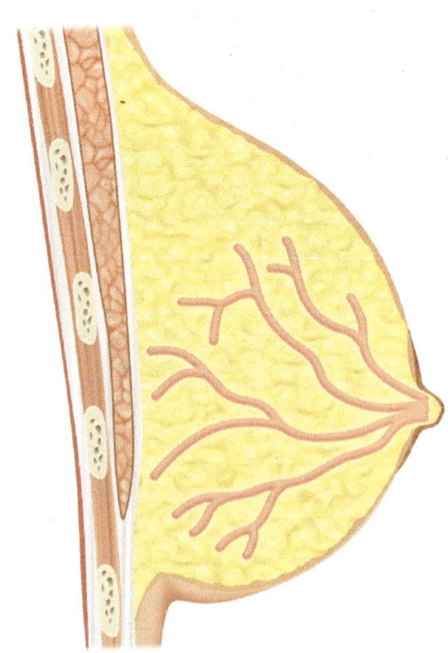

Fig. 28: Normal ductal anatomy on ductogram with smooth walls and branching appearance of ducts.

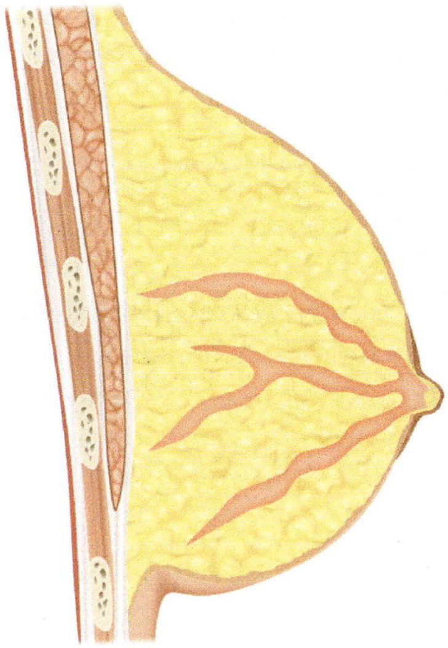

Fig. 29: Duct ectasia with a pruned appearance.

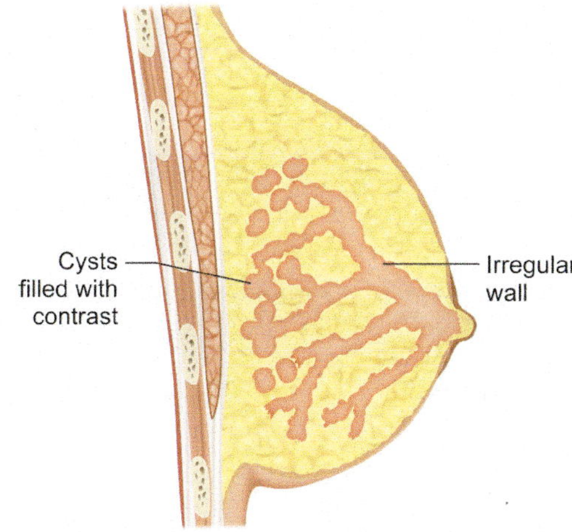

Fig. 31: Multiple cysts communicating with the ducts having irregular wall in fibrocystic disease on ductography.

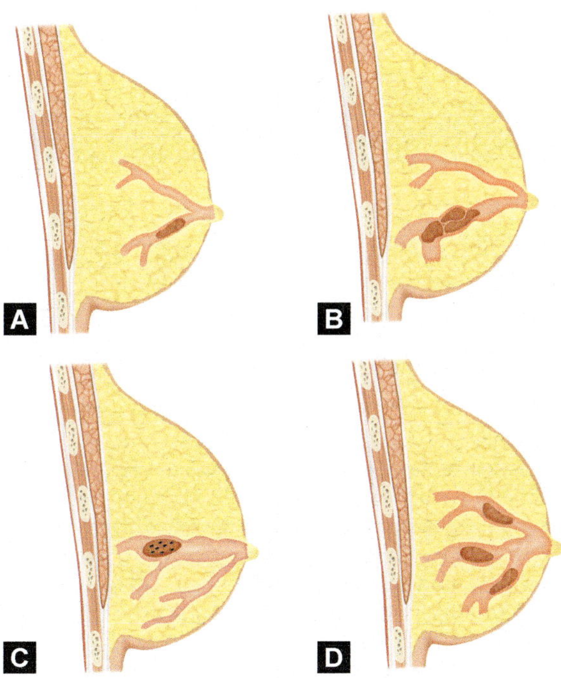

Figs. 30A to D: Multiple appearances of papilloma on ductogram: (A) Circumscribed filling defect; (B) Multilobulated filling defect; (C) Circumscribed filling defect with microcalcifications; (D) Multiple papilloma in multiple ducts.

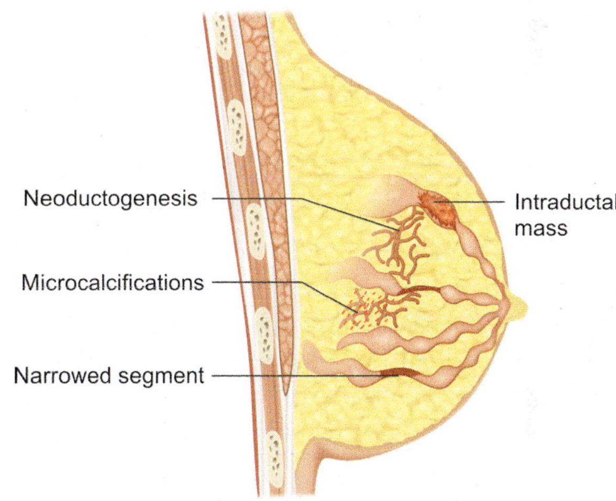

Fig. 32: Ductography findings in a malignant mass.

multiple papilloma in branching ducts (Figs. 30A to D). They may also cause an "amputated duct" due to complete obstruction.

Fibrocystic disease is seen as dilated ducts with irregular walls and cysts filled with contrast material communicating with the ducts (Fig. 31).

DCIS with invasive cancers is seen as multiple duct distortions and narrowing of ducts, neoductogenesis, microcalcifications and irregular filling defects (Fig. 32).

Ductography is relatively underused and if performed properly can really be beneficial for the patients.

MRI AND MR DUCTOGRAPHY

Magnetic resonance imagin (MRI) may be helpful when ultrasound and mammogram are normal in patient with a serous or serosanguineous discharge. Sometimes, a papilloma may be detected as a circumscribed, oval, or irregular enhancing mass. Kinetic assessment using time intensity curves may show a progressive, type 2 or type 3 wash out curve. DCIS may be seen along with invasive

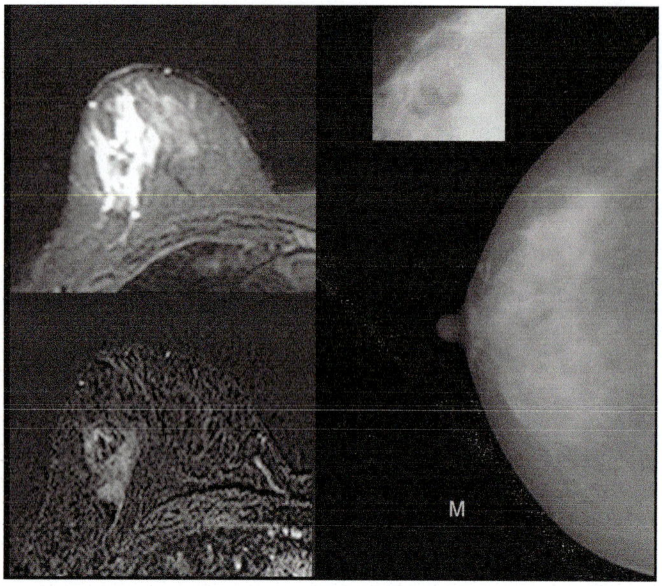

Fig. 33: MRI of breast in a patient with histopathological proven DCIS showing diffusion restriction and clumped non-mass like focal enhancement which correlated with focal pleomorphic calcifications on mammogram. (DCIS: ductal carcinoma in situ).

cancer. The imaging findings in DCIS include clumped or non-mass like enhancement (Fig. 33) in a ductal, segmental, focal or regional distribution. Invasive cancer and DCIS show enhancing mass in 76% cases.[18] Therefore, contrast enhanced MRI can be used in cases where basic imaging work up is negative in a patient presenting with nipple discharge to ascertain its cause.

MR ductography: This is done using 3D fat suppressed heavily T2 weighted fast spin echo sequence without the use of intravenous contrast.[19] A three-dimensional image is produced of the abnormal duct with the lesion where duct is seen as dilated tubular structure while intraductal lesion is seen as a filling defect. Other findings like duct irregularity and obstruction can also be noted. Its fusion with MR mammography shows enhancing lesion within the duct on one image.

It also does not show the duct when it is filled with blood or proteinaceous material where high signal intensity is seen on conventional MRI on non-contrast T1W imaging.

INTERVENTIONS IN DUCTAL PATHOLOGY

For interventions in the nipple-areolar region, it is important to give additional local anesthesia in a radial manner in the retroareolar region because of discomfort or burning pain. The lesions are usually smaller than 1 cm in size; hence, instead of using a spring loaded biopsy device which decompresses the duct after the first pass, a vacuum-assisted device should be used to sample intraductal pathology.

In conclusion, nipple discharge is a very common problem; however, evaluation of ductal disease is still an overlooked area in breast imaging often leading to delayed diagnosis and treatment. The list of differential diagnosis is broad and includes both benign and malignant pathologies. Imaging evaluation should include a combination of modalities like mammogram, ultrasound, ductography and MRI to arrive at a diagnosis. Whenever required a percutaneous biopsy should be done, preferably with vacuum assisted devices for accurate sampling.

Flowchart 1: Algorithm for evaluation and management of nipple discharge

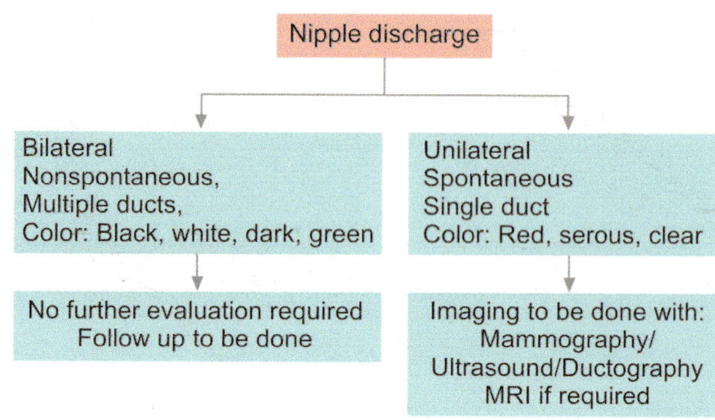

REFERENCES

1. Gulay H, Bora S, Kilicturgay S, et al. Management of nipple discharge. J Am Coll Surg 1994;178:471-4.
2. Chang SW, Kerlikowske K, Napoles-Springer A, et al. Racial differences in timeliness of follow-up after abnormal screening mammography. Cancer 1996;78:1395-402.
3. Cabioglu N, Hunt KK, Singletary SE, et al. Surgical decision making and factors determining a diagnosis of breast carcinoma in women presenting with nipple discharge. J Am Coll Surg 2003;196:354-64.
4. Ito Y, Tamaki Y, Nakano Y, et al. Non-palpable breast cancer with nipple discharge: how should it be treated?. Anticancer Res 1996;17(1B):791-4.
5. Sickles EA. Mammographic features of "early" breast cancer. AJR Am J Roentgenol 1984;143:461-4.
6. Cardenosa G, Eklund GW. Benign papillary neoplasms of the breast: mammographic findings. Radiology 1991;181:751-5.
7. Schneider JA. Invasive papillary breast carcinoma: mammographic and sonographic appearance. Radiology 1989;171:377-9.
8. Ballesio L, Maggi C, Savelli S, et al. Adjunctive diagnostic value of ultrasonography evaluation in patients with suspected ductal breast disease. Radiol Med 2007;112:354-65.

9. Thomas Stavros A. Nontargeted Indications: breast secretions, nipple discharge, intraductal papillary lesions. In: Breast ultrasound. Philadelphia, PA: Lippincott Williams & Wilkins; 2004. pp. 173-9.
10. Brookes MJ, Bourke AG. Radiological appearances of papillary breast lesions. Clin Radiol 2008;63:1265-73.
11. Kopans DB. Ultrasound and breast evaluation. In: Breast imaging. 2nd ed. Philadelphia, PA: Lippincott-Raven; 1998. pp. 431.
12. Liberman L, Feng TL, Susnik B. Case 35: intracystic papillary carcinoma with invasion. Radiology 2001;219:781-4.
13. Kim KW, Cho KR, Seo BK, et al. Sonographic findings of mammary duct ectasia: can malignancy be differentiated from benign disease?. J Breast Cancer 2010;13:19-26.
14. Mesurolle B, El-Khoury M, Khetani K, et al. Mammographically non-calcified ductal carcinoma in situ: sonographic features with pathological correlation in 35 patients. Clin Radiol 2009;64:628-36.
15. Tabar L, Dean PB, Pentek Z. Galactography: the diagnostic procedure of choice for nipple discharge. Radiology 1983;149:31-8.
16. Orel SG, Dougherty CS, Reynolds C, et al. MR imaging in patients with nipple discharge: initial experience. Radiology 2000;216:248-54.
17. Manganaro L, D'Ambrosio I, Gigli S, et al. Breast MRI in patients with unilateral bloody and serous-bloody nipple discharge: a comparison with galactography. Biomed Res Int 2015;2015:9. Article ID 806368. http://dx.doi.org/10.1155/2015/806368.
18. Rosen EL, Smith-Foley SA, DeMartini WB, et al. BI-RADS MRI enhancement characteristics of ductal carcinoma in situ. Breast J 2007;13:545-50.
19. Jara H, Barish MA, Yucel EK, et al. MR hydrography: theory and practice of static fluid. AJR Am J Roentgenol 1998;170:873-82.

3.5 Evaluation of Axilla

INTRODUCTION

The evaluation of axilla is essential in women with axillary symptoms and a newly diagnosed breast cancer. There are various causes of axillary pathologies and the radiologist should be able to make an accurate diagnosis based on the imaging features.

One of the commonest axillary pathologies is axillary lymphadenopathy which can be due to both benign and malignant causes.

It is essential to have a robust knowledge of the anatomy of axilla, its boundaries, contents and lymphatic drainage of breast to make an accurate diagnosis. It is also important to understand the image-guided procedures in the axilla to establish a diagnosis and guide patient management.

ANATOMY OF AXILLA

Axilla is a pyramidal space situated beneath the gleno-humeral joint at junction of the upper limb and the thorax. It is a passageway for neurovascular and muscular structures to enter and leave the upper limb.

Its **boundaries** consist of four walls and a base (Fig. 1) with an opening at the apex as described below:

Apex: Also known as the axillary inlet and is formed by lateral border of the first rib, superior border of scapula and the posterior border of the clavicle.

Lateral wall: Formed by intertubercular groove of the humerus, coracobrachialis and short head of the biceps muscle.

Medial wall: Formed by serratus anterior muscle and first four ribs and intercostal muscles.

Anterior wall: Formed by pectoralis major and pectoralis minor muscles.

Posterior wall: Formed by subscapularis, teres major and latissimus dorsi muscles.

CONTENTS

The clinically important contents of the axilla (Fig. 2) include muscles, nerves, vessels and lymphatics.

- **Axillary artery**: It is the main artery supplying the upper limb and has three parts which are seen in medial, posterior and lateral relation to pectoralis minor muscle. The medial and posterior parts course through the axilla.
- **Axillary vein**: It is the main vein draining the upper limb with two larges tributaries: cephalic and basilic veins.
- **Brachial plexus**: Formed by spinal nerves which lead to the peripheral nerves of the upper limb.
- **Biceps brachii and coracobrachialis**: These tendons also traverse through the axilla, where they attach to the coracoid process of the scapula.

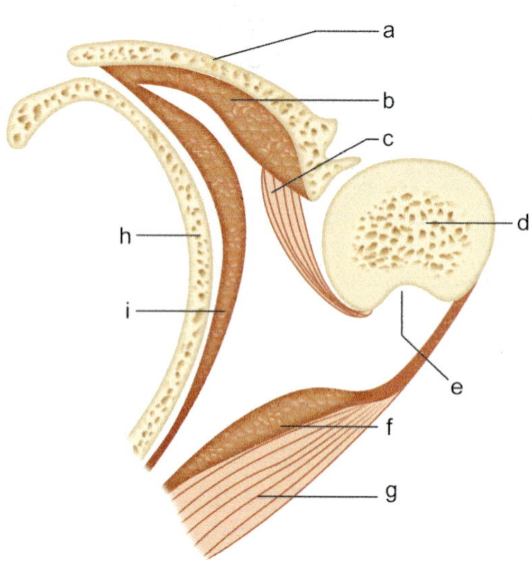

Fig. 1: Anatomy of axilla including its boundaries. (a) Scapula; (b) Subscapularis; (c) Lattisimus dorsi; (d) Humerus; (e) Inter-tubercular sulcus; (f) Pectoralis minor; (g) Pectoralis major; (h) rib; (i) Serratus anterior.

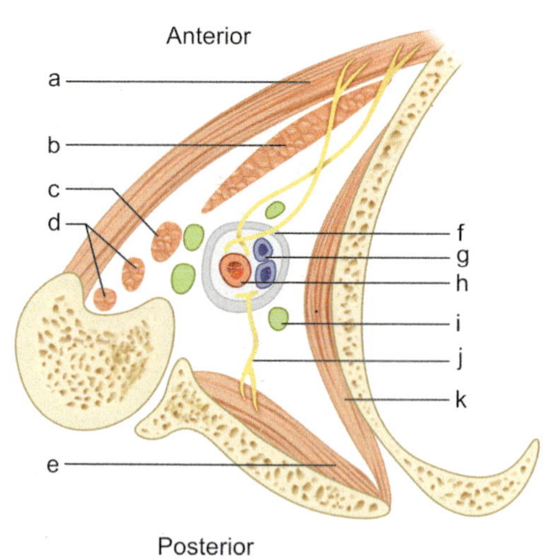

Fig. 2: Contents of axilla. (a) Pectoralis Major; (b) Pectoralis Minor; (c) Coracobrachialis; (d) Short and long head of biceps; (e) Sub-scapularis (f) Axillary sheath; (g) Axillary vein; (h) Axillary artery; (i) Lymph node; (j) Long thoracic nerve; (k) Serratus anterior.

- **Axillary lymph nodes**: The axillary lymph nodes filter lymph that has drained from the upper limb and pectoral region.
- **Fibrofatty tissue**
- **Axillary tail of Spence**

LYMPHATIC DRAINAGE OF BREAST

Lymph from the breast drains into:
- Axillary lymph nodes
- Internal mammary lymph nodes
- Some of the lymph also reaches supraclavicular, cephalic, intercostal, subdiaphragmatic and subperitoneal lymph nodes.

Axillary lymph nodes (Fig. 3): They are arranged into five groups within the axillary fat (Fig. 4).

1. *Anterior*: Lies on the pectoralis minor along lateral thoracic vessels
2. *Posterior*: Lies on posterior wall of axilla on lower border of subscapularis along subscapular vessels
3. *Lateral*: Lies on lateral wall of axilla along third part of axillary vessels
4. *Central group*: Lies in axillary fat at the base of axilla
5. *Apical group*: Lies at apex of axilla

The central and lateral parts of the breast (75%) drain into pectoral group of axillary lymph nodes while upper part of the breast drains into apical group of axillary lymph nodes.

The lymphatics that drain the medial part of breast perforate the pectoral and intercostal muscles and enter the internal mammary lymph nodes which lie along the lateral edge of sternum and form a chain along the internal thoracic vessels. The internal mammary nodes and lymphatics lie in the intercostal spaces along the margins of the sternum and are usually present from the fifth intercostal space to the clavicles. The second and third intercostal spaces should be examined routinely to look for metastatic involvement of these nodes.

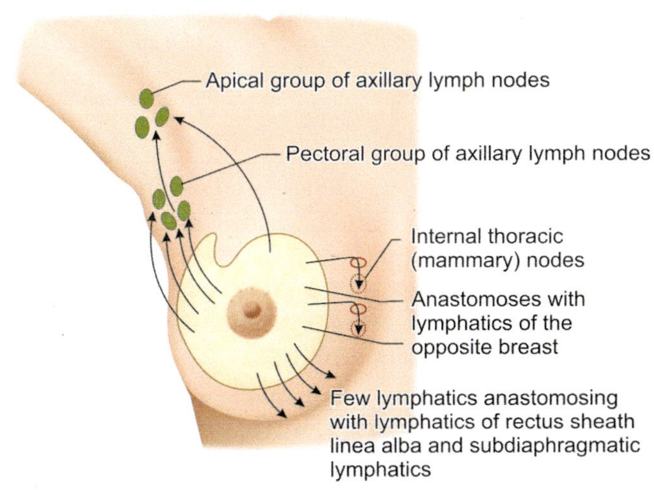

Fig. 3: Lymphatic drainage of breast.

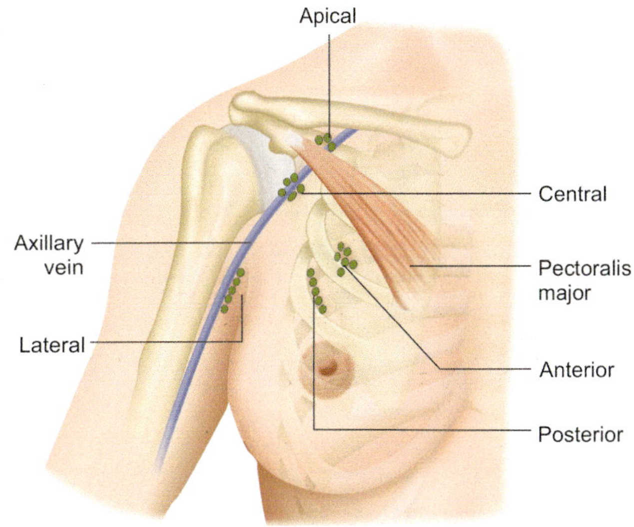

Fig. 4: Axillary lymph node groups.

Some lymphatics from the medial part of the gland pass across the front of sternum to anastomose with opposite side. The lymphatics from the inferomedial part of breast anastomose with lymphatics of rectus sheath and linea alba and some pass deep to anastomose with the subdiaphragmatic and subperitoneal lymphatics.

The skin of the breast drains to the axillary, inferior deep cervical and infraclavicular nodes. The nipple and areola drains into the subareolar lymphatic plexus.

Approximately 75% of lymph from the breast drains into the axillary lymph nodes. In case of carcinoma of one breast, the contra-lateral breast and the opposite axillary lymph nodes may be affected because of the anastomosing lymphatics between both breasts**.** When tumor obstructs normal lymphatic flow, collateral pathways open. These include contralateral internal mammary and mediastinal lymphatics. Spread through the rectus abdominis muscle sheath to the subdiaphragmatic and subperitoneal plexus may lead to spread to the liver and retroperitoneal nodes.

IMAGING OF AXILLA

Mammogram: The axilla is partially imaged on Mammography in the mediolateral oblique (MLO) view and may show a variety of findings (Figs. 5A to E). Accessory breast

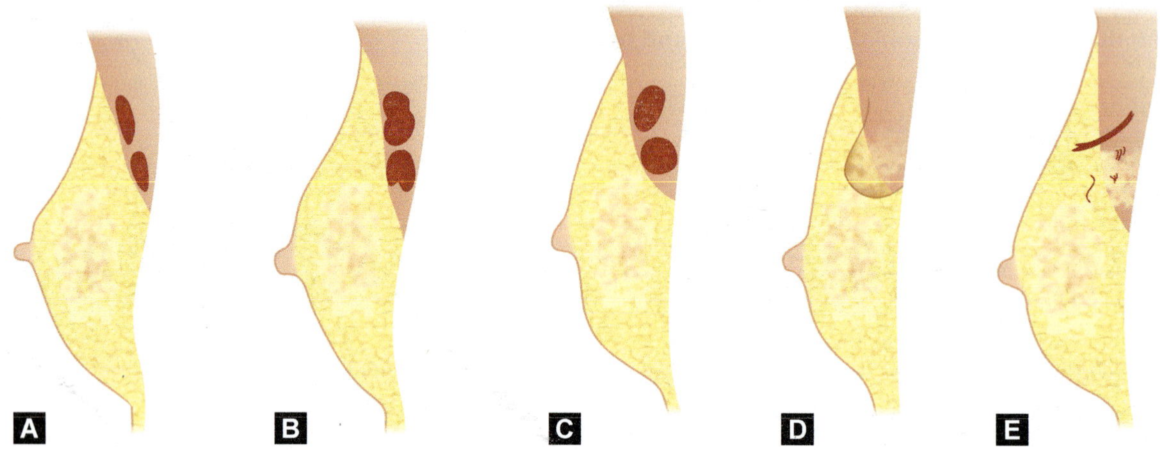

Figs. 5A to E: Mammogram—MLO view showing various findings in axillary region: (A) Normal axillary lymph nodes; (B) Enlarged lymph nodes due to inflammatory pathology; (C) Metastatic lymph nodes; (D) Accessory breast tissue; (E) Normal postoperative findings in axilla showing scars and surgical clips.

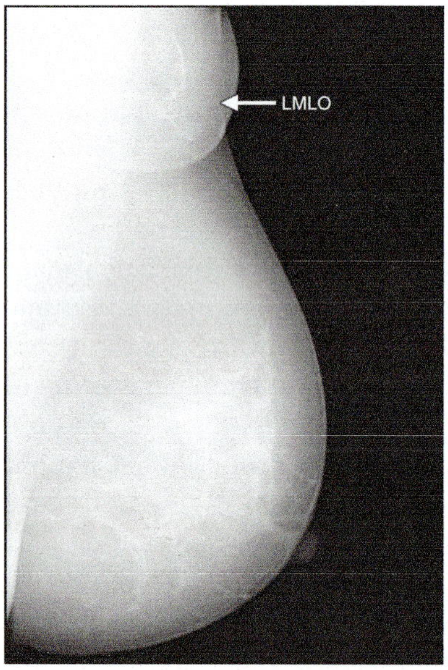

Fig. 6: Mammogram of left breast—MLO view showing accessory breast tissue.

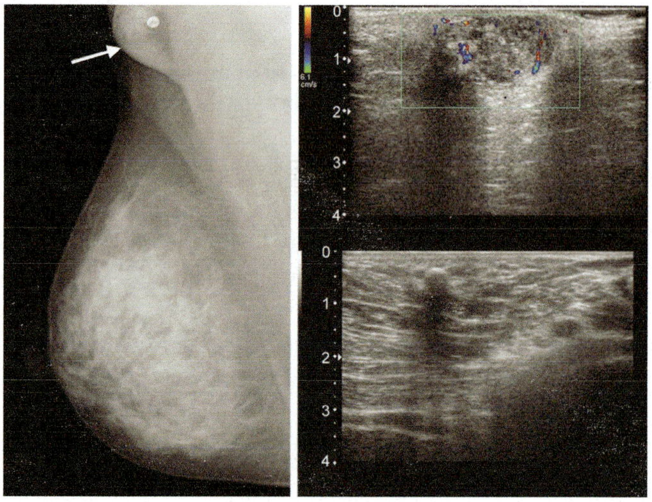

Fig. 7: Mammogram of right breast—MLO view showing a circumscribed soft-tissue density (arrow) with a round calcific focus in the axilla. Targeted ultrasound showed a circumscribed mass with heterogeneously hypoechoic echotexture and a small calcific focus in the adjacent tissue. Histopathology was s/o epidermal inclusion cyst.

tissue can be seen on mammogram (Fig. 6) and may have a glandular component in addition to fatty tissue. Sometimes, a fibroadenoma or cyst may develop in accessory breast tissue in axilla and skin lesions may also be seen (Fig. 7).

Lymph nodes may have a variety of appearances on mammogram. The normal axillary lymph nodes are seen overlying the pectoralis muscle high in the axilla. They are lobulated or oval, dense sharply marginated lesions <2 cm in size and have a radiolucent fatty hilum (Fig. 8). In the clinical setting of a malignant mass in breast, the lymphnodes may enlarge in size and assume a rounded shape with loss of fatty hilum which is highly suggestive of metastatic involvement (Figs. 9A and B). The lowest level 1 lymph node may be seen on MLO view. Intramammary lymph nodes may also be seen sometimes with a typical oval shape and lucent fatty hilum.

In those with history of tuberculosis, calcification may be seen in axillary lymph nodes (Fig. 10).

The **differential diagnosis for calcified lymph nodes** includes prior granulomatous infection, gold therapy in patients with rheumatoid arthritis, collagen vascular

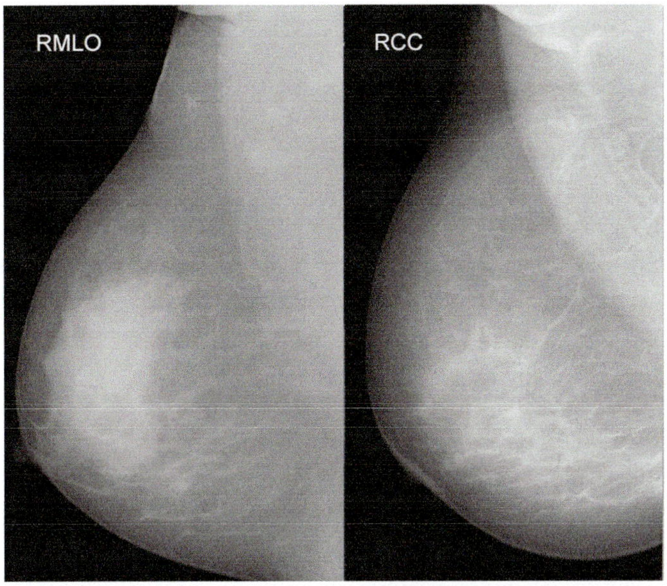

Fig. 8: Mammogram of right breast in two different patients showing normal lymph nodes—Oval-shaped lymph nodes with a radio-lucent fatty hilum. (Please remember that all the normal lymph nodes may not show a fatty hilum).

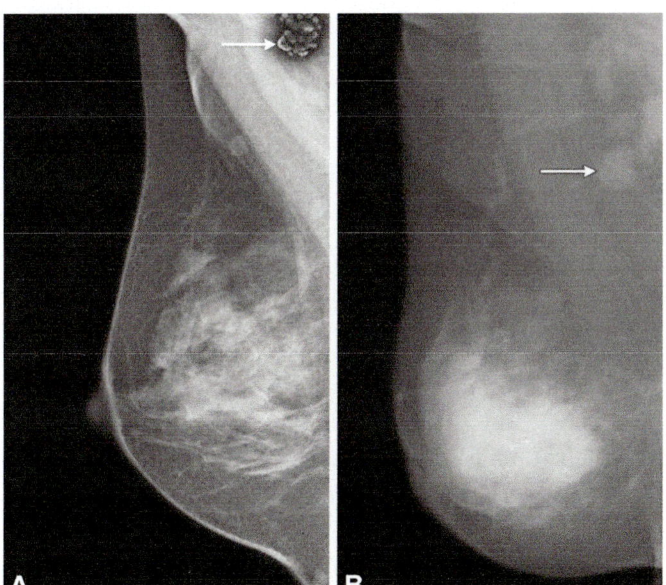

Figs. 9A and B: Mammogram MLO in two different patients: (A) axillary lymph node calcification noted which was proven to be a granulomatous infection; (B) Pleomorphic calcification seen in breast parenchyma with axillary lymph node calcification. Histopathology was s/o invasive ductal carcinoma with lymph node metastases.

disease and metastasis from breast, thyroid or ovarian cancer. At times, massive lymphadenopathy is seen in tuberculosis on a mammogram (Figs. 11A and B) in the MLO view.

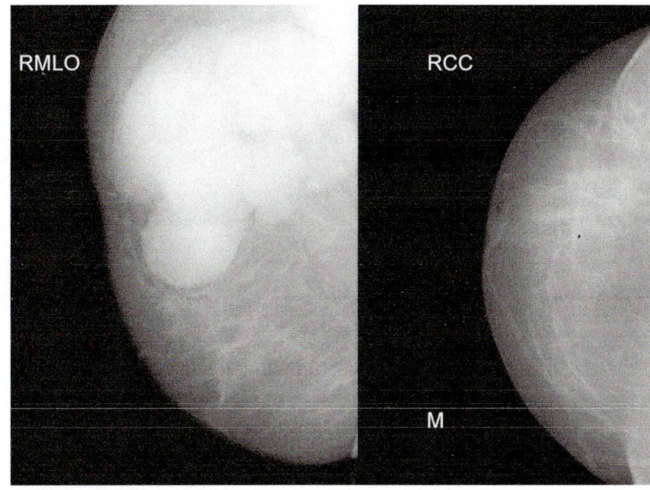

Fig. 10: Mammogram MLO and CC view in a patient presenting with axillary lump showed multilobulated soft-tissue density with smooth margins overlying the axillary tail region and upper quadrant s/o lymph nodal mass. Histopathology was s/o tubercular lymph nodes.

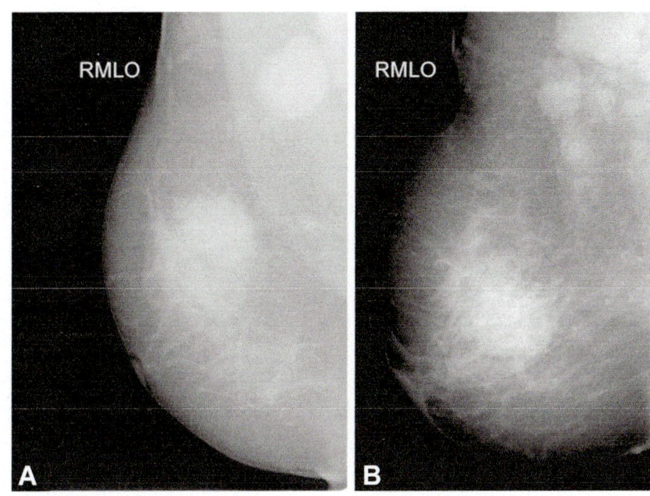

Figs. 11A and B: Mammogram in two different patients (A and B) showing a primary breast mass and enlarged lymph nodes which are round and shape with loss of fatty hilum s/o metastatic lymphadenopathy.

Postoperative changes in axilla in patients who have undergone breast surgery and who present with unilateral arm swelling include skin thickening, fluid collections, fat necrosis, abscess and hematoma. Residual lymph nodes may be seen in axilla if incomplete surgery is done (Fig. 12). Some patients may also have recurrent carcinoma in previously unresected lymph nodes.

Soft-tissue masses like lipoma, neurofibroma, schwannoma may also be found in axillary region.

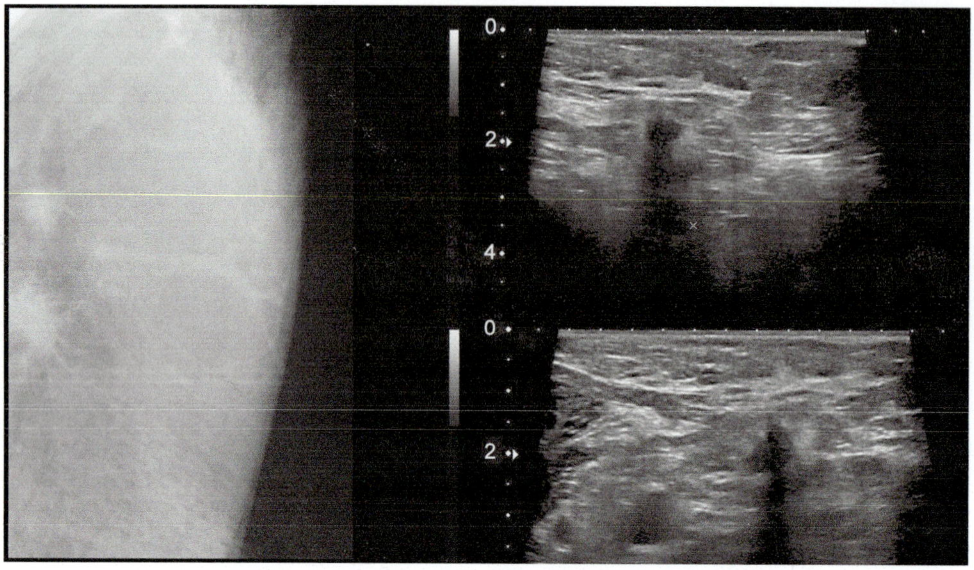

Fig. 12: A 39-year-old female who had undergone lumpectomy for breast lump was referred for mammogram which showed two irregular spiculated masses in axillary tail region and axilla. Targeted ultrasound showed two hypoechoic masses with irregular margins and posterior acoustic shadowing. A re-excision and axillary clearance was done. Histopathology revealed axillary tail, level 1 and level 2 lymph nodes with metastasis from invasive ductal carcinoma. However no residual tumor was seen in sections from lumpectomy defect.

ULTRASOUND

Ultrasound is an extremely useful modality to assess the axilla and make an accurate diagnosis. There are many pathologies confined to the axilla; hence, the list of indications for assessing the axillary region is also long.

Indications

- To characterize a clinically detected axillary mass
- Skin lesions (epidermal inclusion cyst, sebaceous cyst)
- Visualize accessory breast tissue
- Diagnose soft-tissue lesions (lipoma, liposarcoma), nerve pathology (neurofibroma, schwannoma), vascular lesions (hematomas, axillary vein thrombosis, thrombophlebitis)
- Staging of newly diagnosed breast cancer
- Follow-up of locoregional relapse of breast cancer
- Guidance for intervention in suspicious findings in the axilla.

Ultrasound Examination Technique

The ultrasound of axilla is done with a high-frequency linear transducer (7.5–17 MHz). If the patient has large breasts and more axillary fat then a 5–7-MHz probe can be used but the spatial resolution will be less.

Position

The patient should lie down in supine oblique position with hand kept above the head and arm abducted and externally rotated. Low wall filter and low velocity settings should be used while doing Doppler. The color gain should be increased high enough to detect subtle flow without causing a color noise artifact or aliasing.

Ultrasound Findings

A number of findings can be seen while performing ultrasound of axilla. These include skin lesions (sebaceous cyst, epidermal inclusion cyst), accessory breast tissue with or without a focal mass like fibroadenoma or cyst, tuberculous lymph nodes, metastatic lymphadenopathy (from breast, ovary), inflammatory pathologies like breast abscess and postoperative changes like seroma, lymphocele, etc.

Accessory breast tissue occurs in 2%–6% of women[1] and can be appreciated on mammography, ultrasound and MRI. It occurs due to failure of involution of the milk line and is seen most commonly in the axilla, but it can occur anywhere from the axilla to the inguinal region. When accessory breast tissue is present both benign and malignant breast lesions can be seen within (i.e. cysts, fibroadenomas, pseudoangiomatous stromal hyperplasia - PASH, breast cancer).

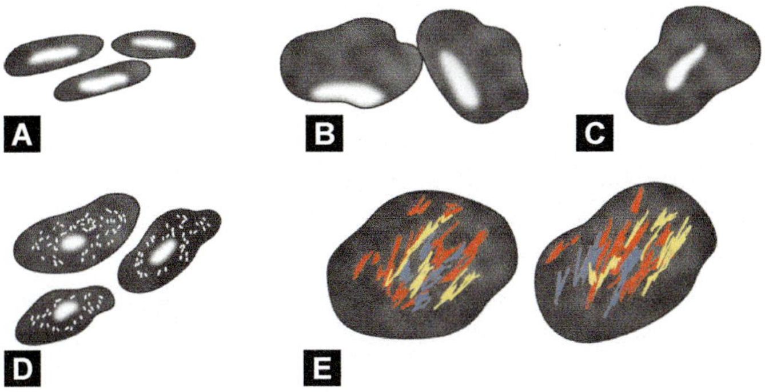

Figs. 13A to E: Varied appearances of axillary lymph nodes on ultrasound: (A) Normal oval lymph nodes with fatty hilum; (B) Enlarged lymph node with eccentric fatty hilum and increased cortical thickness; (C) Diffusely enlarged lymph node with central fatty hilum which is thinned out; (D) Lymph node with calcifications; (E) Lymph node with central and peripheral vascularity.

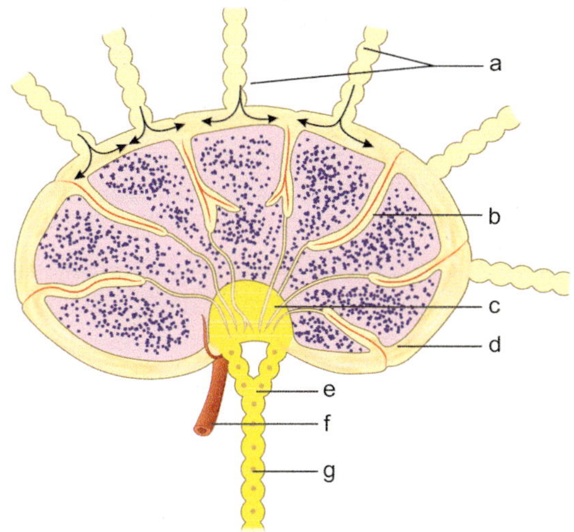

Fig. 14: Normal anatomy of lymph node: (a) Afferent lymph vessels; (b) Trabeculae; (c) Medullary sinus; (d) Subcapsular sinus; (e) Lymphocytes in outflowing lymph; (f) Blood flowing into hilum; (g) Efferent lymph vessel.

If there is a malignant mass in breast, ultrasound of axillary lymph nodes has a high sensitivity and specificity. It is rare to find axillary lymph node metastases with occult breast cancer, defined as metastatic cancer with undetected primary at presentation.

Axillary lymph nodes have a variety of appearances on ultrasound as shown (Figs. 13A to E).

Causes of axillary lymphadenopathy: The causes of axillary lymph node enlargement are as follows:

- Lymph node metastases from breast cancer. Other cancers which can cause axillary lymph node metastases are stomach, ovarian or melanoma
- Infectious diseases like tuberculosis, HIV
- Inflammatory and infectious conditions of the arm or breast (mastitis, breast abscess)
- Lymphoproliferative disorders (lymphoma, leukemia)
- Connective tissue disorders like rheumatoid arthritis, Systemic lupus erythematosus (SLE), etc
- Silicone droplets in lymph nodes secondary to silicone breast implant rupture

ANATOMY OF LYMPH NODE

Lymph node is an or oval or kidney shaped structure (Fig. 14) which ranges in size from a few millimeters to about 1–2 cm. Each lymph node is surrounded by a fibrous capsule, which extends inside the lymph node to form trabeculae.

It is divided into outer cortex and inner medulla. The cortex of the lymph node is located underneath the capsule and the subcapsular sinus. The medulla contains large blood vessels, sinuses and medullary cords that contain antibody-secreting plasma cells. B cells are found in cortex and T cells are found in medulla. The cortex is continuous around the medulla except where the medulla comes into direct contact with the hilum.

Lymph enters the lymph node through multiple afferent lymphatic vessels and flows through spaces called sinuses which include the subcapsular sinus. After the lymph is filtered, it drains into the medullary sinus and leaves the node through efferent lymphatic vessels.

ULTRASOUND FEATURES OF NORMAL LYMPH NODES

A normal lymph node on ultrasound appears hypoechoic, oval or lobulated in shape and has smooth margins. There is a uniform hypoechoic cortex (<3 mm in thickness) and an echogenic fatty hilum. The concurrent constriction and bulges due to cortex and fatty hilum leads to lobulated shape. This appearance has a high negative predictive value for excluding metastases.[2] The lymph node is supplied by a single artery and drained by a single vein that enter and exit through the hilar notch and can be demonstrated by color Doppler.

The ultrasound appearance of lymph nodes varies (Figs. 15A to C) with the relative size of the cortex and hilum and degree of fatty infiltration in hilum.

The fatty infiltration in hilum and cortical thinning increases with age and with repeated episodes of inflammation, scarring and atrophy (Figs. 16A to C). In younger individuals, there is a uniform cortical thickness and small echogenic hilum as there are fewer episodes of inflammation. As the patient's age advances, there is atrophy and scarring of the cortex seen as cortical irregularity and thinning because of repeated episodes of inflammation. With aging, there is also increased deposition of fat in the hilum along with thinning of cortex, so much so that the cortex is barely seen. It is also important to remember that with cortical atrophy and increase in fat in hilum, the size of the node also increases reaching almost up to 2 cm in short axis diameter which is normal and of no clinical or radiological concern.

Ultrasound features of abnormal lymph nodes (Figs. 17A to G and 18A to F): Malignant lymph nodes have a focal cortical thickness >3 mm, increased concentric cortical thickening, round shape, hypoechoic cortex and effaced, eccentric or absent fatty hilum. Table 1 shows ultrasound features of abnormal lymph nodes.

Focal cortical bulge or thickening: It is the earliest detectable morphologic change in lymph node. A truly abnormal cortical bulge is distinctly hypoechoic and there is focal or eccentric thickening of the cortex which does not follow the margin of the echogenic hilum.[1,3] This is because malignant cells enter the lymph node through the afferent lymphatics and lodge in subcapsular and cortical sinuses of lymph node giving rise to eccentric thickening and hypoechoic cortex. Later on, it may involve the entire cortex giving rise to uniform compression of the hilum.

Sometimes, the metastatic cells lodge in deep cortical sinusoids rather than the subcapsular sinusoids which

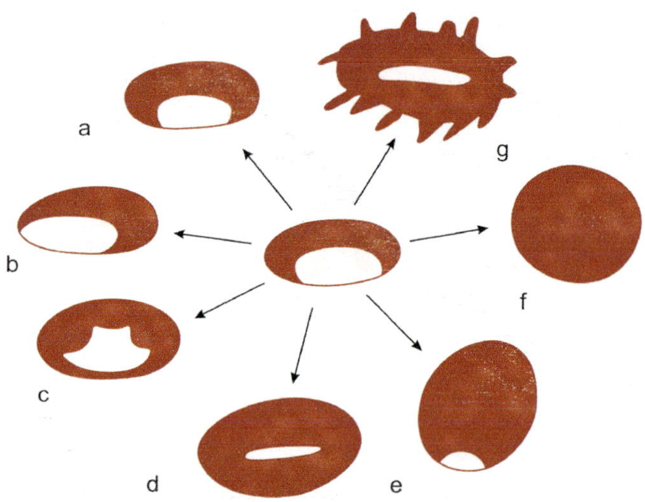

Figs. 17A to G: Spectrum of abnormal lymph nodes: (A) Mildly uniformly thickened cortex as in reactive nodes; (B) Eccentric cortical thickening commonly seen in metastatic lymph nodes; (C) Convex indentations on medulla (rat bites) favoring metastatic disease; (D) Severe compression of medulla leading to slit like configuration seen in metastases or inflammatory disease; (E) Severe eccentric compression of medulla with displacement to periphery; (F) Rounding of lymph node with complete obliteration of medulla which favors metastatic disease but also can be seen in necrotizing and suppurative lymphadenitis; (G) Perinodal invasion with angular margins.
Source: Adapted from Stavros—Ref. [4].

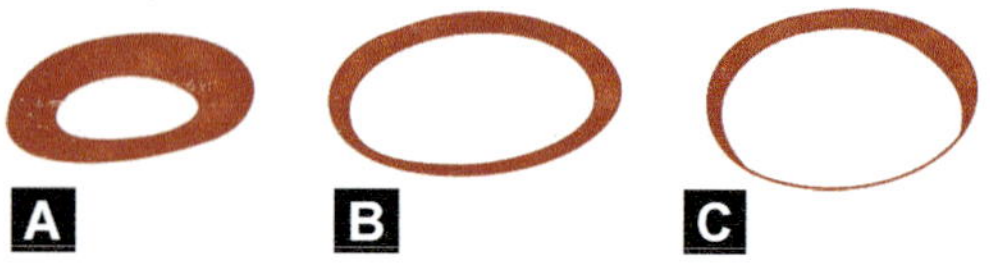

Figs. 15A to C: Spectrum of normal appearance of lymph node on ultrasound: (A) Lymph node with normal cortical thickness in a young female; (B) Enlarging hilum due to fatty infiltration with thinning of cortex as aging process goes on; (C) Severe cortical atrophy and extensive fatty infiltration of hilum.
Source: Adapted from Stavros—Ref. [4].

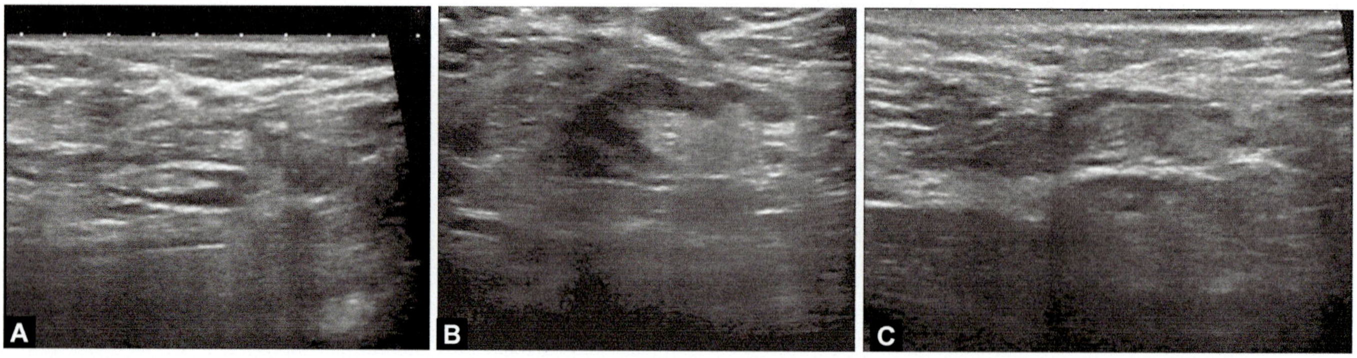

Figs. 16A to C: (A) Normal lymph node; (B) Lymph node with increased fatty infiltration, irregular cortical thickness and scarring due to inflammation; (C) Grossly increased fatty infiltration of hilum with a thin cortex.

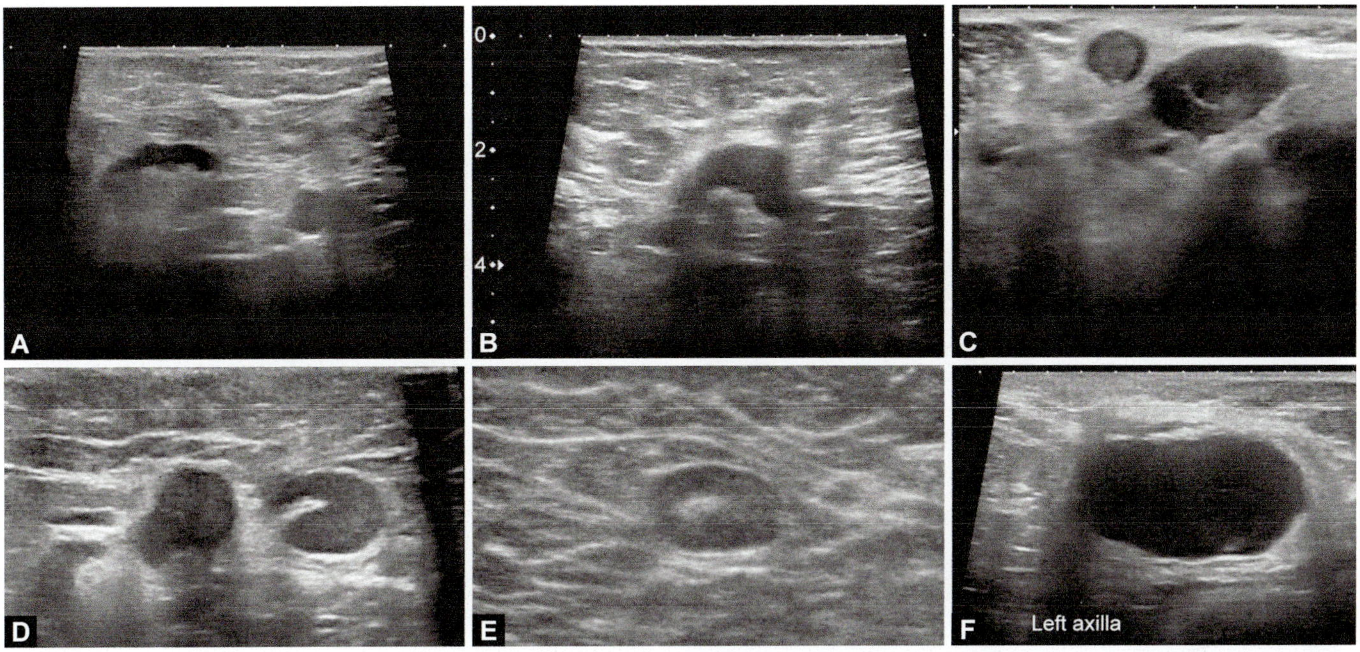

Figs. 18A to F: Ultrasound showing abnormal lymph nodes: (A) Lymph node with mild cortical thickening seen in reactive lymph nodes; (B) Eccentric cortical thickening in metastatic lymph node; (C) Metastatic lymph node showing severe compression of medulla with a slit like appearance (note that similar appearance can be seen in acute inflammatory nodes); (D) Round and hypoechoic lymph node with eccentric displacement of fatty hilum in metastatic lymph node; (E) Lymph node with uniformly thickened cortex typically seen in a reactive or inflammatory node; (F) Enlarged lymph node with complete obliteration of medulla in metastatic disease.

Table 1: Sonographic features of abnormal lymph nodes

1.	Focal cortical bulge or eccentric cortical thickening which does not follow the margin of the echogenic hilum
2.	Diffuse cortical thickening
3.	Hypoechoic cortex
4.	Partial or complete effacement of the fatty hilum
5	Loss of echogenic capsule and presence of irregular or angular margins
6.	Shape (length-to-width ratio <2)
7.	Peripheral vascular flow at the cortex

causes focal thickening of inner cortex. This is seen as convex inward indentation of mediastinum and fatty hilum by the hypoechoic cortex typically seen as "rat bites".[4] Occasionally, an inflamed lymph node with previous scarring may show an eccentrically thickened cortex and may be extremely difficult to distinguish from malignant lymph nodes on ultrasound.

Diffuse or concentric cortical thickening: It may be seen in both inflammatory and neoplastic lymph nodes. An inflammatory lymph node tends to enlarge proportionately, while a neoplastic pathology causes a disproportionate enlargement with abnormal rounding and nearly spherical appearance of lymph node.

Therefore, it is important to remember that both focal and diffuse cortical thickening may be seen in both reactive and malignant lymph nodes and requires further evaluation. Since metastatic involvement is a subcapsular and cortical process, hence morphological assessment of cortex is more important than only assessing the shape of lymph node.

Echogenicity of cortex: It is also important with hypoechoic appearance of the cortex seen more commonly in metastatic involvement though it can also be seen in necrotizing lymphadenitis. The hypoechoic appearance is due to high cellularity which can be due to lymphoid hyperplasia or due to metastatic tumor cells.

Eccentric or effaced hilum: It is because of severe eccentric cortical thickening that displaces the hilum to one edge of lymph node or even outside it. This is a specific finding of metastatic involvement as inflammatory process rarely causes such displacement except in severe necrotizing lymphadenitis.

Perinodal invasion: There is loss of echogenic outer capsule and presence of irregular and angular margins, which is seen in metastatic involvement (Fig.19). Once there is perinodal invasion, the node becomes fixed and cannot be compressed or moved by sonographic compression.

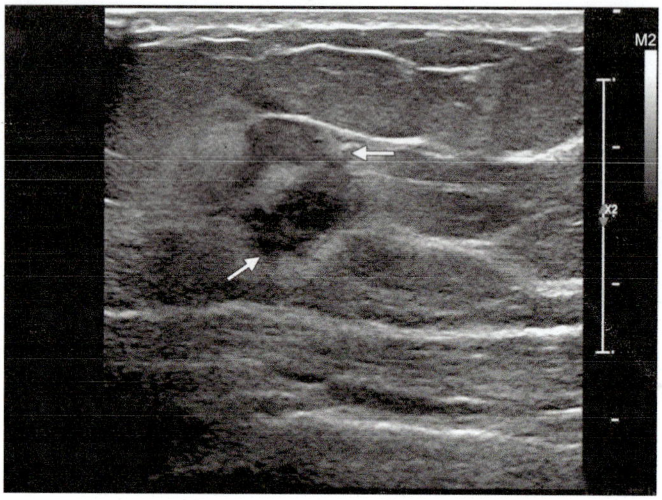

Fig. 19: Ultrasound of intramammary node showing loss of echogenic capsule s/o perinodal invasion and angular margins (arrows).

Asymmetrical involvement of axillary lymph nodes is more common in metastatic infiltration than inflammation; however, if there is unilateral mastitis, there can be unilateral reactive lymphadenopathy which is indistinguishable sonologically from metastatic involvement. In such cases, the clinical context is very important and therefore the clinical history should always be asked.

Findings having a high positive predictive value for malignancy include round shape, effaced fatty hilum, hypoechoic cortex, replacement of a portion of node by an irregular mass, microcalcifications and presence of cortical and transcapsular flow along with hilar flow on color Doppler.

Doppler in metastatic lymph node shows increased vascularity (Figs. 20A to D) with usually high systolic peak velocities, sharp systolic peaks, high resistive index and low diastolic flow. Reactive or inflammatory lymph nodes have lower systolic velocities, rounded systolic peaks and lower impedance.

Adjacent lymph nodes: Involvement of lymph node in malignancy is a step by step process and initially only one lymph node is involved which is called the sentinel lymph node. A perfectly normal uninvolved lymph node may be

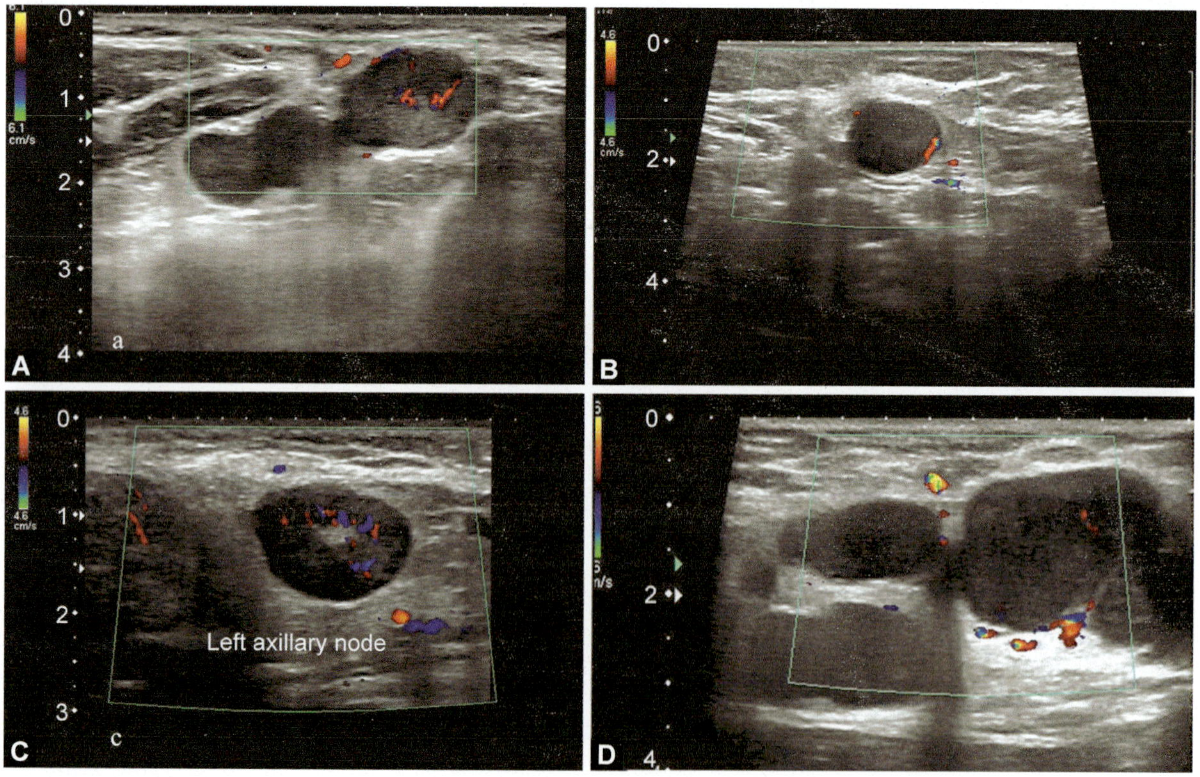

Figs. 20A to D: Color Doppler findings in metastatic lymph nodes showing central and /or peripheral vascularity.

seen adjacent to it. In such a situation, malignancy should be considered as the first differential and not inflammatory pathology. Over a period of time, other adjacent lymph nodes may also get involved. In contrast to malignancy, all the lymph nodes in a regional chain are involved at the same time in inflammatory process.

OTHER FINDINGS IN AXILLA

In a patient with silicone breast implant, a snowstorm appearance on ultrasound is pathognomonic for extracapsular rupture of implant because of deposition of silicone in lymph node (Fig. 21). The deposition of silicone begins in the hilum making it appear more echogenic. Silicone can deposit in intramammary lymph node that lie adjacent to implant but can accumulate in axillary lymph nodes also.

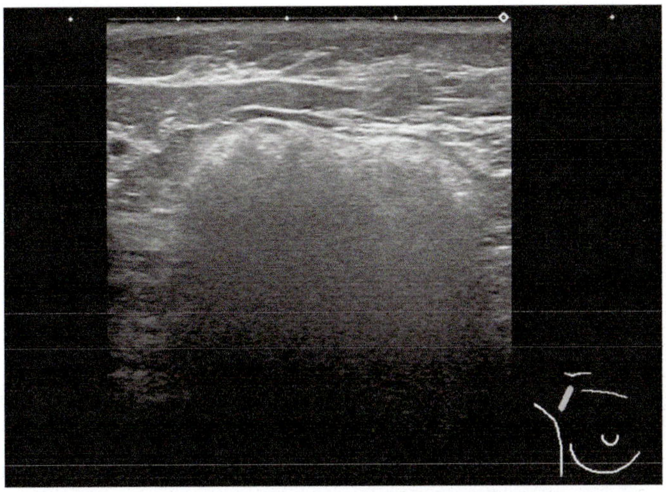

Fig. 21: Ultrasound of axilla in extracapsular rupture of breast implant showing the typical snowstorm appearance of lymph node due to deposition of silicone.

EVALUATION OF LYMPH NODES IN BREAST CANCER

Axillary Lymph Nodes

The axillary lymph nodes are divided into three levels by their relation to pectoralis minor (Figs. 22A and B).[5]

Level I or low axillary lymph nodes: Lymph nodes peripheral and inferolateral to the pectoralis minor muscle (Fig. 23).

Level II: Lie between the medial and lateral borders of the pectoralis minor and include the interpectoral nodes of Rotter.

Level III or high axillary lymph nodes: Lymph nodes proximal and superomedial to medial border of the pectoralis minor muscle. They are also called infraclavicular nodes.

Intramammary nodes or nodes within the breast parenchyma are regarded as axillary nodes for staging purposes.

Ultrasound can demonstrate level 1 lymph nodes. Normal level 2 lymph nodes are difficult to demonstrate but if they are enlarged they can be seen.

Internal Mammary Lymph Nodes

The internal mammary lymph nodes are smaller than axillary lymph nodes (4-6 mm in diameter) and their morphology and internal structure is difficult to demonstrate

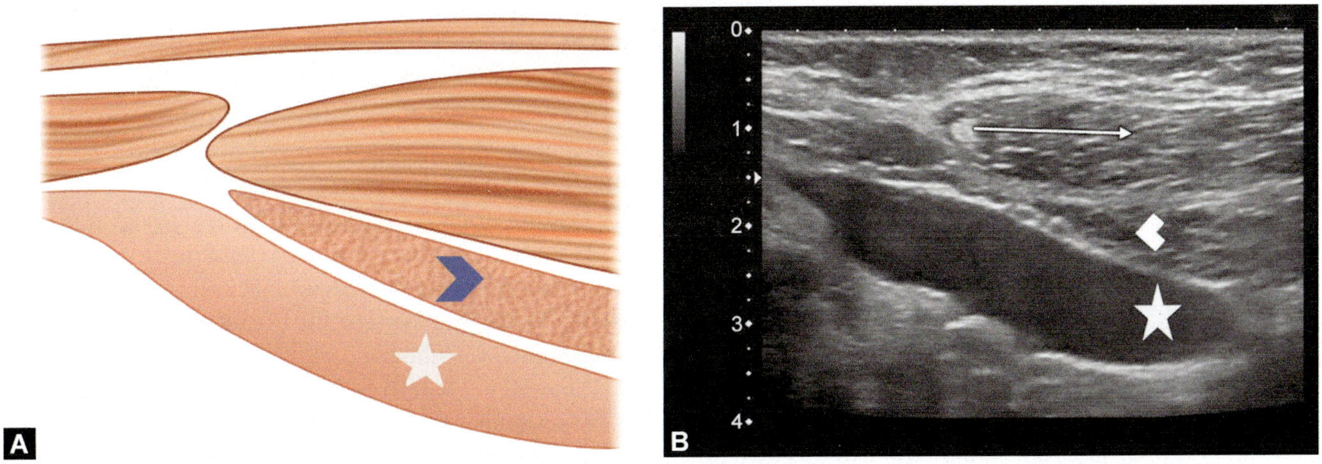

Figs. 22A and B: (A) Line diagram and (B) Ultrasound of axilla showing the landmarks for assessing levels of lymph nodes: arrow—pectoralis major, arrowhead—pectoralis minor and star—axillary vein. The lymph nodes inferolateral to pectoralis minor are level 1 lymph nodes.

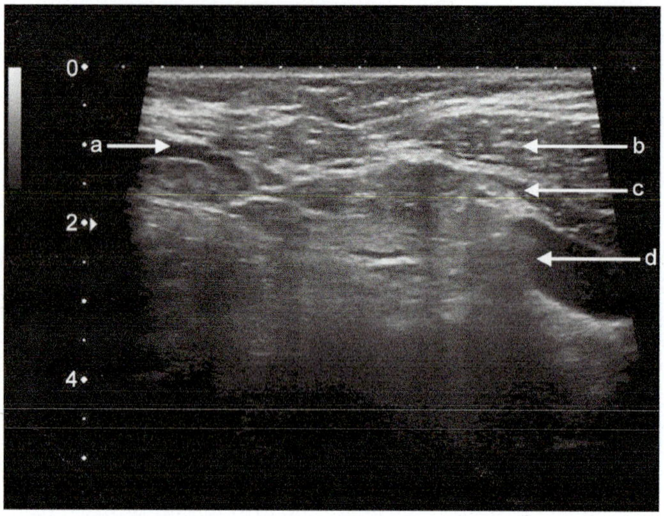

Fig. 23: Ultrasound of axilla showing (a) Level 1 lymph node; (b) Pectoralis major; (c) Pectoralis minor; (d) Axillary vein.

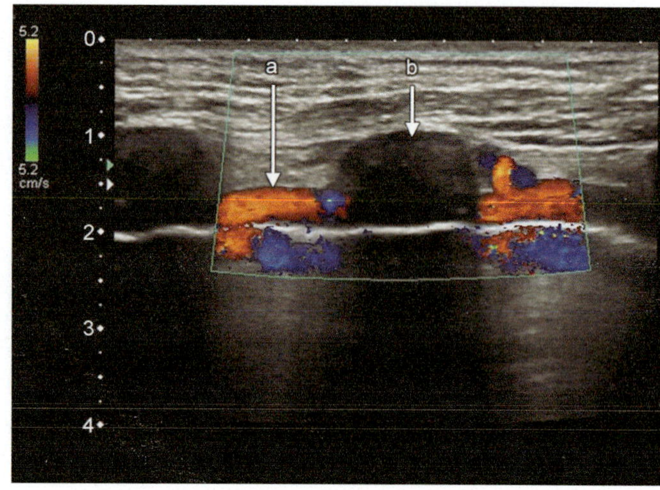

Fig. 24: Ultrasound showing location of internal mammary lymph nodes adjacent to internal mammary vessels (a) between the costal cartilages (b) in second intercostal space in a craniocaudal direction.

because of depth and small size. They lie between the costal cartilages in the craniocaudal direction and normal sized nodes are most frequently seen along the upper edge of third costal cartilage in second intercostal space (Fig. 24). Since these lie close to internal mammary vessels, color Doppler is used to identify the vessels lateral and deep to sternum.

The internal mammary nodes are involved in large medial masses in breast and deep lesions involving chest wall. It is however important to remember that they are most frequently involved in masses in upper outer quadrant associated with extensive lymph nodes which block the normal route of lymphatic drainage and cause collateral drainage through internal mammary lymph nodes.

Intramammary Lymph Nodes

These are seen as incidental findings on mammogram and if fatty hilum is seen, no further evaluation is necessary. They are most common in upper outer quadrant or in axillary tail region but can be seen in any quadrant. On ultrasound, a common site is medial aspect near the lateral edge of sternum close to internal mammary nodes. It is important to remember that an intramammary node may be a sentinel lymph node and at times can show a pseudocystic appearance if the primary is a high-grade invasive ductal carcinoma.

Supraclavicular Lymph Nodes

These are evaluated when enlarged and are taken as distant metastases as there is no direct drainage to them and it must pass through level 1, 2 and 3 or internal mammary lymph nodes before reaching supraclavicular lymph nodes.

Sentinel Lymph Node

Lymphatic drainage from a tumor is first received by a node which is called "sentinel lymph node" and it is important to identify it accurately. This is done by injecting a radioactive colloid or blue dye in the intradermal location around the tumor.

If the sentinel node is involved, then it is assumed that all other nodes in the basin are also involved and the surgeon proceeds with axillary lymph node dissection.

If the sentinel lymph node is not involved, it is assumed that the other nodes in the basin are also free and then axillary lymph node dissection is not done which reduces morbidity and lymphedema.

Usually the sentinel lymph node is a level 1 lymph node, though sometimes it can bypass level 1 lymph node and go to level 2 lymph node. Surgical dissections involve both level 1 and level 2 lymph nodes.

Contrast-enhanced ultrasonography can be used to visualize enhancing abnormal nodes after periareolar injection of microbubble and can be used to identify sentinel lymph node.

Lymph node status is one of the most important prognostic factors in breast cancer.

The **TNM staging system** for breast cancer classifies the lymph nodes as follows:

1. No regional lymph node metastases
2. Metastases in mobile axillary nodes (N1 disease requires chemotherapy and/or hormone therapy in addition to surgery)
3. Metastasis in fixed ipsilateral axillary nodes

4. Metastasis in an internal mammary node. (N2 disease requires chemotherapy and radiation therapy in addition to surgery.)
5. Metastasis in ipsilateral infraclavicular and axillary nodes
6. Metastasis in ipsilateral internal mammary and axillary nodes
7. Metastasis in an ipsilateral supraclavicular. (Preoperative or neoadjuvant chemotherapy is necessary in cases of N3 disease)

INTERVENTIONS IN AXILLA

FNAC: It relies on cytology instead of histology and has considerable false-negative findings. Though it is still practiced in a lot of hospitals in Indian setting, appropriate follow-up and treatment may require a further evaluation with biopsy.

CORE NEEDLE BIOPSY

An axillary core biopsy helps in pretreatment staging and planning treatment in patients with breast cancer. It strongly correlates with tumor burden and number of lymph nodes involved.[6] Biopsy of lymph node is also indicated in recurrence and in lymphoma patients with involved lymph nodes.

Sentinel lymph node procedure: Ultrasound is used to inject radionuclide for the procedure. It may be injected in deep subcutaneous plane superior, inferior, medial and lateral to the primary mass in breast.[7] Alternatively, it can be injected subdermally over the tumor in periareolar area. In this way, the radionuclide is placed adjacent to tumor with an anatomic region rich in lymphatics.

Lymphoscintigraphy is then performed after 1 hour of injection of radionuclide and focal activity in axilla corresponding to the sentinel node is identified and overlying skin is marked in axilla. A hand held scintillation counter is used to confirm skin mark.

Ultrasound of the axilla is subsequently performed over the skin mark and sentinel lymph node is visualized. Needle localization of the sentinel lymph node is done under ultrasound guidance making it easier for surgeon to remove it during surgical procedure. The surgeon can check radioactivity with intraoperative scintillation counter after node is removed. The axillary bed should then be checked by surgeon for any further "hot" nodes which may be present in the vicinity of sentinel node.

Since the introduction of sentinel lymph node biopsy, there has been increase in interest in metastatic internal mammary node (IMN) as it is the most important drainage outside axilla.[8] Metastasis to the IMN has been reported in about 27% patients with primary breast cancer, with about 7% having metastasis only to the IMN without involving axillary nodes.[9]

In **conclusion**, ultrasound evaluation of axilla is an important area that every radiologist must be aware of with an emphasis on lymph node assessment. He or she must know the range of normal findings while evaluation lymph nodes. If a grossly abnormal lymph node is seen at the time of detection of primary breast mass, both should undergo biopsy at the same sitting. Ultrasound also plays a role in performance of sentinel lymph node procedures and can be used to evaluate internal mammary lymph nodes.

REFERENCES

1. Choi YJ, Ko EY, Han BK, Shin JH, Kang SS, Hahn SY. et al. High-resolution ultrasonographic features of axillary lymph node metastasis in patients with breast cancer. Breast 2009;18(2):119-22.
2. Shetty MK, Carpenter WS. Sonographic evaluation of isolated abnormal axillary lymph nodes identified on mammograms. J Ultrasound Med 2004;23(1):63-71.
3. Deurloo EE, Tanis PJ, Gilhuijs KG, Muller SH, Kröger R, Peterse JL, Rutgers EJ, et al. Reduction in the number of sentinel lymph node procedures by preoperative ultrasonography of the axilla in breast cancer. Eur J Cancer 2003;39(8):1068-73.
4. Stavros T. Evaluation of regional lymph nodes in breast cancer patients. In: Breast ultrasound. Philadelphia, PA: Lippincott Williams & Wilkins; 2004. pp. 834-76.
5. Greene FL, Page DL, Fleming ID, et al. eds. AJCC cancer staging manual. 6th ed. New York, NY: Springer-Verlag; 2002. pp. 91-124.
6. Cools-Lartigue J, Sinclair A, Trabulsi N, Meguerditchian A,Mesurolle B, Fuhrer R, et al. Preoperative axillary ultrasound and fine-needle aspiration biopsy in the diagnosis of axillary metastases in patients with breast cancer: predictors of accuracy and future implications. Ann Surg Oncol 2013;20(3):819-27.
7. Stavros T. Ultrasound guide needle procedures. In: Breast ultrasound. Philadelphia, PA: Lippincott Williams & Wilkins; 2004. pp. 769-75.
8. Noguchi M. Relevance and practicability of internal mammary sentinel node biopsy for breast cancer. Breast Cancer 2002;9(4):329-36.
9. Van der Ent FWC, Kengen RAM, van der Pol HAG van der Pol HAG, Hoofwijk AGM., et al. Halsted revisited: internal mammary sentinel lymph node biopsy in breast cancer. Ann Surg 2001;234(1):79-84.

3.6 Newer Techniques

The major recent advances in ultrasound technology include elastography: strain and shear wave (SW) and automated breast volume ultrasound.

ELASTOGRAPHY

Introduction

Elastography is an effective and useful technique which when used along with gray scale ultrasound can improve its specificity. Basically, it measures the compressibility of a lesion which helps in distinguishing between benign and malignant lesions.

The malignant lesions are stiffer than surrounding parenchymal tissue while benign lesions are more compressible on elastography with few exceptions.

Technique: Elastography uses a dynamic compressing force to measure the elasticity of the tissues by assessing the deformity achieved. Lesions that are soft deform more than those that are stiff. There are two types of elastography techniques: Strain wave elastography and Shear wave elastography.

Strain Wave Elastography

These days elastography software is present in most state of art ultrasound machines. Once elastography mode is activated, the lesion is displayed and an external compression is applied with the transducer. The pressure applied on the probe must always be vertical and as low as possible. While applying external compression, lateral movements should be avoided. A qualitative variable scale (usually in color) denotes the tissue stiffness within the imaging field.[1]

Malignant lesions are stiffer compared to benign lesions and the resultant tissue deformity is less as compared to the benign lesions. In other words, that malignant tissues require high compressible force to achieve the same deformity when compared to the benign lesion.

Real-time elastography is performed by manual freehand compression. The region of interest (ROI) for control is kept in the normal glandular tissue in the plane of the lesion. The ROI for lesion is moved throughout the lesion and the largest numerical value of tissue–lesion ratio (TLR) also called strain ratio is taken. The strain ratio has different values for benign and malignant lesions. It is higher for malignant lesions which are stiffer (Figs. 1 and 2) though some benign lesions like sclerosing adenosis (Fig. 3) can also show high values. Benign masses like fibroadenoma have low value for strain index (Fig. 4) as compared to malignant masses.

With the use of strain elastography, malignant lesions appear larger in the elastogram while benign lesions appear smaller. The limitation of strain wave elastography is that it depends on the observer for external compressive force which is different for different observers.

Shear wave elastography: In this an ultrasound push pulse (acoustic radiation force impulse or ARFI) is used to generate shear waves (SW) which are perpendicular to the push pulse. The SW velocity (Vs) in the tissue

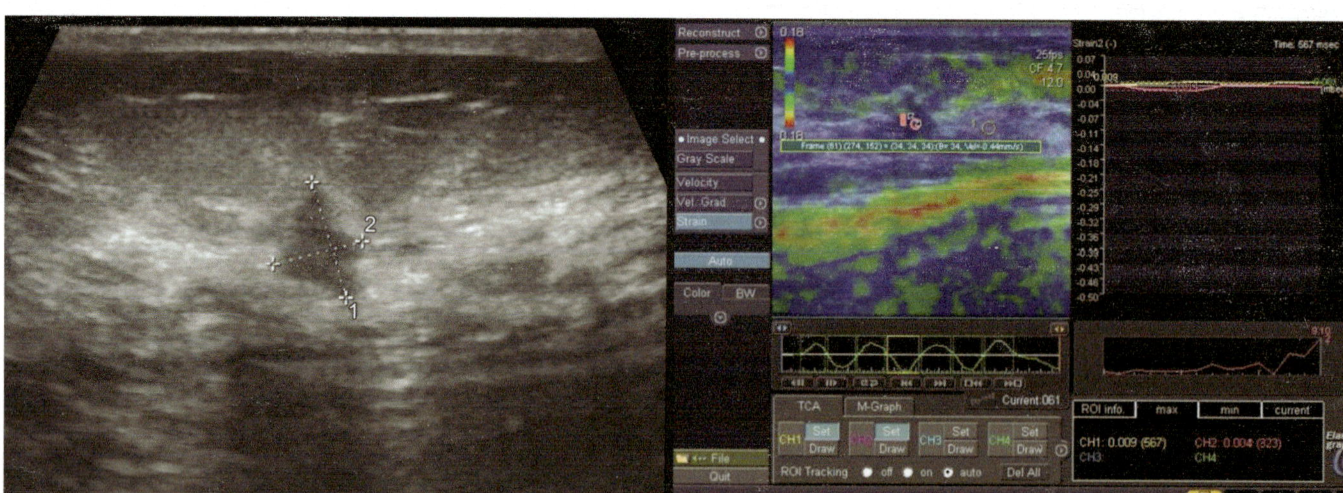

Fig. 1: A 46-year-old female, a postoperative case of lobular carcinoma of right breast presented for a routine follow-up evaluation. Ultrasound showed a new irregular hypoechoic lesion in left breast—BI-RADS 5. High TLR value was seen on elastography. Histopathology was s/o lobular carcinoma. (BI-RADS: breast imaging reporting and data system; TLR: tissue–lesion ratio).

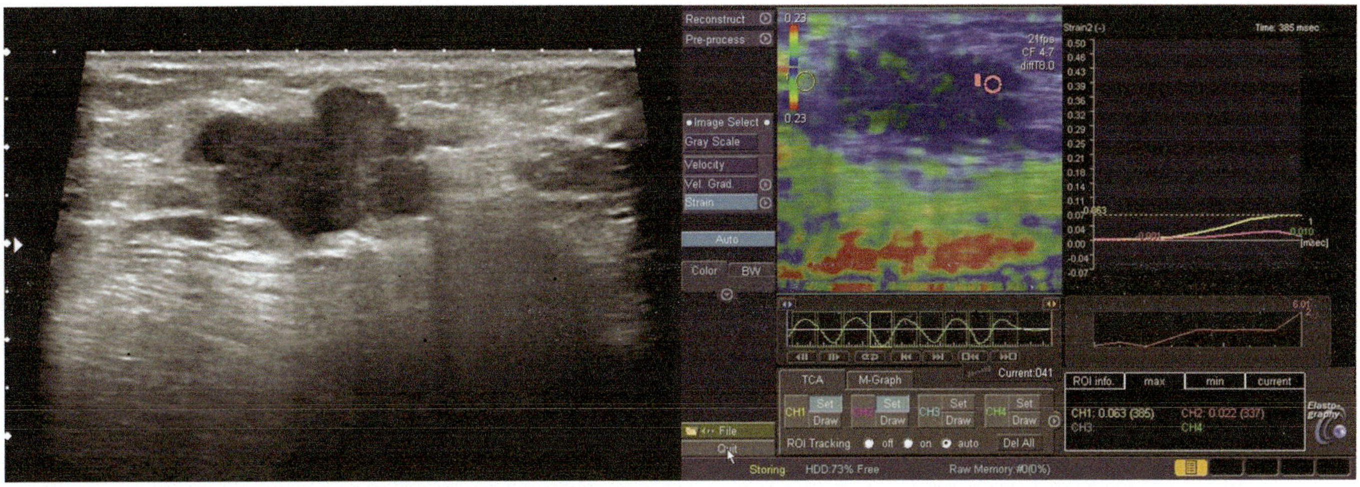

Fig. 2: A 37-year-old female presented with a palpable lump in right breast which on ultrasound was hypoechoic and showed microlobulations s/o BI-RADS 4C. Elastography showed high strain index. Histopathology was s/o invasive ductal carcinoma. (BI-RADS: breast imaging reporting and data system).

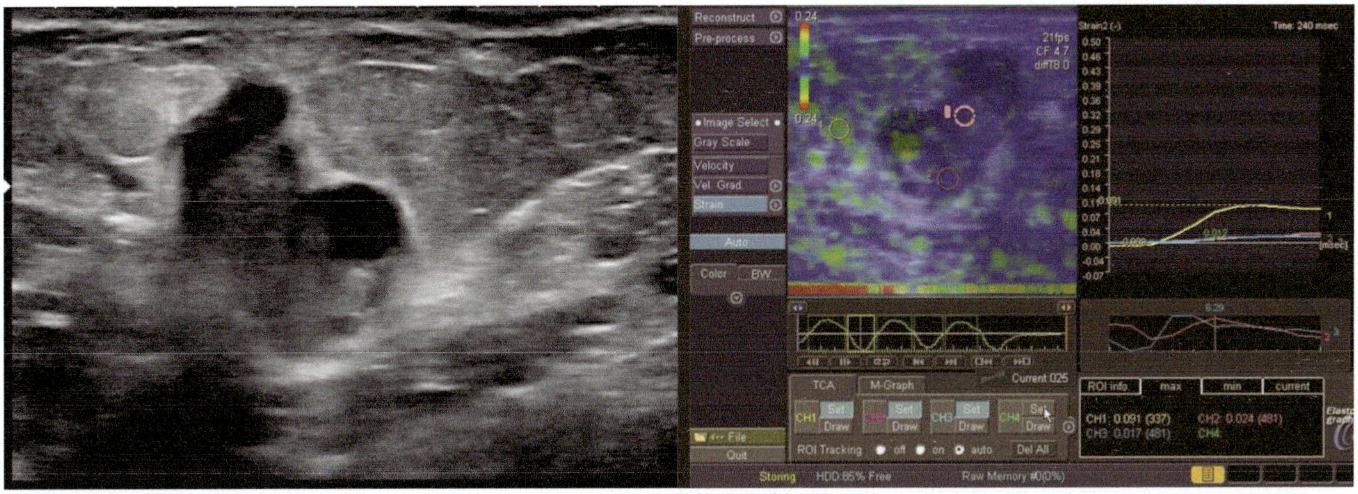

Fig. 3: An elderly woman showed a circumscribed hypoechoic lesion with obscured margins on ultrasound which was suspicious for malignancy—BI-RADS 4B. High TLR values were noted on elastography. Histopathology was s/o sclerosing adenosis. (BI-RADS: breast imaging reporting and data system; TLR: tissue–lesion ratio).

is proportional to the square root of stiffness (Young's modulus) of the lesion measured in units of kilopascals. Dynamic SW elastography produces **quantitative** elasticity values for different tissue types.

A color coded map of tissue elasticity is generated which is laid on gray scale image. Fibroadenoma shows low elasticity values <30 Pa with a blue color map. Since malignant lesions are stiffer as compared to benign lesions, they show higher elasticity values >120 kPa and appear red.

Elastography is a promising method of improving ultrasound's ability to characterize benign and malignant lesions. Elastography is more accurate than ultrasound and can be used as a complementary imaging modality along with ultrasound. This will helps in reducing the number of breast biopsies for benign lesions.

It is important to correlate elastography with B-mode, color Doppler and subsequent histology and follow-up. Elastography combined with B-mode and color Doppler has a high sensitivity for invasive cancers as they are stiff and appear larger on strain imaging with better demonstration of tumor extent. Benign lesions appear significantly smaller.

It has been proposed that SW elastography be used to upgrade or downgrade breast imaging reporting and data system (BI-RADS) category 3 and 4a lesions. Using this algorithm, Berg et al.[2] demonstrated an increase in specificity without a loss of sensitivity.

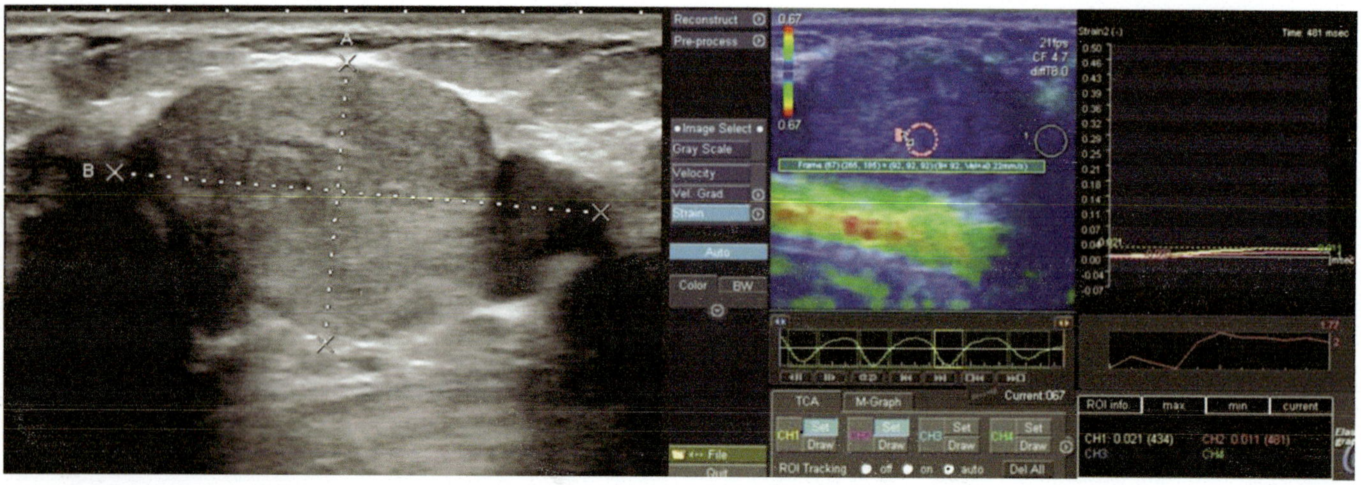

Fig. 4: A 29-year-old female presented with a palpable lump in left breast. Ultrasound showed a circumscribed hypoechoic mass with gentle lobulations—BI-RADS 3. Low TLR was seen on elastography. Lumpectomy was done. Histopathology was s/o fibroadenoma. (BI-RADS: breast imaging reporting and data system; TLR: tissue–lesion ratio).

AUTOMATED BREAST VOLUME ULTRASOUND (ABUS)

It is a well-known fact that denser the breast, the more difficult it is to see underlying breast masses on mammogram as they get obscured. The dense breast is a nightmare for the interpreting radiologist and a cause of anxiety for patients. In addition, dense breast is an independent risk factor for development of breast cancer; therefore, they need to be evaluated adequately.

Automated breast ultrasound (ABUS) is a newer advancement in which there is improved consistency and reproducibility of images, minimum operator dependence and full-field volumes of the breast are obtained in 3-D.

In ABUS, 3-D volumetric images are obtained using high-frequency sound waves and images are available at various angles making it easier for interpretation. Once the images are acquired, a complete and comprehensive analysis is done on the workstation. With the help of multiplanar reconstructions, coronal, sagittal and axial images are obtained.

There are two types of ABUS:

1. A standard ultrasound transducer is mounted onto an articulating arm and scanning is done by mechanically moving the articulating arm over the breast, in a way similar to the way in which hand-held ultrasound is performed. Imaging data is acquired continuously throughout the scanning process and stored. Interpretation is done later on a workstation by a radiologist.
2. A dedicated transducer paddle is placed over the breast, with a small amount of compression and routinely 3 scans are taken for a normal size breast excluding axilla. Once the imaging data are obtained, the data is processed using computer algorithms and stored to be reviewed on a standard workstation in coronal, axial and sagittal planes. Images are displayed in typical gray scale.

Currently, neither Doppler applications nor elastography is available for automated ultrasound. In the coronal view, the entire breast anatomy and architecture is seen clearly. Normally the acquisition time is 15 min, but with larger breasts more than standard views are required, and aquisition time may be increased. The operator dependence is less as the transducer automatically scans the breast.

Advantages of ABUS:

- Consistency and reproducibility
- Does not require a radiologist or ultrasound technologist
- Time to acquire the raw data is more consistent in ABUS.
- Concerns related to false positives have been limiting factor preventing for widespread adoption and implementation of screening breast ultrasound.
- Call back (ACRIN 6666 multi-institutional trial) rate from ultrasound screening was 5.4%.

REFERENCES

1. Barr RG, Zhang, Z. Shear-wave elastography of the breast: value of a quality measure and comparison with strain elastography. Radiology 2015;275(1):45-53.
2. Berg WA, Cosgrove DO, Doré CJ, et al. Shear-wave elastography improves the specificity of breast US: the BE1 multinational study of 939 masses. Radiology 2012;262(2):435-49.

Magnetic Resonance Imaging

CHAPTER

4

4.1 Image Acquisition and Indications

INTRODUCTION

Overall, mammography is considered the single most effective screening tool and has been credited with reducing breast cancer-related mortality by 20%–30%. Indeed, mammography is an extremely cost-effective modality for screening of breast malignancy; however, its sensitivity is 67.8% and specificity is 75%. Also, ionizing radiation as well as lower spatial resolution (in comparison to MRI) are considered as disadvantages in younger women and in those with dense breasts. Ultrasonography, in conjunction with mammography, has become the norm when working up a lesion. However, its efficacy is limited when used for screening. The most evident disadvantages are ultrasound's inability to detect microcalcifications and the heavy reliance on skill of the operator. MRI can play a great role to overcome some of these limitations of mammography and ultrasonography.

MRI of breast can be performed either for screening purpose or diagnostic purpose. The American Cancer Society (ACS) guidelines for using breast MRI for screening purpose is given below:[1]

AMERICAN COLLEGE OF RADIOLOGY GUIDELINES FOR USING BREAST MRI FOR CANCER SCREENING

- Women with a BRCA 1 or BRCA 2 mutation
- A first degree relative of a BRCA carrier who has not been tested
- A lifetime risk of breast cancer >25% as defined by risk-assessment models
- Women who received radiation to the chest between ages 10 and 30 years.
- Women with Li-Fraumeni, Cowden and Bannayan-Riley-Ruvalcaba syndromes and their first-degree relatives

Screening breast MRI can also be considered in the following populations:

- A lifetime risk of breast cancer between 15% and 20% as defined by risk-assessment models
- Women with lobular carcinoma in situ (LCIS) or atypical lobular hyperplasia
- Women with atypical ductal hyperplasia (ADH)
- Women with heterogeneous or extremely dense breasts on screening mammography
- Women with a personal history of breast cancer or ductal carcinoma in situ (DCIS)
- The evaluation of patients with breast augmentation via saline or silicone implants.

INDICATIONS OF BREAST MRI FOR DIAGNOSTIC PURPOSES

- **Detection of occult primary breast cancer in women with axillary metastases:** MRI has been found to detect 64%–75% of occult breast malignancies, with the average tumor size being 15 mm at detection.[2]
- **Preoperative evaluation of newly diagnosed breast cancer patients:** A preoperative breast MRI for women who carry a deleterious mutation in BRCA 1, BRCA 2 or other high-risk genetic syndromes may be useful for detection of an ipsilateral or contralateral cancer.
- **Evaluation of a suspected breast cancer:** A breast MRI may be helpful in the clinical setting of a doubtful clinical or mammographic/sonographic examination in a patient that is not an operative candidate.
- **Evaluation of inconclusive clinical or imaging findings:** Breast MRI can be used for the evaluation of equivocal findings on mammography and ultrasound, such as focal asymmetry or a mammographic abnormality seen on only one view. MRI may be helpful as

an adjunct study to provide guidance for targeted ultrasound or core biopsy when localization would be difficult with conventional imaging alone. However, a negative MRI does not preclude biopsy for suspicious findings on conventional imaging or physical examination. *There is no data to support the use of breast MRI to evaluate patients with breast pain or patients with palpable lumps who have had normal mammography and sonography. Palpable breast lumps require biopsy for diagnosis.*

- **Measurement of response to neoadjuvant chemotherapy:** Neoadjuvant systemic therapy, also referred to as primary or preoperative systemic therapy, is an established treatment modality for women with locally advanced breast cancer to reduce the size of the cancer and possibly allow for breast conservation. In most cases, response to treatment can be assessed with physical examination along with the breast-imaging technique that most clearly showed the cancer at the time of diagnosis. There is increased interest in using breast MRI for assessment of the response to chemotherapy since reduction in lesion size and changes in enhancement kinetics correlate with pathologic response. *However, MRI has been shown to both overestimate and underestimate the size of residual tumor after neoadjuvant chemotherapy.*[3] For patients receiving neoadjuvant therapy, assessment of enhancement pattern, tumor distribution pattern, tumor size and background enhancement may improve the MRI specificity to monitor cancer response to therapy.
- **Differentiating postoperative changes from recurrence:** Approximately 10%–15% of patients with breast cancer develop a locoregional recurrence within 10 years of breast-conserving surgery. Breast MRI is useful in distinguishing surgical scarring and radiation changes from breast cancer recurrence in cases where the clinical examination, mammography and/or ultrasound are difficult to interpret. Enhancement in the prior surgical site is suggestive of recurrence and merits core biopsy, while the absence of enhancement in the biopsy bed suggests fibrosis. However, false-positive readings can arise from fat necrosis that can also enhance avidly.
- **Assessment of breast implants:** Breast MRI is useful for detection of silicone implant rupture and diagnosis of masses caused by free silicone injection. Breast MRI is the most useful imaging test for detecting both intracapsular and extracapsular ruptures of a silicone breast implant with a sensitivity and specificity of over 90%. The most important risk factor for silicone breast implant rupture is time duration since placement, since 50% of implants rupture after 12 years. The United States Food and Drug Administration (US FDA) recommends that regular MRI screening be performed for asymptomatic women with silicone implants 3 years after implantation and every 2 years thereafter. However, there is little evidence to support a recommendation for regular MRI screening, which is expensive and may lead to anxiety and false-positive results and result in unnecessary surgery. Therefore, most experts agree that breast MRI should be used as a confirmatory diagnostic test and not be used to screen asymptomatic women for implant rupture.

MRI BREAST IMAGING PROTOCOL

Prior to acquiring the MRI images, it is desirable to have a questionnaire prepared to know about the present hormonal status (menopause, day of the menstrual cycle, pregnancy, breastfeeding), personal history of breast cancer (specifying the date of surgery, the date of the end of radiotherapy, history of axillary lymph node dissection, chemotherapy or hormone treatment) and any family history. **To minimize the effects of physiologic glandular enhancement occurring during the natural menstrual cycles, premenopausal patients or patients on cyclic hormone replacement therapy should be imaged between days 7 and 14 of their menstrual cycle.**

Ideally, breast MRI should be performed on a magnet having a field strength of 1.5 T or greater. Also, a dedicated breast coil should be used for breast MRI. The breast coil is designed to receive signals from the breast tissue and allows imaging of both breasts together.

Surface coils are important to get adequate spatial resolution while maintaining a high signal-to-noise ratio.

Patients are positioned prone over the breast coil, which has openings for the patient's breasts. The patient must be in a comfortable position with her arms above her head to limit aliasing artifacts and artifacts relating to phase encoding. Foam wedges may be used inside the coil when the breast volume is low, so as to minimize respiratory motion artifacts. Any skin fold that could form when the breast is abnormally compressed by the edge of the coil should be avoided. Care should also be taken to position the nipple directly below the breast, so as to enable localizing lesions and also to enable better correlation with the mammogram and ultrasound. Some centers image the patient with the breasts in mild compression, which minimizes motion artifact and aids in planning biopsy.

Intravenous gadolinium contrast must be used to maximize cancer detection and highlights the neovascularity associated with cancers. Contrast is not necessary when the study is performed to evaluate silicone implant integrity.

The commonly used sequences for morphological assessment include the following:

- T2-weighted sequences to look for cysts or microcysts, which suggest benign nature. These can be performed without fat saturation, since a T2 signal higher than that of non-saturated fat has very good predictive value for a cyst being benign. T2-weighted sequences with fat saturation are useful for MRI ductography-in case of nipple discharge, and in order to optimize the detection of small cancers. Fibroadenomas are also most commonly hyperintense on T2W imaging with hypointense septations.
- T1-weighted sequences without fat saturation are useful for detecting the presence of a fatty component within a lesion, which also predicts its benign nature. They also allow detection of metal markers that may have been placed following biopsy of the lesion.
- Dynamic sequences must be acquired with good temporal resolution of ≤2 min and good spatial resolution of isotropic pixel size of 1 mm. 3D T1 gradient-echo sequences with a moderate flip angle are ideal as they allow acquisition of thinner slices with a better signal-to-noise ratio as compared to 2D sequences.
- The maximum intensity projection (MIP) can be used as a basic overview but should not be relied on solely to interpret the images as it excludes non-enhancing lesions. Both pre and postcontrast images are acquired, which can be subtracted based around the same principles as digital subtraction angiography. Fat does not enhance on postcontrast sequences. Using subtraction essentially cancels out all of the bright fat signal on the T1 images leaving behind the truly enhancing areas, namely, masses, lymph nodes, and blood vessels. The T1 images are also excellent to look for intraductal blood and lymph node morphology, identifying the benign fatty hilum of normal lymph nodes.

BASIC BREAST IMAGING PROTOCOL

- T1W axial without fat suppression
- T2W axial without fat suppression
- T2W axial, sagittal and coronal planes with fat suppression
- Short tau inversion recovery (STIR) axial and sagittal
- Axial diffusion weighted imaging using $b = 0$, $b = 600$
- Precontrast axial 3D T1 with fat suppression (mask images for subtraction)
- Postcontrast axial dynamic multiphase 3D T1W sequence with fat-suppression (60–90 s acquisitions, one pre and four to five postcontrast acquisitions) followed by subtraction.
- Dynamic contrast curve evaluation: The kinetic curve assessment involves description of the initial peak—slow, medium, rapid. The delayed phase—persistent, plateau, or washout of contrast enhancement—assists in lesion differentiation.
- High-resolution postdynamic 3D scan Sagittal or Axial
- Spectroscopy at the lesion.

Multiparametric analysis of a lesion also emphasizes on deriving the contrast enhancement kinetics from the dynamic postcontrast scan, by placing ROIs within the lesion.

KINETIC CURVES (FIG. 1)

A benign lesion shows a progressive enhancement pattern (type 1 curve), while a typical malignant lesion shows an early rapid enhancement with either a plateau phase (type 2 curve) or a washout pattern (type 3 curve). Apart from

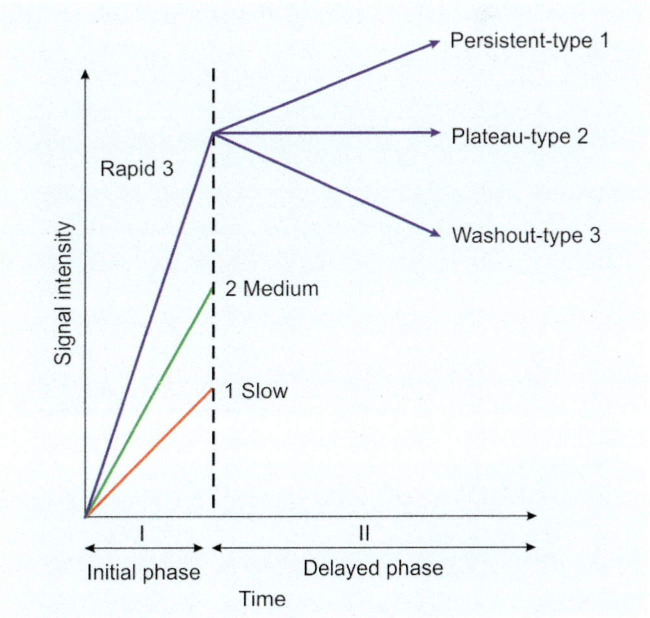

Fig. 1: Line diagram showing time intensity curve showing the various types of curves—type 1: progressive/persistent enhancement pattern; type 2: plateau pattern; type 3: washout pattern.

descriptive analysis, semiquantitative and quantitative analysis can also be performed by deriving maps of wash-in/washout, time-to-peak or area under the curve.

Certain special conditions require specific sequences to gain more information, for example, implant imaging requires acquisition of selective water and fat suppressed T2-weighted images, in which the silicone appears bright or a noncontrast or direct contrast-injected MR ductography in the case of nipple discharge.

Additional sequences like diffusion-weighted MRI and MRI spectroscopy are also being commonly employed for characterization of a breast lesion. Diffusion-weighted imaging works on the principle that cellular tumors prevent free diffusion of molecules, thereby showing restricted diffusion and bright signal. It has a disadvantage of poor spatial resolution and, as such, is recommended for lesions >1 cm in size. Diffusion-weighted imaging and ADC values are of value for assessing response to neoadjuvant chemotherapy[4] and postoperative recurrence.[5]

MR-spectroscopy works on the principle of molecular imaging, where elevation of choline peak at 3.2 ppm is considered to be a sign of a malignant lesion. Point-resolved spectroscopy sequence (PRESS) or stimulated echo acquisition mode (STEAM) sequence is used, with the former providing a better signal-to-noise ratio. A single voxel or multivoxel acquisition may be performed.

Recent studies are targeted toward lesser sequences and more efficient and cost and time-effective strategy and hence an abbreviated protocol is suggested which takes between 3 and 6 min instead of the usual 30–40-minutes span. This consists of only a precontrast T1-weighted image with fat saturation and a single postcontrast T1-weighted image with fat saturation. This abbreviated protocol shows similar diagnostic accuracy with reduction in the time of the scan and can be useful in wider screening operation by MRI.[6]

REFERENCES

1. Saslow D, Boetes C, Burke W, et al. American Cancer Society guidelines for breast screening with MRI as an adjunct to mammography. CA Cancer J Clin 2007;57: 75-89.
2. De Bresser J, de Vos B, van der Ent F, et al. Breast MRI in clinically and mammographically occult breast cancer presenting with an axillary metastasis: a systematic review. Eur J Surg Oncol 2010; 36:114-9.
3. Martincich L, Montemurro F, Cirillo S, et al. Role of magnetic resonance imaging in the prediction of tumor response in patients with locally advanced breast cancer receiving neoadjuvant chemo-therapy. Radiol Med 2003; 106:51.
4. Iacconi C, Giannelli M, Marini C, et al. The role of mean diffusivity (MD) as a predictive index of the response to chemotherapy in locally advanced breast cancer: a preliminary study. Eur Radiol 2010;20:303-8.
5. Rinaldi P, Giuliani M, Belli P, et al. DWI in breast MRI: role of ADC value to determine diagnosis between recurrent tumor and surgical scar in operated patients. Eur J Radiol 2010;75:e114-23.
6. Jain M, Jain A, Hyzy MD, et al. FAST MRI breast screening revisited. J Med Imaging Radiat Oncol 2016.

4.2 Breast Imaging-reporting and Data System (BI-RADS) Lexicon

INTRODUCTION

BI-RADS lexicon has been used for mammography, ultrasound and MRI so that a common language is spoken as far as the lesion description is concerned, thereby avoiding ambiguity. This not only includes lesion description but also the composition of breast that varies in individual and depends upon factors like age, hormonal influence, use of medications, etc.

BREAST COMPOSITION

Visual estimation of fibroglandular tissue (FGT) determines the four categories of breast composition (Figs. 1A to D). If the breasts have unequal amounts of FGT, the breast with the larger amount of FGT should be considered to categorize. At present, quantification of breast FGT volume on MRI is not recommended.

The following BI-RADS terminology is used instead of numbers to classify breast FGT in order to eliminate any possible confusion with the BI-RADS assessment categories on Mammogram and is classified as follows:

- Almost entirely fat
- Scattered FGT
- Heterogeneous FGT
- Dense FGT.

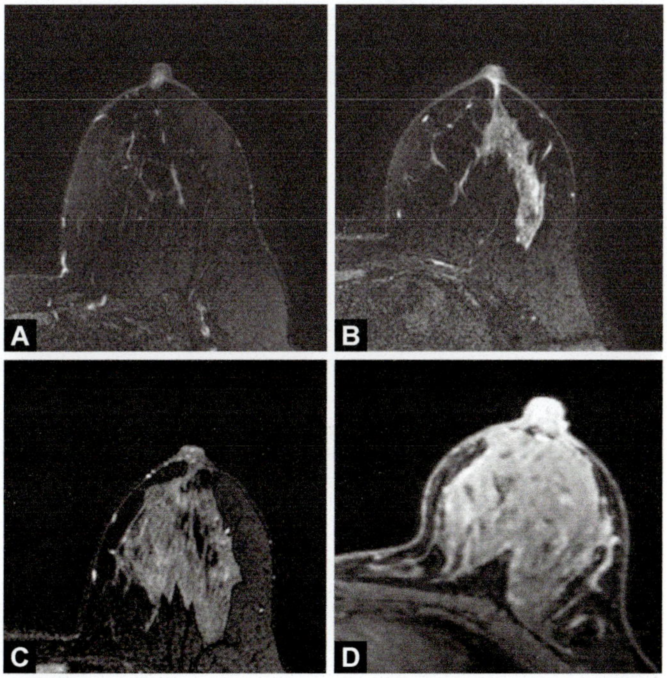

Figs. 1A to D: Four categories of breast composition on MRI: (A) Almost entirely fatty involuted; (B) Scattered fibroglandular tissue; (C) Heterogeneous fibroglandular tissue; (D) Dense fibroglandular tissue.

BACKGROUND PARENCHYMAL ENHANCEMENT

There are four categories of background parenchymal enhancement (BPE), defined by the visually estimated enhancement of the FGT of the breast or breasts. These may be unequal and the breast with the most BPE should be used to categorize BPE. If treatment has altered BPE in one or both breasts, this can be reported.

At present, BPE refers to the volume of enhancement and the intensity of enhancement and is categorized as:

- Minimal
- Mild
- Moderate
- Marked

BPE can be symmetrical or asymmetrical.

CLEAR DESCRIPTION OF ANY IMPORTANT FINDINGS

The following descriptors should be used to describe the mass:

- Side
- Location (Breast quadrant and clock-face position or central, retroareolar and axillary tail descriptors)
- Size
- Distance from nipple, skin or chest wall in centimeters (if applicable)

DESCRIPTORS FOR ABNORMAL ENHANCEMENT

- **Artifacts:** That affect interpretation
- **Focus:** A tiny dot of enhancement that does not clearly represent a space-occupying lesion or mass and does not clearly show a mass on precontrast imaging.
- **Masses:** Space-occupying lesions that may displace or retract surrounding breast tissue

DESCRIPTORS—MODIFIERS DESCRIBING A MASS

- **Shape:** Describes the overall morphology of the enhancement
  - Oval (includes lobulated) (Fig. 2)
  - Round
  - Irregular
- **Margin:** Describes the borders
  - Circumscribed
  - Not circumscribed
    - Irregular
    - Spiculated (Fig. 3)
- **Internal enhancement characteristics:**
  - Homogeneous
  - Heterogeneous
  - Rim enhancement (Fig. 4)
  - Dark internal septations (Fig. 5)
- **Intramammary lymph node (Fig. 6)**
- **Skin lesion (rarely important)**
- **Non-mass enhancement (NME):** Modifiers describing enhancement patterns with a specific MRI pattern
  - Distribution
    - Focal
    - Linear
    - Segmental

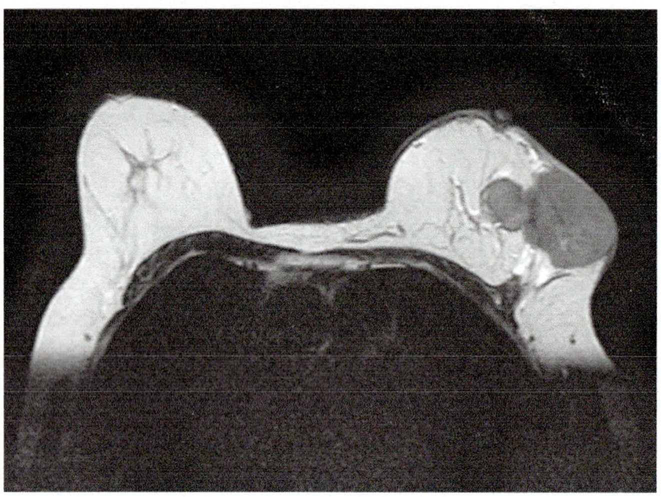

Fig. 2: MRI T2W sequence, axial sections show a well-defined lobulated mass in left breast.

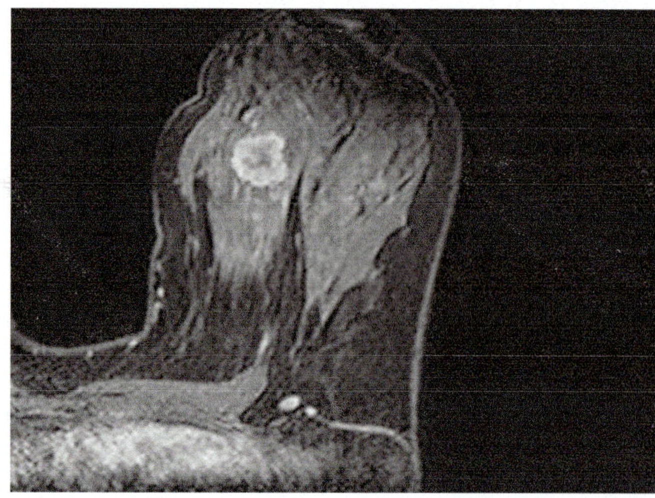

Fig. 4: MRI T1W postcontrast study shows mass with rim enhancement.

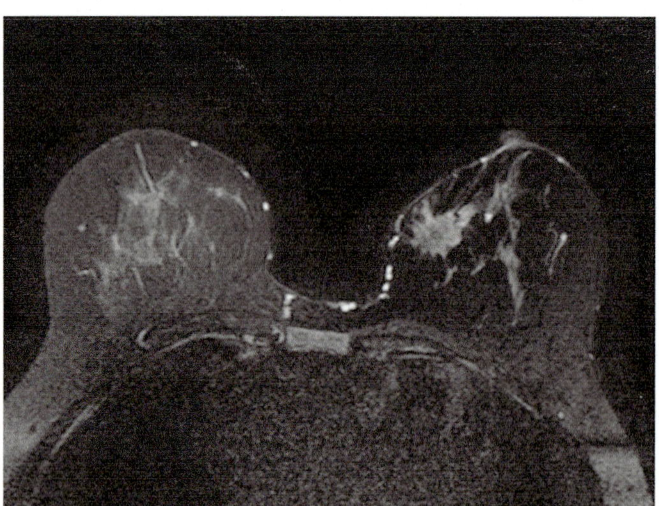

Fig. 3: MRI axial sections shows a mass with spiculated margins in left breast.

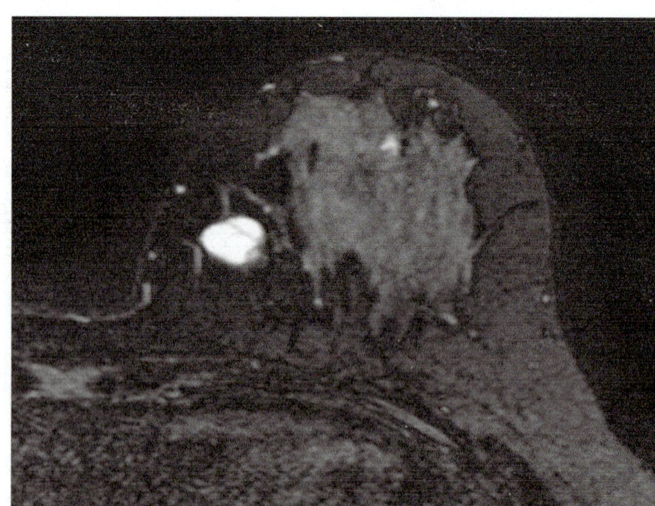

Fig. 5: MRI breast shows a circumscribed hyperintense mass with hypointense internal septations on T2W.

- o Regional
- o Multiple regions
- o Diffuse
- – Internal enhancement patterns (for all other types)
  - o Homogeneous
  - o Heterogeneous
  - o Clumped
  - o Clustered ring
- **Non-enhancing findings**
  - – Ductal precontrast high signal on T1W
  - – Cyst
  - – Postoperative collections (hematoma/seroma)
  - – Post-therapy skin thickening and trabecular thickening
  - – Non-enhancing mass
  - – Architectural distortion
  - – Signal void from foreign bodies, clips, etc.
- **Associated features**
  - – Nipple retraction
  - – Nipple invasion
  - – Skin retraction
  - – Skin thickening
  - – Skin invasion
- **Fat-containing lesions**
  - – Lymph nodes
    - o Normal
    - o Abnormal
  - – Fat necrosis
  - – Hamartoma
  - – Postoperative seroma/hematoma with fat

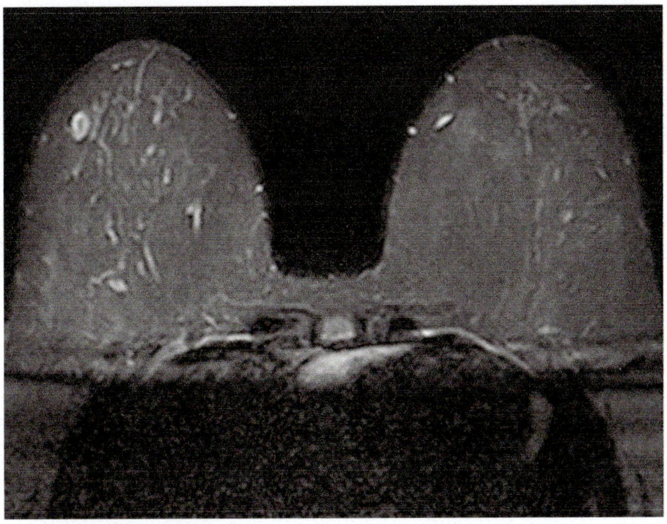

Fig. 6: MRI non-contrast T1W fat suppressed image showing intramammary lymph node with fatty hilum

- **Stability:** It describes how the enhancement changed (if new, stable or changed in size from previous examination)
- **Kinetic curve assessment (if applicable)**
  - – The fastest enhancing portion of the lesion or the most suspicious washout curve pattern in the lesion should be assessed
    - o Sample fast enhancing areas
    - o Sample for and report on the worst looking kinetic curve shape
  - – Signal intensity/time curve
    - o **Initial enhancement phase**—describes the enhancement pattern within the first 2 min or when the curve starts to change
      - ▪ Slow
      - ▪ Medium
      - ▪ Fast
    - o **Delayed phase**—describes the enhancement pattern after 2 min or after the curve starts to change
      - ▪ Persistent
      - ▪ Plateau
      - ▪ Washout
- **Implants** (Discussed in detail in chapter on implants)
  - – Implant material and lumen type
    - o Saline
    - o Silicone
    - o Other implant material (such as soy oil, polypropylene, polyurethane and sponges)
    - o Lumen type
  - – Implant location
    - o Retroglandular
    - o Retropectoral
    - o Submuscular
  - – Abnormal implant contour
    - o Focal bulge
  - – Intracapsular silicone findings
    - o Radial folds
    - o Subcapsular line
    - o Keyhole sign (teardrop, noose)
    - o Linguine sign
  - – Extracapsular silicone
    - o Breast
    - o Lymph nodes
  - – Water droplets
  - – Peri-implant fluid.

BI-RADS ASSESSMENT CATEGORIES

The assessment categories are based on BI-RADS categories developed for mammography (Table 1).

Assessment is Incomplete

Category 0: Incomplete—Need Additional Imaging Evaluation

This category is for a finding that needs additional imaging evaluation. This may be used for a technically unsatisfactory scan or when more information is needed to interpret the scan, for example, a repeat MRI with satisfactory technique or obtaining information with other imaging modalities (mammographic views, ultrasound, etc.). The radiologist should use judgment in how vigorously to pursue previous studies.

Every effort should be made not to use category 0 on MRI. If a category 0 assessment is given at MRI, detailed recommendations should describe the subsequent diagnostic imaging workup and the level of suspicion (pertinent in case the additional imaging does not establish benignity). When additional studies are completed, a final assessment is given.

For example, if a suspicious mass is seen on MRI but there is a possibility that it may represent a benign finding, such as an intramammary lymph node, then a category 0 assessment may be made, with the recommendation for targeted US (that might demonstrate characteristically benign features) to possibly avert biopsy.

Another example would be when one suspects fat necrosis, in which mammography should be recommended (that might demonstrate characteristically benign features) to possibly avert biopsy.

Assessment is Complete—Final Assessment Categories

Category 1: Negative

This is a normal examination with no abnormal enhancement; hence, a routine follow-up is advised. The breasts are symmetric and no enhancing masses, architectural distortion or suspicious areas of enhancement are present.

Category 1 includes a normal description of breast composition (amount of FGT) and the degree of parenchymal enhancement.

Category 2: Benign

This is a normal assessment, but a benign finding is described in the breast MRI report. These include intramammary lymph node, implants, metallic foreign bodies (such as core biopsy and surgical clips), enhancing and non-enhancing fibroadenomas, cysts, old non-enhancing scars or recent scars, postoperative collections, fat-containing lesions (such as oil cysts, lipomas, galactoceles and hamartomas).

Both category 1 and 2 assessments indicate that there is no evidence of malignancy. The difference is that category 2 should be used when describing one or more specific benign MRI findings in the report, whereas category 1

Table 1: BI-RADS categories of cancer: assessment, management and likelihood

Assessment	*Management*	*Likelihood of Cancer*
Category 0: incomplete—need additional imaging evaluation	Recommend additional imaging: mammogram or targeted US	N/A
Category 1: negative	Routine breast MRI screening if cumulative lifetime risk ≥20%	Essentially 0% likelihood of malignancy
Category 2: benign	Routine breast MRI screening if cumulative lifetime risk ≥20%	Essentially 0% likelihood of malignancy
Category 3: probably benign	Short-interval (6-month) follow-up	≥0% but ≤2% likelihood of malignancy
Category 4: suspicious	Tissue diagnosis	>2% but <95% likelihood of malignancy
Category 5: highly suggestive of malignancy	Tissue diagnosis	≥95% likelihood of malignancy
Category 6: known biopsy-proven malignancy	Surgical excision when clinically appropriate	N/A

should be used when no such findings are described (even if such findings are present).

For categories 1 and 2, an annual follow-up MRI and mammography is recommended, which is in line with established guidelines for high-risk screening.

Category 3: Probably Benign

This category should have a ≤2% likelihood of malignancy, but >0% likelihood of malignancy. A probably benign finding is not expected to change over the suggested period of imaging surveillance, but the interpreting physician feels that it is better to establish stability of the finding before recommending routine breast screening.

The use of a probably benign (category 3) assessment is reserved for specific findings that are separate from the BPE and are very likely benign. There are several studies[1-3] that specifically address rates of malignancy and to a very limited extent, types of lesion and several of them were able to demonstrate a ≤2% malignancy rate demonstrating the feasibility of using category 3 assessments at MRI. However, none of the studies provided PPVs for specific types of lesions; so, the use of category 3 assessment at MRI remains intuitive for radiologists who lack extensive personal experience with any given specific type of lesion.

If a probably benign finding is smaller or less prominent (i.e., less contrast enhancement) on follow-up examination, the finding should be assessed as benign (category 2), eliminating the need for continued surveillance imaging. When a finding with probably benign imaging criteria is either new or has increased in size, extent, or conspicuity then biopsy should be recommended and a further follow-up is not rendered.

If MRI findings cannot be ascribed to normal variation of BPE and there is a question whether observed enhancement could be transient and related to the hormonal status of the patient, then a probably benign (category 3) assessment with a recommendation to return for very short-interval follow-up (2–3 months) may be appropriate.

The follow-up MRI examination should be scheduled for the optimal (week 2) phase of her cycle. Additionally, a category 3 assessment may be used for the postmenopausal patient who is on hormone replacement therapy (HRT) and in whom probable hormonal enhancement is observed. Stopping HRT for several weeks and repeating the scan may be warranted. *It should be emphasized that unexplained areas of enhancement that are demonstrated to be due to HRT are uncommon.* As with mammography, if the finding is smaller or less prominent (i.e., less contrast enhancement) at follow-up examination the finding is benign.

Follow-up of foci: Foci are small dot-like enhancement, which are different from BPE and stand out separately. Because of their small size, they cannot be accurately assessed for internal or marginal enhancement. If there is an increase in size of foci or new foci are seen, then they should be viewed with suspicion.

These foci should be compared with T2W imaging or short tau inversion recovery (STIR) sequence and if they are bright on these like a cyst, then it should be considered as a benign finding. Many of these may represent lymph nodes or a myxomatous fibroadenoma. It is important to remember that if focus does not have a very high signal on bright-fluid imaging (T2W or STIR), then the focus may or may not be benign. These foci may be followed or biopsied. If the finding is new or increased in size, the focus always should be biopsied. It is important to note that malignant foci may be brighter than the surrounding FGT, although they do not usually appear cyst-like.

Follow-up of masses: Masses that enhance and are identified on an initial MRI examination should be assessed based on morphology and kinetics. Sometimes malignancy may demonstrate benign-appearing MRI features, such as an oval or round shape with a circumscribed margin and homogeneous internal enhancement. These will need periodic surveillance imaging depending on various factors that affect the probability of malignancy (age, cancer risk, etc.) as well as the patient's willingness to accept surveillance imaging as an alternative to biopsy. If surveillance imaging is undertaken, an increase in size of the mass should prompt immediate biopsy.

Follow-up of NME: Non-mass enhancement that is unique and separate from the overall background enhancement should be assessed based on morphology and kinetics. Bright-fluid imaging sequences (T2W and STIR) are helpful to demonstrate any associated cysts, which may support a diagnosis of focal fibrocystic change and a benign (category 2) assessment. However, limited data on linear, clumped and segmental enhancement indicate that these findings should not be followed up, as the malignancy rate appears to be >2%.[4] At this time, the literature is not sufficiently robust to endorse the use of a category 3 assessment for NME.

Timing of follow-up on MRI: Category 3 is best used for a unique focal finding and managed with an initial short-interval follow-up (6 months) examination followed by additional examinations until long-term (2- or 3-year) stability is demonstrated. The recommended 2- or 3-year follow-up in these cases is 6 months, 1 year, 2 years and optionally, 3 years from the date of first detection. After 2–3 years of stability, the finding should be assessed as benign (category 2). This is what is followed on mammography too but sometimes biopsies are done instead (patient preference or overriding clinical concern). With a properly worded report, the assessment category should be given as what the current reader feels is appropriate.

It appears that the ≤2% malignancy rate already demonstrated at mammographic follow-up also may be achieved at MRI. Several studies have demonstrated that focal lesions assigned to category 3 had a ≤2% malignancy rate, albeit without use of specific BI-RADS MRI descriptors for the lesions included in the studies.[5-7] It should be noted that a ≤2% malignancy rate may be difficult to achieve in the high-risk population that usually is studied by MRI (higher than average prior probability of cancer).

A desirable goal for the frequency of making category 3 assessments at MRI is <10%. Over time, this rate should decrease to the point that a mature program should demonstrate a rate much closer to the approximately 1%–2% rate currently achieved at mammography.

Category 4: Suspicious

This category is reserved for findings that do not have the classic appearance of malignancy but are sufficiently suspicious to justify a recommendation for biopsy. The ceiling for a category 3 assessment is a 2% likelihood of malignancy and the floor for a category 5 assessment is 95%; so, category 4 assessments cover the wide range of likelihood of malignancies in between. Thus, almost all recommendations for breast interventional procedures will come from assessments made using this assessment category. *In breast MRI, assessment category 4 is not currently divided into subcategories 4A, 4B and 4C.*

Category 4 is used for the majority of findings prompting breast intervention, which can be performed by percutaneous biopsy by US or stereotactic guidance or by MRI guidance for lesions not visible at either US or mammography. As cysts rarely pose a problem in interpretation at MRI, diagnostic aspiration is not commonly performed. In many patients with a suspicious abnormality at MRI, targeted US will identify a corresponding abnormality so that US-guided biopsy can be performed. US-guided biopsies are faster, more comfortable for the patient and more cost-effective than MRI-guided biopsies. In general, patients with masses larger than 5 mm should be examined by targeted US (second look US) if the MR appearance is suspicious. Areas of NME may be evident on US as well, thus bringing the radiologist's judgment into play. Factors that may limit visibility at US include fatty breasts, extremely complex breasts with multiple cysts, very large breasts and very deep lesions. *If there is any question about whether a presumed sonographic correlate actually is the same as the suspicious MRI lesion, MR-guided biopsy is advised.*

Category 5: Highly Suggestive of Malignancy

These lesions have a very high probability (≥95%) of malignancy. The current oncologic management involves tissue diagnosis of malignancy via percutaneous tissue sampling. This facilitates treatment options, such as when sentinel node biopsy is included in surgical management or when neoadjuvant chemotherapy is administered prior to surgery. Therefore, the current rationale for using category 5 assessment is to identify lesions for which any non-malignant percutaneous tissue diagnosis is considered discordant, resulting in a recommendation for repeat (usually surgical) biopsy. There is no single MRI descriptor which is sufficiently predictive of malignancy to produce the ≥95% probability required for a category 5 assessment. Just as in mammography and US, an appropriate combination of suspicious findings is needed to justify a category 5 assessment at MRI.

Category 6: Known Biopsy-proven Malignancy

This category is for examinations performed after biopsy proof of malignancy (imaging performed after percutaneous biopsy) but prior to surgical excision, in which there are no abnormalities other than the known cancer that might need additional evaluation.

This category should not be used after successful lumpectomy or mastectomy (margin of resection free of tumor). In the event that the breast with known cancer has a separate suspicious MRI finding that requires biopsy for diagnosis, the appropriate category 4 or 5 assessment should be given, and this would be the overall assessment because it leads to more prompt intervention.

REFERENCES

1. Weinstein SP, Hanna LG, Gatsonis C, et al. Frequency of malignancy seen in probably benign lesion at contrast-enhanced breast MR imaging: findings from ACRIN 6667. Radiology 2010;255:731-7.
2. Eby PR, DeMartini WB, Peacock S, et al. Cancer yield of probably benign breast MR examinations. J Magn Reson Imaging 2007;26:950-5.
3. Kriege M, Brekelmans CTM, Boetes C, et al. Efficacy of MRI and mammography for breast-cancer screening in women with a familial or genetic predisposition. N Engl J Med 2004;351:427-37.
4. Liberman L, Morris EA, Dershaw DD, Abramson AF, Tan LK. Ductal enhancement on MR imaging of the breast. AJR Am J Roentgenol 2003;519-25.
5. Mahoney MC, Gatsonis C, Hanna L, DeMartini WB, Lehman CD. Positive predictive value of BI-RADS MR imaging. Radiology 2012;264:51-8.
6. Eby PR, DeMartini WB, Gutierrez RL, Lehman CD. Probably benign lesions detected on breast MR imaging. Magn Reson Imaging Clin N Am 2010;18:309-21.
7. Warner E, Plewes DB, Hill KA, et al. Surveillance of BRCA 1 and BRCA 2 mutation carriers with magnetic resonance imaging, ultrasound, mammography, and clinical breast examination. JAMA 2004;292:1317-25.

4.3 Multimodality Evaluation of Breast Lesions

Breast masses are initially evaluated by either mammography or ultrasound with magnetic resonance imaging (MRI) done in selective cases. There are rapid advances in MRI technology with respect to spatial resolution, higher field strength, new coil technology and improved capabilities for MR-guided biopsy during the past few years.

In this chapter, we will discuss a few cases in which multimodality evaluation of breast masses was done.

CASE 1

A 46-year-old female presented with painless lump in the right breast. Mammogram and ultrasound were followed by MRI.

Findings: Mediolateral oblique (MLO) view of the right breast (Fig. 1A) shows a lobulated high-density lesion in the superior quadrant that appeared as a circumscribed lobulated hypoechoic lesion on ultrasound (Fig. 1B). This lesion was categorized as BI-RADS 4. The lump was excised—lumpectomy with wide local excision was done and histopathology was s/o low-grade invasive papillary carcinoma. Figures 1C and D are axial short tau inversion recovery (STIR) and T1W contrast enhanced MRI sections respectively, which showed the lesion in the superior quadrant of right breast as well as the scar tissue, just anterior to the pectoralis muscle. Figure 1E shows the kinetic curves obtained from the lesion as well as the scar tissue color of ROIs not seen, which show type 3 and 1 patterns, respectively.

The patient came for a follow-up after 2 months and since clinically a thickening was felt in the same breast, a mammogram was done again. Follow-up mammogram (MLO view) of right breast showed scar tissue in the axillary tail region. Another round high-density lesion was seen in the superior quadrant, which was retrospectively also detected in the initial mammogram as it had increased in size. (Please remember to always compare with previous mammogram if available. In this case, a small lesion

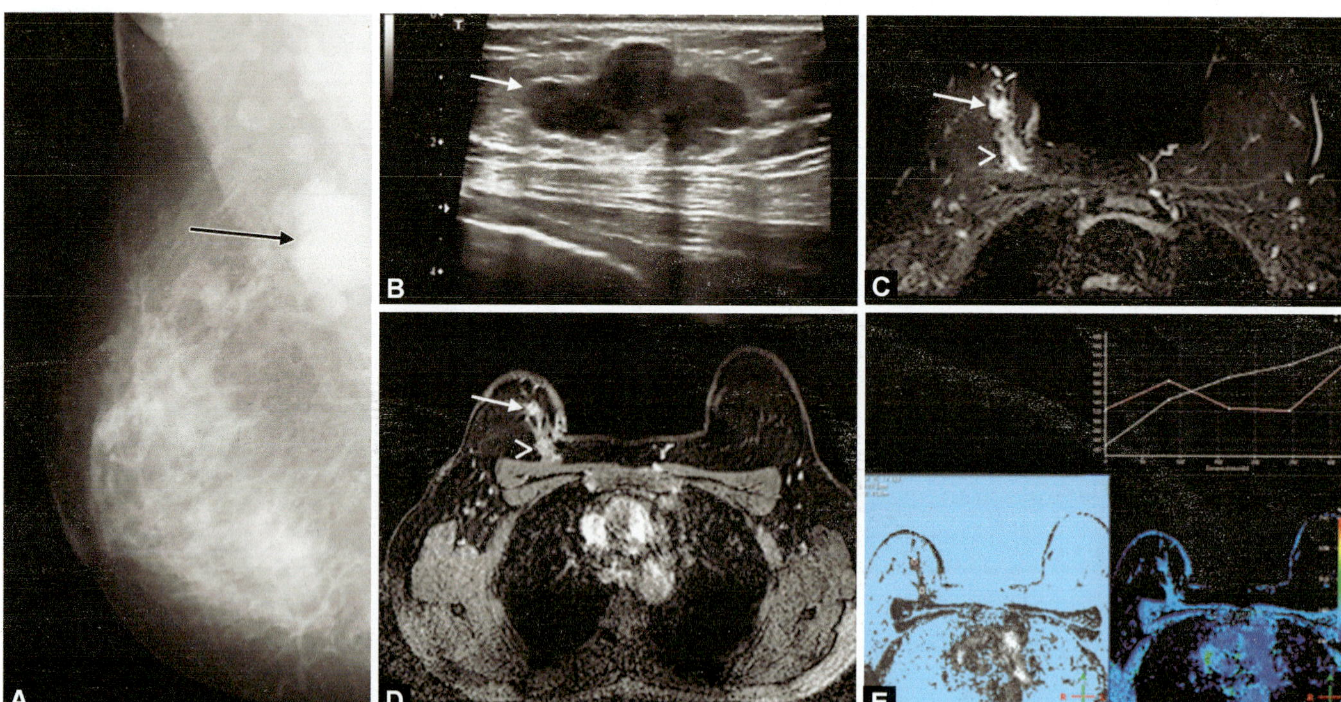

Figs. 1A to E: (A) A lobulated high-density lesion in the superior quadrant of the right breast (MLO view); (B) The lesion appears as a circumscribed lobulated hypoechoic mass on ultrasound (white arrow); (C and D) Axial STIR and contrast enhanced MRI sections of the breast show the lesion in the superior quadrant (white arrow) of right breast as well as the scar tissue, just anterior to the pectoralis muscle (white arrowhead); (E) Kinetic curves obtained from the lesion (pink ROI) as well as the scar tissue (white ROI) show types 3 and 1 patterns, respectively. (MLO: mediolateral oblique; STIR: short tau inversion recovery; ROI: region-of-interest).

was present in previous mammogram that was missed and not mentioned in the report. It was noticed on follow-up mammogram when there was an increase in size.)

The patient underwent an MRI breast examination to look for a residual lesion.

The patient underwent modified radical mastectomy. Histopathology confirmed the lesion to be residual tissue, while the scar tissue showed areas of fat necrosis.

Comments: MRI is especially useful to look for residual lesion once lumpectomy or conservative surgery is done and distinguish it from postoperative changes.

CASE 2

A 28-year-old woman presented with lump in right breast since 5 months. The lump was painless and firm to hard in consistency. There was no family history of breast cancer. The patient underwent ultrasound followed by MRI of breast.

Findings: Figure 2A is an ultrasound image showing an microlobulated, hypoechoic mass in the right breast at 12 o'clock position. Figures 2B and C are the axial STIR and diffusion-weighted images (DWIs), respectively, showing an oval hyperintense lesion having irregular margins in the superior quadrant of right breast, which showed diffusion restriction. Postcontrast study showed rim-enhancement (Fig. 2D). Kinetic curves obtained from various ROIs in the lesion (Fig. 2E) show type 2 pattern. A biopsy was done under ultrasound guidance which is suggestive of medullary carcinoma. The patient underwent modified radical mastectomy.

Comments: Medullary carcinoma of the breast is a rare subtype of invasive ductal carcinoma. Medullary carcinoma does not grow quickly and usually does not spread to the lymph nodes. For this reason, it is typically easier to treat than other types of breast cancer. Always pay attention to morphology of the lesion apart from kinetic curves as there are more important.

CASE 3

A 34-year-old woman came with complaint of thickening in right breast that she noticed 2 months back.

Findings: Figure 3A is the mammography image of both breasts—CC view, which shows asymmetric density in the left breast. Figure 3B is the ultrasound image of right breast that shows an irregular hypoechoic lesion having spiculated margins at 9–10 o'clock position. Figure 3C is the ultrasonography image of the left breast showing a small circumscribed round lesion showing posterior acoustic shadowing at 2 o'clock position. Figure 3D is the axial contrast-enhanced MRI showing heterogeneous

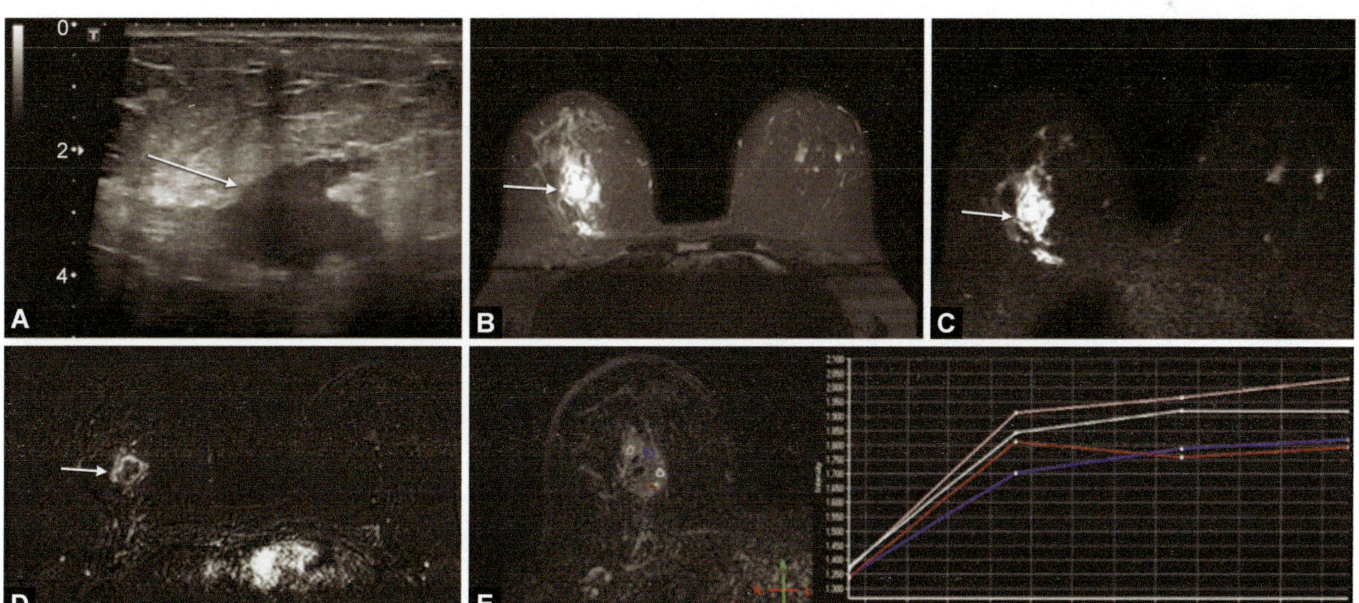

Figs. 2A to E: (A) US image shows a microlobulated, hypoechoic mass in the right breast at 12 o'clock position (long white arrow); (B and C) Axial STIR and diffusion-weighted images show an oval hyperintense lesion having irregular margins in the superior quadrant of right breast; (D) Postcontrast study was done and the lesion shows rim-enhancement; (E) Kinetic curves obtained from various ROIs in the lesion show type 2 pattern (STIR: short tau inversion recovery; ROI: region-of-interest).

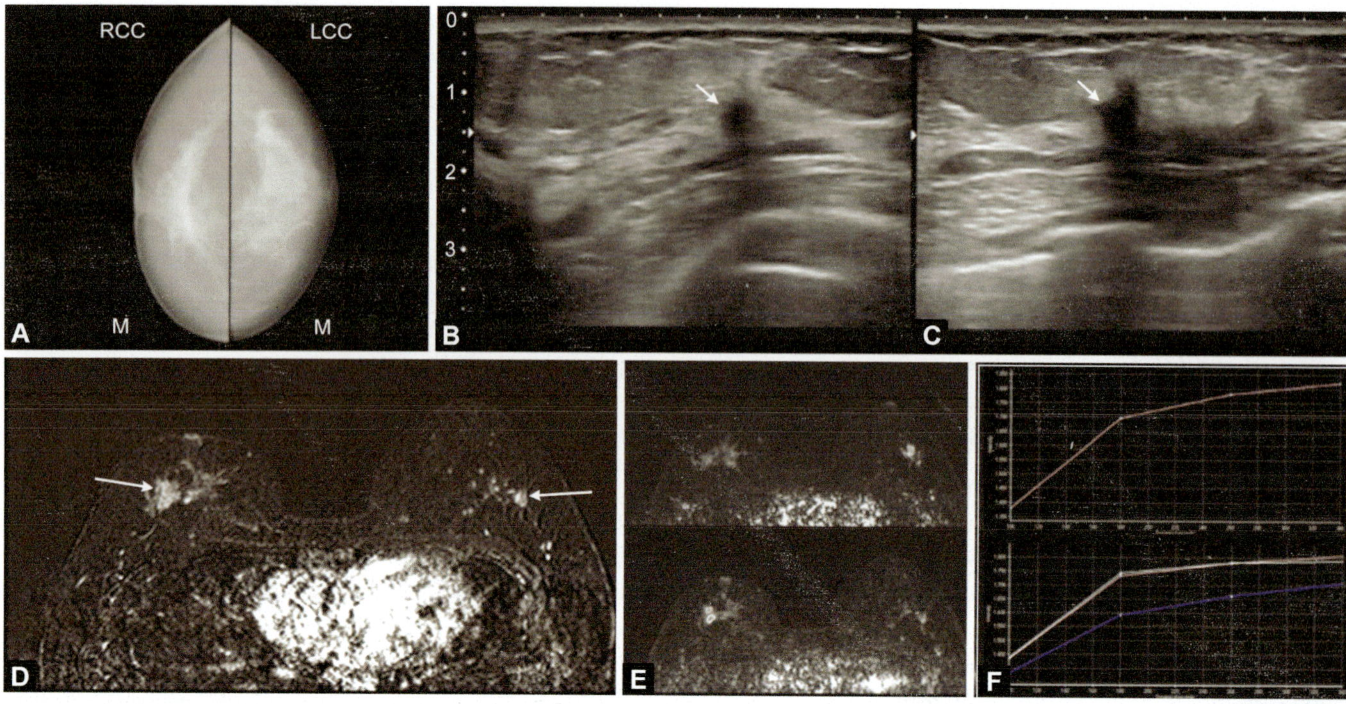

Figs. 3A to E: (A) Mammograph of both breasts (CC view) shows asymmetric density in the left breast. (B) Ultrasound image of right breast shows an irregular hypoechoic lesion having spiculated margins at 9–10 o'clock position (white arrow); (C) Ultrasound image of the left breast shows a small circumscribed round lesion showing posterior acoustic shadowing at 2 o'clock position (white arrow); (D) Axial contrast-enhanced MRI shows heterogeneous enhancement of both lesions (white arrows); (E and F) Kinetic curves obtained from both lesions show type 2 pattern (CC: craniocaudal; MRI: magnetic resonance imaging).

enhancement of both lesions. Figures 3E and F are kinetic curves obtained from both lesions, showing type 2 pattern in both lesion.

The patient underwent an ultrasound-guided biopsy from right breast that showed features of lobular carcinoma.

Since a diagnosis of lobular carcinoma was made histopathologically, the patient underwent. biopsy from left breast which also showed lobular carcinoma.

Comments: For lobular cancers, MR-imaging detection and sizing accuracy have been shown to be superior to physical examination, mammography and ultrasound. Additional ipsilateral disease is reported approximately 50% of the time, while synchronous contralateral disease is reported in 13% of cases. Preoperative MR imaging for lobular cancers changes surgical management.

CASE 4

A 58-year-old woman presented with complaint of lump in right breast since 6 months.

Finding: Figures 4A to D are the axial T1W, T2W, STIR, and contrast-enhanced MRIs of the breasts showing an irregular spiculated mass in the retroareolar region of the right breast with heterogeneous enhancement associated with nipple retraction and skin thickening.

Ultrasound-guided biopsy was s/o invasive ductal carcinoma of right breast. The patient underwent modified radical mastectomy.

CASE 5

A 57-year-old patient underwent breast conserving surgery for left breast carcinoma and she is on annual follow-up.

Findings: Figure 5A is the mammogram of left breast in craniocaudal projection showing a low (fat) density lesion in the region of the surgical scar, surrounded by surgical clips. There is associated architectural distortion and nipple retraction. Figure 5B is the ultrasound of the same lesion that shows a circumscribed oval iso- to hypoechoic lesion that is parallel in orientation. Figure 5C is the axial STIR MRI of the breasts showing that the lesion is completely suppressed on STIR. These findings are s/o fat necrosis.

Comments: Fat necrosis has variable appearances ranging from typically benign to that which is worrisome for

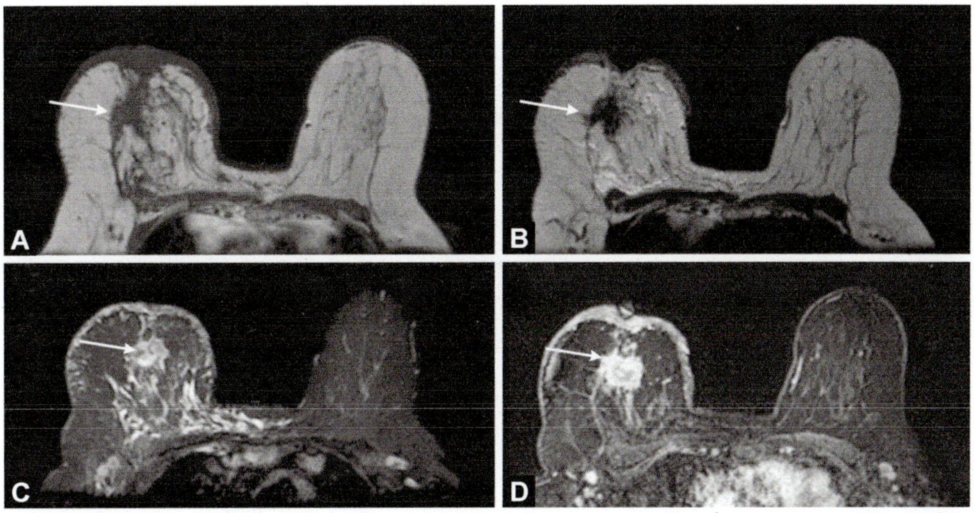

Figs. 4A to D: Diagnostic images of the both breasts show an irregular spiculated mass in the retroareolar region of the right breast (white arrows). The mass shows heterogeneous enhancement and is associated with nipple retraction and skin thickening. (A) Axial T1W image; (B) Axial T2W image; (C) STIR-MRI scan; (D) Contrast-enhanced MRI (STIR: short tau inversion recovery; MRI: magnetic resonance imaging).

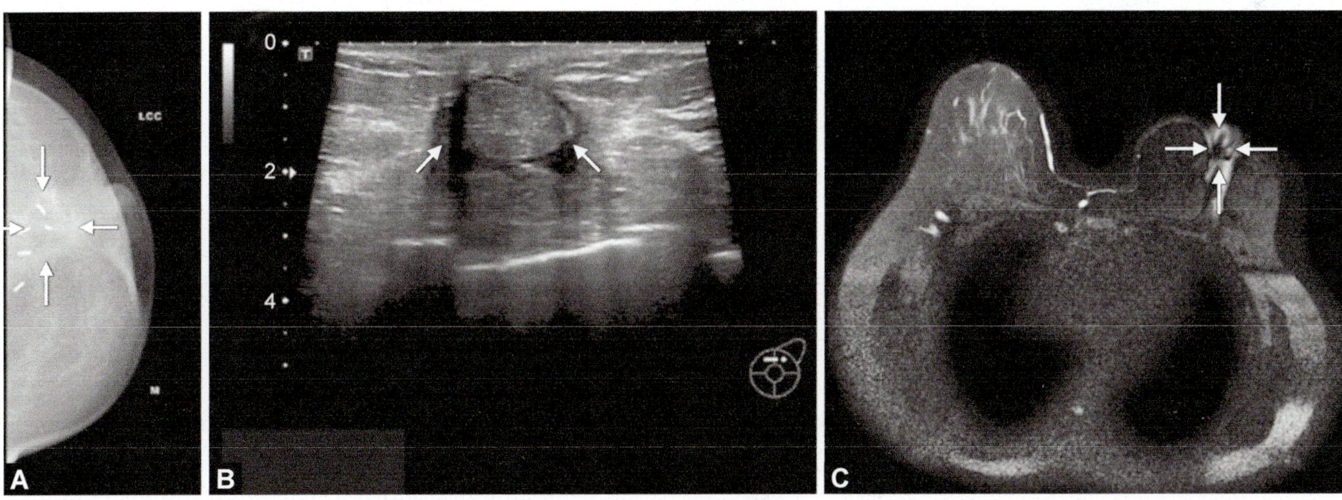

Figs. 5A to C: (A) Mammogram of left breast (CC view) shows a low (fat) density lesion in the region of the surgical scar (white arrows), surrounded by surgical clips; (B) Ultrasound image of the same lesion shows a circumscribed oval iso- to hypoechoic lesion that is parallel in orientation (white arrows); (C) Axial STIR-MRI scan of the breasts shows that the lesion is completely suppressed on STIR (white arrow). (CC: craniocaudal; STIR: short tau inversion recovery; MRI: magnetic resonance imaging).

malignancy. MRI has a wide spectrum of findings for fat necrosis due to inflammatory reaction, the amount of liquefied fat and the degree of fibrosis. The most common appearance of fat necrosis on MRI is a lipid cyst, round or oval mass with hypointense T1-weighted signal on fat saturation images. "Black hole" sign has been described as another characteristic on MRI to help diagnose fat necrosis, marked central hypointensity of the lesion on short tau inversion recovery (STIR) images when compared with surrounding fat.

CASE 6

A 32-year-old female underwent lumpectomy with wide excision for a mass in left breast that on histopathology turned out to be ductal carcinoma in situ with microinvasion. MRI breast was done to look for residual mass.

Findings: Figure 6A is mammogram of left breast showing postoperative changes in the form of architectural distortion, increased density and skin thickening. Figures 6B and C are STIR and T2W sequence showing a circumscribed

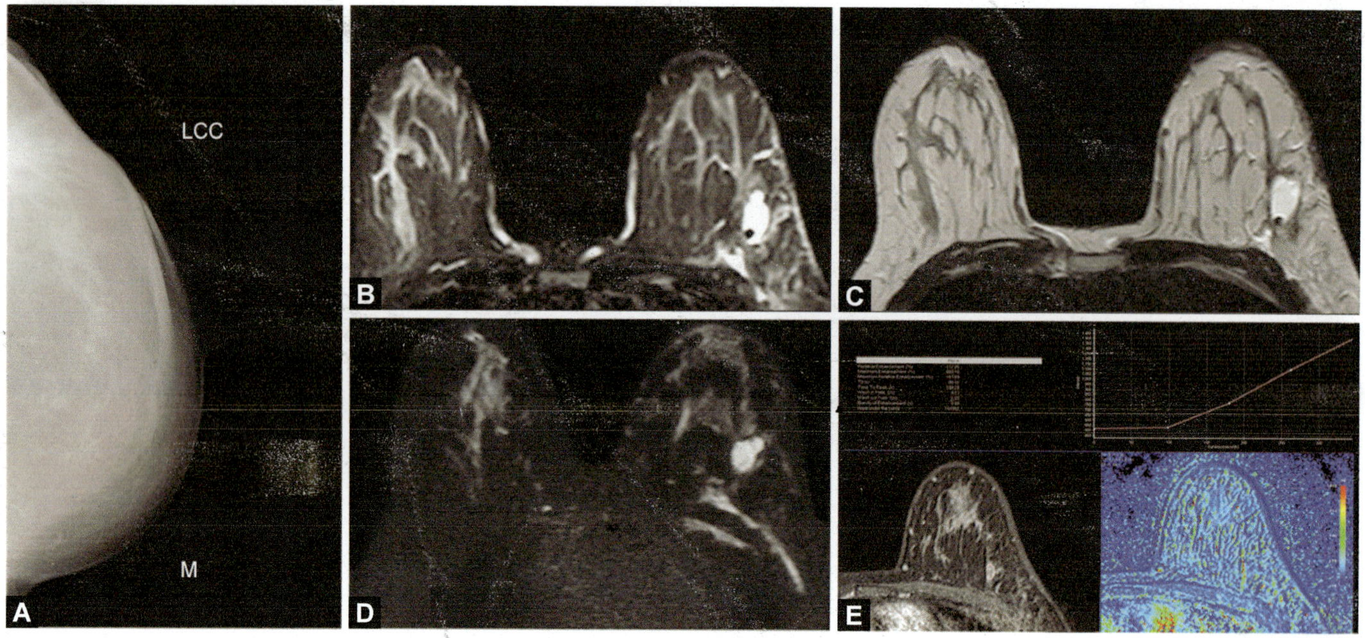

Figs. 6A to E: (A) Mammogram of left breast shows postoperative changes in the form of architectural distortion, increased density and skin thickening; (B and C) STIR and T2W sequence shows a well-defined hyperintense collection; (D) Hypointense collection is showing restriction on DWI; (E) Postcontrast dynamic image shows peripheral enhancement with a type 1 curve (STIR: short tau inversion; DWI: diffusion-weighted image).

hyperintense collection showing restriction on DWI (Fig. 6D). Postcontrast dynamic image (Fig. 6E) shows peripheral enhancement with a type 1 curve. These features represent postoperative seroma. There is no enhancing residual mass in this case.

Comments: As breast conservative surgery is increasing and becoming a common form of treatment in women, the patients who undergo MRI are also increasing in order to look for residual lesion and differentiate it from postsurgical changes. It is a challenge to assess postoperative breast and has a learning curve.

CASE 7

A 58-year-old female was diagnosed with peritoneal malignancy and underwent surgery followed by chemotherapy. The histopathology from the peritoneal lesions showed adenocarcinoma deposits that were morphologically similar to lobular carcinoma of breast.

Therefore, mammogram was done to evaluate the breasts which was followed by MRI.

Findings: Figure 7A is mammogram—craniocaudal view of both breasts which shows an asymmetric density in left breast. Figure 7B is ultrasound image in the medial quadrant of left breast that showed posterior acoustic shadowing. The patient then underwent MRI. Figure 7C is T2W sequence that extended hypointense architectoral deformity in the medial quadrants of left breast. Figure 7D is DWI that shows a hypointense area in the corresponding portion. Figure 7E is dynamic postcontrast sequence showing irregular area of non-mass enhancement in the medial quadrant extending posteriorly. Figure 7F is the time intensity curve showing type 2 curve. An ultrasound-guided biopsy was done from the hypoechoic area with posterior shadowing in the left breast.

Histopathology showed infiltrating tumor composed of "Indian file" pattern of monotonous neoplastic cells with scant neoplasm, round to oval hyperchromatic nuclei and desmoplastic fibrous stroma. The findings were s/o invasive lobular carcinoma.

Comments: Lobular carcinoma frequently metastasizes to unusual sites, including the gastrointestinal tract, peritoneum and adnexa. Gastrointestinal tract involvement is as frequent as liver involvement, appearing as bowel wall thickening on computed tomography (CT) scan. It is not uncommon for patients to first present with symptoms associated with their gastrointestinal metastatic disease, like early satiety, epigastric pain and weight loss, as their initial presentation of their breast cancer rather than from mammogram findings or palpatory findings on physical examination of the breast.

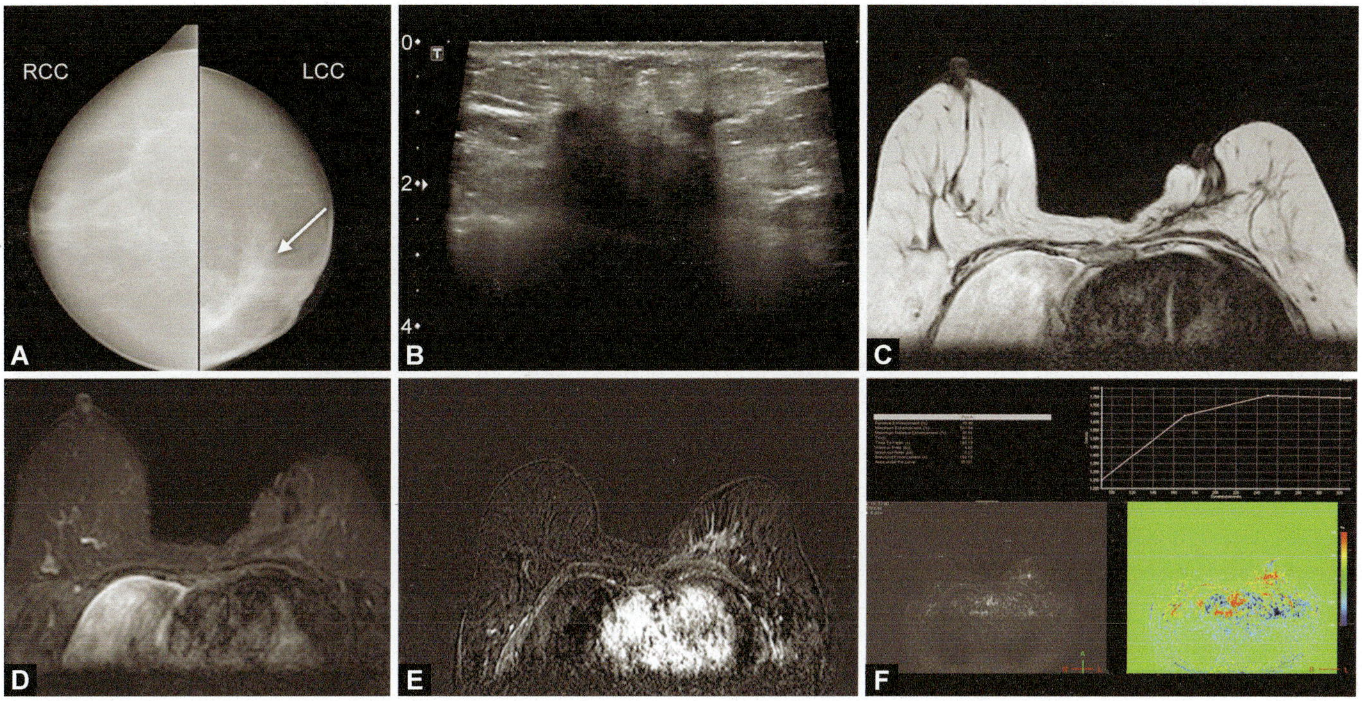

Figs. 7A to F: (A) Mammogram (CC view) of both breasts shows an architectoral deformity in left breast; (B) Ultrasound image in the medial quadrant of left breast shows irregular hypoechoic mass with posterior acoustic shadowing; (C) T2W sequence shows hypointense architectoral deformity in the medial quadrants of left breast; (D) DWI shows a hypointense area in the corresponding portion; (E) Dynamic postcontrast sequence shows irregular area of non-mass enhancement in the medial quadrant extending posteriorly; (F) Time intensity curve shows type 2 curve (CC: craniocaudal; DWI: diffusion-weighted image).

CASE 8

A 46-year-old woman underwent breast conservative surgery for carcinoma left breast followed by chemotherapy and radiotherapy 1 year back. She now presented with right nipple discharge. There was no palpable lump. Ultrasound of right breast was normal.

Mammogram of both breasts was done followed by MRI.

Findings: Figure 8A is mammogram-craniocaudal view of left breast showing increase breast density and skin thickening. Figures 8B and C are T2W and STIR sequence showing skin thickening and coarsened trabecular pattern with hyperintensity in left breast due to postsurgical and postradiation breast edema. There is also irregular hyperintensity in left pectoralis muscle likely due to postradiation changes. Figure 8D is DWI showing mild restriction in superomedial quadrant of left breast. Figure 8E is postcontrast T1W sequence showing non-mass-like enhancement at the surgical site.

There was no focal lesion or abnormal enhancement in right breast.

The above findings represent post-radiation treatment changes and should not be confused with recurrence.

Comments: Post-treatment changes include edema, skin thickening, seroma and enhancement at the lumpectomy site which progressively decrease over time. Lumpectomy site enhancement may be seen in one third of women till first 12 months after treatment and may persist in 15% of women at 5 or more years.

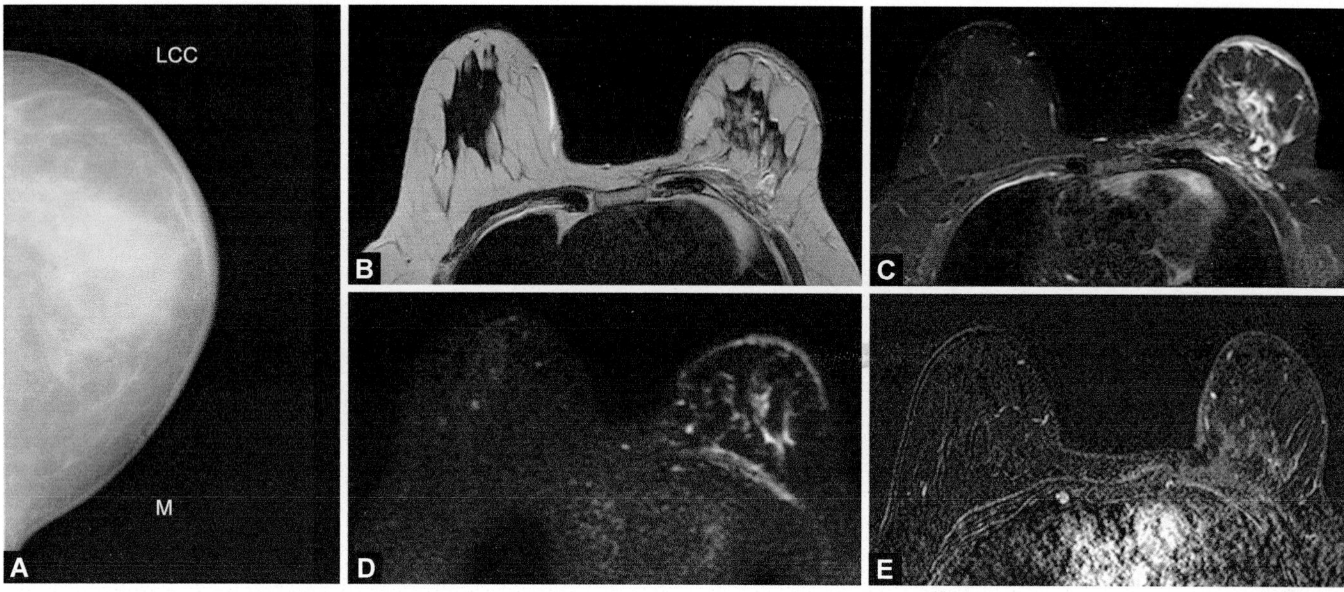

Figs. 8A to E: (A) Mammogram (CC view) of left breast shows increase breast density and skin thickening; (B and C) T2W and STIR sequence show skin thickening and coarsened trabecular pattern with hyperintensity in left breast due to postsurgical and postradiation breast edema; (D) DWI shows mild restriction in superomedial quadrant of left breast; (E) Postcontrast T1W sequence shows non-mass-like enhancement at the surgical site (CC: craniocaudal; STIR: short tau inversion recovery; DWI: diffusion-weighted image).

Inflammatory Conditions of Breast

CHAPTER 5

INTRODUCTION

Breast inflammation has a wide spectrum of etiologies, ranging from infection to the dreaded inflammatory cancer. The history, clinical presentation and imaging features are often non-specific and cause a diagnostic dilemma. The context in which the inflammation arises and how and where it occurs should be clearly defined by proper clinical examination, since these are essential for proper radiologic diagnosis of the inflammatory process and for monitoring its evolution/resolution.

Inflammatory diseases of breast include mastitis (puerperal and non-puerperal), breast abscess, idiopathic granulomatous mastitis (IGM), tuberculosis, plasma cell mastitis, sarcoidosis, fungal infections, etc. Secondary infection of sebaceous cysts, hidradenitis and infectious complications after plastic surgery or radiotherapy may also be encountered.

According to the WHO, **mastitis** is defined as an inflammation of the breast, which may or may not be accompanied by an infection. An **abscess** is a complication of mastitis, although it may not be necessarily preceded by symptomatic mastitis. The diagnosis and treatment of breast abscess, both puerperal and non-puerperal is challenging and the radiologist plays an important part in the multidisciplinary team that manages these patients.

Idiopathic granulomatous mastitis is a diagnosis of exclusion in patients who are referred for imaging after repeated course of antibiotics, multiple unsuccessful attempts at drainage and incomplete response to treatment for mastitis. A core needle biopsy is needed in these cases to establish the diagnosis.

Primary breast tuberculosis is rare even in India, and its imaging features overlap with other infections and malignancy. Its diagnosis needs a high index of suspicion and histopathological evaluation that demonstrates acid fast bacilli since the course of treatment is long and completely different from other inflammatory pathologies.

Considering that there is often an overlap between the clinical and imaging findings of various forms of breast inflammation/infection and inflammatory cancer, *whenever there is a clinical suspicion of malignancy or an atypical clinical course of mastitis, core needle biopsy is imperative for diagnosis.*

DISEASES

Mastitis

Puerperal or nonpuerperal mastitis is the inflammation of breast parenchyma. Puerperal mastitis may be seen in 1–24% of breast feeding women[1] and is an important cause of morbidity. Non-puerperal mastitis is seen in women following rupture of underlying ectatic ducts or cysts, producing chemical inflammation.

Clinical Features

Puerperal mastitis is infectious mastitis, generally seen within the first postpartum week. Patients present clinically with tender, red, hot, indurated and painful breast with nipple retraction or axillary node enlargement. There may be associated symptoms like fever, nausea or lethargy. The underlying cause is generally bacterial infection by a skin contaminant, commonly staphylococcus aureus, staphylococcus epidermidis or streptococcus pyogenes. *It is important to encourage breastfeeding during this period to reduce duct engorgement*, unless antibiotics contraindicated in breastfeeding are given for management.

Infectious mastitis should be distinguished from congestive or non-infectious mastitis which is due to engorgement of breast on second or third day of breastfeeding. The latter presents clinically with tenderness or swelling of both breasts without any inflammation or edema and has a self-limiting course.

Imaging

Ultrasound is the imaging modality of choice. An ill-defined irregular heterogeneous hypoechoic area with (Fig. 1) or without vascularity is noted within parenchyma associated with increased echogenicity of surrounding fat lobules (Fig. 2).[1] The pertinent role of ultrasound specifically in this

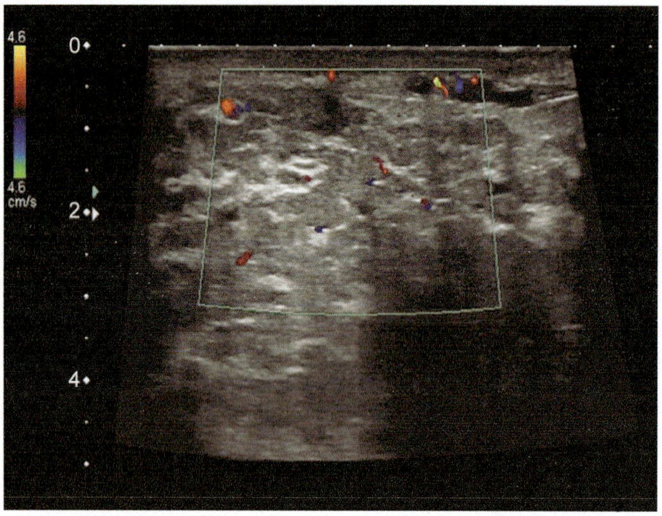

Fig. 1: Ultrasound of breast in a 31-year old female shows increased echogenicity of fat with increased vascularity s/o mastitis.

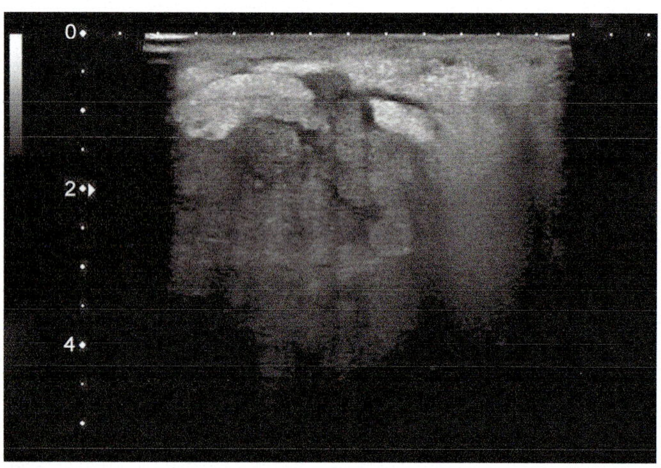

Fig. 2: A 26-year old lactating female presented with pain and tenderness in right breast since 1 week. Ultrasound of the right breast showed an irregular heterogeneous area with increased vascularity s/o mastitis. Patient was managed conservatively.

situation is to look for underlying abscess (Figs. 3 and 4) which is a well-known complication of mastitis. Other associated ultrasound features include skin thickening, prominent lymphatic vessels or enlarged axillary lymph nodes.

Breast Abscess

Breast abscess is the outcome of uncontrolled inflammatory mastitis and generally occurs in young women. Puerperal abscesses have a better outcome and a shorter clinical course as compared to non-puerperal abscesses.

Earlier, these were managed by incision and drainage, but now management has changed with active participation by radiologist in managing and following up these patients.

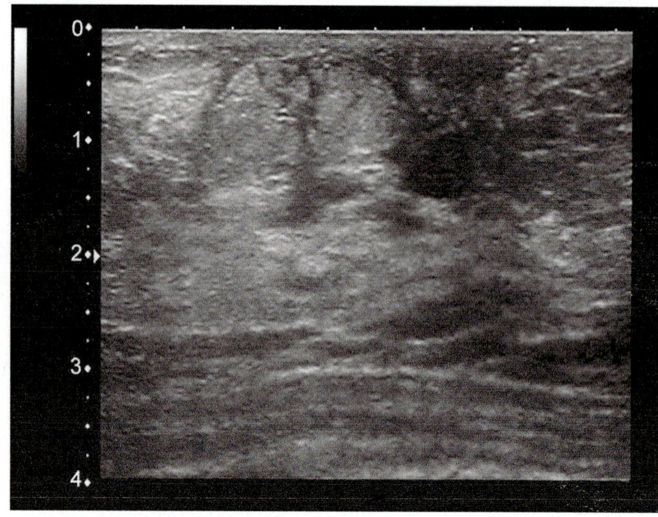

Fig. 3: Ultrasound of breast in a 18-year old female showing inflamed echogenic fat with evolving abscess.

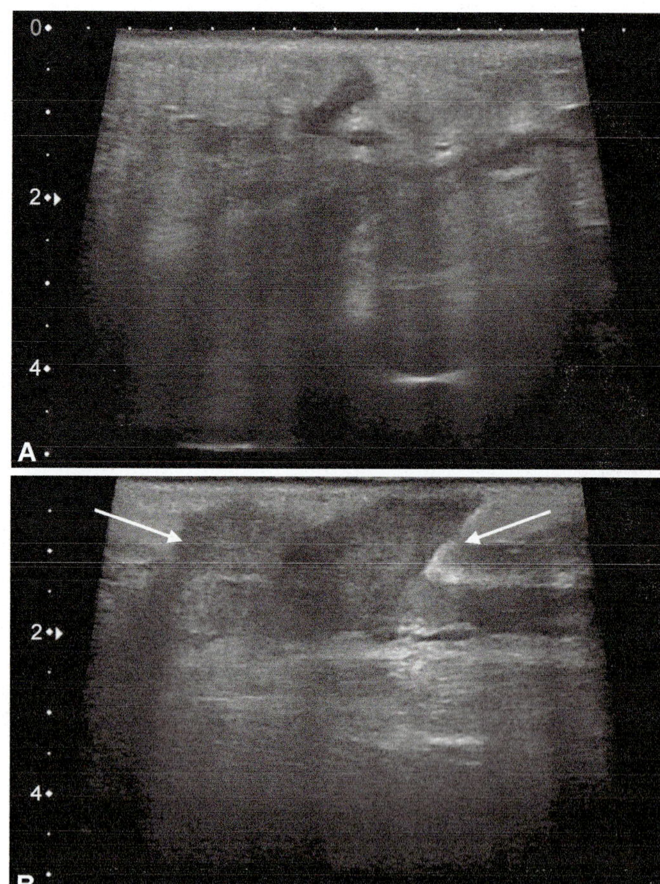

Figs. 4A and B: A 62-year old woman presented with painful and inflamed right breast. Ultrasound of right breast (A and B) showed inflamed echogenic fat with a hypoechoic collection (arrows). Ultrasound-guided aspiration was done which showed thick pus consistent with abscess and moderate growth of *Staphylococcus* was seen on culture.

Clinical Features

The patient presents with breast edema, pain, warmth and redness in a localized portion of breast; though a larger area may be involved. Associated symptoms like fever, nausea, vomiting and spontaneous discharge from nipple may also be present.

Imaging

Ultrasound allows accurate localization and assessment of extension, number of abscess cavities, communicating pockets and consistency. It also provides information regarding amenability for percutaneous drainage under imaging guidance and eventually allows follow-up to look for resolution.

Ultrasound features depend upon the stage of abscess, whether it is liquefied or has become organized. The ultrasound findings range from ill-defined or well-defined heterogeneous hypoechoic collections with low-level echoes, heterogeneous mass with a hypoechoic necrotic central component having peripheral vascularity or anechoic to hypoechoic collection with multiple septations (Figs. 5 to 8). Posterior acoustic enhancement is usually present. The surrounding parenchyma is echogenic because of inflamed fat lobules with increased vascularity on color Doppler. In addition, enlarged hypoechoic axillary lymph nodes with a thickened cortex may also be present. Sometimes, there may be a chronic, partially-treated abscess which appears well defined and heterogeneous (Fig. 9).

Mammography can be performed in older women but should be withheld until the acute episode gets over as it can add to the discomfort, while the examination itself is difficult due to inflammation-induced increased breast density and corresponding decrease in compressibility. Mammographic findings are nonspecific and include skin thickening, asymmetric density, architectural distortion or mass. If suspicious microcalcifications are present, core needle biopsy should be performed to rule out an underlying malignancy. The features differentiating between breast abscess and inflammatory carcinomas are discussed later.

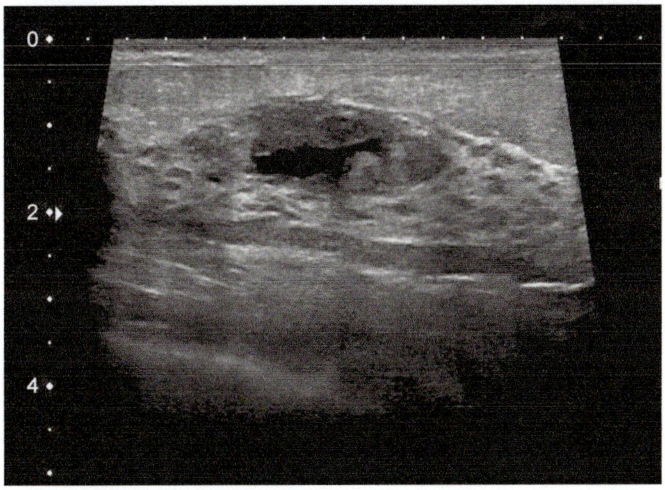

Fig. 5: A 21-year old female presented with pain and tenderness in left breast. Ultrasound of breast showed a thick-walled cystic mass. Ultrasound-guided aspiration showed thick pus.

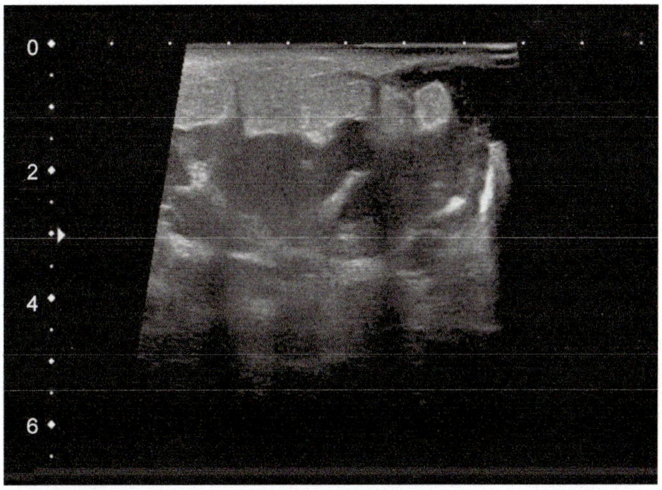

Fig. 6: A 42-year old female presented with pain in the left breast and fever. Ultrasound showed an irregular hypoechoic collection with low-level echoes. Surrounding fat appears echogenic s/o inflammation. Thick pus was aspirated out.

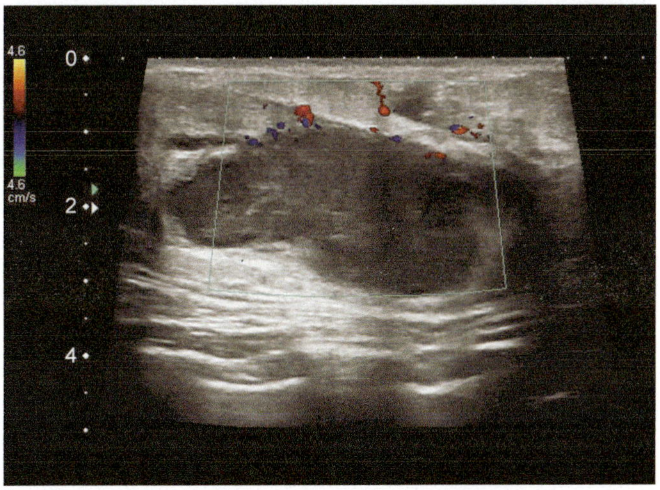

Fig. 7: A 23-year old female presented with complaint of pain and tenderness in left breast along with a palpable lump. The patient had undergone irregular treatment with antibiotics. A possibility of antibioma was considered clinically. Ultrasound showed a hypoechoic lesion with closely packed echoes without internal vascularity and thick pus was aspirated out.

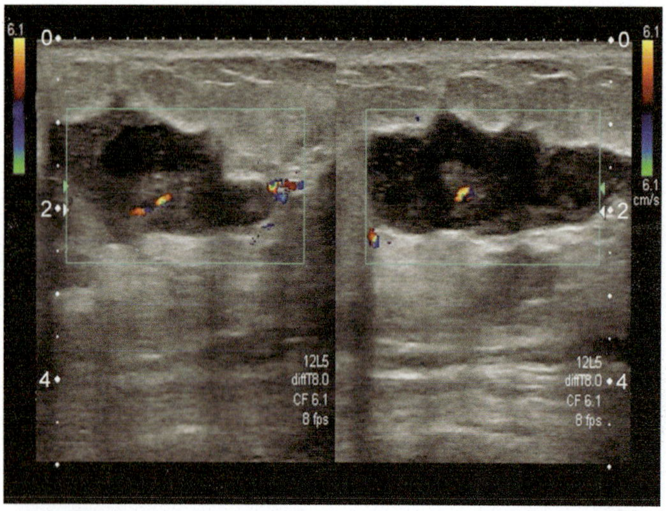

Fig. 8: A 25-year old female presented with breast pain on right side. Ultrasound of breast showed an irregular hypoechoic lesion having a hyperechoic area showing vascularity and a cystic component within. Features were s/o abscess and pus was aspirated.

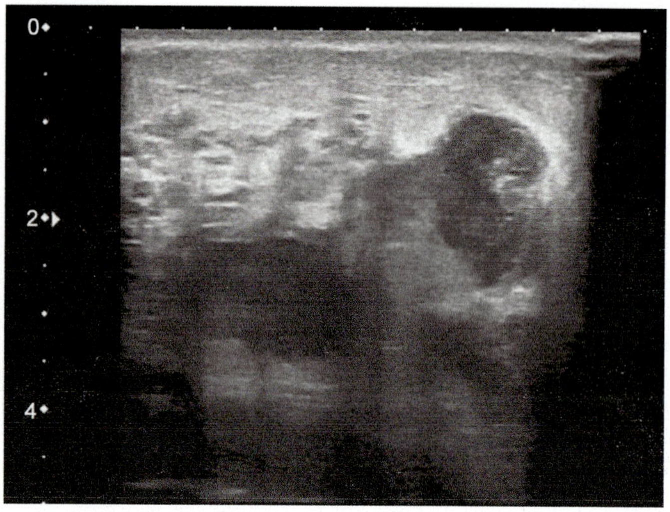

Fig. 10: A 28-year old female who was breast feeding her child came with a complaint of pain and redness in left breast. Ultrasound showed multiple pockets of collections communicating with each other. Thick pus was aspirated s/o lactational abscess and microbiological examination showed growth of *Staphylococcus aureus*.

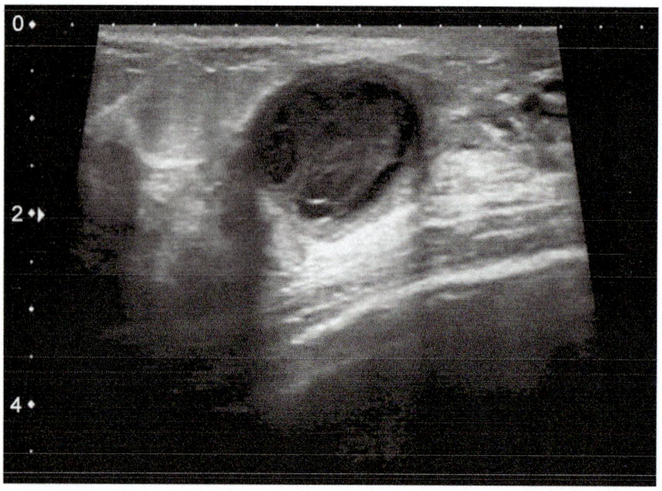

Fig. 9: A 36-year old female presented with painful lump in right breast for 4 weeks which reduced in size after a course of antibiotics. Ultrasound of the breast showed a circumscribed hypoechoic lesion with multiple septations. Aspiration showed chronic abscess.

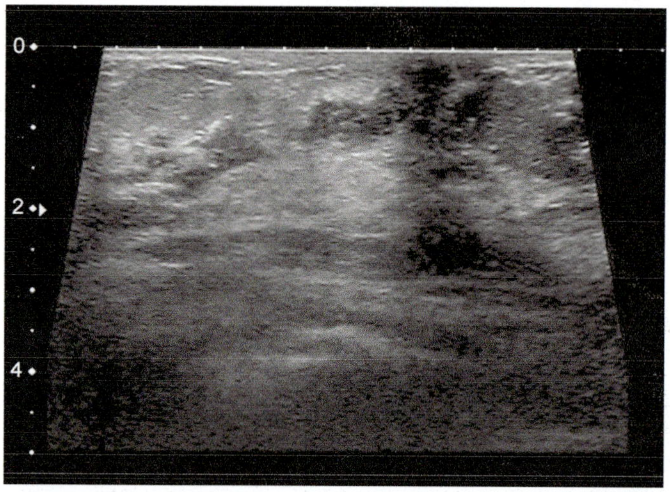

Fig. 11: A 33-year old female who is breast feeding her child came with complaint of pain and tenderness in right breast. Ultrasound of breast showed thick walled collection having low-level echoes with surrounding echogenic fat. Features were s/o lactational breast abscess. Thick pus was aspirated and organism isolated was *E. coli*.

Types of Breast Abscess

Breast abscesses are clinically divided into two types: Puerperal and non-puerperal.

Puerperal abscess: Also known as lactational abscesses, they are seen as a complication of mastitis in 5-11% of cases and occur within the first 12 weeks of childbirth or at the time of weaning.[2] The most common organism involved is staphylococcus aureus which enters via skin lacerations and proliferates in stagnant lactiferous ducts. An appearances are variable, ranging from heterogeneous masses to well-defined hypoechoic masses with low-level echoes (Figs. 10 to 13). These abscesses respond well to drainage and antibiotic treatment and have a shorter clinical course.

Nonpuerperal abscess: They occur outside the breast-feeding period and can be central or peripheral in location. Smoking and obesity are risk factors for development of these abscesses.[3]

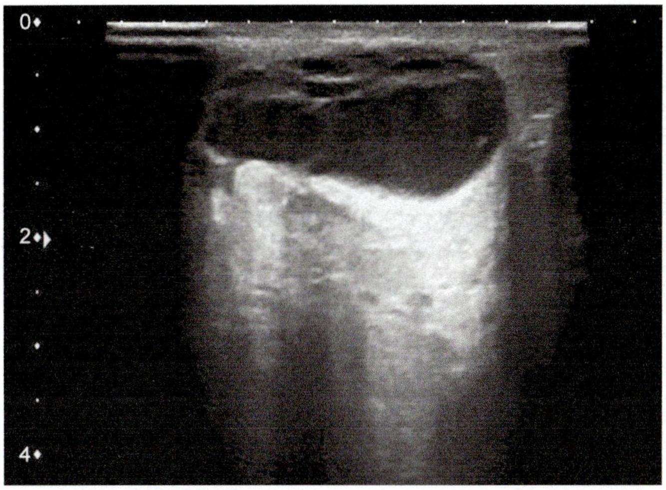

Fig. 12: A 28-year old female who was breastfeeding her child came with a complaint of pain and tenderness in the lower quadrant of left breast. Ultrasound showed a circumscribed hypoechoic collection in lower quadrant having multiple septations.

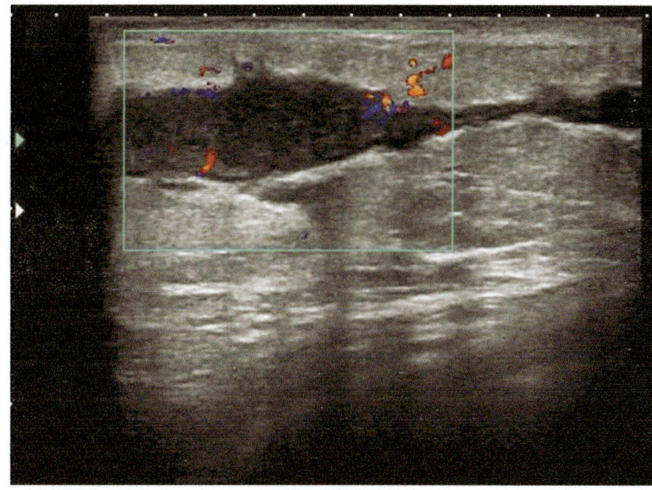

Fig. 14: A 28-year old female presented with painful right breast lump for last 3 months. Ultrasound of right breast showed multiple circumscribed hypoechoic lesions interconnecting with each other. Histopathology was s/o granulomatous mastitis.

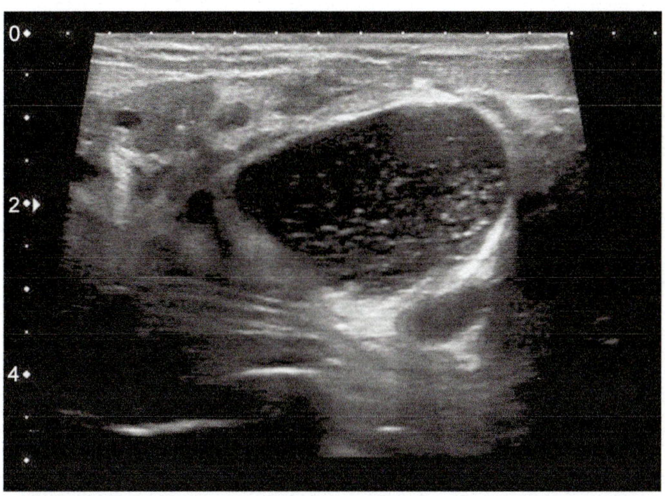

Fig. 13: A 35-year old female who was lactating presented with a lump in left breast with pain. Ultrasound revealed a circumscribed hypoechoic lesion with refractile echoes. No vascularity was seen. Thick milky fluid was aspirated s/o galactocele.

Central or periareolar abscesses: These occur in young women due to periductal mastitis, resulting from acute inflammation and cellular infiltrates in the retroareolar region which blocks the lactiferous ducts and causes duct dilatation. The dilated ducts get secondarily infected and form an abscess with or without cutaneous fistulae. "Zuska disease" is the term given to recurrent central abscesses with cutaneous fistulas. The abscesses have a chronic course and are difficult to treat. Staphylococcus, streptococcus and sometimes anaerobes are found and treatment is by percutaneous drainage and antibiotics.

Table 1: Difference between nonpuerperal and puerperal abscess.

S.No	*Nonpuerperal abscess*	*Puerperal abscess*
1.	**Age range:** Midteens to eighth decade	Reproductive age group
2.	Associated with smoking	Association with lactation
3.	**Younger patients:** (1) More pain due to acute inflammation and periductal mastitis. (2) Nipple discharge is thinner **Older patients:** (1) Less pain due to less acute inflammation and more fibrosis. (2) Nipple discharge is viscous	Pain and inflammation
4.	Recurrences more common	Recurrences are less
5.	Require multiple drainage or surgical procedure	Does not require multiple drainage
6.	Fistula formation between abscess cavity and skin surface is more common.	Fistula formation is less common

Peripheral: These abscesses are found in slightly older women, especially those with chronic medical conditions and those who have undergone surgery or radiotherapy. The common pathogens are *Staphylococcus aureus*, *Streptococcus* and anaerobes. As there is good response to antibiotics, recurrences are rare (Table 1).

Flowchart 1: Algorithm for diagnosis and treatment of breast abscess.

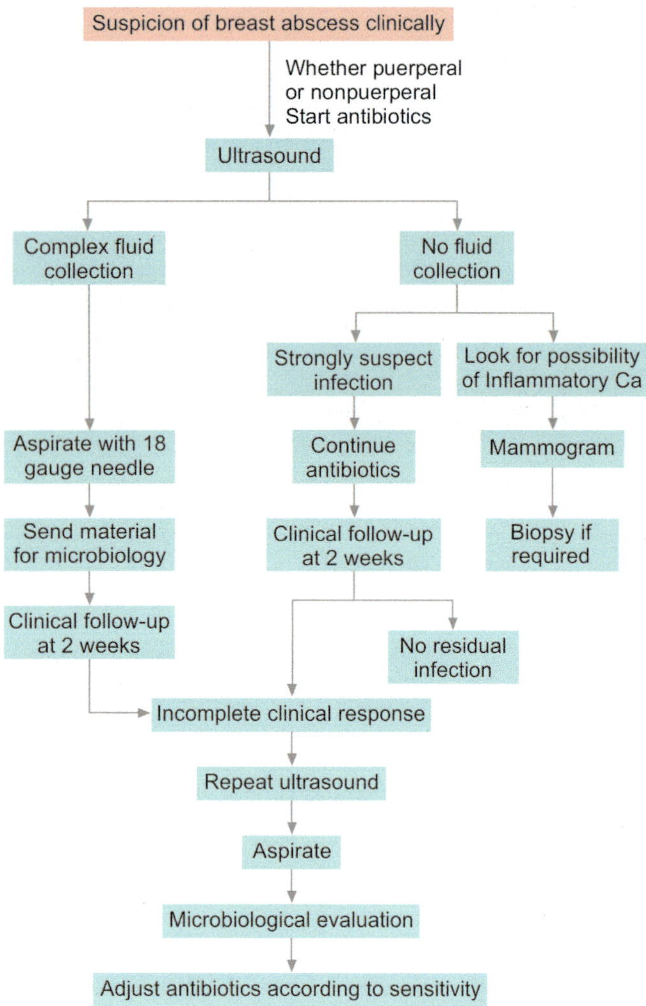

Treatment: Algorithm for diagnosis and treatment of breast abscess is given in flow chart 1.

Idiopathic Granulomatous Mastitis

IGM is due to chronic inflammation of the breast tissue, first described by Kessler and Wolloch in 1972.[4] Its diagnosis is made after other causes are excluded. It is common in Asian women.

It is commonly seen in women of childbearing age with history of recent child birth, ranging from 2 to 9 months after delivery and in those using oral contraceptives.

It often causes a diagnostic dilemma and shows overlapping imaging and clinical findings with malignancy and other inflammatory conditions like plasma cell mastitis, tuberculosis, histoplasmosis, Wegener granulomatosis, etc.[5] On histopathology, there is non-necrotizing granulomatous inflammation of lobules[6] and no microorganisms are found.

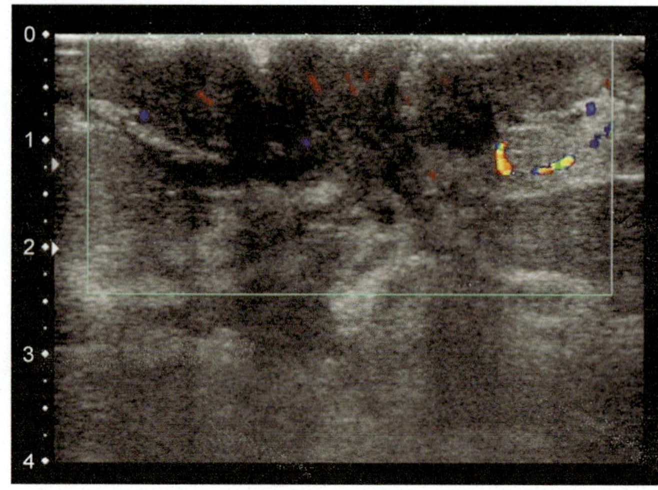

Fig. 15: A 33-year old female presented with on and off pain in right breast. Ultrasound showed an ill-defined hypoechoic lesion showing minimal vascularity and a suspicion of malignancy was considered. Histopathology was s/o granulomatous mastitis.

Clinical Features

IGM presents most commonly with a breast lump which may be unilateral and firm to hard in consistency on palpation. Sometimes, bilateral involvement is seen. The other presenting symptoms include mastalgia, nipple retraction, draining sinus or axillary lymphadenopathy.

Etiopathogenesis

The etiology is not known properly but since it responds to steroids, it is hypothesized that it can be autoimmune in origin. It is seen in reproductive age women and there is an association with lactation. During lactation damage to ductal epithelium occurs due to local trauma[6] which in turn leads to accumulation of secretions and their extravasation. This causes a granulomatous response.

The other causes are oral contraceptives[7] and duct ectasia where there is duct dilatation and rupture causing periductal mastitis.[8] An autoimmune origin is also hypothesized.

Imaging

Ultrasound There are varied appearances of granulomatous mastitis on ultrasound which include parenchymal heterogeneity, multiple hypoechoic masses with tubular extension connecting with nearby masses (Fig 14), irregular heterogenously hypoechoic area or mass (Fig 15), mass with abscess formation with low-level echoes (Fig. 16), and hypoechoic mass with tubular extension

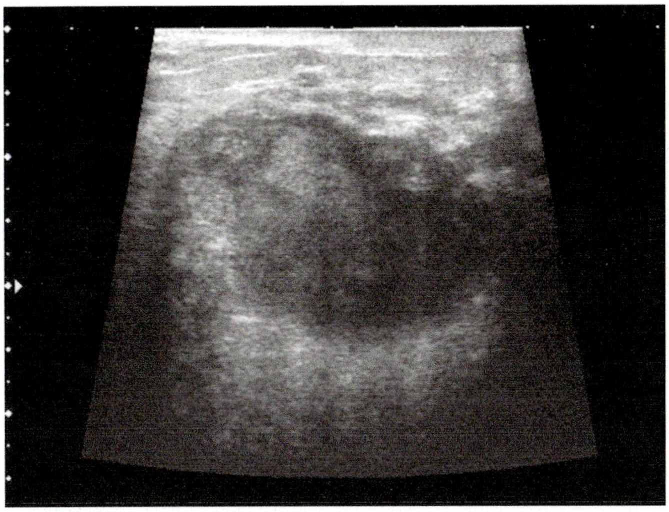

Fig. 16: A 42-year old female presented with a painless, hard mass for last 4 months and clinically a suspicion of malignancy was considered. Ultrasound showed a well-defined heterogeneous mass with thick echoes at places which turned out to be idiopathic granulomatous mastitis on histopathology.

to subcutaneous tissue and skin surface (Figs. 17A and B). According to Kiyak et al.,[9] if there is abscess formation with parenchymal heterogeneity and axillary nodes, a possibility of inflammatory process should be considered which should be confirmed by histopathology. Other synchronous findings include subcutaneous fat obliteration and skin thickening.

The appearance of irregular heterogeneous mass (Fig. 18) on ultrasound simulates carcinoma and causes a diagnostic dilemma, hence biopsy is indicated. An increase in vascularity in the involved area on color doppler may also be seen in some cases.

Mammogram: It is not possible to distinguish granulomatous mastitis with other inflammatory conditions on mammography. Findings include focal asymmetric density (Figs. 19A and B) architectural distortion, increased density due to diffuse inflammation, skin thickening and benign axillary lymph nodes.[10] Unilateral involvement is common though bilateral involvement has also been reported.

Differential Diagnosis

Malignancy should always be ruled out on histopathology and when there is diffuse involvement of breast, it is important to rule out **inflammatory carcinoma**.

The common mammography findings in inflammatory carcinoma include enlarged breast with prominent

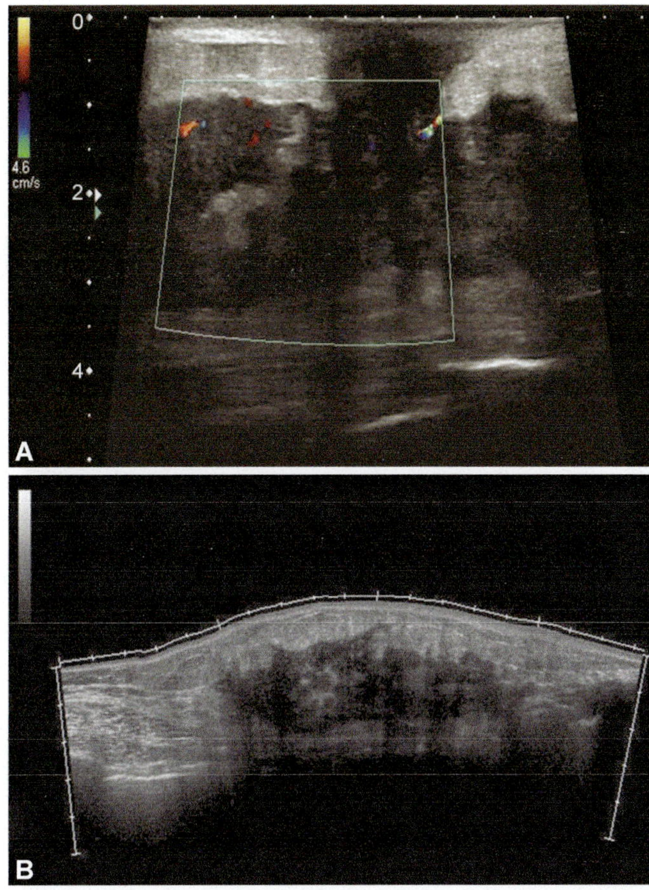

Figs. 17A and B: A 31-year old female presented with pain and swelling in the left breast with h/o fever off and on. Ultrasound (A and B) showed a large irregular heterogeneously hypoechoic lesion in the left breast with increased vascularity in some areas and extension to skin surface. Histopathology was s/o granulomatous mastitis.

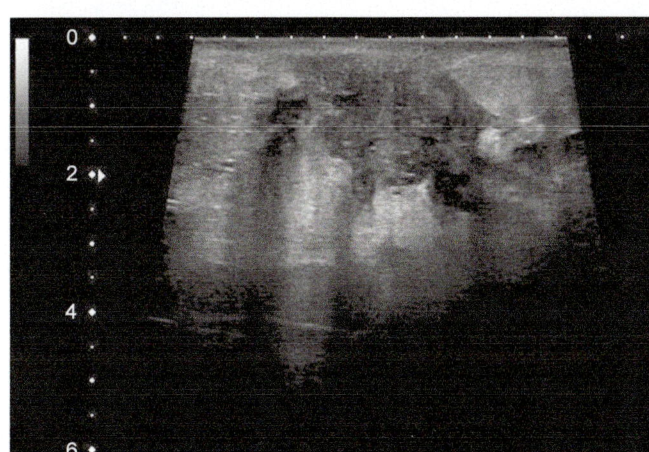

Fig. 18: A 38-year old female presented with pain and tenderness in right breast for which she had been on antibiotics. Ultrasound of the right breast showed a heterogeneous area with irregular margins. No collection was seen. Ultrasound guided biopsy was done which was s/o granulomatous mastitis.

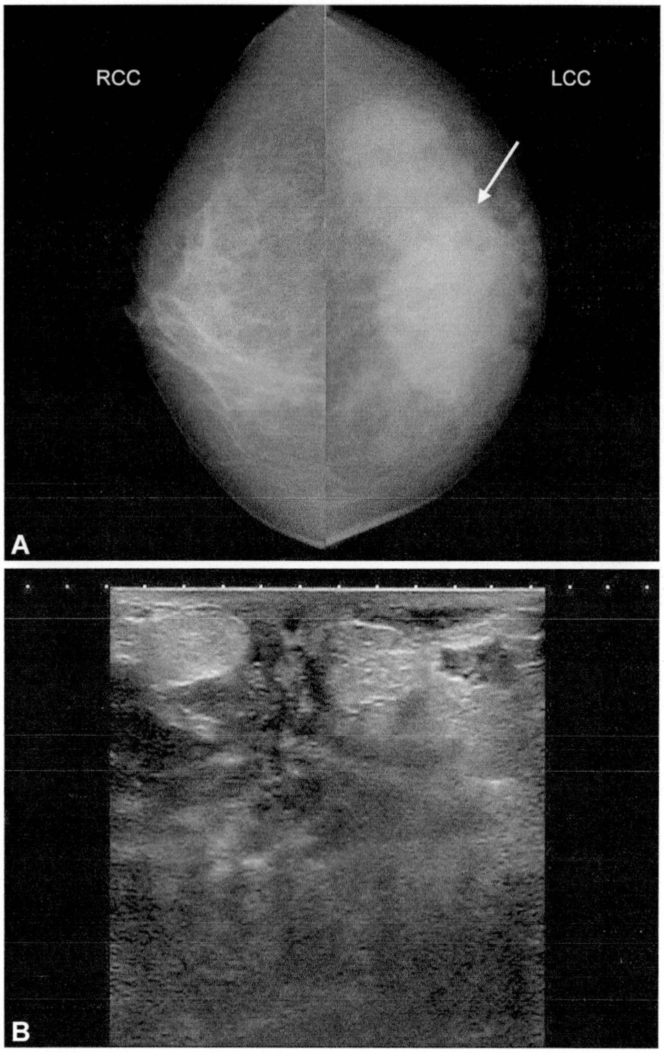

Figs. 19A and B: A 45-year old female presented with lump in left breast for two months. (A) Mammogram (Cranio-caudal view) showed an asymmetric density in left breast which on (B) Ultrasound was seen as irregular hypoechoic areas with low-level echoes extending up to the subcutaneous plane. Histopathology was s/o granulomatous mastitis.

trabeculae because of edema, architectural distortion and skin thickening.

Microcalcifications may be present as opposed to IGM where the lesions almost never calcify.

Tubercular Mastitis: This is another differential diagnosis of an inflammatory condition affecting young parous women that has overlapping imaging features with IGM. One must differentiate these two because they require completely different treatment. Histopathological and microbiological evaluation is essential to make a definitive diagnosis of tuberculous mastitis over IGM.

Microscopically: IGM is a diagnosis of exclusion. It shows chronic lobulitis with granulomatous inflammation and polymorphonuclear leucocytes, giant cells and epitheloid cells. There may be predominant neutrophils with absence of caseous necrosis.

Tuberculosis is the most important differential diagnosis and shows AFB (Acid fast bacilli) in sections or positive culture for acid-fast bacilli.

Management

The treatment of IGM remains controversial with options ranging from conservative management with antibiotics to wide local excision and corticosteroid therapy. Treatment must be tailored to the patient's clinical presentation.

Breast Tuberculosis

Tuberculosis of breast is a rare disease and is more common in developing countries as compared to the western countries. It is important to be aware of the imaging findings of breast tuberculosis as it may mimic a carcinoma. Sir Astley Cooper described the first case of breast tuberculosis in 1829 and called it "scrofulous swelling of the bosom."[11]

The incidence of breast tuberculosis in western countries is <0.1%,[12,13] but with increase in HIV patients, its incidence has increased. In India, there is increased incidence of pulmonary and extrapulmonary tuberculosis, still breast tuberculosis is uncommon with an incidence of 0.64–3.59%.[14] There is an overlap in clinical features of carcinoma and pyogenic abscess; hence, there has to be a high index of suspicion.

Clinical Features

The most common clinical presentation is a lump more commonly in upper outer quadrant with axillary lymph node involvement. The lump may be painful, hard, irregular and sometimes fixed to the chest wall. Clinically it is difficult to distinguish from carcinoma. Another presentation can be skin ulceration with discharging sinuses and underlying abscess formation.[15] Fever may or may not be present.

Breast tuberculosis typically affects young lactating multiparous women, possibly because the breast in this period is more prone to trauma and infection due to increased hormonal activity, increased vascularity and dilated ducts.[16,17] Males and elderly patients are rarely affected.

Routes of infection: Breast is generally resistant to tuberculosis; hence, primary tuberculosis is rare. Most often it is due to secondary involvement from active focus elsewhere.

It can spread through a hematogeneous route or via lympatics, direct inoculation, contiguous spread or through infection of the ducts.[18]

The most commonly accepted theory is spread from the lungs through lymphatic pathway involving trachea-bronchial, paratracheal, mediastinal and internal mammary nodes. There can be a retrograde spread to the breast from axillary lymph nodes according to Cooper.[19]

Classification of Tuberculosis

Breast tuberculosis is classified as either primary or secondary type. In primary tuberculosis which is extremely rare, there is no tubercular focus elsewhere in the body, whereas in secondary tuberculosis, there is a known tubercular infection elsewhere.

Breast tuberculosis was first classified by McKeown and Wilkinson into five types[18]: (1) nodular tubercular mastitis, (2) disseminated or confluent tubercular mastitis, (3) sclerosing tubercular mastitis, (4) tuberculous mastitis obliterans and (5) acute miliary tubercular mastitis.

The terms Sclerosing tubercular mastitis, tuberculous mastitis obliterans and acute miliary tubercular are not used now.

The sclerosing form with excessive fibrosis was seen in elderly women with involuting breast. In tuberculous mastitis obliterans, there was proliferation of ductal epithelium due to duct infection leading to periductal fibrosis and occluded ducts producing cystic spaces (cystic mastitis). Acute miliary tubercular mastitis was a part of generalized miliary tuberculosis and is not seen these days.

With the change in clinical presentation, tuberculosis is now reclassified as:

- Nodulocaseous tubercular mastitis
- Disseminated/confluent tubercular mastitis
- Tubercular breast abscess.

In nodulocaseous tuberculosis, there may be an abscess, painless mass with involvement of skin and subcutaneous tissue and formation of sinuses in later stages. When there is dissemination of tuberculosis, the individual foci coalesce and caseate and lead to sinus formation.

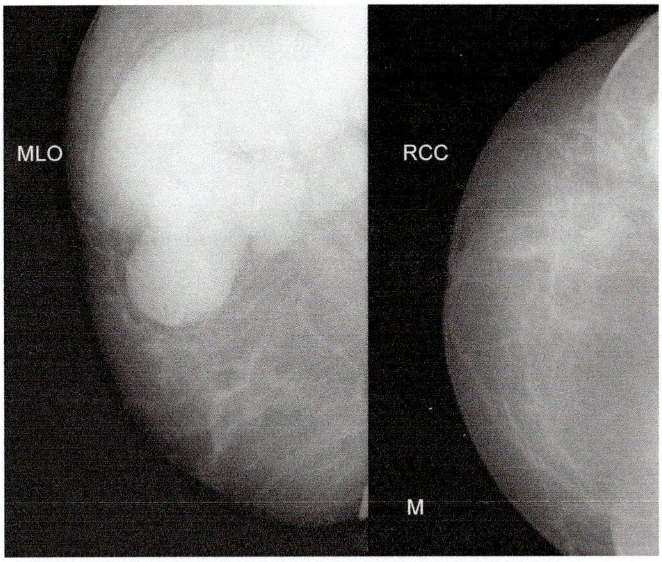

Fig. 20: A 42-year-old female presented with lump in right axillary region. Mammogram-Mediolateral oblique view showed a multilobulated mass in right axillary region which was extending down to the upper quadrant s/o axillary lymphadenopathy. Histopathology from axillary nodes was s/o tuberculosis.

Imaging

Mammography: It is of limited value because of overlapping features with carcinoma, both in nodulocaseous and disseminated forms. The nodular form can be seen as a circumscribed density, whereas disseminated form may show increased density and overlying skin thickening—similar to inflammatory cancer. There may be asymmetric density, macrocalcifications, nipple retraction and axillary lymphadenopathy (Fig. 20).

Ultrasound: Since tuberculosis occurs in a younger age group (20–40 years), ultrasound is more informative and is the modality of choice. The nodulocaseous form can be seen as circumscribed or irregular hypoechoic mass(es) (Fig. 21) or complex cystic mass(es). There may be thickening of subcutaneous tissues or fistula formation. In disseminated form, there are multiple irregular or circumscribed hypoechoic masses, some communicating with each other. The tubercular abscess has the same imaging features as pyogenic abscess and cannot be differentiated on ultrasound. It may appear heterogeneously hypoechoic or may show low-level internal echoes (Figs. 22A to D). Sometimes, an abscess in the retromammary area may show fistulous communication with thoracic wall or an intramuscular abscess in pectoralis may present as a breast mass (Fig. 23). Other findings in tuberculosis include axillary lymphadenopathy, duct ectasia and fistula formation with the skin.

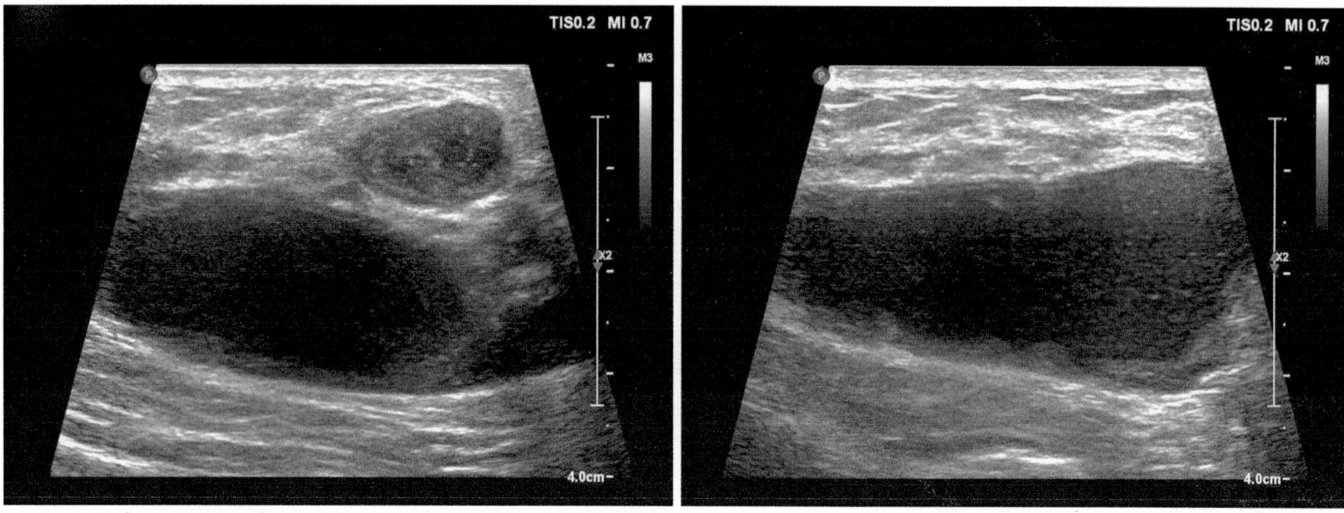

Fig. 21: A middle-aged woman presented with a lump in left breast. There was no history of fever or weight loss. Ultrasound revealed a circumscribed collection with low-level echoes and thickened wall with similar smaller collection adjacent to it. Aspiration was done from the larger lesion which was s/o tuberculosis.

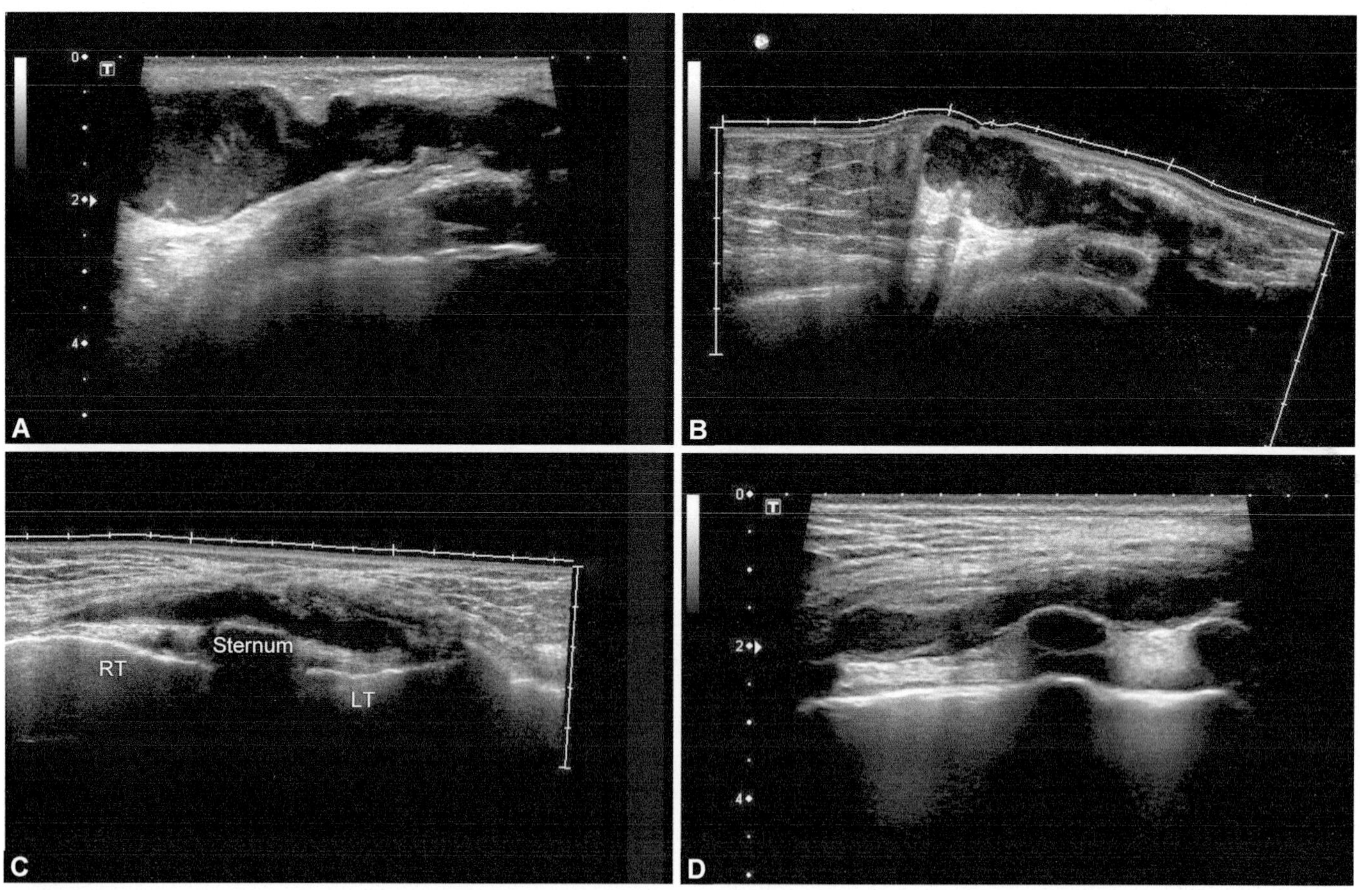

Figs. 22A to D: A 39-year old female presented with pain and swelling in right breast. Ultrasound of right breast (A–D) showed a collection with mobile internal echoes at 3–4 'o clock position with extension medially, anterior to sternum and further in to bilateral chest wall deep to pectoralis major. The fluid was aspirated under ultrasound guidance and was s/o tuberculosis.

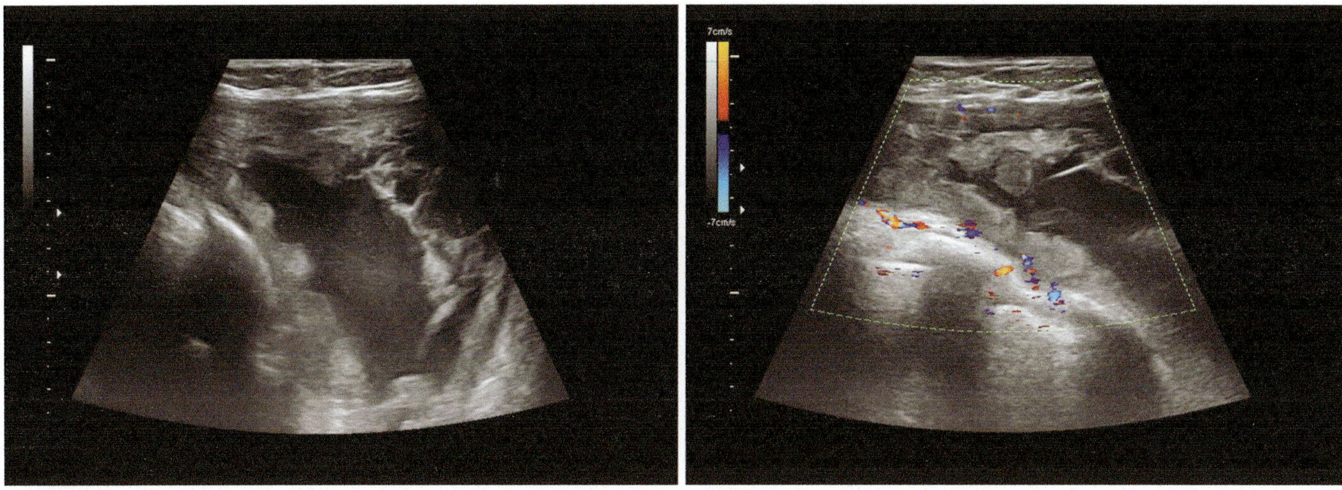

Fig. 23: A 27-year old female presented with pain and swelling in right breast along with history of fever since 1 month. Ultrasound showed a collection with low-level echoes with thickened wall in pectoralis major from second to fifth intercostal space. Aspiration of fluid was done and findings were s/o tuberculosis.

Diagnosis and Treatment

Since most of these imaging features are nonspecific, tubercular mastitis can be very difficult to distinguish from carcinoma and pyogenic abscess. Fine needle aspiration or biopsy is necessary to establish the diagnosis. In Fine needle aspiration cytology, often acid-fast bacilli cannot be demonstrated and only acute inflammatory exudates are seen. AFB negative abscesses which do not heal in spite of drainage and prolonged antibiotic treatment should raise a suspicion of underlying tuberculosis, with biopsy from the abscess wall showing epitheloid cell granulomas with caseous necrosis. Other laboratory tests include mycobacterial culture or polymerase chain reaction (PCR). The treatment consists of antitubercular chemotherapy (ATT). Surgical procedures are indicated in specific cases, including scraping of sinuses in the breast, incisional or excisional biopsy.

Diabetic Mastopathy

Diabetic mastopathy presents with benign tumor like masses in the breasts in women with long-standing type 1 or type 2 diabetes. The prevalence in such women is up to 13%, although it is also seen in men.[19] Pathologically, there is dense fibrosis and predominantly B-cell lymphocytic infiltrate surrounding the ducts, lobules and vessels. There is lobular atrophy and presence of characteristic myofibroblastic epithelioid cells.

Clinical Features

The common findings are enlarged breast or hard and painless mass and there may be involvement of both breasts.

Imaging findings: On mammography, there is either increased breast density, asymmetric density, or irregular masses.

Ultrasound shows irregular or hypoechoic masses with posterior acoustic shadowing though circumscribed masses can also be seen rarely. On FNAC, inadequate material is usually obtained and a definitive diagnosis cannot be made; hence, a core biopsy should be done to establish the diagnosis. Diabetic mastopathy is usually a self-limiting disease and no treatment is required.

Inflammatory Breast Carcinoma

Inflammatory breast cancer (IBC) is type of invasive carcinoma which is relatively uncommon, grows rapidly and metastasizes early. It presents clinically with a rapid onset signs of inflammation like erythema, warmth and edema.[20]

It is difficult to distinguish acute mastitis from IBC and therefore, if the symptoms do not regress even after administration of antibiotics for 8–10 days, further evaluation should be done in all cases of mastitis to exclude inflammatory carcinoma.

Clinical Features

The patient presents clinically with an enlarged edematous breast with induration, increased temperature, tenderness, pain, peau d'orange or cutaneous edema and redness of the skin. Pathologically, dermal lymphatic vessels are involved.[21]

Imaging

Mammography: Compared to infectious mastitis, mammography is relatively less painful in inflammatory carcinoma and can be tolerated by the patient. Findings are non-specific and include skin and trabecular thickening because of breast edema, more diffuse than expected for infectious mastitis (Fig. 24).

The other findings are focal area of asymmetry, architectural distortion, microcalcification or irregular mass.[22] Axillary lymph nodes may be present.

Ultrasound: A large heterogeneous hypoechoic mass with irregular margins may be seen or there may be parenchymal heterogeneity with thickened skin, breast edema and enlarged lymph nodes. The nodes show marked cortical thickening and hilar displacement as is commonly seen in metastatic nodes.

Magnetic resonance imaging (MRI) may not always help in differentiating infections from IBCs (inflammatory breast carcinoma) and the radiologic diagnosis still remains a challenge. The morphological features may be similar in both conditions—including skin thickening, edema, mass or non-mass like enhancement. However, following findings are more in favour of inflammatory carcinoma:

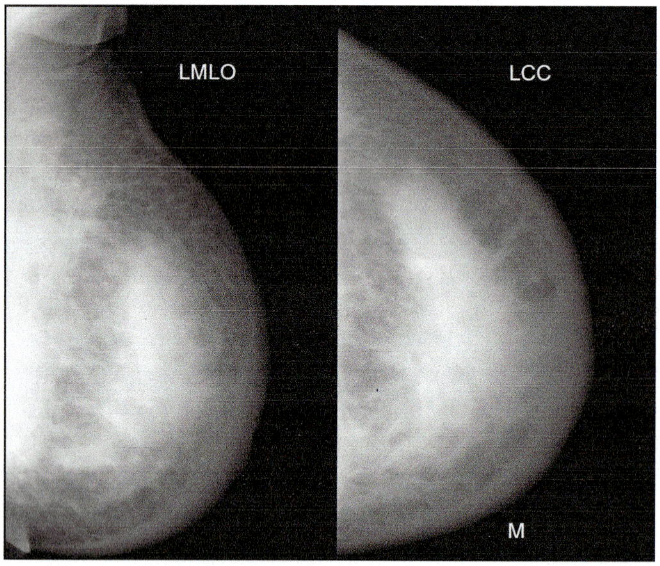

Fig. 24: A 49-year-old female presented with pain, redness and enlargement of left breast since 2 months. Mammogram showed diffuse increase in breast density with trabecular and skin thickening. Histopathology was s/o inflammatory carcinoma.

- Irregular masses located in central and deep parenchyma that are hypointense on T2W images due to desmoplastic fibrous reaction
- Early intense punctiform enhancement in the cutaneous layer due to tumoral emboli to lymphatic vessels of the skin
- Edema in pectoral muscles (hyperintense on T2W images or T2 weighted images)
- Axillary lymphadenopathy

The enhancement kinetics in IBC and acute mastitis may also be similar because of both tumoral and angiogenesis phenomena. Non-mass like enhancement and intense early phase enhancement is seen in both conditions; however, washout is seen more commonly in IBC with type 3 kinetics, whereas a type 2 plateau curve is generally seen in subareolar mastitis.[23]

If symptoms of acute mastitis do not subside with a course of antibiotics, additional imaging with ultrasound and mammography should be followed by biopsies from axillary lymph nodes, skin and the breast mass if any. MRI is helpful in assessing the extent of tumor and to look for contralateral lesions (Table 2).

Table 2: Differences between inflammatory breast cancer and subareolar mastitis.

Inflammatory breast cancer	*Subareolar mastitis*
Age: Older women, at least one decade older than in subareolar mastitis	**Age:** Younger women
Clinical presentation Peau d'orange or erythema Palpable mass most commonly in upper and outer quadrant	**Clinical presentation:** Skin thickening, edema and retroareolar mass
Mammography Skin thickening Prominent trabeculae or edema Asymmetric density Or normal mammography findings	**Mammography:** Findings similar to inflammatory carcinoma
Ultrasound Skin thickening Mass: Solid	**Ultrasound** Skin thickening Subareolar mass: Mixed cystic and solid
MRI **Morphological features:** Mass or non-mass like enhancement Skin thickening Edema Location: Deep, central **Kinetic curve:** Type 3 curve may be seen	**MRI:** **Morphological features:** Mass or non-mass like enhancement Skin thickening Edema Location: Subareolar **Kinetic curve:** Type 2 curve

MRI: magnetic resonance imaging.

REFERENCES

1. Ulitzsch D, Nyman MK, Carlson RA. Breast abscess in lactating women: US-guided treatment. Radiology 2004;232:904-9.
2. Thomsen AC, Espersen T, Maigaard S. Course and treatment of milk stasis, noninfectious inflammation of the breast, and infectious mastitis in nursing women. Am J Obstet Gynecol 1984;149:492-5.
3. Benson EA. Management of breast abscesses. World J Surg 1989;13:753-6.
4. Kessler E, Wolloch Y. Granulomatous mastitis: a lesion clinically simulating carcinoma. Am J Clin Pathol 1972;58: 642-6.
5. Imoto S, Kitaya T, Kodama T, Hasebe T, Mukai K. Idiopathic granulomatous mastitis: case report and review of the literature. Jpn J Clin Oncol 1997;27:274-7.
6. Akcan A, Akyildiz H, Deneme MA, Akgun H, Aritas Y. Granulomatous lobular mastitis: a complex diagnostic and therapeutic problem. World J Surg 2006;30:1403-9.
7. Bani-Hani KE, Yaghan RJ, Matalka II, Shatnawi NJ. Idiopathic granulomatous mastitis: time to avoid unnecessary mastectomies. Breast J 2004;10:318-22.
8. Thomas Stavros A. Breast ultrasound, edition. Colorado: Lippincott William and Wilkins; 2004. Chapter 11, Non-malignant breast disorders that have complex cystic phases. pp. 372-4.
9. Kiyak G, Dumlu EG, Kilinc I, et al. Management of idiopathic granulomatous mastitis: dilemmas in diagnosis and treatment. BMC Surg 2014;14:66, 1-5.
10. Lee JH, Oh KK, Kim EK, et al. Radiologic and clinical features of idiopathic granulomatous lobular mastitis mimicking advanced breast cancer. Yonsei Med J 2006;47:78-84.
11. Cooper A. Illustrations of the diseases of the breast. Part I. London: Longman, Rees, Orme, Brown and Green; 1829. pp.73.
12. Kalac N, Ozkan B, Bayiz H, Dursun AB, Demirag F. Breast tuberculosis. Breast 2002;11:346-9.
13. O'Reilly M, Patel KR, Cummins R. Tuberculosis of the breast presenting as carcinoma. Mil Med 2000;165:800-2.
14. Dharkar RS, Kanhere MH, Vaishya ND, Baisarya AK. Tuberculosis of the breast. J Indian Med Assoc 1968;50: 207-9.
15. Shukla HS, Kumar S. Benign breast disorders in nonwestern populations: Part II—Benign breast disorders in India. World J Surg 1989;13:746-9.
16. Mukerjee P, George M, Maheshwari HB, Rao CP. Tuberculosis of the breast. J Indian Med Assoc 1974;62: 410-2.
17. Shinde SR, Chandawarkar RY, Deshmukh SP. Tuberculosis of the breast masquerading as carcinoma: a study of 100 patients. World J Surg 1995;19:379-81.
18. McKeown KC, Wilkinson KW. Tuberculous diseases of the breast. Br J Surg 1952;39:420.
19. ShaffreyJK, Askin FB, Gatewood OM, Brem R. Diabetic fibrous mastopathy: case reports and radiologic-pathologic correlation. Breast J 2000;6:414-7.
20. Kushwaha AC, Whitman GJ, Stelling CB, Cristofanilli MC, Buzdar AU. Primary inflammatory carcinoma of the breast: retrospective review of mammographic findings. AJR Am J Roentgenol 2000;174:535-8. CrossRef, Medline.
21. Ellis DL, Teitelbaum SL. Inflammatory carcinoma of the breast: a pathologic definition. Cancer 1974;33:1045-7. CrossRef, Medline.
22. Apple SK, Bassett LW, Poon CM. Invasive ductal carcinoma. In: Bassett LW, Mahoney MC, Apple SK, D'Orsi CJ, eds. Breast imaging expert radiology series. Philadelphia, PA: Saunders Elsevier; 2011. 423-82.
23. Hook GW, Ikeda DM, Treatment of breast abscesses with US-guided percutaneous needle drainage without indwelling catheter placement. Radiology 1999;213: 579-82.

Male Breast

CHAPTER

6

INTRODUCTION

Evaluation of the male breast is done commonly for breast enlargement, tenderness or a palpable lump. The most common cause of male breast enlargement is gynecomastia. Benign neoplasms of breast include papilloma, lipoma, myofibroblastoma and angiolipoma while common non-neoplastic pathologies are sebaceous cyst, epidermal inclusion cyst, subareolar abscess and venous malformation. Primary cancer in males is uncommon, seen in only 0.7% cases. Ductal carcinoma in situ (DCIS), invasive ductal carcinoma and papillary neoplasms are also rare and are due to ductal and stromal proliferation.[1]

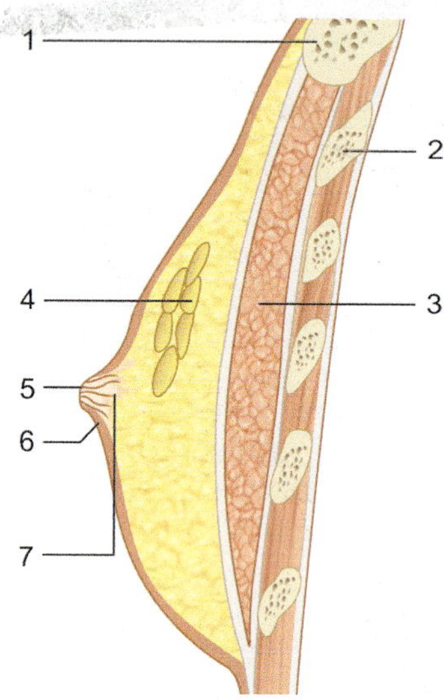

Fig. 1: Clavicle 2. First rib 3. Pectoralis major 4. Suporting fibro-adipose tissue 5. Nipple 6. Areola 7. Blind ducts extending for a short distance below the areola.

ANATOMY OF MALE BREAST

The normal adult male breast consists of skin, adipose tissue, stromal elements and subareolar lactiferous ductal tissue with blind ending ductal elements restricted to the areolar region (Fig. 1). In contrast to the female breast (Fig. 2), there is absence of Cooper ligaments and lack of lobular development, hence lobular pathologies like fibrocystic change, adenosis, fibroadenoma, phyllodes tumor, lobular carcinoma in situ and invasive lobular carcinoma are extremely rare in males.

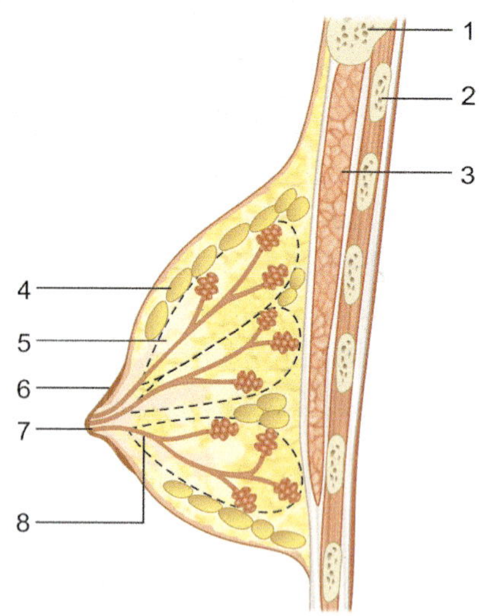

Fig. 2: Line diagram showing anatomy of female breast: 1. Clavicle 2. First rib 3. Pectoralis major 4. Adipose tissue 5. Lobe 6. Areola 7. Nipple 8. Sub-areolar duct each leading to a lobe.

Vascular Supply and Lymphatic Drainage

The arterial supply of male breast is from external artery of Solomon which originates from axillary artery, internal thoracic artery and branches of third, fourth and fifth intercostal arteries. Venous drainage is by superficial and deep veins which converge and empty into the intercostal veins. Lymphatic drainage is mainly by axillary lymph nodes, supraclavicular and internal thoracic nodes.

Imaging

Mammography, ultrasound (Figs. 3A and B) and rarely MRI are used as imaging modalities for evaluation of male breast. Common indications include breast enlargement, breast lump, tenderness and erythema.

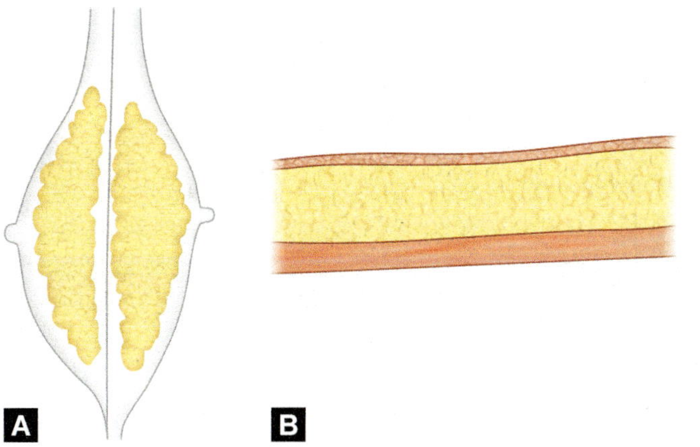

Figs. 3A and B: Line diagram showing (A) Mammogram and; (B) Ultrasound findings in males breast which is composed of predominantly fat lobules.

Mammography

The male breast is positioned in the same way as a small female breast. The Medio-lateral oblique MLO view is done from lateral aspect.[2] The CC projection can be done as a craniocaudal or caudocranial view. It shows skin, nipple and diffuse fatty tissue with a small area of increased density in subareolar region due to fibrous connective tissue and remnant ductal tissue.

Ultrasound

It shows skin, nipple and isoechoic fat lobules which represent subcutaneous fat. The nipple is seen as a hyperechoic nodule with mild posterior attenuation and the pectoralis muscle shows linear echogenic fibrillar pattern.

MRI

These features of pathologies in the male breast are similar to those seen in females.

GYNECOMASTIA

This is the most common cause of breast enlargement due to benign proliferation and hyperplasia of stromal and/or ductal elements.

Clinical Features

It presents as a soft, compressible, mobile and often tender mass in the subareolar region that is unilateral in the majority of patients; however, bilateral and asymmetrical gynecomastia is also seen. There is a bimodal prevalence, with presentation either at puberty or above the age of 50 years.

Etiology

Gynecomastia may be physiological or pathological.

Physiological Gynecomastia

It is seen in infancy, puberty and senescence. In the perinatal period, it is because of transplacental exposure of maternal estrogen, in puberty, it is because of imbalance between blood levels of estrogen and testosterone; while in senescence, it is because of reduced androgen secretion or diminished inactivation of estrogen in liver.

Pathological Causes of Gynecomastia

Pathological causes include cirrhosis, hyperthyroidism, chronic renal disease, neoplasms (germ cell tumor, pituitary tumors) and drugs like cimetidine, thiazide diuretics, antihypertensives, antidepressants, narcotics and steroids. A detailed history of drug consumption is important to ascertain its cause. **Idiopathic gynecomastia** is a diagnosis of exclusion.[3]

Imaging

Three patterns of gynecomastia are recognized on both, imaging and histopathology: nodular, dendritic and diffuse. The nodular pattern is seen in florid phase with proliferation of stromal and ductal elements, periductal inflammation and edema. The dendritic pattern is seen in the fibrotic phase with dilated ducts and moderate epithelial proliferation along with fibrosis. In diffuse gynecomastia, commonly seen in patients taking exogenous hormones, epithelial proliferative changes are present. It has a characteristic pattern on mammography and ultrasound that allows differentiation from malignancy.

The patterns of gynecomastia on mammogram and ultrasound are as depicted in line diagram in Figures 4 and 5, respectively.

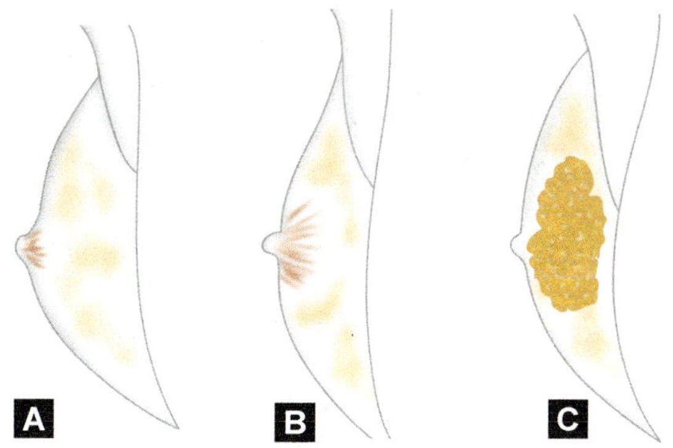

Figs. 4A to C: Line diagram showing (A) nodular; (B) dendritic and; (C) diffuse gynecomastia on mammogram.

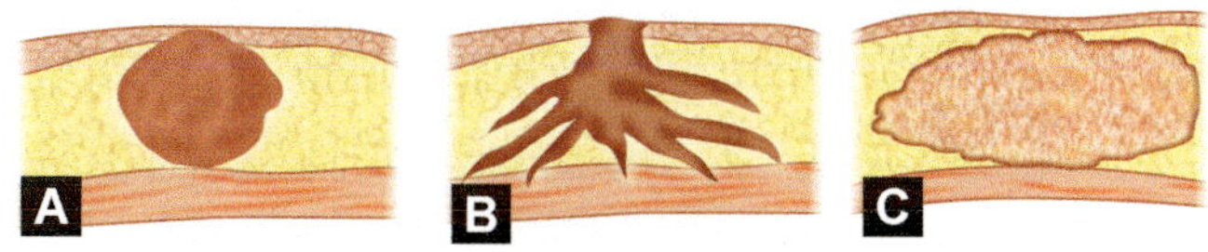

Figs. 5A to C: Line diagram showing (A) nodular; (B) dendritic and; (C) diffuse gynecomastia on ultrasound.

Nodular Pattern

On mammography, a fan-shaped retroareolar density (Fig. 6) is seen blending into the surrounding fat tissue,[3] while ultrasound shows a discrete and well-marginated subareolar round or oval hypoechoic mass (Figs. 7 and 8). It is usually reversible when primary cause is removed.

Dendritic Pattern

On mammography, it is seen as flame-shaped retroareolar glandular tissue radiating from the nipple into deeper adipose tissue (Fig. 9A), while on ultrasound, a triangular hypoechoic retroareolar mass with finger-like projections (Fig. 9B) is seen extending from the nipple into

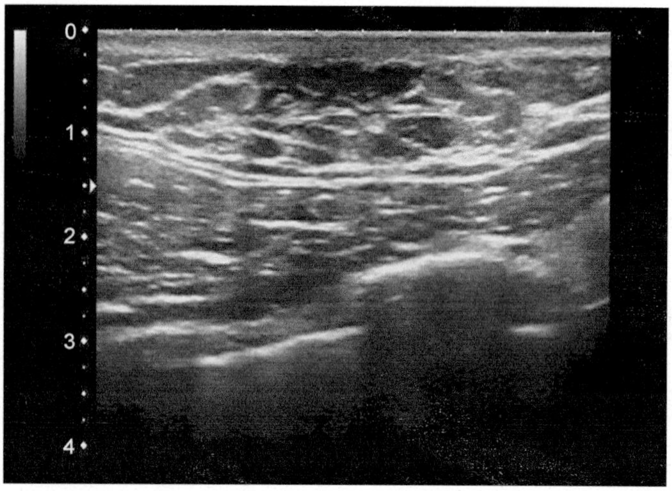

Fig. 8: Ultrasound of left breast in a young male patient shows a well defined oval hypoechoic lesion in sub-areolar region s/o Nodular Gynecomastia.

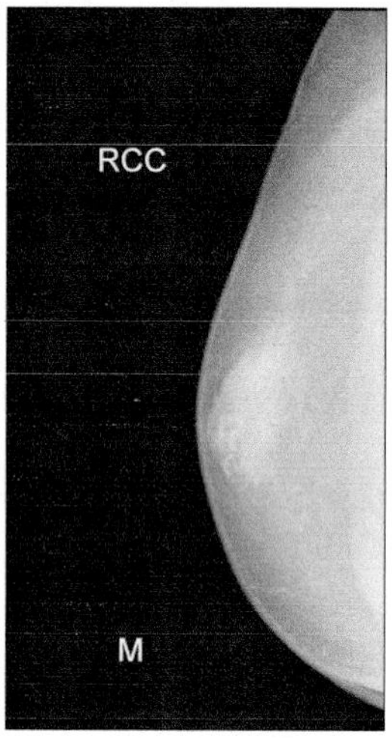

Fig. 6: Mammogram right cranio-caudal (CC) view in a 32-year-old male showing a fan shaped radio-opacity blending into the retroareolar region s/o Nodular Gynecomastia.

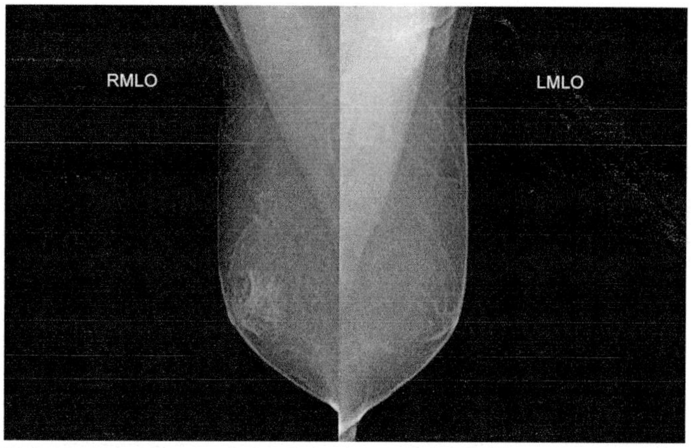

Fig. 9A: Mammogram of right breast (MLO) view in a 38 year male presenting with right breast lump shows finger like opacities in the sub-areolar region.

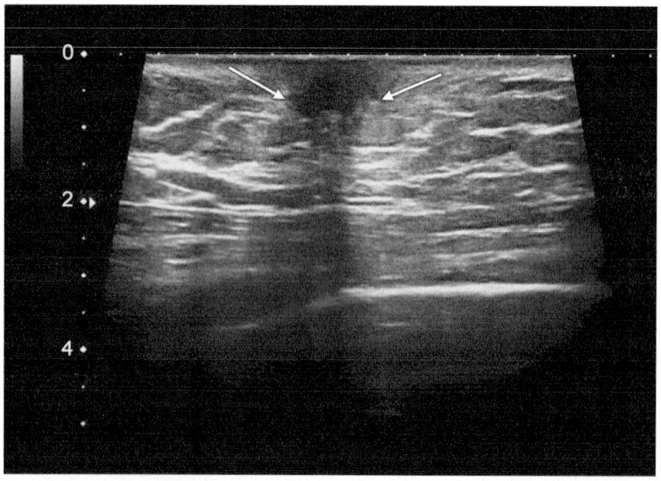

Fig. 7: Ultrasound of right breast in a 29-year-old male presenting with right breast lump shows a well defined round hypoechoic lesion in the right sub-areolar region s/o Nodular Gynecomastia

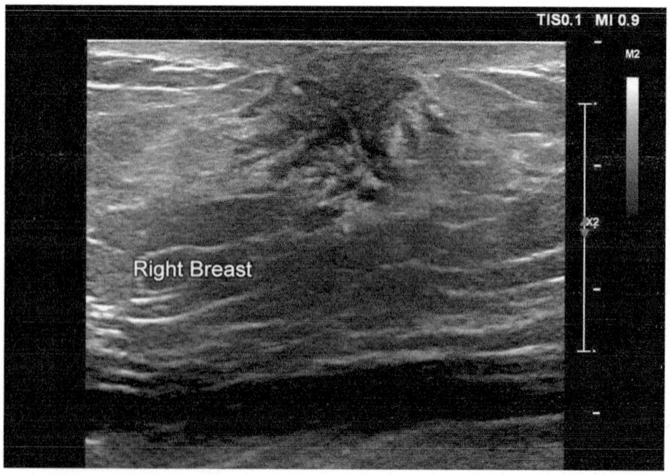

Fig. 9B: Ultrasound of patient in 9A showing irregular hypoechoic lesion in the sub-areolar region. Features are s/o dendritic gynecomastia.

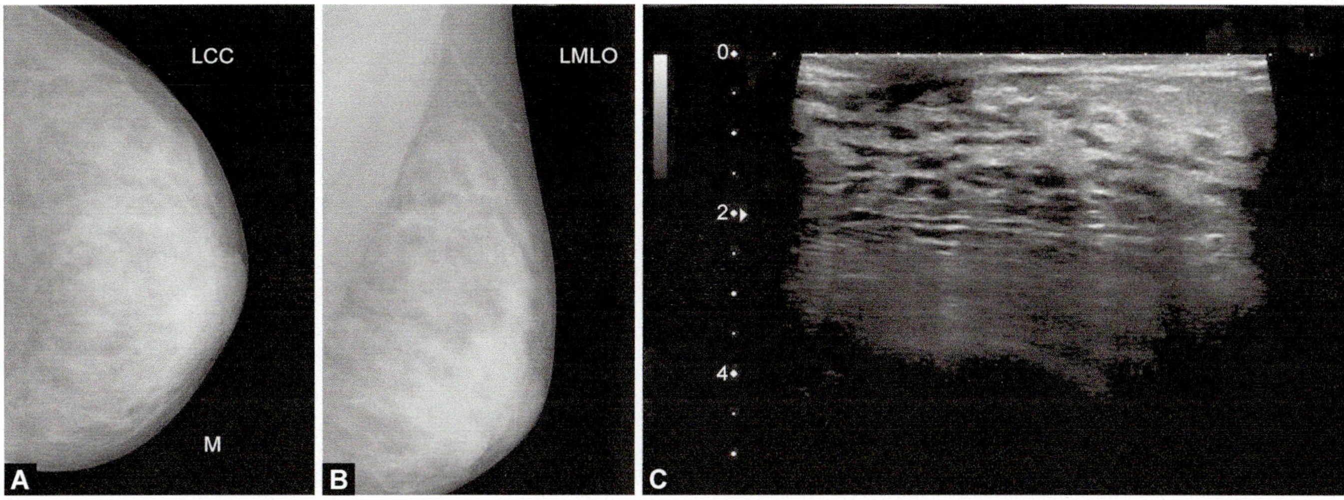

Figs. 10A to C: Mammogram CC and MLO view (A, B) in a 45-year-old male with diffuse left breast enlargement showed diffuse increase in breast density; (C) Ultrasound showed a heterogenously echogenic parenchyma. Features are s/o Diffuse Gynecomastia.

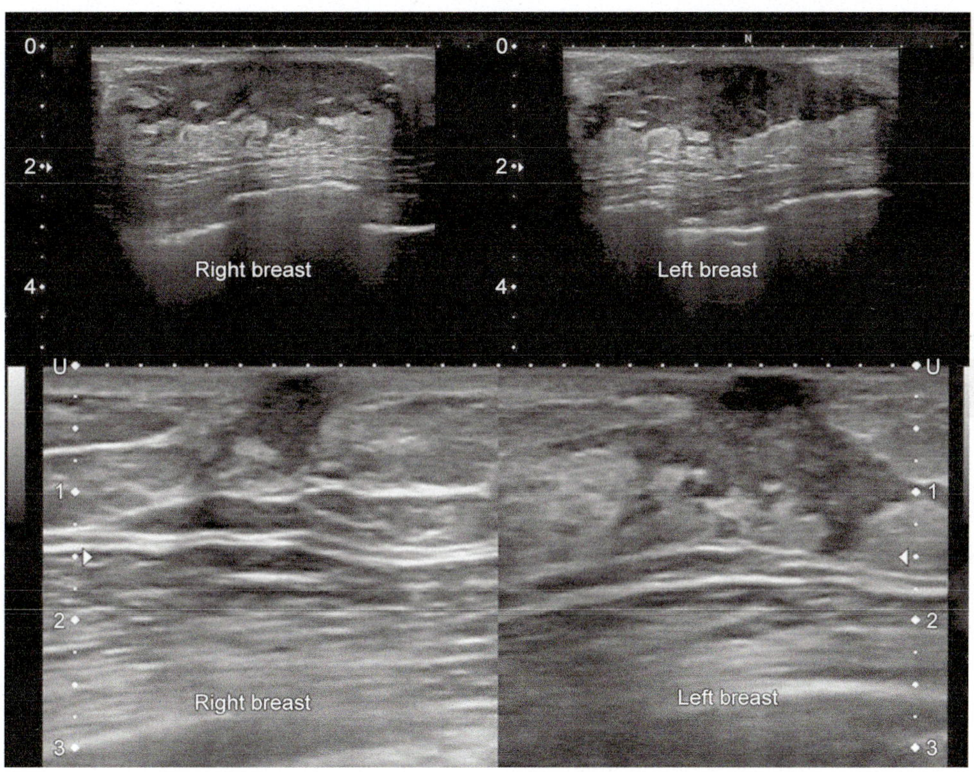

Fig. 11: Ultrasound of male breast in two different patients with bilateral breast enlargement showing bilateral symmetrical dendritic gynecomastia.

the surrounding tissue. The clinical and mammographic features in this phase are irreversible.

Diffuse Pattern

Mammogram shows heterogeneously dense and enlarged breast with both nodular and dendritic components almost looking similar to female breast (Figs. 10A to C), while ultrasound shows prominent glandular tissue distributed diffusely within the fatty tissue.

Gynecomastia can be unilateral or bilateral (Fig. 11) and may be asymmetrical. Sometimes ductal elements can also be seen within (Fig. 12). In addition, another appearance may be seen where there is increased depth (>1 cm) of breast tissue at the nipple, appearing isoechoic, hypoechoic or hyperechoic in appearance.[4]

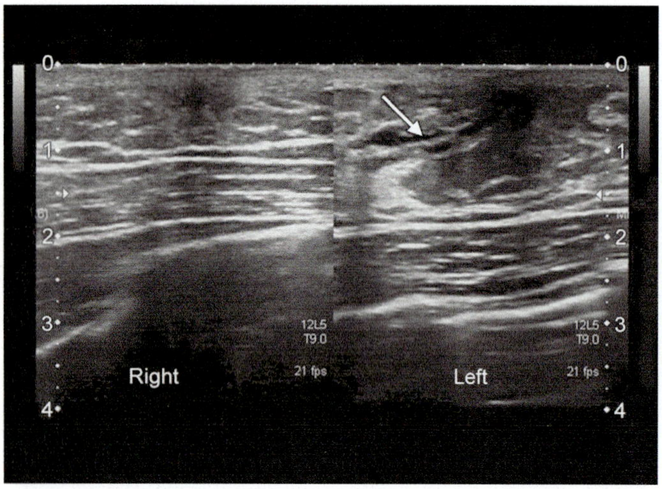

Fig. 12: A young man with asymmetrical breast enlargement shows dendritic gynecomastia on left with ductal elements (Arrow).

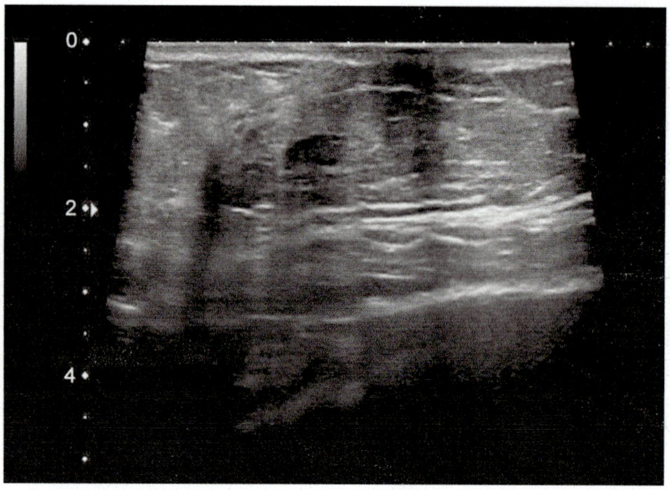

Fig. 13: Ultrasound of breast in a young male shows diffuse fatty tissue s/o pseudogynecomastia

Treatment

The treatment of gynecomastia depends upon the causative condition. Hormonal and physiological causes are responsible during puberty with spontaneous regression in most cases. Gynecomastia due to medications is reversible once the inciting drug is stopped or substituted, while that due to an underlying condition like cirrhosis, malnutrition, etc. requires treatment of the underlying condition. Sometimes surgery may be needed to remove the extra breast tissue.

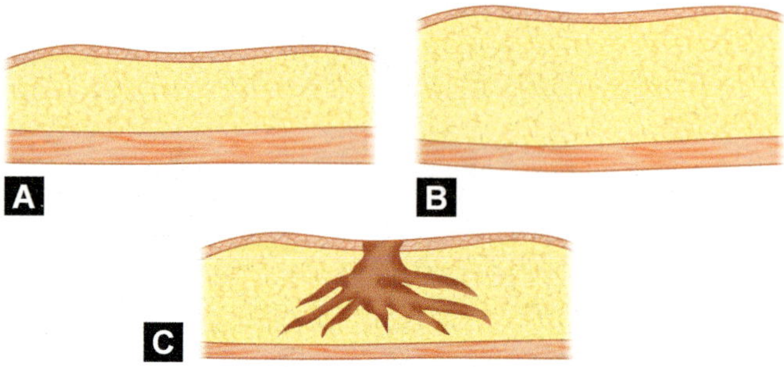

Figs. 14A to C: Line diagram showing (A) normal male breast; (B) Pseudogynecomastia and; (C) Dendritic Gynecomastia on ultrasound.

PSEUDOGYNECOMASTIA

In pseudogynecomastia, there is unilateral or bilateral breast enlargement due to excessive proliferation of fat especially in obese individuals with no palpable or discrete mass. Mammography reveals excessive fat with absence of retroareolar densities (seen in true gynecomastia), while ultrasound shows multiple fat lobules separated by thin hyperechoic fibrous tissue (Fig. 13).

It is important to differentiate imaging findings in normal male breast, gynecomastia and pseudogynecomastia to avoid unnecessary intervention (Figs. 14A to C).

BENIGN BREAST NEOPLASMS

Myofibroblastoma

This is a stromal tumor, predominantly seen in older men and menopausal women. It is a rare and benign lesion, which shares similarities with other mesenchymal tumors as solitary fibrous tumor, leiomyoma and benign fibrous histiocytoma. It presents clinically as a solitary, mobile, palpable and firm mass with a mean age of presentation at 50 years.

On mammography, a circumscribed encapsulated heterogeneous mass is seen without microcalcifications. On ultrasound, the tumor is well-demarcated and lobulated with heterogeneous echotexture and may show peripheral vascularity.

The differential diagnosis includes hamartoma, fibroadenoma and lipoma.

Granular Cell Tumor

It is a benign tumor of neural origin, typically seen in men in their 30s and usually presents as a circumscribed mass but may have a spiculated appearance on imaging.

Lipoma

It is the second most common benign lesion and presents clinically as a small palpable soft mass. On mammogram,

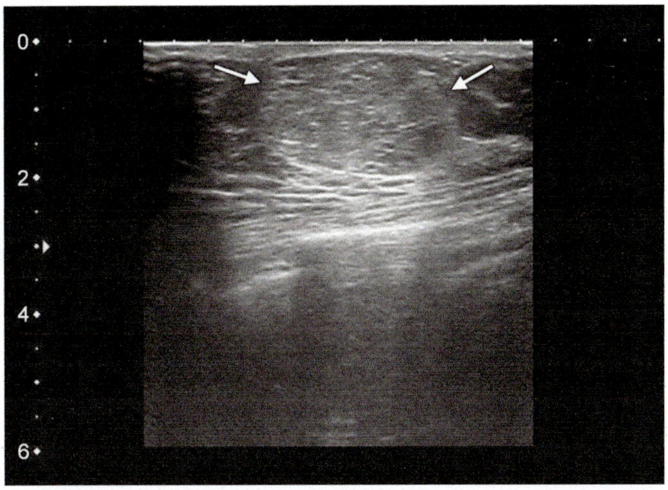

Fig. 15: Ultrasound of male breast showing a well defined encapsulated heterogeneously isoechoic mass s/o lipoma.

it is seen as a well-encapsulated, radiolucent, fat density that is sometimes difficult to distinguish from normal breast tissue. On ultrasound, a circumscribed homogeneously or heterogeneously isoechoic (Fig. 15), echogenic or hypoechoic mass is seen having a thin echogenic capsule without posterior acoustic shadowing or enhancement.

Angiolipoma

It is a benign tumor, typically seen as a mixed fat and soft-tissue density on mammography and as a heterogeneous echogenic mass on ultrasound.

Papilloma

An intraductal (or intracystic) papilloma is an extremely rare benign lesion in the male breast that presents clinically with nipple discharge or a solitary well-defined palpable subareolar mass. It is formed by benign epithelial proliferation with a fibrovascular core and uniformly distributed myoepithelial cells. On ultrasound, a circumscribed eccentric subareolar hypoechoic mass may be seen within an enlarged duct or adjacent to a cyst which is actually an ectatic duct, while on mammography a well-defined subareolar mass is seen if the mass is clinically palpable.

Schwannoma

It presents clinically as a smooth, soft and painless mass. It has non-specific imaging findings, appearing as a circumscribed round or oval mass on mammogram and a hypoechoic solid mass with variable acoustic enhancement on ultrasound.

BENIGN NON-NEOPLASTIC CONDITIONS

These include intramammary lymph node, sebaceous cyst, epidermal inclusion cyst, subareolar abscess and venous malformations.[5] Salient features of these conditions allow accurate imaging interpretation and avoid unnecessary invasive treatment.

Intramammary Lymph Node

These are seen as circumscribed oval or reniform lesions with dense peripheral margins and central lucency because of fatty hilum on mammography (Figs. 16A and B). Ultrasound shows a well-defined oval hypoechoic mass with central echogenic fatty hilum.

Epidermal Inclusion Cyst

It is a skin lesion that presents as a small superficial palpable mass. On mammogram, a well-defined opacity is seen close to the skin (Figs. 17A and B). On ultrasound, a circumscribed hypoechoic oval lesion is seen with a tract that may be contiguous with the skin.

Sebaceous Cyst

It is a typical intradermal lesion, usually smaller than epidermal inclusion cyst and is seen as a well-defined, hypoechoic mass with smooth margins on ultrasound.

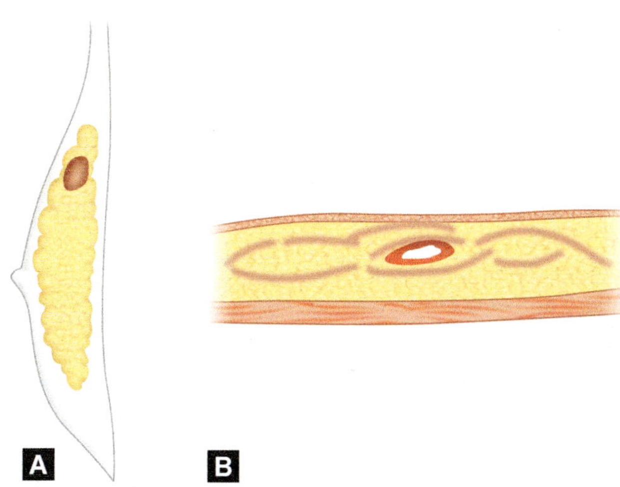

Figs. 16A and B: Line diagram showing a well defined Intramammary lymph node with fatty hilum on Mammography and ultrasound.

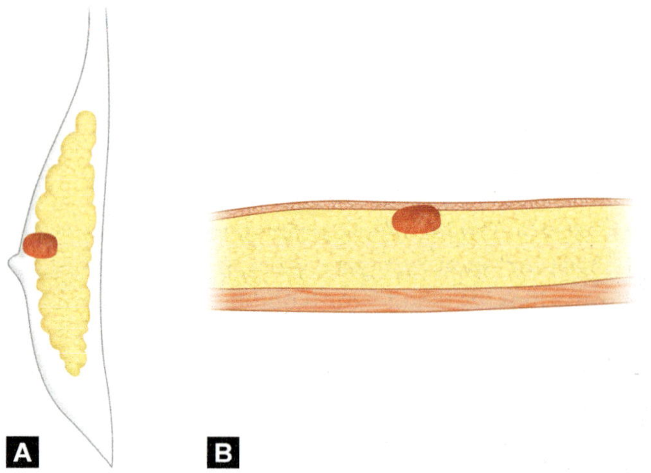

Figs. 17A and B: Line diagram showing a well defined mass in superficial plane on Mammogram and ultrasound s/o epidermal inclusion cyst.

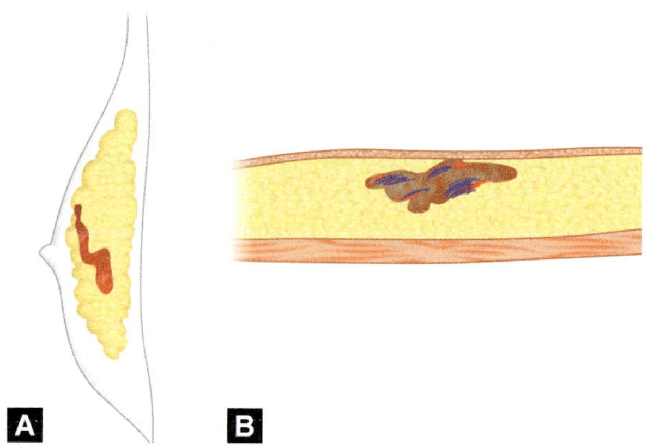

Figs. 18A and B: Line diagram of venous malformation—elongated density on mammogram which is seen as heterogeneously hypoechoic mass with venous flow.

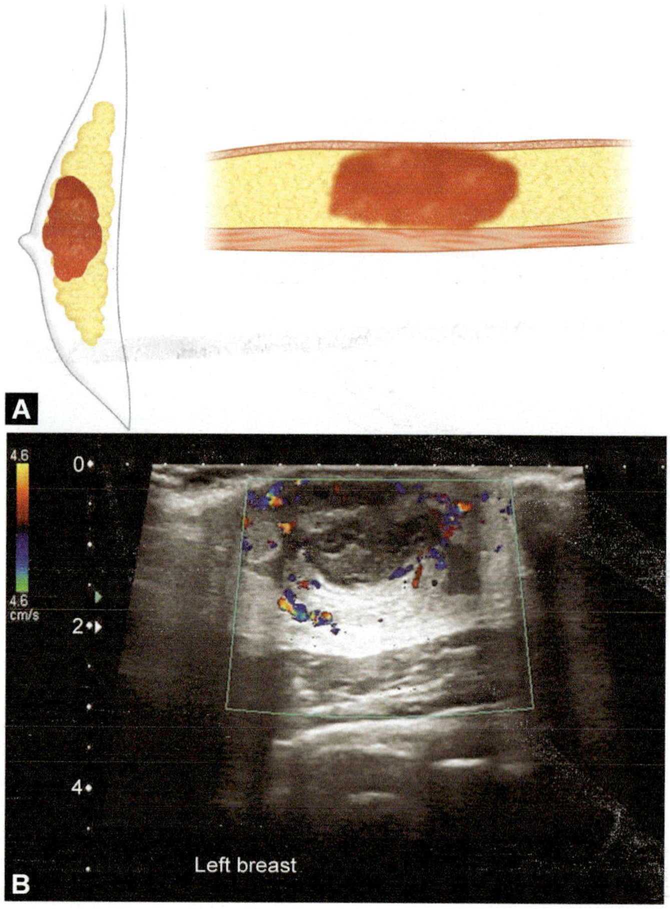

Figs. 19A and B: (A) Line diagram showing subareolar abscess which is seen on Mammogram as an ill-defined mass or density which on ultrasound shows increased peripheral vascularity (red and blue lines); (B) Ultrasound of breast in a young male presenting with painful mass showed a heterogeneously hypoechoic mass in sub-areolar region with peripheral vascularity and surrounding inflammation. Pus was aspirated.

Venous Malformation

It is the most common vascular malformation of the male breast, presenting clinically as unilateral non-tender breast enlargement. On mammography, a tubular soft-tissue density is seen with or without a phlebolith, while ultrasound shows multiple well-defined cystic spaces with slow flow on color Doppler (Figs. 18A and B).

Subareolar Abscess

It represents localized infection secondary to ductal ectasia, chronic obstruction and inflammation, commonly due to chronic mastitis. The abscess tends to recur if not adequately treated and may require surgical excision. Clinically, it presents with pain, nipple swelling, local inflammation, thickened skin and nipple discharge.

On mammogram, it is seen as an ill-defined subareolar mass with indistinct margins and surrounding trabecular thickening. Ultrasound shows an irregular heterogeneously hypoechoic mass with increased peripheral vascularity (Figs. 19A and B) and inflammation in surrounding tissues.

Hematoma

It is suspected clinically when a new palpable abnormality presents after a recent history of trauma. A poorly defined subtle density is seen on the mammogram underlying the

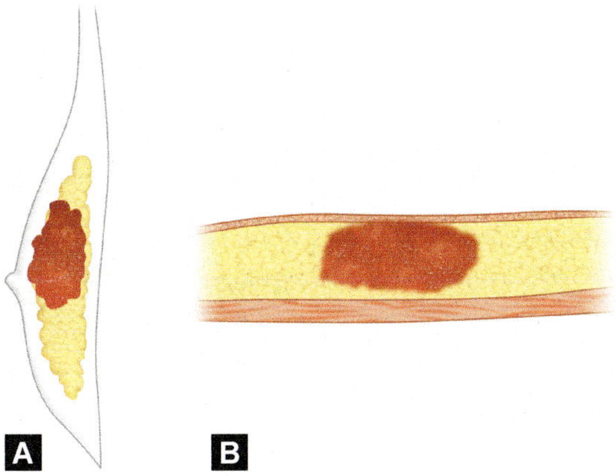

Figs. 20A and B: Line diagram showing a hematoma which appears as irregular density on Mammogram and an ill-defined heterogenous mass on ultrasound. A history of trauma must be asked for.

site of injury. On ultrasound, the typical feature is of a fluid collection that is hypoechoic or of mixed echogenicity and has irregular margins (Figs. 20A and B).

Fat Necrosis

It is seen as coarse or rim calcification on mammography and a circumscribed hypoechoic to anechoic oval lesion with echogenic foci on ultrasound.

MALIGNANT BREAST LESIONS

Carcinoma

Carcinoma is rare in the male breast compared to females, accounting for 0.7% of all male cancers, with the female-to-male ratio for breast cancer being 100:1 in whites and 70:1 in blacks.[6] It is usually an invasive ductal carcinoma in 80% cases, while in 5% cases, it may be a papillary carcinoma that is predominantly intracystic. DCIS may be rarely seen. Since there are very few lobules in the male breast, lobular cancer is very rare except in the case of estrogen exposure. The differentiating features between Gynecomastia and Malignancy are shown in Table 1.

Risk Factors

Risk factors for male breast cancer are advanced age, family history, chest wall irradiation, hyperestrogenism, hyperthyroidism, undescended testicles, *BRCA2* gene mutation, liver dysfunction, prostate cancer, orchiectomy and Klinefelter syndrome.

Clinical Features

It presents as a painless, palpable, eccentric retroareolar mass with or without nipple retraction, bloody nipple discharge, skin thickening and palpable axillary lymph nodes.

Imaging

Mammography is highly sensitive and specific for breast cancer in men. A well-defined retroareolar eccentric mass is seen, which may sometimes be spiculated (Fig. 21A). Microcalcifications are rare and coarser than in females. All circumscribed masses in males should raise a high index of suspicion for carcinoma and all cysts should be rigorously imaged to exclude an intracystic neoplasm.

On ultrasound, a malignant mass appears as a circumscribed or irregular eccentrically placed mass in the subareolar region (Fig. 21B). Vascularity may or may not be present. Ultrasound guided core needle biopsy confirms the diagnosis.

Sometimes a malignant mass may be difficult to distinguish from gynecomastia and imaging findings should be correlated with the clinical presentation.

Table 1: Comparison between clinical and imaging features of gynecomastia and carcinoma in male breast.

	Gynecomastia	*Carcinoma*
Clinical	• Diffusely enlarged breast or a soft, mobile, tender, subareolar mass • May be bilateral and symmetric • Secondary signs like nipple retraction are absent	• Subareolar mass eccentric to the nipple • Unilateral • Secondary signs like nipple retraction may be seen
Mammography	• Subareolar central density • Fan- or flame-shaped density with indistinct lateral and deep margins blending into surrounding fat • Enlarged breast with diffuse increase in density	• Often eccentric, lobulated or circumscribed mass but may be spiculated • Coarse calcification may be present • Secondary signs like nipple retraction may be seen • Axillary lymphadenopathy may be present
Ultrasound	• Discrete round, oval, poorly defined or irregular hypoechoic area in retroareolar region • Extends or blends into surrounding fatty tissue	• Irregular hypoechoic or complex mass, with or without vascularity • Axillary lymphadenopathy may be present

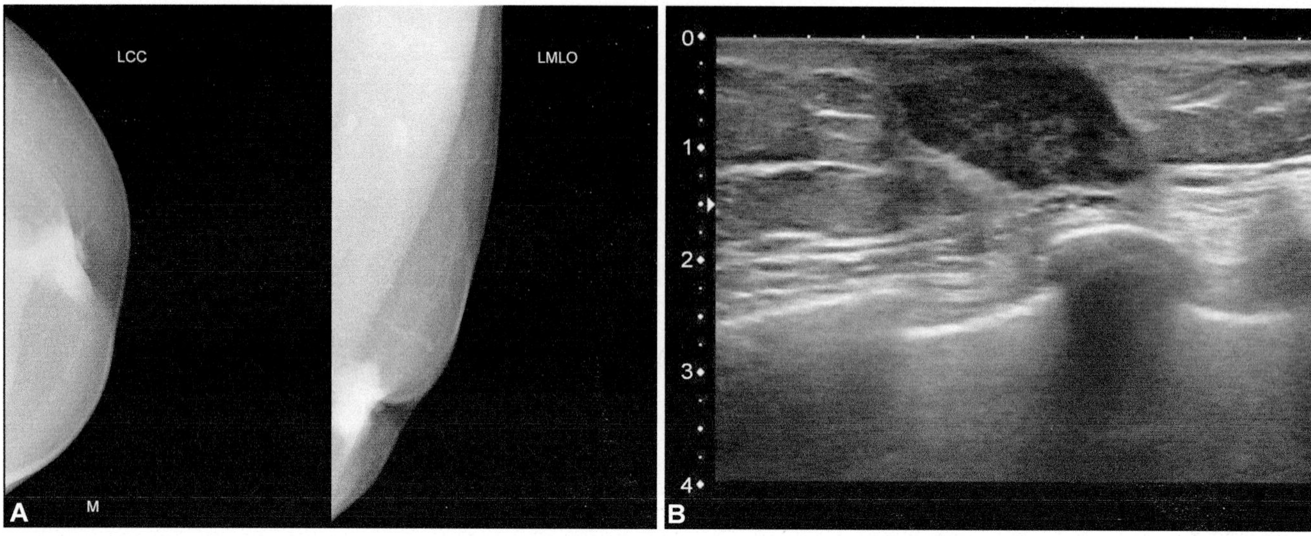

Figs. 21A and B: (A) Mammogram in a young patient presenting with a breast lump shows a microlobulated/spiculated high density mass in retro-areolar region with nipple retraction; (B) Ultrasound of the above patient showed a circumscribed hypoechoic mass. Histopathology was s/o Invasive ductal carcinoma.

Intracystic Papillary Carcinoma (IPC)

It is a rare and slow growing malignancy seen from 64 to 84 years of age and represents 5–7.5% cases of male breast cancer. It has an excellent prognosis with a 10-year survival of 100%.[7] The clinical and radiological diagnosis can be challenging as findings are often non-specific and confirmation needs histopathology and immunohistochemistry. It is important to note that cytology can be falsely negative for this lesion; hence an excision biopsy should be done to establish the diagnosis.

Mammography may be normal in small IPCs which are easily missed, though larger lesions are seen as circumscribed subareolar masses (Figs. 22A and 23A). Ductal dilatation may be seen as a tapering band-like density radiating from the nipple toward the parenchyma.

Ultrasound features are highly variable, ranging from a cystic to hypoechoic to a complex cystic mass (Figs. 22B and 23B). This may be associated with dilated ducts or a solid appearing intraductal or intracystic mass. Increased vascularity may be present on Doppler with a central vascular pedicle and branching vessels.[8]

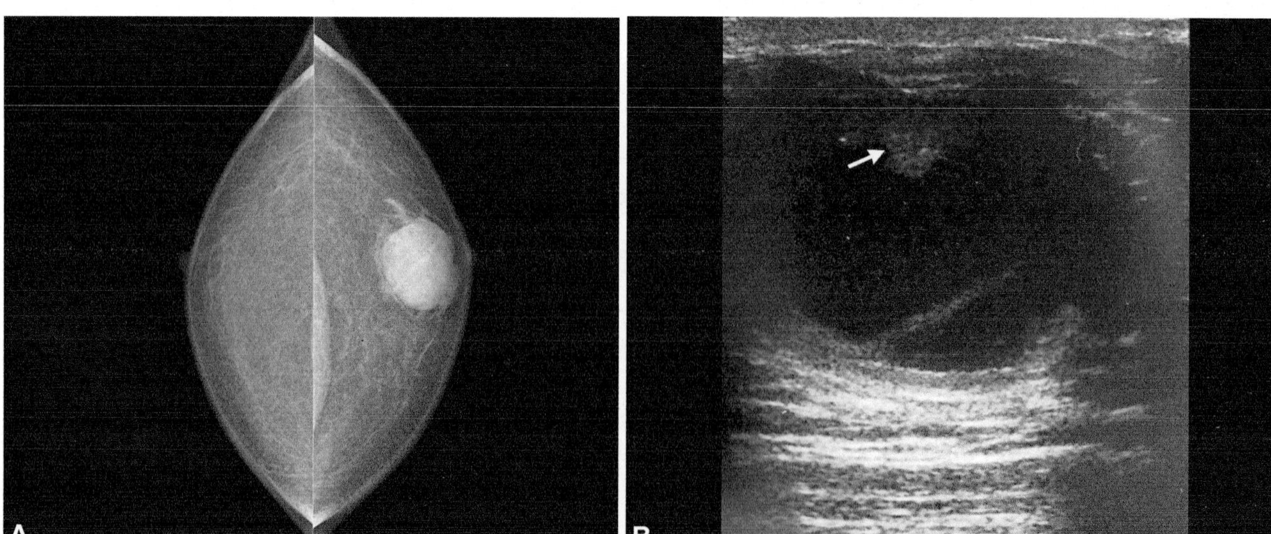

Figs. 22A and B: (A) Mammogram in a 30-year-old male showed a circumscribed sub-areolar mass is left breast; (B) Ultrasound shows a circumscribed cystic mass with a mural nodule and septations. Histopathology was s/o Intracystic papillary carcinoma.

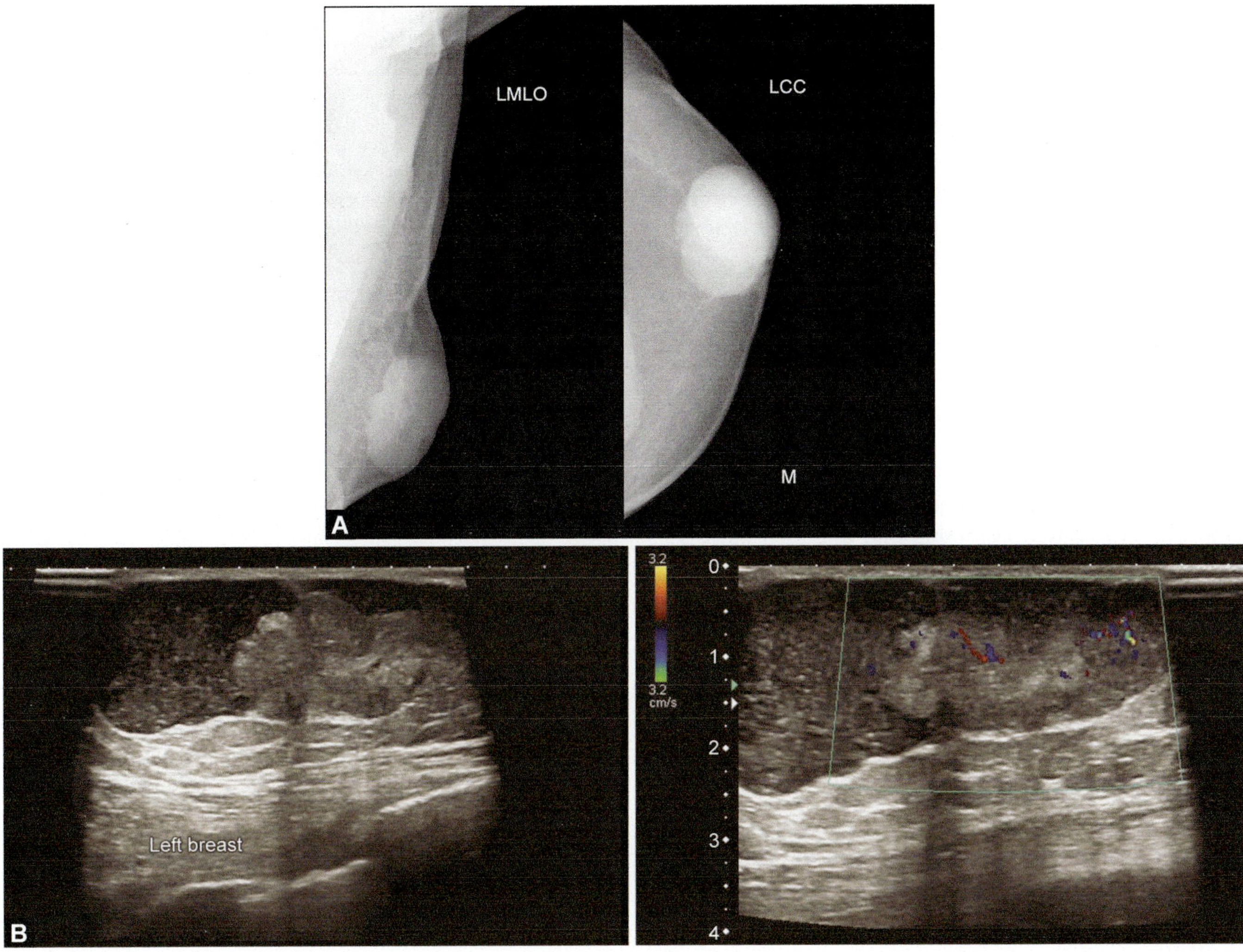

Figs. 23A and B: (A) Mammogram of left breast in a 45 year old male shows a sub-areolar mass in left breast which was seen on; (B) ultrasound as complex cystic mass with low level echoes. Histopathology was s/o Intracystic papillary carcinoma.

On MRI, enhancement of the cyst walls, mural nodules or septations may be present.[9]

Solorzano et al.[10] classified IPC into three categories based on pathological findings: (1) IPC alone, (2) IPC with DCIS and (3) IPC with an invasive carcinoma. The prognosis was the same among the three groups irrespective of the type of surgery done and whether or not adjuvant therapy was given.

Liposarcoma

Liposarcomas are extremely rare, accounting for only about 0.06% of all breast malignancies.[11] They tend to extend into both stromal tissues and pectoral muscles. They may arise from preexisting benign tumors, including lipomas, fibroadenomas and phyllodes tumors[12] and typically present in the fifth through seventh decades as soft, slowly growing masses that may or may not be painful. Mammography shows a circumscribed water-density mass with lucent areas and ultrasound shows a hypoechoic lesion.

Metastases

Metastases to the male breast are extremely rare, and represent hematogenous spread in patients with widespread disease, mostly from prostate cancer. Clinical presentation is with a round or lobulated palpable mass. On ultrasound, a hypoechoic mass with irregular margins is noted and a biopsy is necessary for diagnosis.

Lymphoma

Lymphoma of the breast is uncommon, constituting 0.04–0.5% of malignant male breast neoplasms.[13] Both primary and secondary lymphoma of the breast are known, with most of B cell origin. Primary lymphoma of the breast is defined as a tumor localized to the breast with or without ipsilateral axillary lymph node metastases (seen in 50% of cases of primary lymphoma).[14] Clinically, a painless breast mass or breast edema with erythema or axillary lymphadenopathy is noted. On mammography, a circumscribed mass surrounded by thin radiolucency is noted. Ultrasound shows a circumscribed hypoechoic mass with or without microlobulated margins suspicious for malignancy. Confirmation needs biopsy for histopathology and immunohistochemistry.

In conclusion, some of pathologies in male breast have characteristic mammographic, ultrasonographic and magnetic resonance imaging findings while others require biopsy to establish a diagnosis. When a patient presents with a clinically palpable mass, mammography should be done first followed by a targeted ultrasound and a guided biopsy, if needed. Gynecomastia is the most common cause of male breast enlargement with typical imaging features. *Male breast cancers are very rare but often present at a more advanced stage than in women.* Familiarity with salient features of classic male breast conditions will allow accurate imaging interpretation and avoid unnecessary and often invasive treatment.

REFERENCES

1. Chen L, Chantra PK, Larsen LH, et al. Imaging characteristics of malignant lesions of the male breast. Radiographics 2006;26:993-1006.
2. Kopans DB. Breast imaging. Philadelphia, PA: Lippincott Williams & Wilkins; 2007. p. 311.
3. Braunstein GD. Clinical practice: gynecomastia. N Engl J Med 2007;357:1229-37.
4. Dialani V, Baum J, Mehta TS. Sonographic features of gynecomastia. J Ultrasound Med 2010;29:539-54.
5. Nguyen C, Kettler MD, Swirsky ME, et al. Male breast disease: pictorial review with radiologic-pathologic correlation. Radiographics 2013;33:763-9.
6. Giordano SH. A review of the diagnosis and management of male breast cancer. Oncologist 2005;10:471-9.
7. Lefkowits M, Lefkowits W, Wargots ES. Intraductal (intracystic) papillary carcinoma of the breast and its variants: a clinicopathological study of 77 cases. Hum Pathol 1994;25:802-9.
8. Ganesan S, Karthik G, Joshi M, Damodaran V. Ultrasound spectrum in intraductal papillary neoplasms of breast. Br J Radiol 2006;79:843-9.
9. Soo MS, Williford ME, Walsh R, Bentley RC, Kornguth PJ. Papillary carcinoma of the breast: imaging findings. Am J Roentgenol 1995;164:321-6.
10. Solorzano C, Middleton LP, Hunt KK, et al. Treatment and outcome of patients with intracystic papillary carcinoma of the breast. Am J Surg 2002;184:364-8.
11. Dei Tos AP. Liposarcoma: new entities and evolving concepts. Ann Diagn Pathol 2000;4:252-66.
12. Jeong JY, Park HJ, Lee JH, et al. Liposarcoma of the chest wall: a case potentially transformed from a recurrent lipoma. Gen Thorac Cardiovasc Surg 2011;59:310-1.
13. Takemura A, Mizukami Y, Takayama T, Taniya T, Okumura H. Primary malignant lymphoma of the breast. Jpn J Radiol 2009;27:221-4.
14. Garg NK, Bagul NB, Rubin G, Shah EF. Primary lymphoma of the breast involving both axillae and bilateral breast carcinoma. World J Surg Oncol 2008;6:52.

Imaging of Postoperative Breast

CHAPTER 7

INTRODUCTION

Breast cancer treatments continue to evolve and prognosis treatment options are generally based on tumor-node metastasis staging. Historically, modified radical mastectomy (MRM) was the surgical treatment; however, as the treatment protocols have evolved, breast conservation surgeries have become more widely accepted.

Conservative surgical procedures are performed for both benign and malignant pathologies and include excision biopsy, lumpectomy, segmentectomy, etc. The term "treated" breast is used for breast cancer patients who have undergone breast conservative therapy–BCT (breast conservative surgery and radiation therapy) and the mammogram shows several changes that evolve over a period of time. Women who have already been treated for breast cancer are at risk for second breast cancers, such as ipsilateral recurrence or contralateral metachronous breast cancer and should be evaluated carefully. Over the years, the number of breast cancer survivors has increased; hence, surveillance after treatment has also increased. Evaluation of the treated breast is a challenge for the breast radiologist due to many overlapping features between benign post-treatment changes and tumor recurrence.

BCT: It involves surgical removal of the tumor with a margin of normal surrounding tissue followed by tangential beam irradiation to the whole breast. This makes interpretation of follow-up mammograms difficult because of breast edema, focal skin thickening, decreased compressibility and increased density. BCT is the standard treatment for early cancers as survival rates of patients treated with BCT[1] are equivalent to that of patients treated with mastectomy. Combining conservative surgery with radiation therapy does offer an additional advantage of preserving the breast, usually with a satisfactory cosmetic result.

Diagnostic evaluation of the treated breast is challenging because of high variability in the imaging appearances. The radiologist must be aware of the chronological sequence of normal imaging findings in the treated breast, requiring both experience and expertise in distinguishing treatment-related changes from breast cancer recurrence.

MRM: Though many patients these days undergo breast conservation; MRM still remains a viable treatment option in a select group of patients of breast cancer. The entire breast is removed, including the skin, areola, nipple and most axillary lymph nodes with sparing of the pectoralis major muscle.

Neoadjuvant chemotherapy: It is an important component in the multidisciplinary treatment of clinical stage II and III breast cancer. Its main advantage is to decrease the tumor size prior to surgery, which allows a large number of patients to undergo breast conservation therapy. It is also a reasonable alternative to upfront surgery in the management of locally advanced breast cancer. The radiological assessment in evaluating response to neoadjuvant chemotherapy drug regimen is done by assessing change in size of the tumor on ultrasound or by comparing sequential mammograms (Fig. 1). The accuracy of mammogram

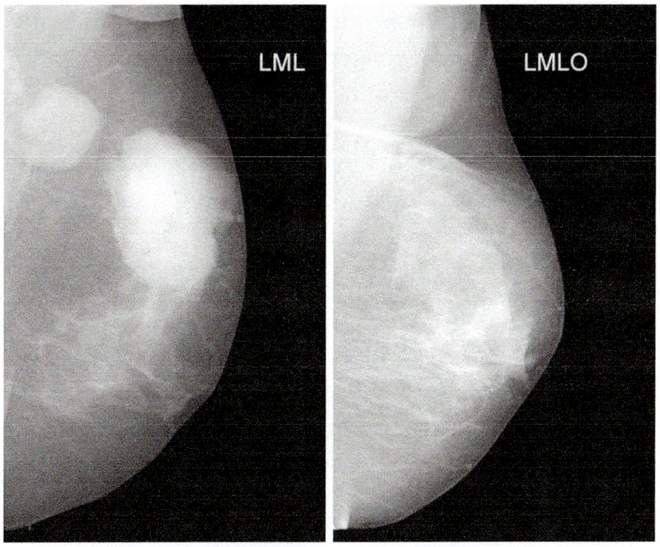

Fig. 1: Mammogram (MLO view) in a 42-year-old patient before and after neoadjuvant chemotherapy showing significant reduction size of mass and lymph nodes. (MLO: mediolateral oblique).

in predicting residual tumor size depends on the initial mammographic appearance of the tumor.

Reduction mammoplasty, breast augmentation and mastopexy (breast lift): They are breast surgeries performed for cosmetic reasons, with an increasing number of women opting for them these days. Hence, it becomes important for the radiologist to be aware of the mammographic findings that differentiate normal from abnormal findings in these cases.

Specimen mammogram: It is another important mammographic examination in which a radiograph of the surgically excised specimen is taken to ascertain the adequacy of margins after lumpectomy or excision biopsy.

BREAST CONSERVATIVE THERAPY

Currently, mammography is the single imaging modality recommended for routine follow-up in women who have been treated for breast cancer. The role of additional imaging modalities, such as US, MRI and PET-computed tomography (CT) has not yet been established, but they are potentially useful and show high sensitivity and accuracy for detecting recurrences or distant metastases. There are no standardized protocols and these practices differ from country to country, institution to institution and the socioeconomic status of patient.

Mammography: What is the ideal time for imaging the treated breast? A "baseline" mammogram can be done after completion of lumpectomy OR after 6–8 months of breast radiotherapy . This time interval allows the immediate postradiation inflammatory changes to resolve significantly. The breast surgeon usually leaves surgical clips to mark the outline of the surgical resection site that is useful for planning radiation therapy. These clips are clearly visible on postoperative mammograms and CT, though not so apparent on ultrasound and MRI.

Ultrasonography: It is widely available and relatively inexpensive, but it involves a steeper learning curve in evaluation of the treated breast. It is useful in assessing and confirming postoperative changes such as seroma, hematoma, scar formation and residual/recurrent mass and also enables guided biopsy when required.

MRI: It is used mainly as a problem solving tool in the postoperative breast when mammographic and sonographic findings are indeterminate. It is also useful in looking for a residual mass if positive surgical margins are found on histopathology. MRI has high sensitivity and specificity for differentiating post-treatment changes from recurrent malignancies, particularly when performed >12 months after treatment.

PET-CT: It is highly sensitive for detecting lesions in the treated breast and in determining whether a recurrence is solitary or disseminated. The information obtained from PET-CT has significant impact on further treatment and post-treatment patient outcome.

Mammography

The treated breast presents a confounding situation for the radiologist. It is equally difficult for the technologist to produce good-quality mammographic images. The greatest difficulty faced by the technologist is optimal positioning of breast due to surgical deformity and/or decreased compressibility due to pain and radiation induced inflammation.[2] Resolution of postoperative changes, skin and trabecular thickening are particularly delayed by postsurgical radiation therapy.

There are no universal guidelines for imaging of the treated breast, ultimately the imaging protocol depends upon the institutional policy. In some institutions, the baseline mammogram is done before starting radiotherapy, while in others it is done 6 months after completion of radiotherapy, following annual follow-up mammograms of both breasts are compared with the baseline. The routine mammographic views are mediolateral oblique (MLO) and craniocaudal (CC) views. Additional views like spot compression and magnification views are done if required.

Chronology of Changes on Mammogram After Breast Conservation Therapy

Findings on serial mammography are shown in Figures 2A to D. The first thing observed is reduction in volume of the operated breast as compared to the normal breast. Other changes that follow, in chronological order, include (1) breast edema and skin thickening, (2) fluid collections or hematoma, (3) scarring, (4) architectural distortion and (5) development of benign dystrophic calcifications (Table 1).

These changes acquire stability over a period of 2–3 years and any new change or increase in density should raise a suspicion of a recurrent tumor, which makes it of utmost importance to interpret sequential mammograms in comparison with previous mammograms.

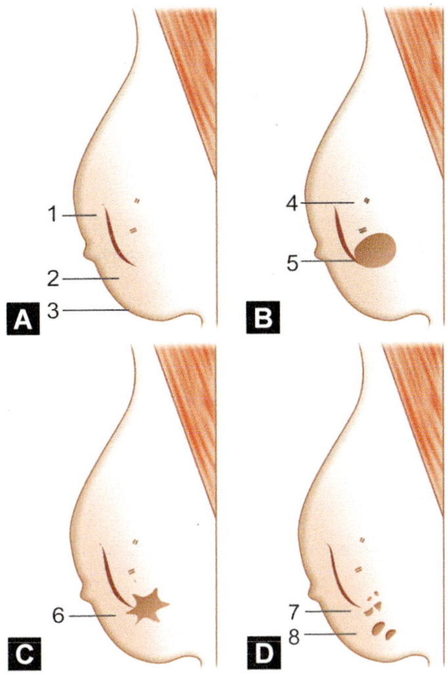

Figs. 2A to D: Evolution of mammogram findings in postoperative breast in patients treated with breast conservation therapy—1. skin fold; 2. increased breast density; 3. skin thickening; 4. surgical staples; 5. seroma; 6. scar; 7. dystrophic calcification; 8. fat necrosis.

Table 1: Mammography findings in post-treated breast.

	Finding	*Appearance on mammogram*
1.	Breast edema	Trabecular thickening and diffuse increase in breast density
2.	Skin thickening	Thickening in periareolar region and dependent portions (≤1 cm)
3.	Seroma/ hematoma	Oval or round opacity/mass at the lumpectomy site
4.	Architectural distortion	Distortion of breast tissue in involved area
5.	Surgical scar	• Poorly marginated soft-tissue mass with interspersed radiolucent areas • Morphology changes in different projections
6.	Calcifications: a. Dystrophic calcifications b. Fat necrosis	• Coarse, large and round calcifications • Radiolucent cyst • Coarse rim calcification • Benign lucent calcification
7.	Recurrence	• **Relative increase** in asymmetry or skin thickening or edema • Enlarging mass or appearance of pleomorphic calcifications near the tumor site

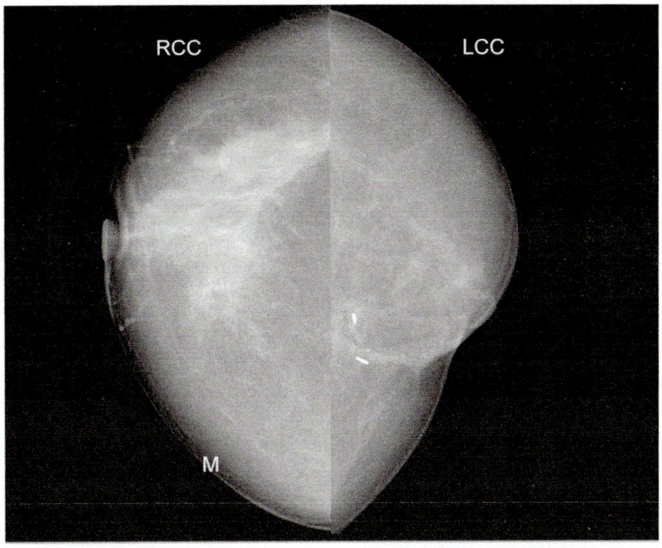

Fig. 3: Mammogram of both breasts CC view in a 41-year-old patient with breast conservative surgery in left breast showing postoperative changes in left breast in the form of volume loss, architectural distortion and surgical staples (CC: craniocaudal).

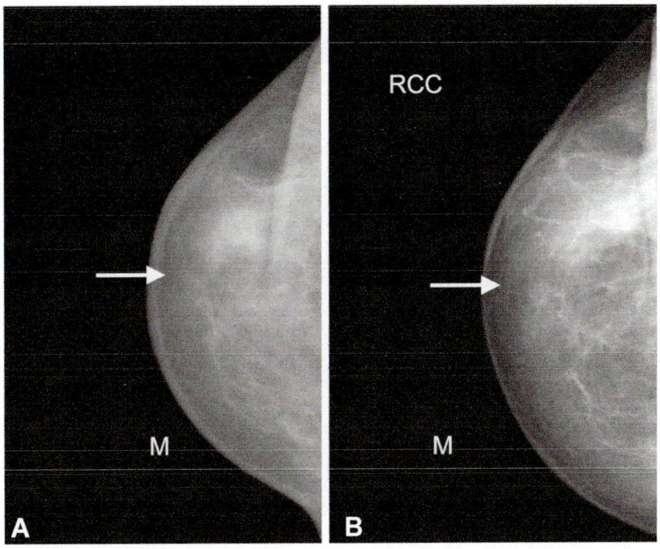

Figs. 4A and B: A 45-year-old female underwent lumpectomy in right breast for infiltrative ductal carcinoma followed by chemotherapy and radiation. Mammogram of right breast—CC view (A) shows skin thickening (arrow) that has reduced thickness in mammogram done after 1 year (B) (CC: craniocaudal).

Breast Edema and Skin Thickening

Edema is commonly seen in the breast treated with radiotherapy. Mammographic features include skin and stromal thickening, trabecular thickening and diffuse increase in breast density[3] (Figs. 3 to 5), which are obviously better

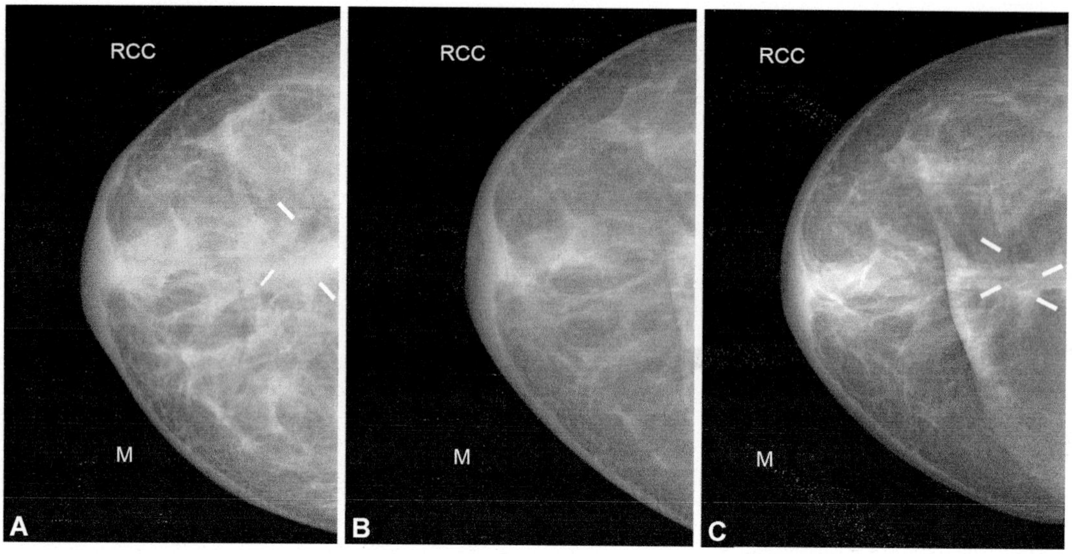

Figs. 5A to C: Serial annual mammograms—CC view (A to C) in a patient who underwent breast conservation therapy shows increased breast density and skin thickening in the initial mammogram (A) that shows reduction with time (B, C). (CC: craniocaudal).

appreciated when compared with the contralateral normal breast. There may be subareolar edema that is due to surgical disruption of lymphatics.[4] Breast density may also increase because of suboptimal compression due to radiation-induced changes.

It is observed that skin thickening is maximum at around 6 months after radiation therapy and may reach a thickness of 1 cm. Later, it gradually decreases and attains stability over a period of 2–3 years. An increase in skin thickening or breast edema once stability is achieved should raise the possibility of lymphatic obstruction due to metastatic spread or obstructed venous drainage.

Fluid Collection

Seromas form in the surgical cavity after lumpectomy, mastectomy or axillary surgery, vary considerably in occurrence and are more common in obese and elder patients.[5] A seroma or fluid collection is seen on the mammogram as an oval or round opacity/mass at the lumpectomy site (Figs. 6 and 7) or in the lower axillary region if axillary clearance is done. Seromas or hematomas can persist from weeks to months but gradually get resorbed and decrease in size over a period of time. Initially, a seroma may be partially obscured by surrounding breast edema and focal skin thickening; however with resolution of the edema, the cavity becomes more apparent. It may completely resolve in some patients in 12–18 months and may only be seen later as a remnant scar or area of fibrosis. In some patients, it may reduce more gradually in size

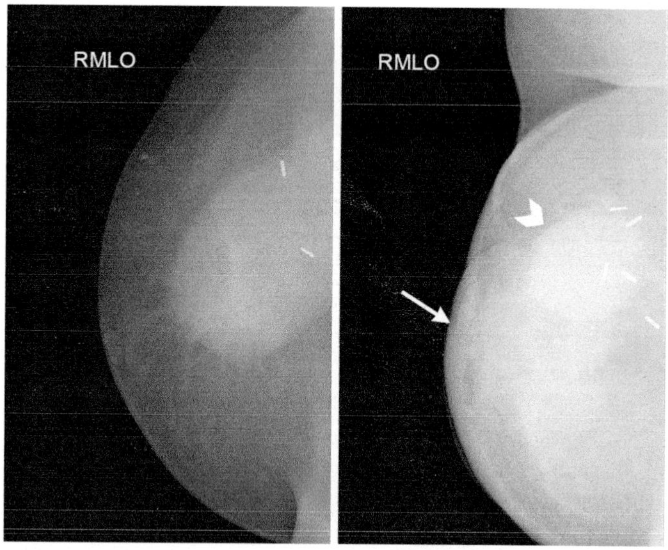

Fig. 6: Postoperative mammogram of right breast in two different patients showing a well-defined opacity at the surgical site s/o seroma. Note the surgical clips.

and persist for a few years. In the study by Mendelson, seromas were seen till 6 months in 25% patients.[6] An increase in size of a seroma after a few years should raise a suspicion of recurrence.

Architectural Distortion

Architectural distortion is noted at the lumpectomy site or in the axillary tail region, if axillary dissection is done, in the form of loss of normal-appearing curvilinear crescentic

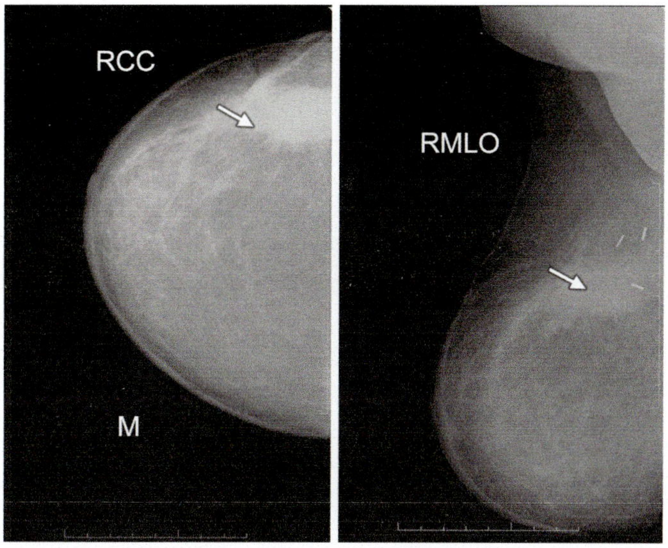

Fig. 7: A 49-year-old female who underwent breast conservation therapy of right breast underwent mammogram after 1 year. Mammogram—CC and MLO views show a circumscribed mass in right breast (arrow) suggestive of seroma. (CC: craniocaudal; MLO: mediolateral oblique).

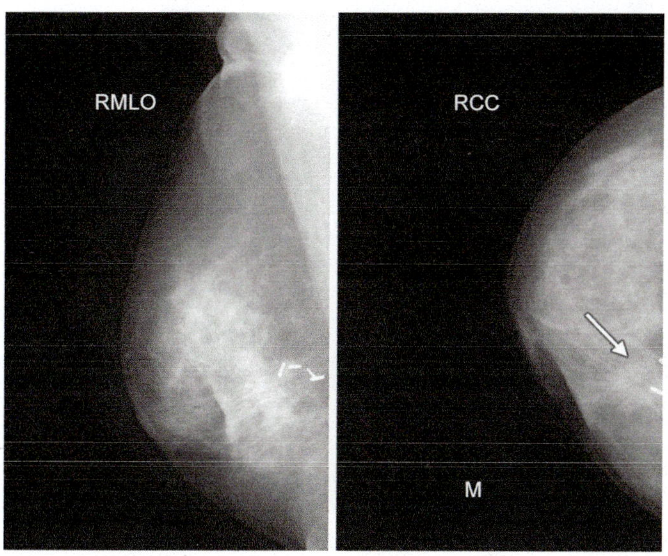

Fig. 8: Mammogram of right breast (MLO and CC view) in a 35-year-old female who underwent lumpectomy for infiltrative ductal carcinoma shows an ill-defined opacity with central area of lucency near the site of surgical staples s/o post surgical scar (arrow) (CC: craniocaudal; MLO: mediolateral oblique).

planes of the breast and "pulling-in" of Cooper ligaments with irregular soft-tissue density giving rise to a spiculated appearance. It is imperative that the parenchymal scarring, architectural distortion and skin retraction at the surgical site due to surgical changes be differentiated from a recurrent carcinoma.

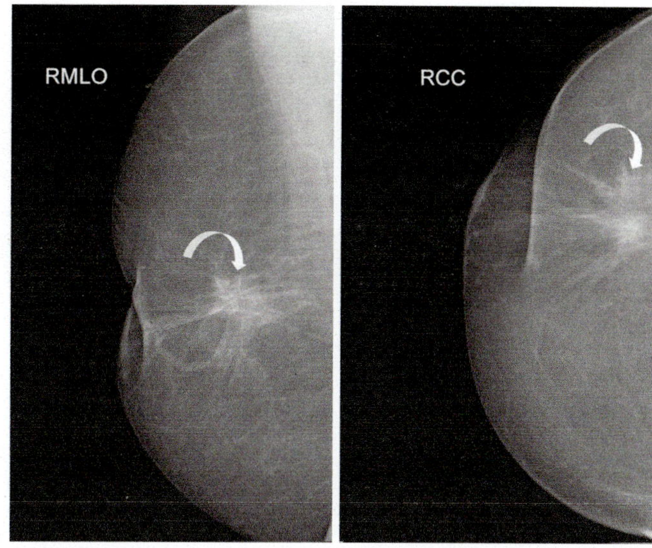

Fig. 9: Mammogram showing scar in right breast in a 48-year-old patient who underwent breast conservative surgery.

Table 2: Comparison of mammographic findings in surgical scar and radial scar.

	Surgical scar	*Radial scar*
1.	History of surgery present	No history of surgery/trauma
2.	Skin thickening and skin retraction	Not palpable, no skin thickening/retraction present
3.	a. Poorly marginated soft-tissue mass with interspersed radiolucent areas b. No change in appearance on different projections	a. Architectural distortion with long thin radiating spicules and central fat—"black star" appearance b. Variable appearance in different projections

Surgical scar: It is a benign finding, seen as an area of architectural distortion with a poorly marginated soft-tissue mass having internal interspersed radiolucent areas of fat entrapped by fibrous tissue (Figs. 8 to 11). It usually has some relation to the cutaneous scar or region of previous surgery. When followed up on annual mammograms, the scar gradually reduces in size, attains stability and eventually fades away. Some patients may heal with little or no mammographic findings, while some may have extensive scarring resulting in keloid formation. A carefully taken history and visualization of placement markers can help prevent misinterpretation of these lesions. It is important to remember that mammographic appearances of a post-surgical scar can mimic a recurrent malignant mass or radial scar and must be differentiated from it (Table 2).

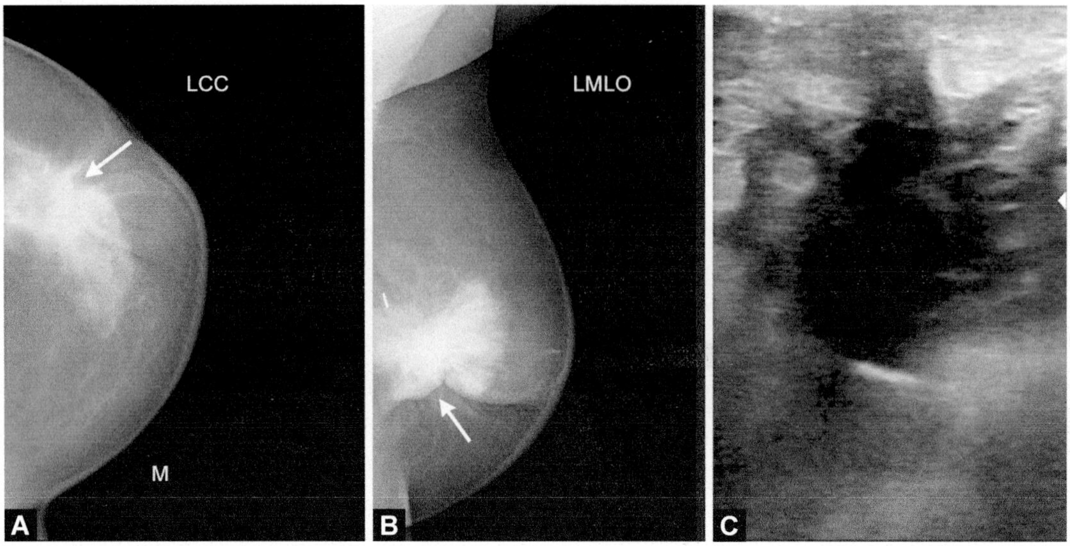

Figs. 10A to C: (A and B) Mammogram of left breast MLO and CC views in a 55-year-old patient with breast conservative therapy shows architectural distortion, skin fold and increased density along with scar tissue; (C) Ultrasound of the region of interest in the same patient shows an irregular hypoechoic lesion with entrapped fat within. There was no vascularity and no mass was seen. These features were suggestive of scar tissue. (CC: craniocaudal; MLO: mediolateral oblique).

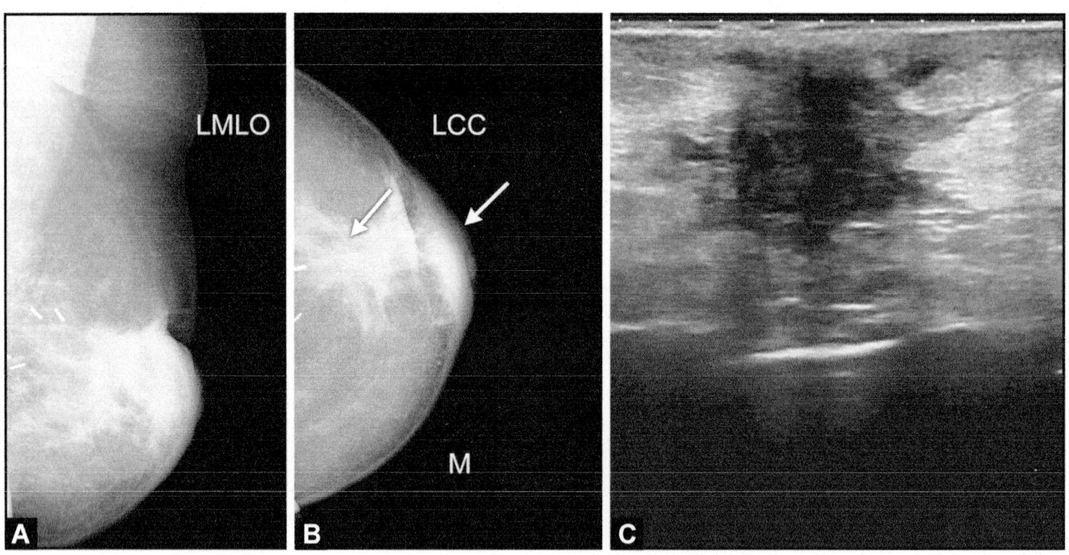

Figs. 11A to C: (A and B) Mammogram of left breast in a patient with breast conservative surgery shows skin thickening and scar tissue; (C) Ultrasound of left breast shows an irregular hypoechoic area, suggesting of scar.

Radial scars: Also known as sclerosing ductal hyperplasia, radial scars are not true scars but complex sclerosing lesions not related to previous surgery or trauma. These are non-palpable clinically and do not cause any skin thickening or skin retraction. However, they mimic malignancy on mammograms and are seen as asymmetric density or architectural distortion with central translucent areas representing fat without a discrete central mass, the appearance varying in orthogonal views. A "black star" appearance is seen because of long, thin radiating spicules against a background of radiolucent fat.[7] Though radial scars are benign entities, they *may be associated with atypical ductal hyperplasia and carcinoma in 31%–50% of cases.*[8] An excision biopsy is necessary to establish a definitive diagnosis.

Mass: If there is no lucency within the area of architectural distortion and a central soft-tissue density is seen, additional views like spot compression and magnification views should be obtained. If the density persists on these views, biopsy should be done from the suspicious area to establish a diagnosis. An increase in size or density of the scar should always raise the possibility of recurrence and warrant further evaluation.

Calcifications

Benign calcifications appear at the operative site after approximately 6–12 months of surgery.

Fat necrosis It is a benign non-suppurative inflammatory process of adipose tissue and imaging appearances depend upon the stage of evolution. In early stages, it is seen as a soft-tissue density mass with partial halo (Figs. 12A and B) that evolves into a well-defined radiolucent cyst with rim calcification. The diagnosis is confirmed on the basis of either serial imaging that shows chronological changes compatible with evolution of fat necrosis or improvement in clinical symptoms. Oil cysts due to fat necrosis have thin peripheral arcs of calcification because of reduction of fat to fatty acids and formation of fibrous capsule, the latter calcify to give a crescentic appearance (Figs. 13 to 16). A fat-fluid level may form due to layering of oil and serosanguinous fluid and benign lucent-centered calcifications may be seen in late stages.

Dystrophic calcifications at the operative site are coarse, large, round and can be seen on sequential mammograms (Figs. 17 to 18A and B). Sutural calcifications, though rare, may also be seen. If indeterminate calcifications are seen (e.g., early rim of calcification in evolving fat necrosis), findings should be compared with previous mammograms. A biopsy is indicated when the calcifications appear suspicious or indeterminate.

Generally, new findings within the first 2 years of follow-up represent benign treatment-related changes.[10]

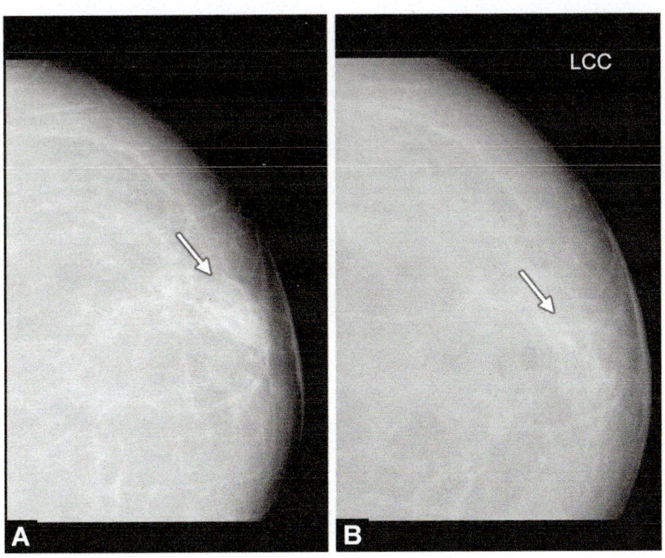

Figs. 12A and B: Serial mammogram of left breast shows fat necrosis as a soft-tissue density (A) that on subsequent image is seen as a radiolucent halo (B) with peripheral rim calcification.

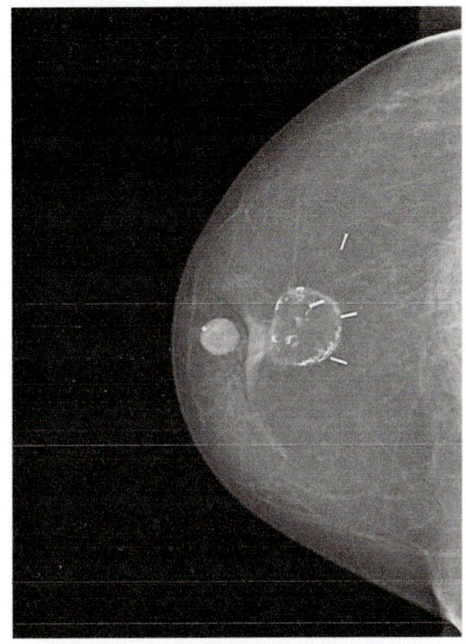

Fig. 13: Postoperative mammogram of right breast—CC view, in a 64-year-old woman shows a circumscribed lucent area with predominantly peripheral calcifications along with a few central calcific densities. Features represent fat necrosis (CC: craniocaudal).

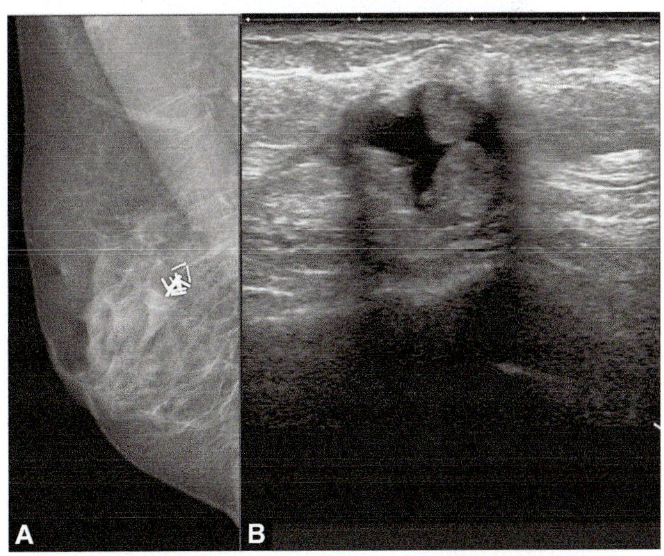

Figs. 14A and B: (A) Mammogram of right breast—MLO view in a 66-year-old female who underwent breast conservation surgery shows surgical staples and a circumscribed rounded lucency with a radiopaque rim suggestive of fat necrosis. (B) Ultrasound of the same region shows a round circumscribed anechoic lesion with peripheral nodularity that was suggestive of fat necrosis (MLO: mediolateral oblique).

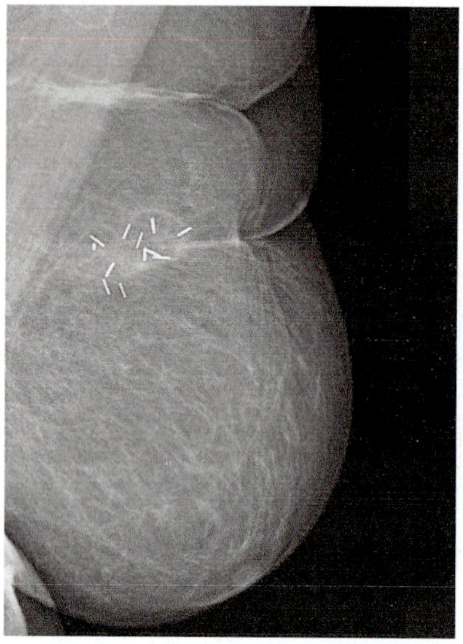

Fig. 15: Postoperative mammogram of left breast—MLO view in a 72-year-old female shows surgical staples and a circumscribed rounded lucency adjacent to it suggestive of fat necrosis (MLO: mediolateral oblique).

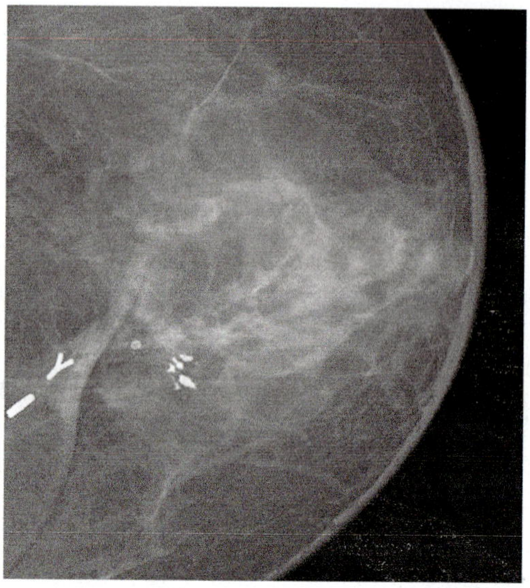

Fig. 17: Mammogram of left breast—CC view of a woman who underwent breast conservation shows surgical staples and multiple large irregular calcific foci suggestive of dystrophic calcification. (CC: craniocaudal).

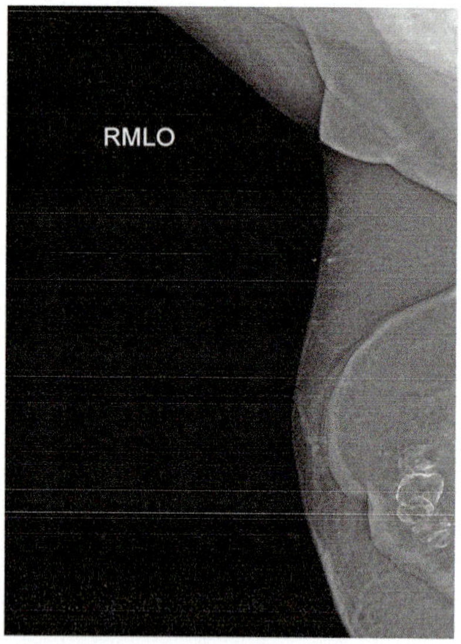

Fig. 16: Mammogram of right breast shows multiple large, circumscribed calcifications at the operative site s/o fat necrosis.

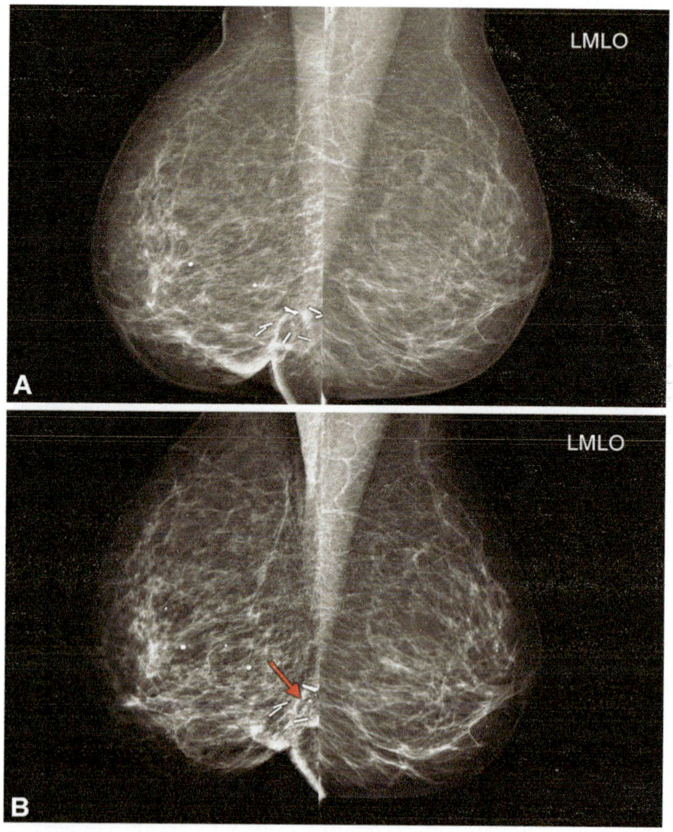

Figs. 18A and B: Sequential mammogram in a post-BCS patient taken at an interval of 1 year shows dystrophic calcifications at the surgical site (arrow).

Ultrasound

Ultrasound is an adjunct to mammography with an important role in the evaluation of the treated breast. Especially in cases where extensive surgery has been done, when the residual breast is too small to be evaluated on mammography or a mammographic finding in the treated breast is suboptimally covered, ultrasound proves to be invaluable.

Not only does it confirm the findings on mammogram, but it may also show a residual or recurrent mass that is not well appreciated on mammogram. Apart from evaluation of the treated breast itself, ultrasound is also an excellent modality to evaluate the chest wall and axillary region. One of the most common sites for post-treatment breast cancer recurrence is the chest wall either from direct extension of the tumor, indirect extension via interpectoral nodes or from undissected lymphatics.

Ultrasound findings in the treated breast include skin thickening (>3 mm), trabecular thickening with blurring of normal structures due to breast edema, seroma, scar and sometimes oil cyst as shown in the line diagram (Fig. 19) and described in Table 3.

Evaluation in the early part of treatment shows more heterogeneous and echogenic parenchyma (Fig. 20) as compared to the contralateral breast. The postoperative cavity (seroma or hematoma) can have a variable appearance as shown in the line diagram (Fig. 21). The ultrasound appearances range from a circumscribed anechoic collection, collection with thick wall or septations, a hypoechoic lesion or a cystic lesion showing an echogenic mesh like appearance, which may reduce in size over a period of time or may persist for a few years (Figs. 22A to F).

The surgical scar is seen as an irregular heterogeneous hypoechoic area that may show entrapped fat and may reach up to the subcutaneous plane (Fig. 23). It typically produces extensive posterior acoustic shadowing and in many cases, may be indistinguishable from shadowing produced by a malignancy. Hence, a biopsy may be necessary for confirmation. On follow-up scans, surgical scars gradually reduce in size and attain stability (Figs. 24A to C).

Fat necrosis may appear as a complex mass that may evolve into either more solid or more cystic appearing lesions. Solid fat necrosis may typically remain solid and be mistaken for residual or recurrent lesion, being a significant false positive finding and prompting biopsy for confirmation. Hemorrhage within the fat may be seen as a well-defined hyperechoic area with the typical appearance

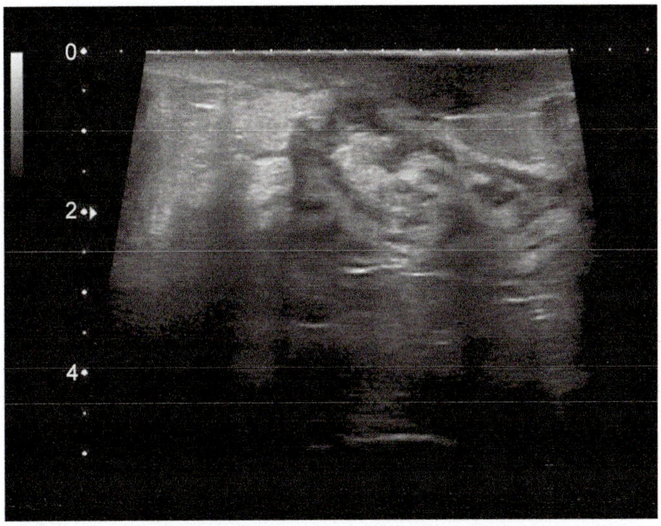

Fig. 20: Ultrasound in patient who underwent breast conservation therapy showing heterogenous and echogenic parenchyma due to breast edema.

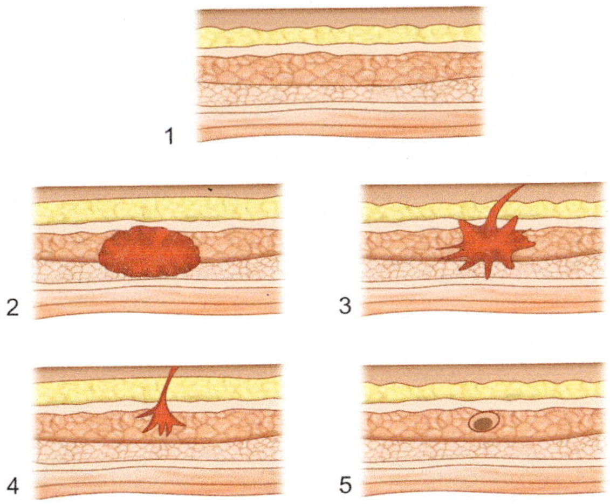

Fig. 19: Line diagram showing ultrasound findings in a breast treated with breast conservative therapy : 1. skin thickening, 2. Seroma 3. Developing scar resembling malignant lesion, 4. Scar tissue becoming smaller in size, 5. Residual tissue.

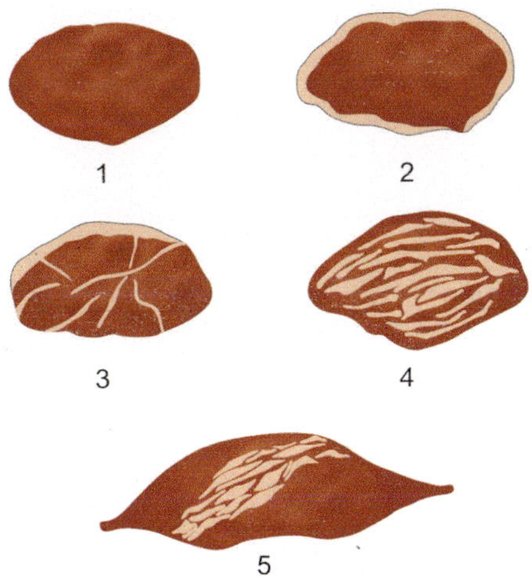

Fig. 21: Various appearances of seroma on ultrasound: 1. round to oval anechoic collection; 2. anechoic collection with thickened wall; 3. cystic collection with septations; 4. cystic collection with multiple closely placed septations; 5. cystic collection with echogenic mesh like appearance centrally.

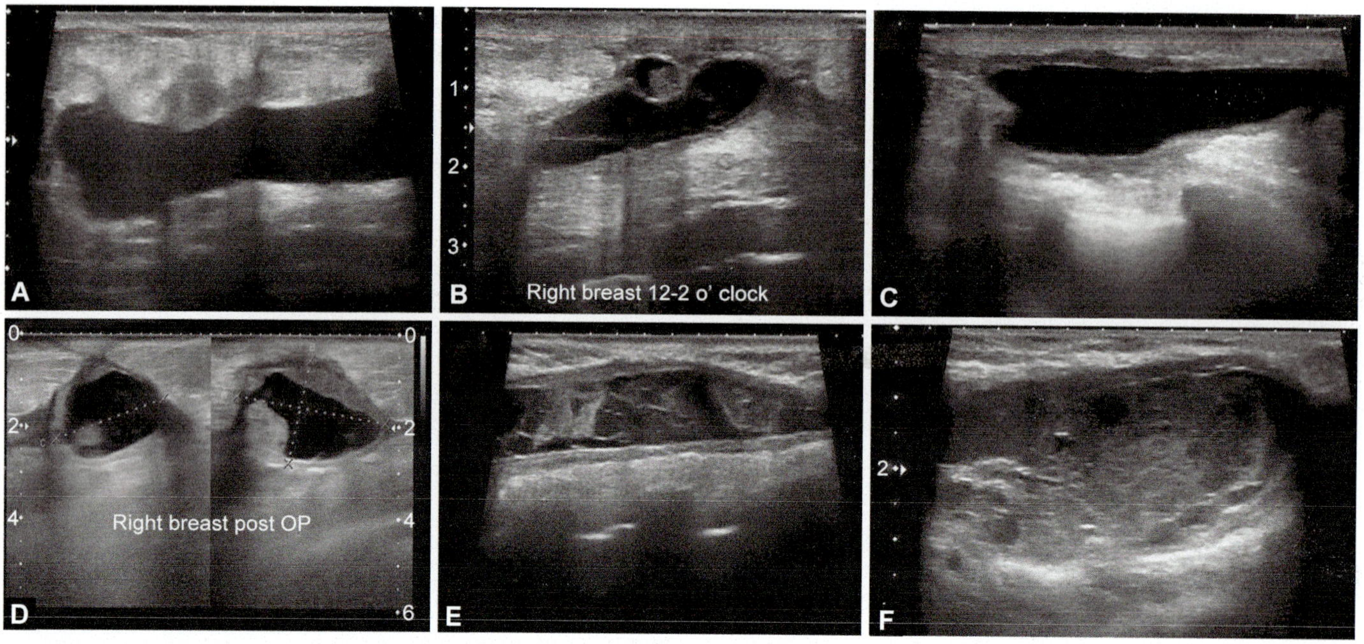

Figs. 22A to F: Various appearances of seroma on ultrasound: (A) Anechoic collection; (B) Anechoic collection with echogenic nodule and septations; (C) Anechoic collection with thickened wall; (D) Anechoic collection with mural nodule; (E) Collection showing echogenic mesh like appearance; (F) Heterogeneous collection with echoes.

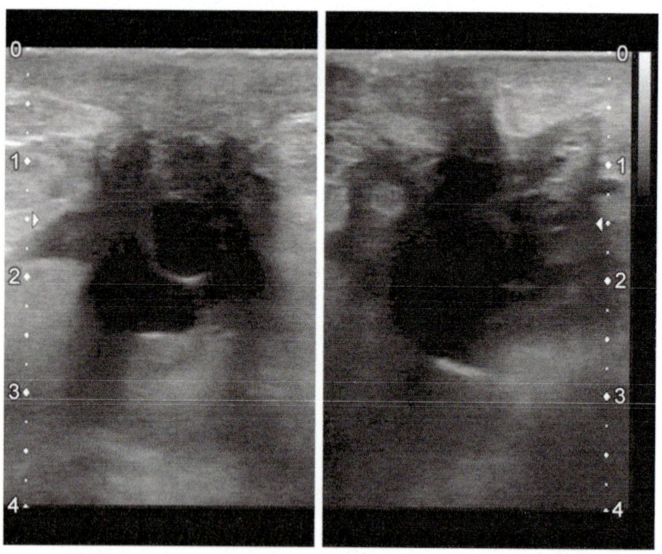

Fig. 23: Ultrasound in a 35-year-old patient showing postsurgical scar at the lumpectomy site as an irregular heterogeneously hypoechoic area reaching up to the subcutaneous tissue.

Table 3: Ultrasound findings in postsurgical breast.

	Finding	*Appearance on ultrasound*
1.	Skin thickening	>3 mm in periareolar region
2.	Trabecular thickening and breast edema	Heterogeneous hyperechoic breast parenchyma
4.	Seroma/ hematoma	Anechoic/hypoechoic lesion with low-level echoes or septations, complex cystic lesion
5.	Surgical scar	Irregular hypoechoic area with posterior acoustic shadowing
6.	Fat necrosis	Anechoic lesion with hyperechoic nodular wall, complex cystic lesion, fat fluid layering, echogenic lesion with peripheral halo
7.	Recurrence	Increase in size of scar, hypoechoic masses away from scar site, axillary lymphadenopathy

of fat necrosis on correlated mammogram (Figs. 25A, B and 26). Fat necrosis may also be seen as circumscribed anechoic cystic lesions with echogenic margins due to calcific rim or as cystic lesions with nodular margins (Figs. 27A and B). The most specific sign of fat necrosis is an echogenic band within an oil cyst that shifts in orientation with change in patient position.

Dystrophic calcifications at the surgical site are seen as multiple echogenic foci with posterior acoustic shadowing.

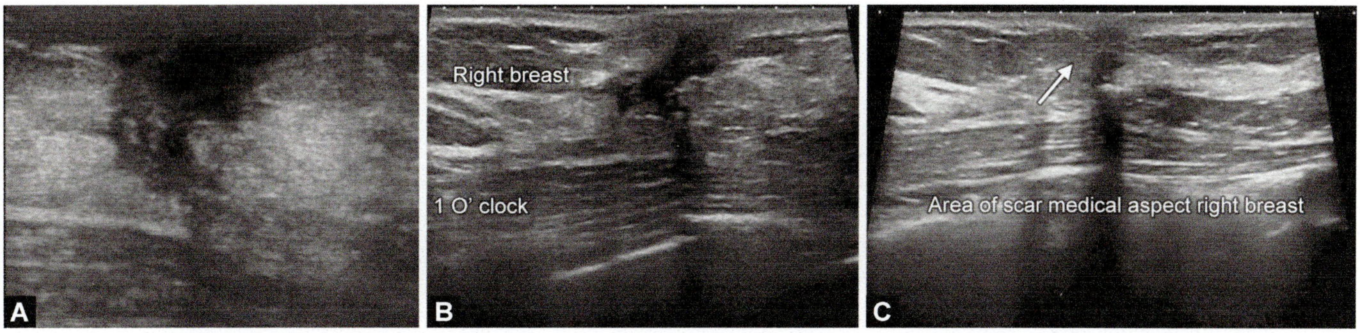

Figs. 24A to C: Sequential ultrasound at the surgical site in a patient with breast conservative therapy shows a postoperative scar that gradually reduces in size and attains stability over a period of time.

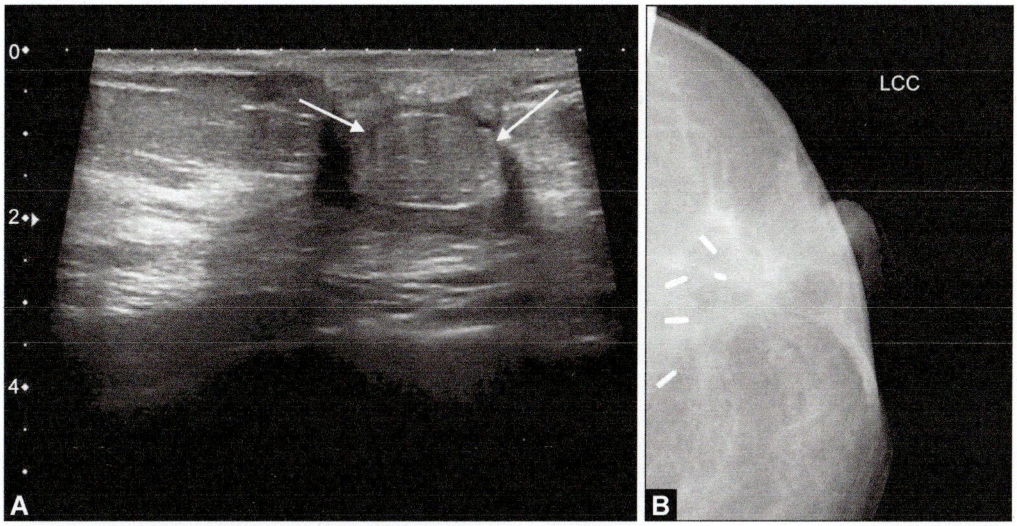

Figs. 25A and B: (A) Ultrasound of the left breast shows a circumscribed round echogenic mass with hypoechoic rim at the scar site in a patient with breast conservation therapy; (B) Mammogram of the left breast in the same patient shows a fat lucency with a calcific rim at surgical site s/o fat necrosis.

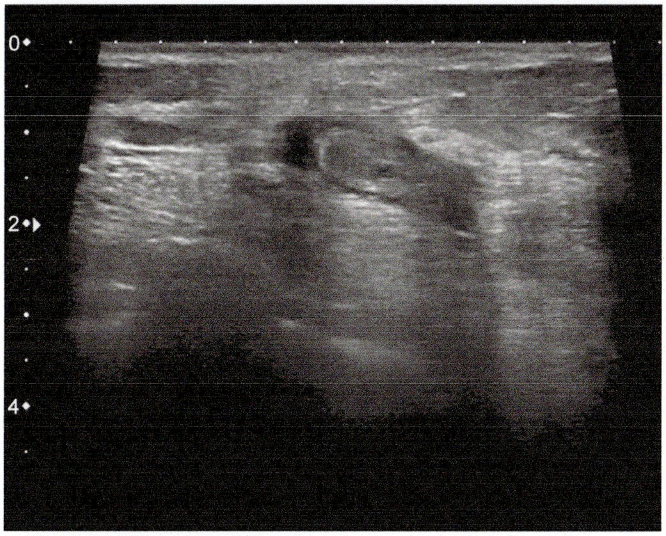

Fig. 26: Ultrasound of breast at the postoperative site shows a circumscribed echogenic mass with anechoic rim s/o fat necrosis.

A residual mass is generally visualized at the operative site as an irregular hypoechoic mass, while a complex fluid collection indicates a seroma or hematoma. Positive tumor margins on histopathology warrant a high index of suspicion for residual lesion and a biopsy should be performed for confirmation. Any lesion increasing in size on either clinical or imaging assessment should be viewed with suspicion, unless it corresponds to a definitively benign mammographic finding, such as fat necrosis.

In a patient who has undergone MRM, the operated side should always be examined on ultrasound. The ultrasound appearance on operated side shows the pectoralis major muscle without any overlying breast tissue as compared to the opposite side (Fig. 28) with normal breast parenchyma. Sometimes a postoperative seroma is present and can persist for a long time (Fig. 29). Any new mass arising at the scar site should be evaluated for malignancy.

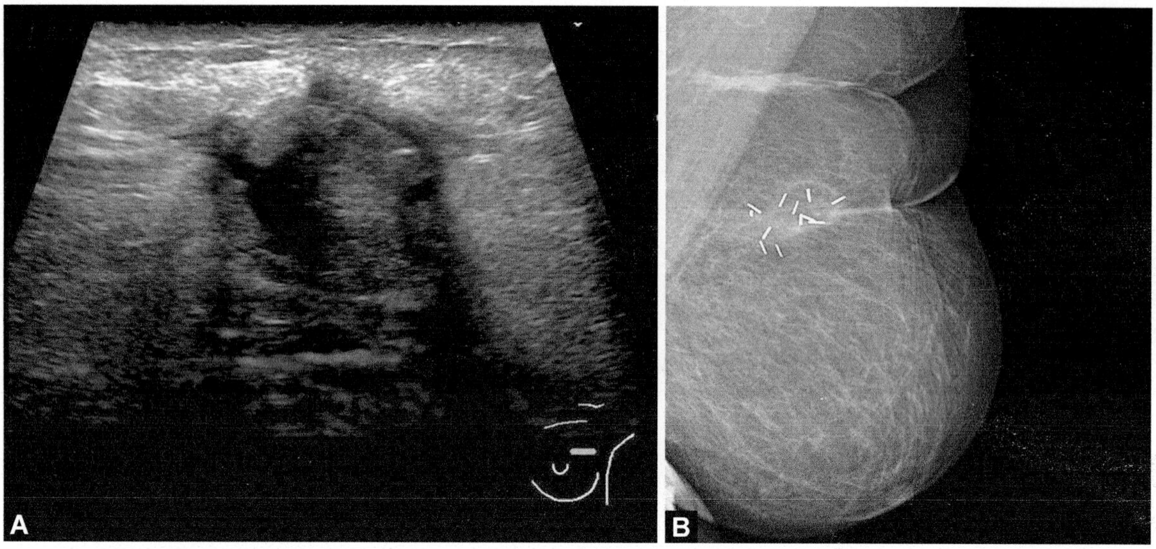

Figs. 27A and B: Ultrasound shows a well-defined cystic lesion with nodular margins in left breast; (B) Mammogram of left breast (CC view) in the same patient shows the surgical site confirming fat necrosis (CC: craniocaudal).

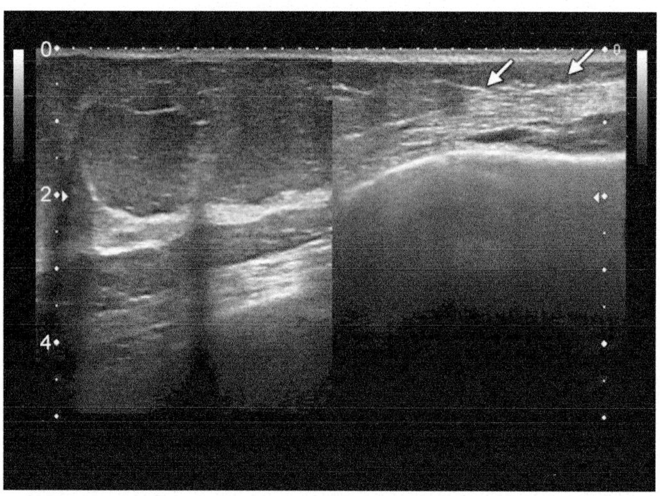

Fig. 28: Ultrasound of breast in a post-MRM patient shows normal breast parenchyma on the contralateral side. Pectoralis muscle (arrows) is seen on the operated side (MRM: modified radical mastectomy).

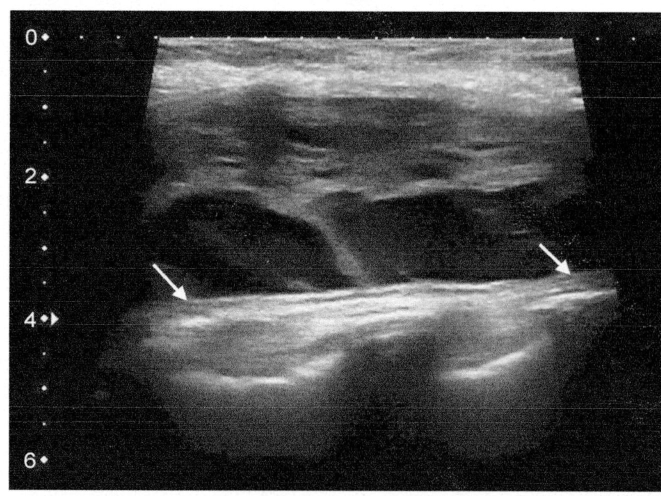

Fig. 29: Ultrasound of right breast in a 52-year-old female who underwent MRM shows seroma (MRM: modified radical mastectomy). Arrows denote the pectoralis muscle.

Computed Tomography

Breast cancer patients often undergo staging or surveillance CT during or after the course of their treatment. The postsurgical changes seen on CT depend upon the type of surgery performed like (lumpectomy, mastectomy, breast reconstruction or axillary surgery). Complications related to surgery like seroma, infections, fat necrosis and lymphedema can be easily evaluated on CT.

Breast conservation therapy: CT shows distortion at the surgical site with overlying skin retraction, surgical clips, skin and trabecular thickening due to radiation therapy.

MRM: Two types of mastectomy are done: skin sparing mastectomy (SSM) and nipple sparing mastectomy (NSM).

In SSM, the breast tissue, nipple and areola are removed keeping the overlying skin intact, so that immediate reconstruction can be done for better cosmetic results. The nipple will not be seen on postoperative CT in these cases. Potential complications are skin necrosis and locoregional recurrence.

NSM is preferred in patients with tumor size <2.5 cm, nipple-to-tumor distance >4 cm and no lymphovascular invasion. The breast tissue is removed keeping the overlying skin, the nipple and areola intact. Nipple necrosis and nipple insensitivity are major complications of NSM. Nipple is seen in these patients on postoperative CT.

Both NSM and SSM are followed by immediate reconstruction, initiated with the placement of an expander at the time of mastectomy.

Breast reconstruction: These include breast prostheses (implants); myocutaneous flaps, such as latissimus dorsi flap and transverse rectus abdominis myocutaneous (TRAM) flap; and muscle-sparing free-flap autologous reconstruction, such as the deep inferior epigastric perforator (DIEP) flap.

Postsurgical Complications

Seroma: Postsurgical seroma (Figs. 30A to D) occurs in 20%–50% patients after MRM compared with 9%–20% of patients after lumpectomy.[11] The seroma appears as a low-attenuation fluid collection without internal enhancement in the surgical bed, chest wall or axilla.

Hematoma: A hematoma is a less common postsurgical complication. The hematoma may have a variable appearance depending on its age. In the initial stages, it usually appears as a low-attenuation mass in the breast, chest wall or axilla but with relatively higher attenuation than a serous fluid collection. Later, it may appear similar to a simple fluid attenuation since contents break down, making it difficult to distinguish from a seroma.

Infection: Postoperative infection may manifest as cellulitis or abscess. Cellulitis appears as diffuse fat stranding in subcutaneous fat along the surgical bed, while an abscess is seen as a low-attenuation fluid collection with peripheral enhancement and often, with thicker walls.

Fat necrosis: Fat necrosis is a sterile inflammation of fat resulting from loss of vascular supply. On CT, the lesion will have fat attenuation centrally with adjacent fat stranding and enhancement.

Magnetic Resonance Imaging

MRI plays an important problem-solving role in the postoperative breast when mammography and ultrasound are difficult to interpret due to postsurgical inflammatory

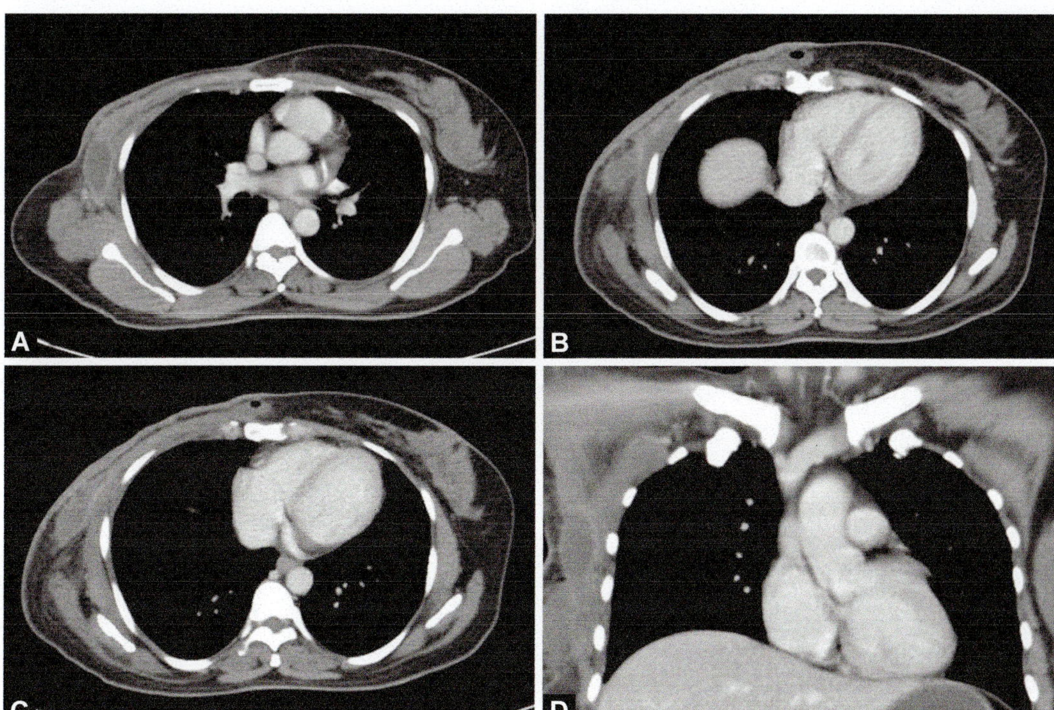

Figs. 30A to D: Contrast enhanced CT axial sections of thorax and coronal reconstruction (D) in post-MRM patient on right side shows pectoralis muscle and seroma formation. (MRM: modified radical mastectomy).

changes, edema, architectural distortion and a recurrence needs to be ruled out. *The operative site can show enhancement on MRI up to 6 months after surgery or up to 18–24 months of radiation therapy.* The optimal time for breast imaging is 4 weeks or more after surgery. The obvious advantage is evaluation of both mammographically visible and occult lesions. Compression is not required. Sensitivity is not limited to lesions with calcifications. It identifies benign lesions also and can help in differentiating lesions that require a close follow-up and those which are suspicious for malignancy/recurrence and require immediate attention.

Breast imaging reporting and data system (BI-RADS) lexicon by the American College of Radiology for MRI is followed while reporting the treated breast also, with the same descriptors and no separate terminologies for the operated breast so far. The BIRADS classification is used but one must keep in mind that *BIRADS category 1 cannot be assigned to the postoperative breast.*

Benign postoperative changes near the lumpectomy site include architectural distortion, edema, signal void or signal flare due to biopsy clips and seroma with thin rim enhancement ≤5 mm. These findings are assigned BIRADS category 2.

Breast edema may persist for a long time (Figs. 31A to D)—even up to 6 years in 25% patients. A seroma is seen as fluid-filled cavity of low or intermediate signal intensity on T1-weighted images and high signal intensity on T2-weighted images. It may or may not show thin rim enhancement (Figs. 32A to D).

Fat necrosis presents a challenge even on MRI, with a spectrum of findings that may be assigned a BIRADS category 2, 3 or even 4 when features are indeterminate. The commonest appearance of a circumscribed lesion at the lumpectomy site is isointense to fat with adjacent contrast enhancement (Figs. 33A to D). T1-weighted images without fat saturation show a central high signal representing spared fat; however, if hemosiderin is present it may be of low signal intensity. T2-weighted fat saturated images show central hypointensity. Rim enhancement is seen on contrast study. Other appearances of fat necrosis are focal or diffuse homogenous or heterogenous enhancement, oil cyst (round or oval mass of fat intensity), calcification seen as signal voids, mass with rim enhancement or irregular mass. Features that appear typically benign are assigned the BIRADS 2 category.

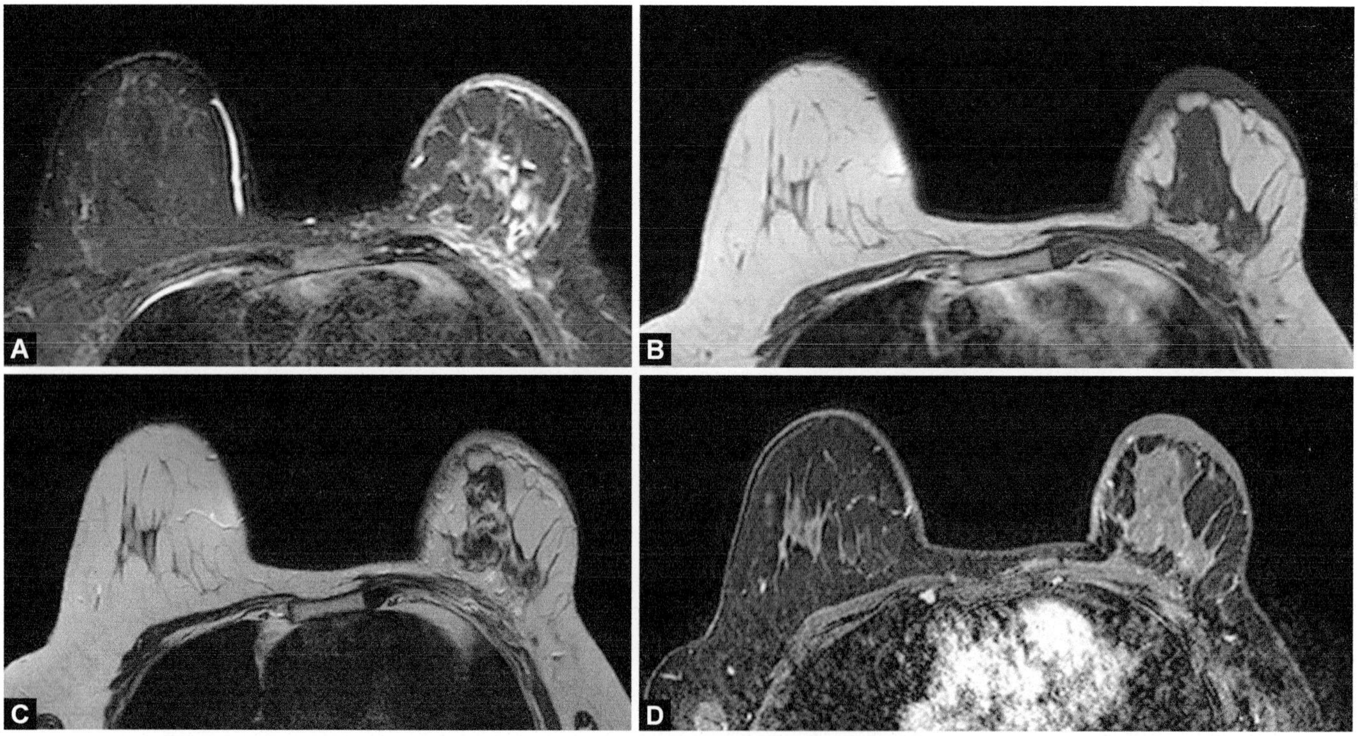

Figs. 31A to D: MRI breast in a 38-year-old female who underwent breast conservative therapy on left side (A)—STIR (Short tau inversion recovery); (B)—T1W; (C)—T2W; and (D)—postcontrast T1W) shows reduced volume in left breast with skin thickening and underlying edema. (T1W: T1 weighted; T2W: T2 weighted).

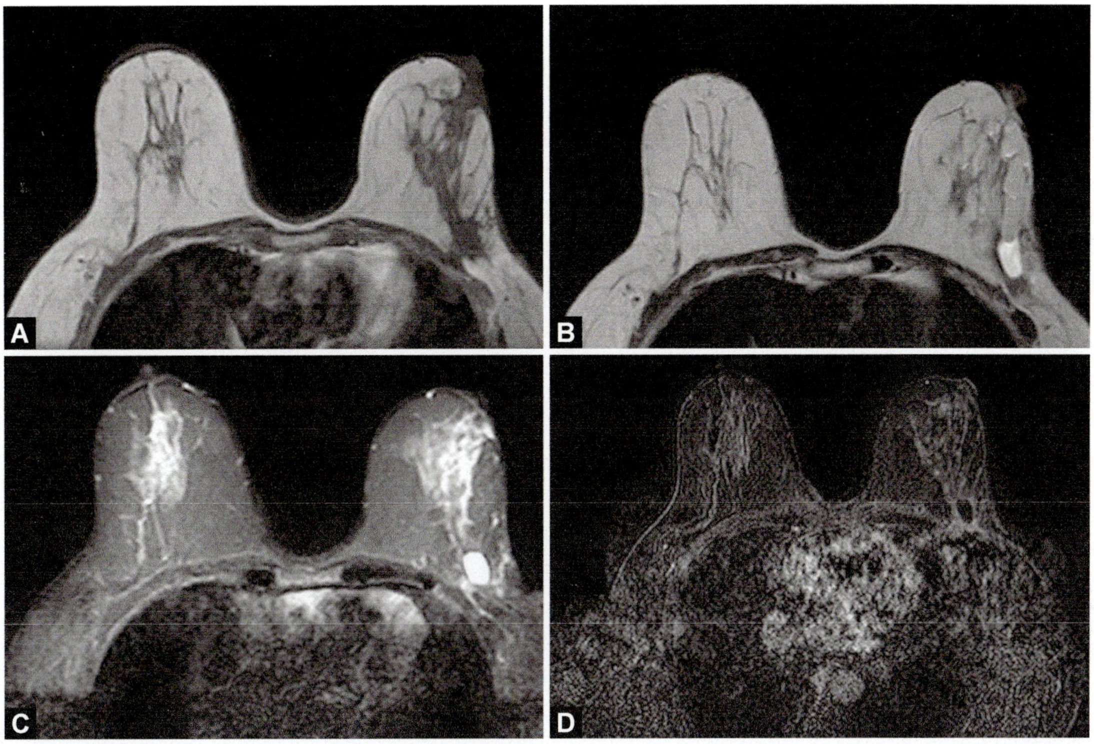

Figs. 32A to D: A 35-year-old female underwent breast conservative surgery. MRI was done to rule out recurrence. Axial sections of MRI left breast show a circumscribed area near axillary tail region that was hypointense on T1W (A), hyperintense on T2W and STIR (B and C) and shows peripheral enhancement on postcontrast dynamic sequence (D) suggestive of seroma. (T1W: T1 weighted; T2W: T2 weighted).

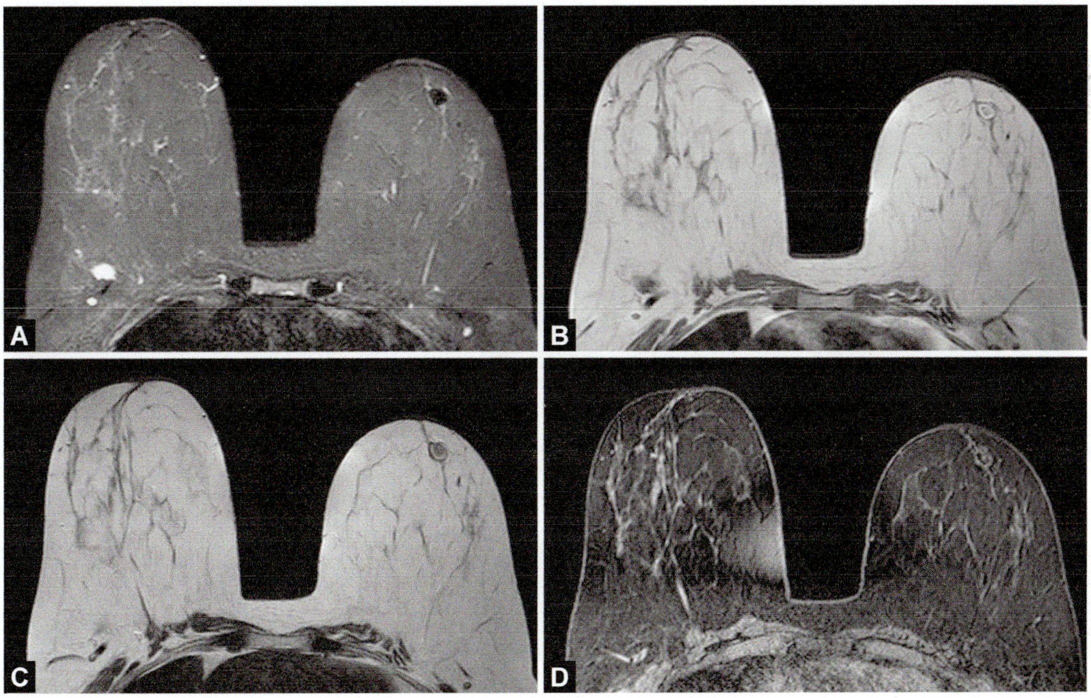

Figs. 33A to D: A 55-year-old female with prior history of breast surgery underwent MRI. (A to D) A circumscribed round mass showing hypointensity on STIR, central hyperintensity on T1W that was isointense to hyperintense on T2W and showed peripheral enhancement on postcontrast T1W sequence s/o fat necrosis. (T1W: T1 weighted; T2W: T2 weighted).

Minimal or small focal area of non-mass-like enhancement (NMLE) or thin linear persistent NMLE at or adjacent to the lumpectomy site is frequently seen and assigned BIRADS category 3, a 6-month follow-up is advised.

Imaging of Recurrence

Approximately 10–15% of patients with stage I/II invasive breast cancer will develop a clinically isolated local recurrence. The standard management of an ipsilateral breast tumor recurrence following breast-conserving surgery and radiation is salvage mastectomy, while local excision and radiation are optimal treatment of a chest wall recurrence following initial mastectomy.

The most important cause for recurrent cancers in a patient with breast conservative surgery at the operative site is because of incomplete surgical clearance. These tumors can be invasive cancers (Fig. 34) or in situ carcinoma (Figs. 35A to C and 36) unrelated to whether the earlier tumor was invasive. According to Roch et al., the risk of local recurrence increases at the rate of 2.5% per year from 2 to 6 years after treatment.[12] Tumors occurring after 10 years generally represent development of a new malignancy.

Once stability is achieved on mammography, appearance of any new findings must put the radiologist on alert. These include increasing asymmetry, skin thickening or edema; an enlarging mass or appearance of pleomorphic calcifications near the tumor site or in the same quadrant. Malignant calcifications in a recurrent lesion can be pleomorphic, branching, linear, coarse or heterogeneous in appearance.

It is important to remember that mammogram of both treated and contralateral breasts should be examined carefully to look for recurrent and metachronous cancers. An additional view like magnification may be required.

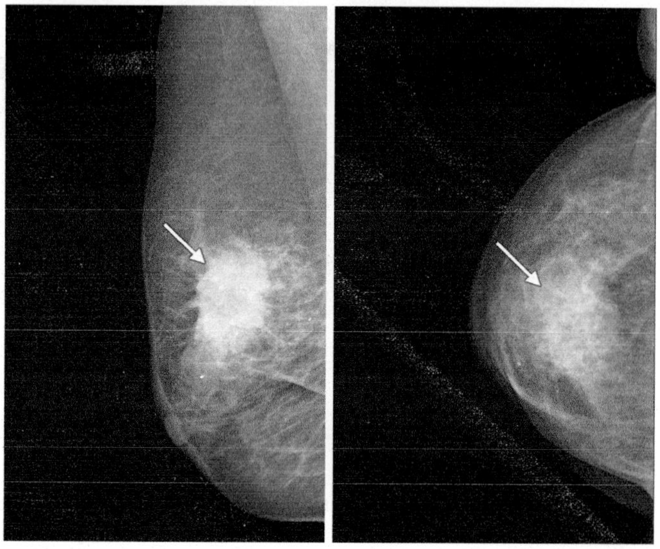

Fig. 34: Postoperative follow-up mammogram of right breast—MLO and CC views show an irregular dense asymmetry (arrow). Biopsy was suggestive of invasive ductal carcinoma. (CC: craniocaudal; MLO: mediolateral oblique).

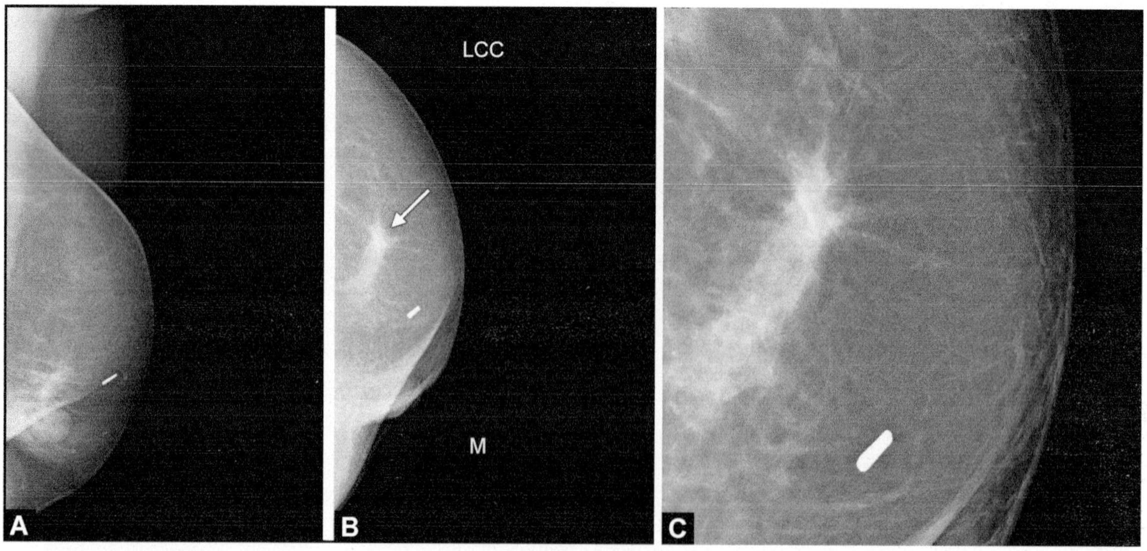

Figs. 35A to C: A 50-year-old patient underwent breast conservative surgery for invasive ductal carcinoma of left breast. Follow-up mammogram—MLO and CC views (A and B) after 1 year show linear/grouped calcification with related irregular soft tissue asymmetry (arrow); (C) Magnification view shows suspicious calcifications. Biopsy from this area was done, which showed invasive ductal carcinoma-suggestive of recurrence. (CC: craniocaudal; MLO: mediolateral oblique).

On ultrasound, a recurrent malignancy should be considered in a treated breast if the postbiopsy scar enlarges or if the edges start to become rounder on ultrasound. New masses that are not located in the surgical bed are also of serious concern and should be biopsied. The axilla should always be evaluated in such cases to look for axillary lymph nodes (Figs. 37A and B).

In post-MRM patients, the axilla and the mastectomy scar site should always be assessed for any new mass or nodule as local recurrences may occur (Fig. 38).

The sensitivity of MRI for detection of residual/recurrent tumor in the treated breast is over 90%.[13] It helps in differentiating scar tissue from tumor recurrence with nonenhancing areas having a high negative predictive value for malignancy (88–96%).[14] MRI findings that should raise the suspicion for recurrent or residual tumor are:

- Mass-like enhancement
- Enhancing thickened wall of a seroma (>5 mm)
- Irregular or enhancing rim or nodularity around resection cavity (>5 mm thickness)
- Segmental or ductal and clumped NMLE

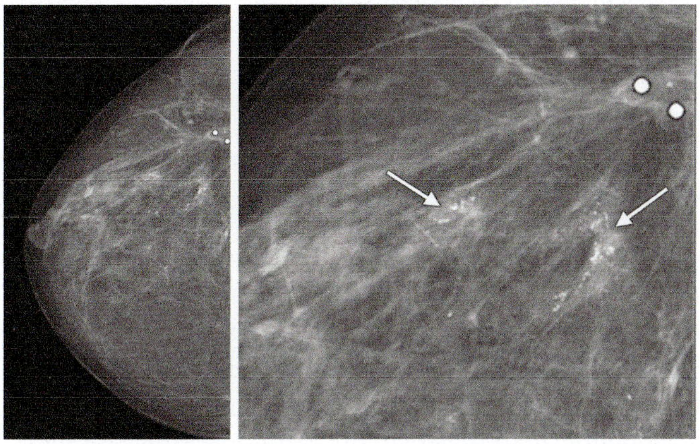

Fig. 36: Follow-up mammogram of right breast in a patient with breast conservative surgery shows linear, branching calcifications at the surgical site s/o recurrence.

Kinetic enhancement curve assessment includes evaluation of initial peak (slow, medium or rapid) and delayed phase (persistent, plateau, or washout). When suspicious features and enhancement are seen on MRI, then local recurrence should be considered (Figs. 39 and 40). Any suspicious findings away from the lumpectomy site should also be described.

If histopathology shows positive margins after excision, MRI is performed to look for residual tumor followed by re-excision or mastectomy. It should be noted that if there is no enhancement in the surgical bed, but the surgical margins are positive on histopathology then also re-excision has to be done.

OTHER BREAST SURGERIES

Reduction Mammoplasty and Mastopexy

Reduction mammoplasty and mastopexy (breast lift surgery) are increasingly common cosmetic surgeries these days; therefore, the breast radiologist must be aware of their characteristic imaging findings.

A preoperative mammogram should be done prior to any cosmetic surgery in women >40 years of age to detect

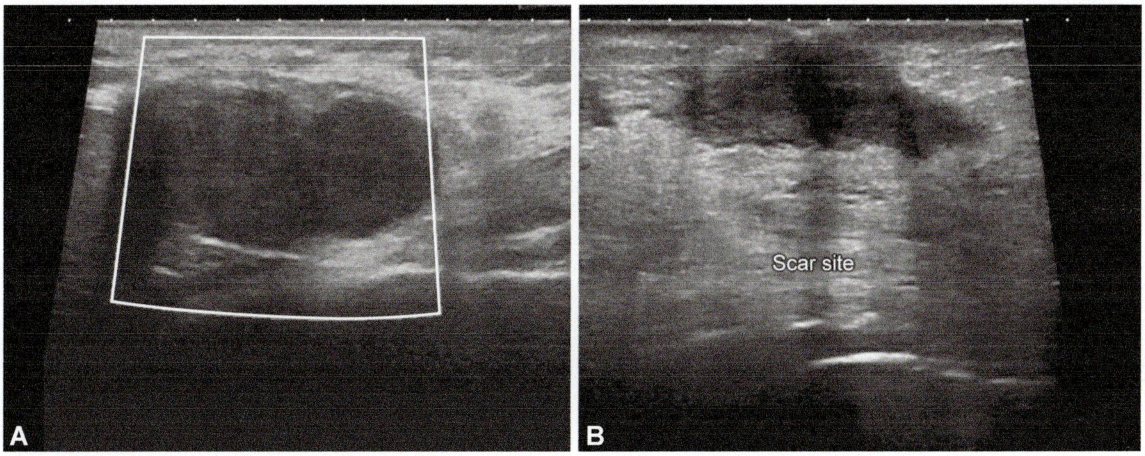

Figs. 37A and B: (A) Ultrasound of the axillary tail region of a patient who had undergone breast conservation surgery a year back shows a circumscribed hypoechoic lobulated mass s/o lymph-nodal mass; (B) Ultrasound at the surgical site shows an irregular hypoechoic area suggestive of scar. Biopsy from the axillary tail lesion was confirmed to be metastatic lymph nodes.

any significant disorder or pathology that may be resolved before or during surgery. A patient with a family history of breast cancer should be counseled about their high-risk status and the possible need for genetic testing prior to any cosmetic procedure surgery.

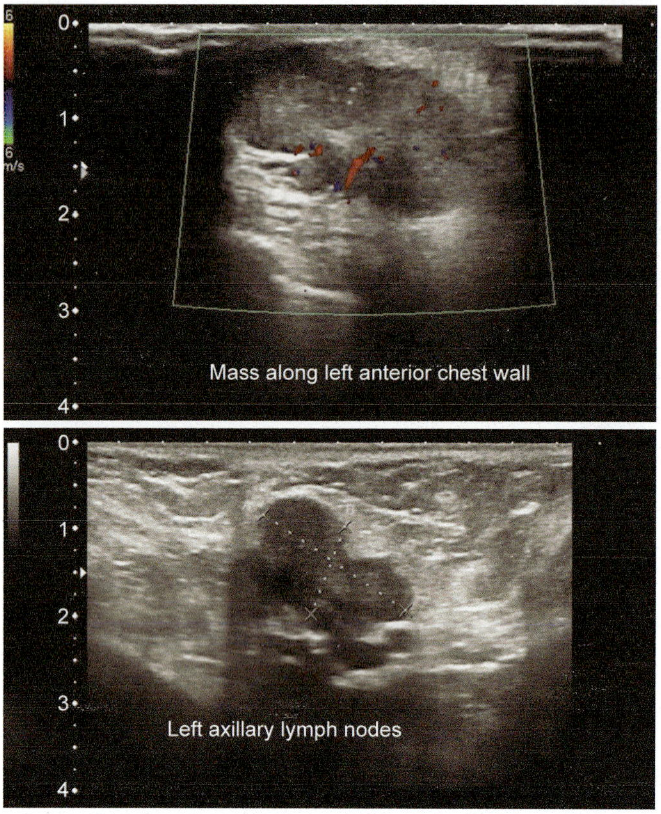

Fig. 38: Ultrasound of left breast in a 52-year-old patient who underwent MRM shows a recurrent mass in left breast at scar site along with axillary lymphadenopathy. (MLO: mediolateral oblique).

Reduction Mammoplasty

Partial removal of breast tissue may result in significant scarring, architectural distortion and calcifications, usually from fat necrosis.[15] Liposuction has been associated with calcifications from fat necrosis. Regardless of the type of procedure performed, changes on mammogram reflect the removal and repositioning of breast tissue and nipple areolar complex. The most common mammographic findings[16] in reduction mammoplasty are shown below, and depicted in line diagram (Figs. 41A and B):

- Elevation of the nipple
- Alteration of breast contour
- Retraction of lower breast
- Downward shifting of breast parenchyma
- Architectural distortion
- Retroareolar fibrotic band
- Skin thickening
- Fat necrosis.

Mastopexy

Mastopexy (breast lift surgery) does not usually disturb the breast parenchyma unless there is some breast tissue reduction. It is mainly a skin reduction with release of the breast from the underlying muscle to reorient the breast into a higher position. Mammographic findings are similar to reduction mastoplasty.[17] The most common finding is skin thickening. Other findings include nipple elevation, areolar skin calcification or lipid cyst, retraction of lower quadrants and retroareolar fibrotic band.

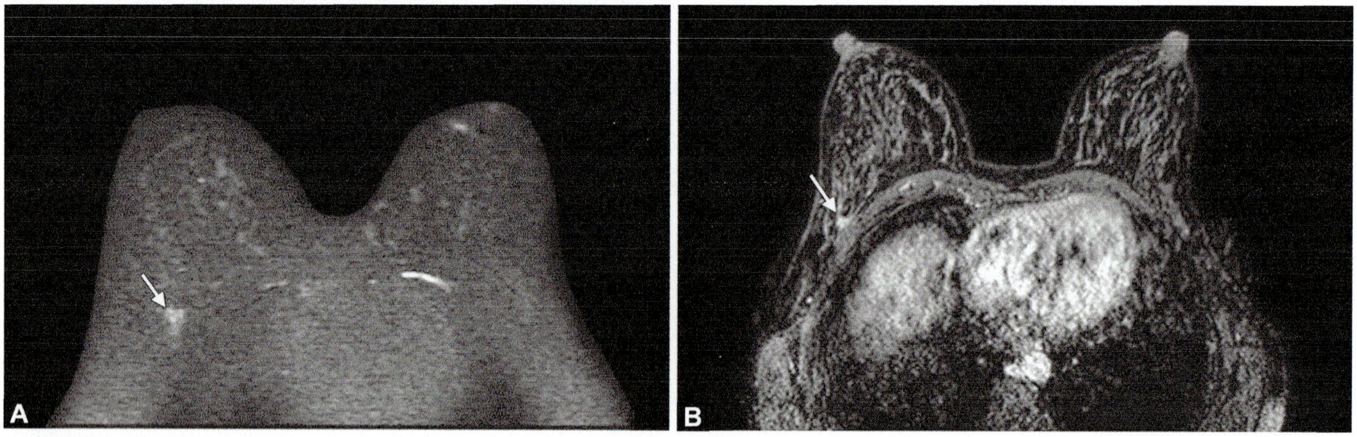

Figs. 39A and B: A 29-year-old female underwent breast conservation surgery for invasive ductal carcinoma of right breast. Since the surgical margins were positive for malignancy, MRI was done to look for residual lesion. MRI axial section (A) DWI shows restricted diffusion; (B) Postcontrast T1W shows a small enhancing mass in operative site. (T1W: T1 weighted).

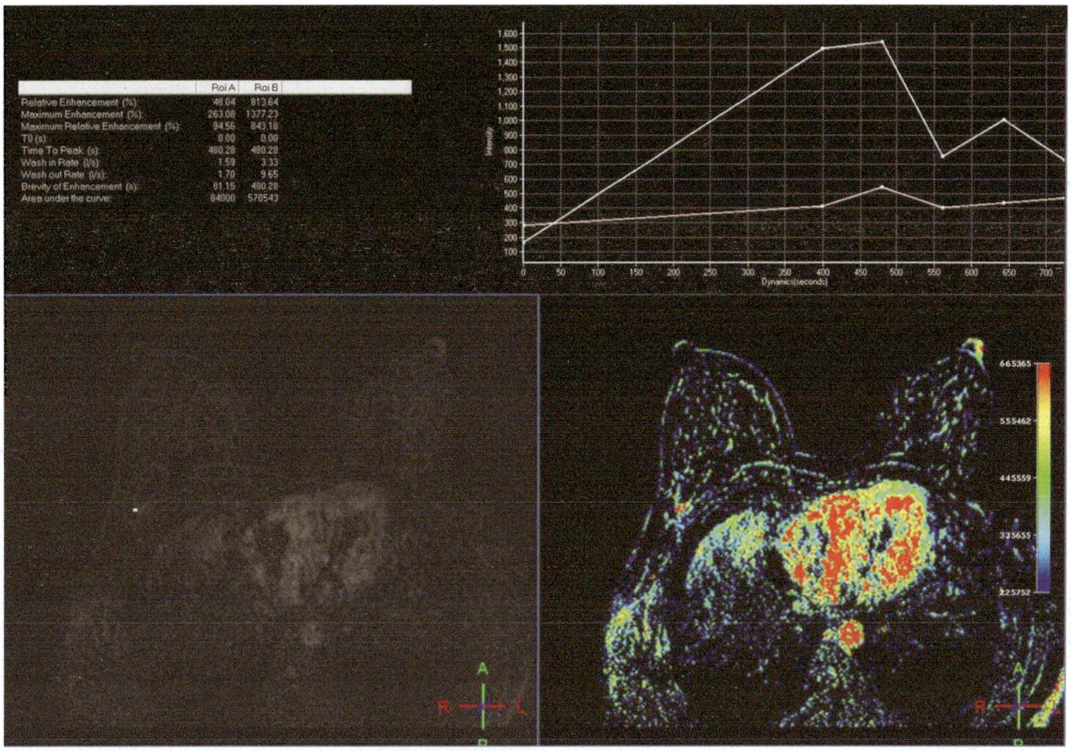

Fig. 40: Postcontrast dynamic sequence and kinetic assessment curve through the region of interest of the same patient as in Figure 39 show a small enhancing mass with subsequent wash out in delayed phase s/o type 3 curve. Patient underwent completion mastectomy and histopathology confirmed it to be residual infiltrative ductal carcinoma.

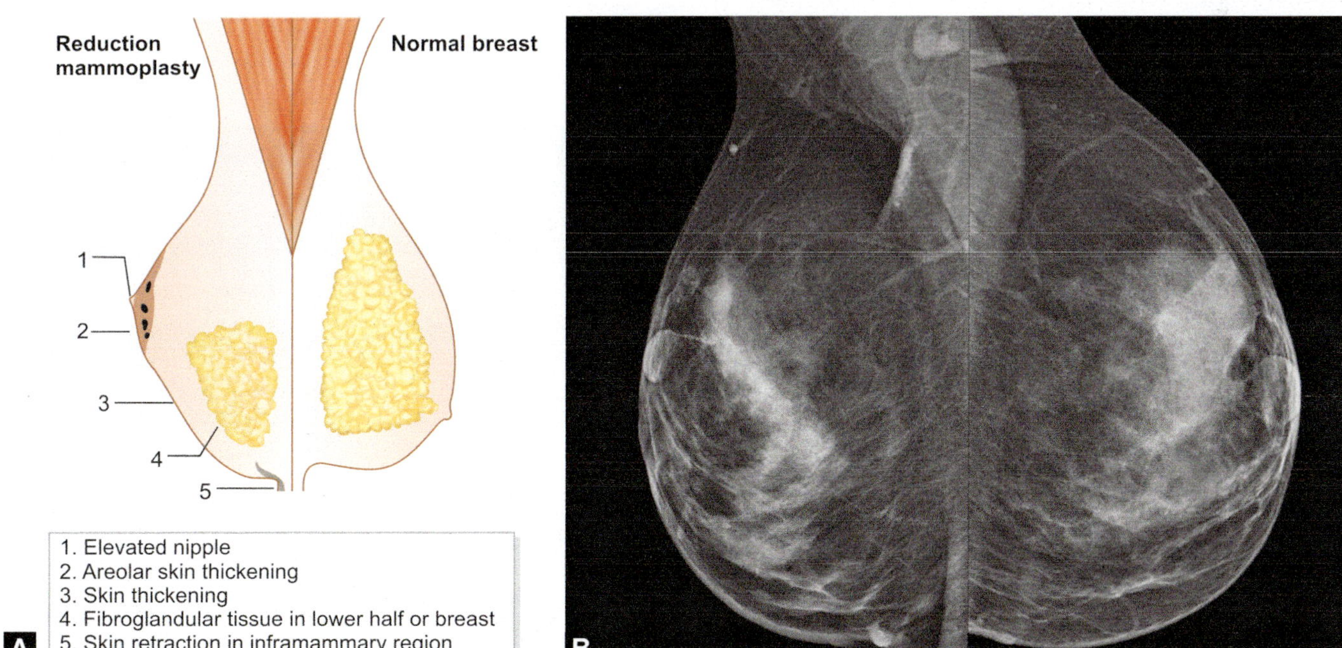

Figs. 41A and B: (A) Line diagram and (B) Mammogram MLO view showing changes seen in reduction mammoplasty. (MLO: mediolateral oblique).

Specimen Mammography

Lumpectomy or excisional biopsies are done for patients with suspicious, indeterminate lesions or masses that are not amenable to image-guided percutaneous biopsy.[18,19] Specimen mammogram is done as a routine procedure for non-palpable lesions that are resected with the help of image-guided localization.

A hook-wire maybe inserted by the radiologist under mammographic or ultrasound guidance that helps the surgeon in accurately identifying and removing non-palpable lesions or abnormal areas with precision (Fig. 42). Sometimes, a skin marking of the mass is done under ultrasound guidance using a skin marker and distance of the lesion from skin surface is measured.

Once the lumpectomy or excision biopsy is done, the specimen is shifted to radiology department for a mammogram to know the adequacy of surgical margins. The margins of the specimen are marked with a different numbers of surgical staples that helps in ascertaining the distance of the mass from a specific margin (Figs. 43A and B). A properly positioned mammogram is obtained in two views perpendicular to each other. The distance of mass from various margins is measured and conveyed to the operating surgeon so that if there are any inadequate margins, it can be taken care off immediately. Sometimes specimen is seen on ultrasound (Figs. 44A to C) also if it is not seen properly on mammogram.

CONCLUSION

In conclusion, interpretation of imaging findings in postoperative breast requires expertise and the breast radiologist plays a crucial role in follow-up of these patients. The normal chronological findings on imaging must be differentiated from a recurrent mass so that the treating surgeon/oncologists can decide further course of management. Being aware of various breast surgeries and their imaging appearances is important to evaluate and assess the postoperative changes accurately.

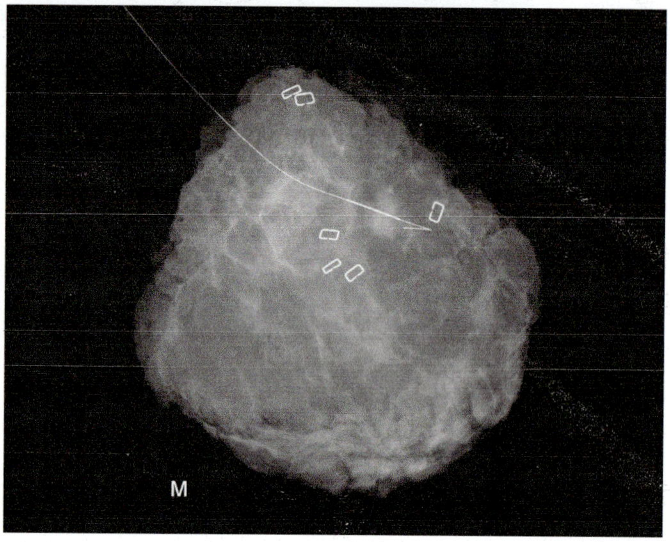

Fig. 42: Specimen mammogram with hook wire in situ showing the thick portion of the wire within the mass.

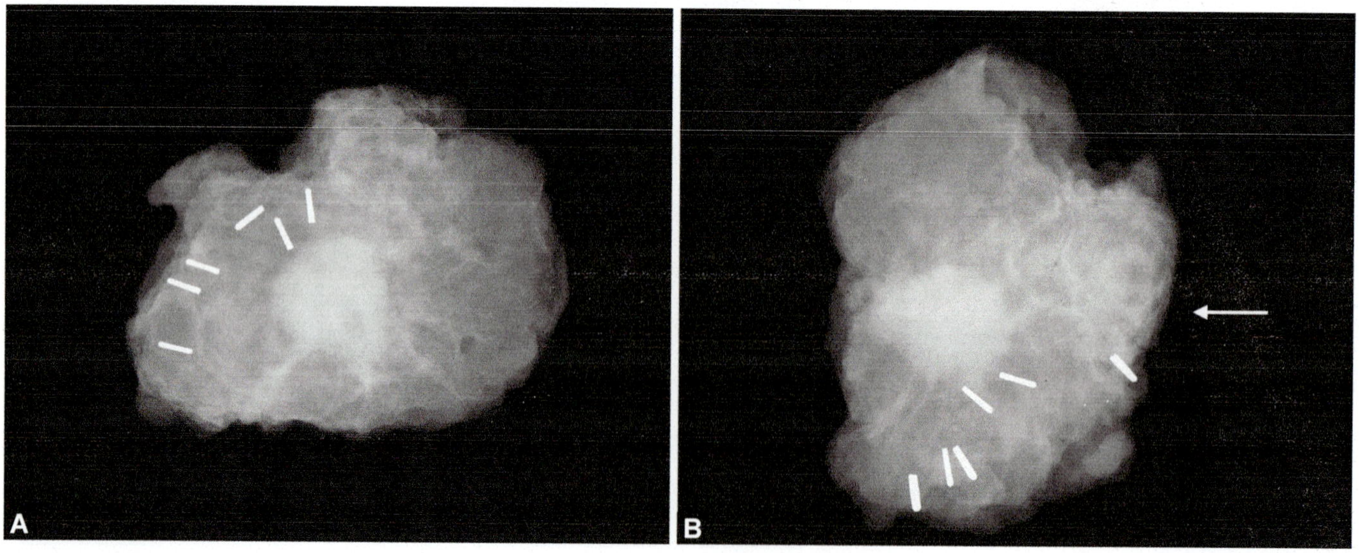

Figs. 43A and B: Specimen mammogram done in two positions perpendicular to each other shows that the mass is well excised and surgical margins are adequate.

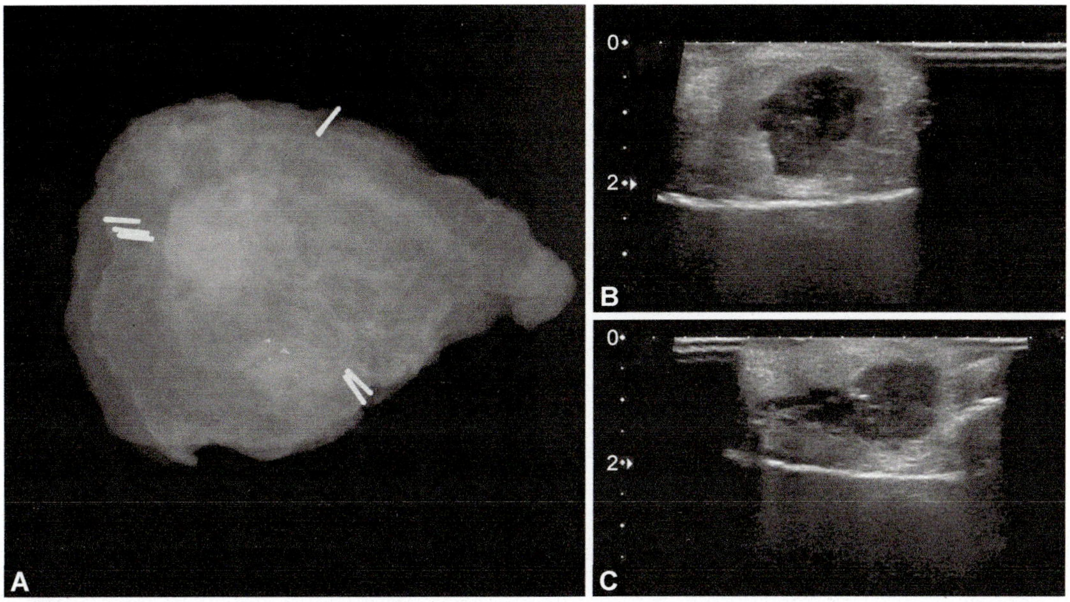

Figs. 44A to C: A 46-year-old female underwent wide local excision for a malignant mass. (A) Specimen mammogram is seen showing the surgical clips; (B and C) Ultrasound of the specimen was also done, which showed a hypoechoic mass.

REFERENCES

1. Veronesi U, Cascinelli N, Mariani L, et al. Twenty-year follow-up of a randomized study comparing breast-conserving surgery with radical mastectomy for early breast cancer. N Engl J Med 2002;347:1227-32.
2. Chansakul T, Lai KC, Slanetz PL. The post conservation breast: Part 1, Expected imaging findings. AJR Am J Roentgenol 2012;198:321-30.
3. Wolfe JN. Xeroradiography of the breast. 2nd ed. Springfield, IL: Charles C Thomas; 1983. pp. 405-35.
4. Peters ME, Fagerholm MI, Scanlan KA, Voegeli DR, Kelcz F. Mammographic evaluation of the postsurgical and irradiated breast. Radiographics 1988;8:873-99.
5. Zieliński J, Jaworski R, Irga N, Kruszewski JW, Jaskiewicz J. Analysis of selected factors influencing seroma formation in breast cancer patients undergoing mastectomy. Arch Med Sci 2013;9:86-92.
6. Mendelson EB. Evaluation of the postoperative breast. Radiol Clin North Am 1992;30:107-38.
7. Huang CC, Sheu CY, Ng SP. Radial scar of the breast. J Radiol Sci 2011;36:41-7.
8. Frouge C, Tristant H, Guinebretière JM, et al. Mammographic lesions suggestive of radial scars: microscopic findings in 40 cases. Radiology 1995;195:623-5.
9. Tabar L, Dean PB. Teaching atlas of mammography. New York, NY: Thieme Stratton; 1985. pp. 172.
10. Dershaw DD, McCormick B, Cox L, Osborne MP. Differentiation of benign and malignant local tumor recurrence after lumpectomy. AJR Am J Roentgenol 1990;155:35-8.
11. Gonzalez EA, Saltzstein EC, Riedner CS, Nelson BK. Seroma formation following breast cancer surgery. Breast J 2003;9:385-8.
12. Recht A, Silen W, Schnitt SJ, et al. Time-course of local recurrence following conservative surgery and radiation therapy for early stage breast cancer. Int J Radiat Oncol Biol Phys 1988;15:255-61.
13. Frei KA, Kinkel K, Bonel HM, et al. MR imaging of the breast in patients with positive margins after lumpectomy: influence of the time interval between lumpectomy and MR imaging. AJR Am J Roentgenol 2000;175:1577-84.
14. Nunes LW, Schnall MD, Orel SG. Update of breast MR imaging architectural interpretation model. Radiology 2001;219:484-94.
15. Shiffman MA. Mammograms in cosmetic breast surgery. Indian J Plast Surg 2005;38:100-4.
16. Thongchai P. The surgically altered breast: imaging technique and findings. Gland Surg 2014;3:48-50.
17. Kim H, Kang BJ, Kim SH, Kim HS, Cha ES. What we should know in mammography after reduction mammoplasty and mastopexy?. Breast Cancer 2015;22:391-8. doi: 10.1007/s12282-013-0494-y.
18. White RR, Halperin TJ, Olson Jr JA, et al. Impact of core-needle breast biopsy on the surgical management of mammographic abnormalities. Ann Surg 2001;233:769-77.
19. American College of Radiology. Practice guideline for the performance of image-guided percutaneous needle biopsy (PNB) in adults. 2008. Available at: http://www.acr.org/w/media/1D9E3F3270CF44F8A2E99-4C94F2F0FAC.pdf [accessed July 13, 2012].

Breast Implants

CHAPTER

8

INTRODUCTION

The augmentation of breast was first described in 1895 when autologous fat transplantation was done for breast reconstruction using a lipoma from the lumbar region of a patient.

Liquid silicone injections were used in 1960s, but because of adverse side effects like skin sloughing, migration of silicone, granuloma formation, granulomatous hepatitits and embolism, these were later banned.

In some Asian countries, liquid silicone is still injected in breast and pectoralis or both.

This leads to formation of fibrous silicone breast masses which are seen as well-defined, rounded, peripherally calcified masses sometimes with spiculated margins which may be difficult to distinguish from cancer.

Silicone gel and saline filled implants were also introduced in 1960s and silicon was preferred over saline because of its natural feel; however, it was banned by the FDA in 1980s because of its toxic effects in case there was rupture of implant. The silicone implants were reapproved in 2006 and have a tougher shell now to prevent implant rupture.

Saline implants were popular in 1980 and were associated with cosmetic problems like wrinkling, shifting and unnatural feel.

Breast implants are commonly used these days for augmentation mainly for cosmetic purpose and reconstruction after mastectomy, therefore radiologists should be aware of imaging findings.

TYPES OF BREAST IMPLANTS

Breast implants are composed of saline, silicone or a combination of the two and can be placed in subglandular or submuscular location (Figs. 1A and B).

The mediolateral oblique (MLO) view is used to see if implant is in subglandular or submuscular location as pectoralis is seen well on this view.

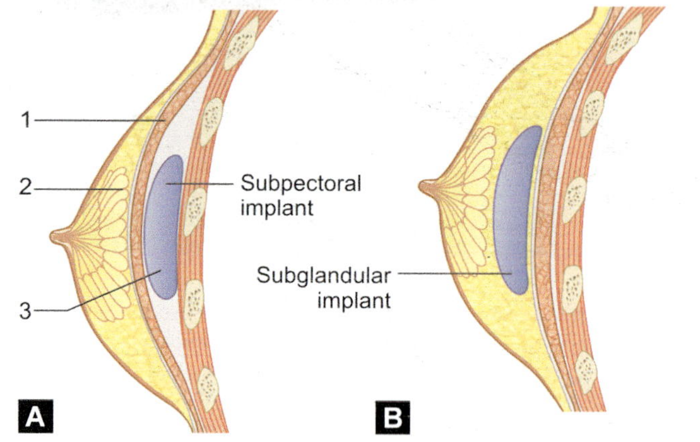

Figs. 1A and B: Mammogram showing (A) subpectoral and (B) subglandular location of implants. 1, Pectoralis; 2, glandular tissue; 3, implant.

The various types of implants[1] are as follows:

- Single-lumen gel: silicone gel-filled
- Single-lumen adjustable: silicone gel-filled, to which can be added a variable amount of saline at time of placement
- Standard double-lumen: silicone gel inner lumen, saline outer lumen
- Reverse double-lumen: saline inner lumen, silicone gel outer lumen
- Reverse-adjustable double-lumen: silicone gel inner and outer lumens, variable amount of saline added to inner lumen at time of placement
- Gel–gel double-lumen: silicone gel inner and outer lumens
- Triple-lumen: silicone gel inner and middle lumens, saline outer lumen

The common types of implant are single lumen (only silicone) or double lumen (silicone with saline) implants (Fig. 2).

TECHNIQUE OF IMPLANT INSERTION

Once it is decided to put a permanent breast implant in the mastectomy site, it is important to place a tissue expander which is inflatable in a pocket which is created under the skin and above the chest muscle. As fluid is inserted in it over a period of weeks, adequate space and volume is created to insert the permanent implant.

Once the implant is placed in position, a thin fibrous tissue forms around the implant which is a normal phenomenon. Sometimes this capsule becomes thickened leading to capsular contracture. Early postoperative complications of breast implant include infection and hematoma formation[2] while implant rupture commonly occurs 10–15 years after implant insertion and is the most common cause of implant removal.[3]

Implant rupture can present clinically as non-specific findings like palpable nodule, tenderness and asymmetry.[4] Sometimes the patients may be asymptomatic and if the implant rupture occurs over a period of time gradually, then there may not be any shape change or deformity.

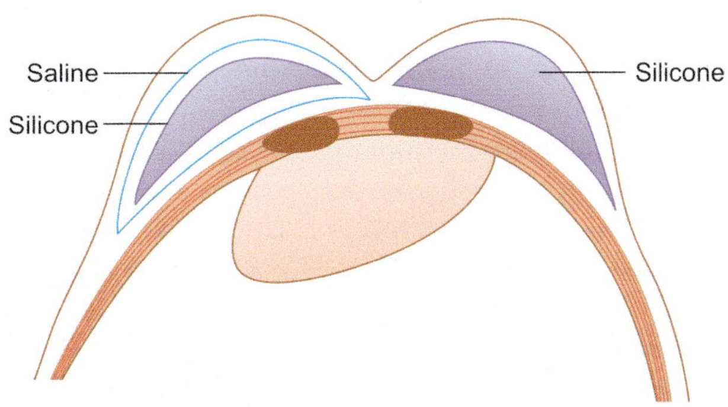

Fig. 2: Line diagram of MRI showing the type of implants—single lumen and double lumen implants.

Breast pain on clinical examination is an important symptom of implant rupture. The other signs and symptoms include contour deformity, mass, displacements and inflammation of breast tissue.

IMAGING OF BREAST IMPLANTS

Mammography and ultrasound are the initial modalities used for evaluation of breast implants but have a lower sensitivity.

MRI characterizes the implants and its types. This is possible because signal from water, fat or silicone can either be suppressed or emphasized. In addition, MRI can assess the integrity of implants if rupture is suspected. It has the highest sensitivity and specificity to assess implant rupture. As the age of implant increases, possibility of rupture increases.

Mammography

The subglandular and subpectoral location of implants can be easily appreciated on mammography (Figs. 3A and B). The standard craniocaudal (CC) and MLO views are done along with implant displaced CC and MLO views (Eklund technique) for routine evaluation of implants.

Eklund view (Figs. 4A and B) or implant displacement views are named after Eklund[5] who introduced this new technique in 1988 to demonstrate more breast parenchyma in patients with implants. In this view, the implant is pushed back against the chest wall posterosuperiorly and breast is pulled forward over it showing more of breast

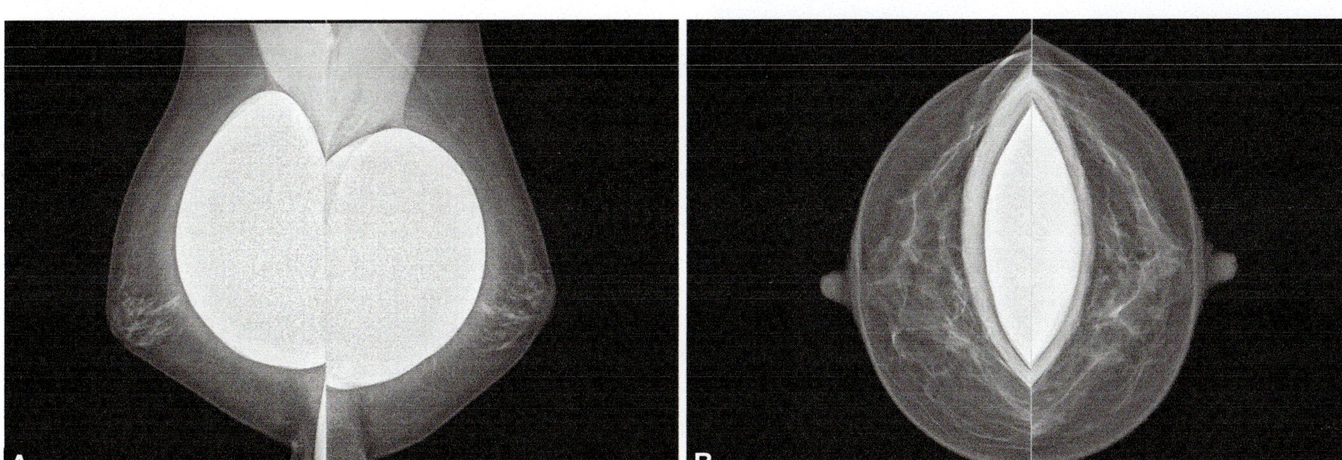

Figs. 3A and B: (A) Mammogram showing location of implants: MLO view showing subglandular implant; (B) CC view showing subpectoral implant. (CC: craniocaudal; MLO: mediolateral oblique).

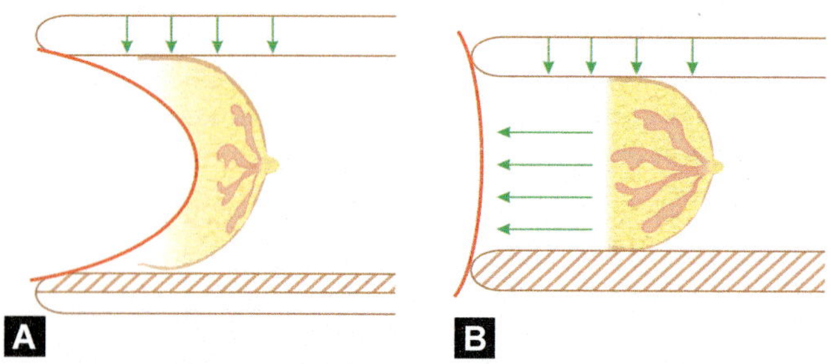

Figs. 4A and B: (A) Normal implant position; (B) Eklund technique—the implant is pushed back against the chest wall and the breast is pulled forward over it so that more of the breast parenchyma is included.

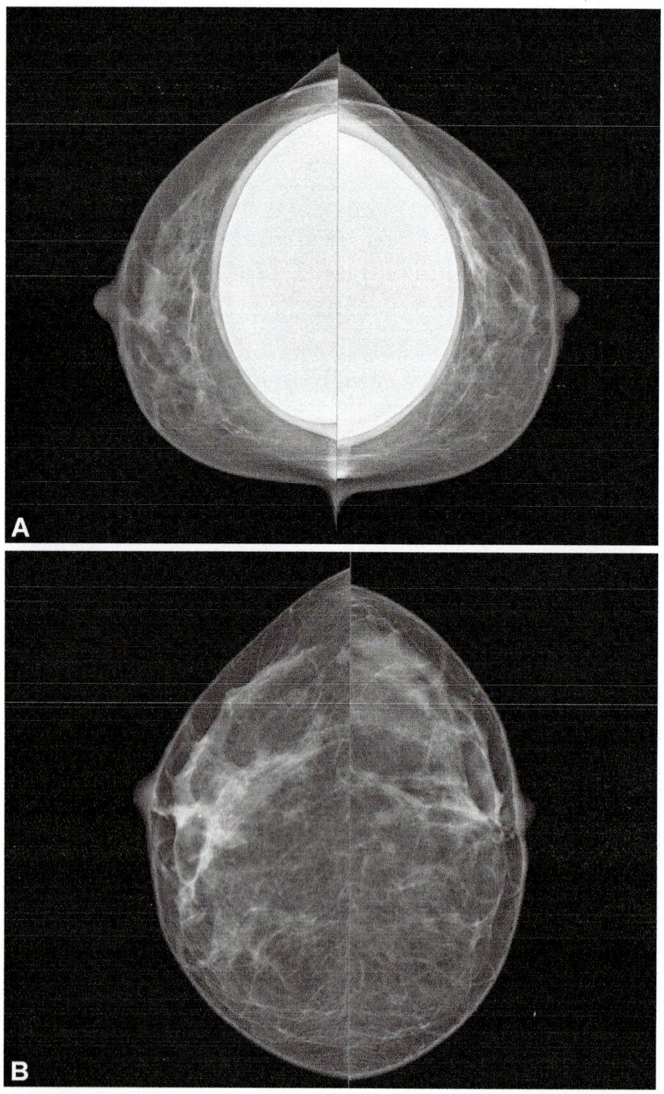

Figs. 5A and B: Mammogram—normal CC view showing more breast parenchyma. (A) Without Eklund technique; (B) With Eklund technique. (CC: craniocaudal).

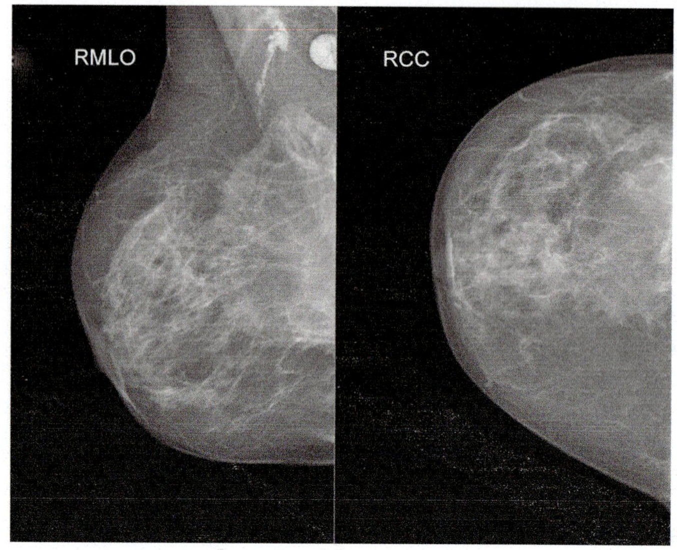

Fig. 6: Post implant removal mammogram of right breast in a 43-year-old female shows a seroma and fibrous capsule. Silicone is noted in right axillary lymph node.

parenchyma (Figs. 5A and B). *This view should not be done in patients with capsular contractures.*

The normal silicone implants are seen as dense oval masses without any separate envelope or accompanying folds. Mammography is used to assess contour deformity of implant, surrounding breast parenchyma, free silicone and periprosthetic calcification. It has limited role in evaluating implant integrity, especially in diagnosing intracapsular rupture. It is, however, an extremely specific method for the diagnosis of extracapsular rupture and can detect silicone gel migration through the glandular parenchyma.[6-9] A seroma may be seen on post implant removal mammograms (Fig. 6).

Ultrasound

This has a steep learning curve in evaluating breast implants, is operator dependent and requires expertise. It is used to evaluate morphology, contour and contents of implants along with examining peri-implant tissue and axilla.[10] The normal implant is anechoic and shows intact shell as a thin and continuous echogenic line at the parenchyma-implant surface. The fibrous capsule is seen as two parallel echogenic lines superficial to the implant (Fig. 7). An intact implant may show simple infolding of the implant shell (Fig. 8A) or a small amount of peri-implant fluid (Fig. 8B). Reverberation artifacts (Fig. 8C) can be noted along the anterior aspect of implants often misjudged as implant rupture and require caution in interpretation. Radial folds are seen as echogenic lines extending from periphery of implant to the interior

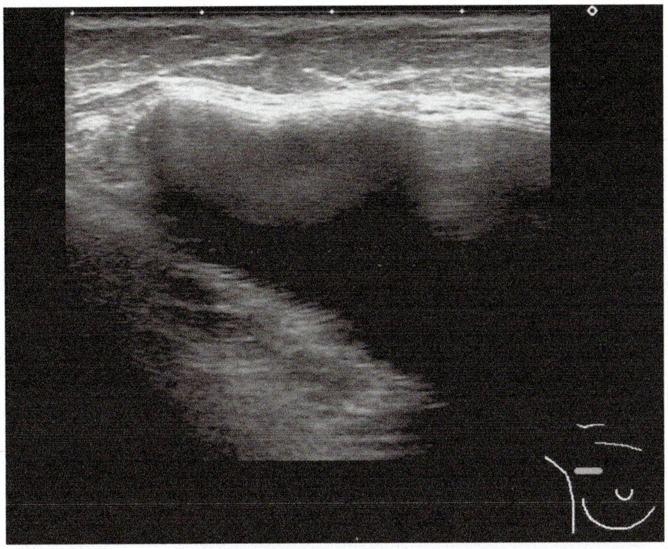

Fig. 7: Ultrasound of right breast in a 37-year-old female shows normal anechoic implant with intact echogenic implant shell seen as echogenic line at implant tissue interface.

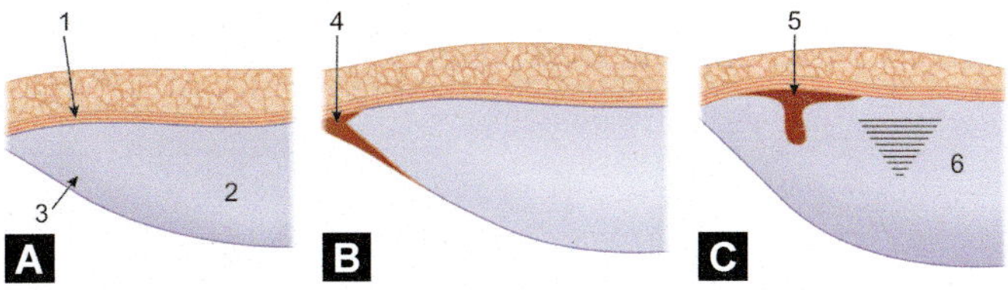

Figs. 8A to C: Normal findings of breast implants. (A) Breast implant located posterior to pectoralis; (B) Implant with peri-implant fluid; (C) Breast implant showing normal radial folds and reverberation artifacts which is a normal finding. 1. Pectoralis, 2. Capsule, 3. Implant 4. Peri-implant fluid 5. Radial fold 6. Reverberation artefact

of implant. Ultrasound has a limitation in evaluating most posterior extent of implants.

Magnetic Resonance Imaging

This plays an important role in assessing implant integrity and has a high sensitivity (80–90%) and specificity (90–70%) in diagnosing implant rupture.[11] A plain MRI is done using a dedicated breast coil to assess the implants; intravenous contrast is required only when there is a suspicion of malignancy in a patient with implants.

The following MRI sequences are done:

- Axial T2 weighted
- Axial T1 weighted
- Axial STIR with fat suppression
- Axial STIR with water suppression
- Axial STIR with silicone suppression.

MRI can ascertain the type of implant-single lumen (Figs. 9A to D) versus double lumen (Figs. 10A to D). The normal variants of implant like peri-implant fluid, radial folds and thickening of fibrous capsule (Figs. 11A to C) can also be seen clearly. The presence of folds (Figs. 12A and B) indicates a certain degree of capsular contraction or tense elastomer.

COMPLICATIONS OF BREAST IMPLANTS

Capsular Contracture

This is due to abnormal constriction of the fibrous capsule that surrounds the breast implant and occurs in the first few postoperative months. It is more commonly seen in implants placed in subglandular location. Clinically the breast may appear distorted, inflamed and tender. On mammography, there is a change in shape of implant with irregularity, crumpling, infolding and peri-implant calcifications (Fig. 13A). Sometimes the residual implant becomes small, wrinkled and partially calcified (Fig. 13B). Ultrasound may show increased thickness of fibrous capsule.

Silicone Granuloma

A silicone granuloma is a type of tissue reaction elicited occasionally by silicone. It can occur in all sizes from microscopic to the clinically recognizable and symptomatic. Calcified capsular silicone granulomas leading to implant rupture have also been described in literature. Cutaneous manifestations due to migration of silicone from ruptured implants are rare.

Implant Rupture

There are two types of implant ruptures—intracapsular and extracapsular (Figs. 14A and B). The various appearances of implant rupture are seen in Figures 15A to E.

Intracapsular Rupture

Intracapsular rupture is more common and is confined within the fibrous capsule and there is no leakage of free silicone beyond it.

It is difficult to diagnose intracapsular rupture on mammogram which may only show a bulge in contour but sometimes linear lucencies with irregularity, redundancy and wrinkled appearance of the implant (Fig. 16) are seen.

The stepladder sign is a predictive sign of intracapsular rupture[12] on ultrasound (Figs. 17A to D) and corresponds to the "linguine sign" in MRI (Figs. 17E to G).

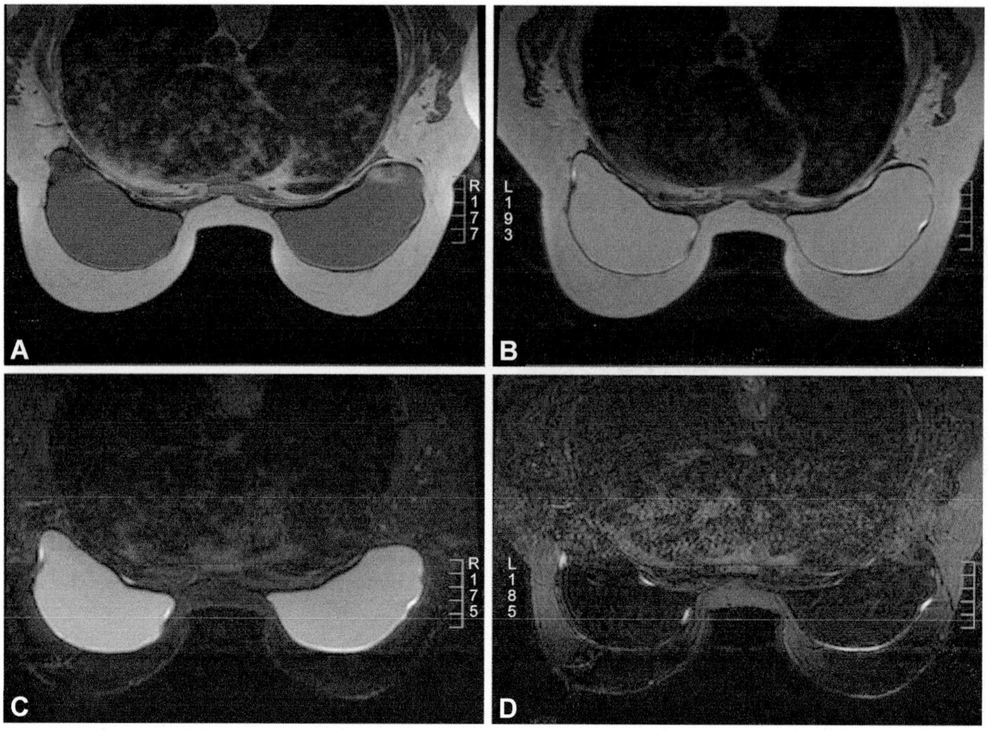

Figs. 9A to D: MRI axial sections of both breasts showing (A) T1W; (B) T2W; (C) STIR and (D) Silicone-suppressed sequences with intact single chambered implants. No signs of rupture seen.

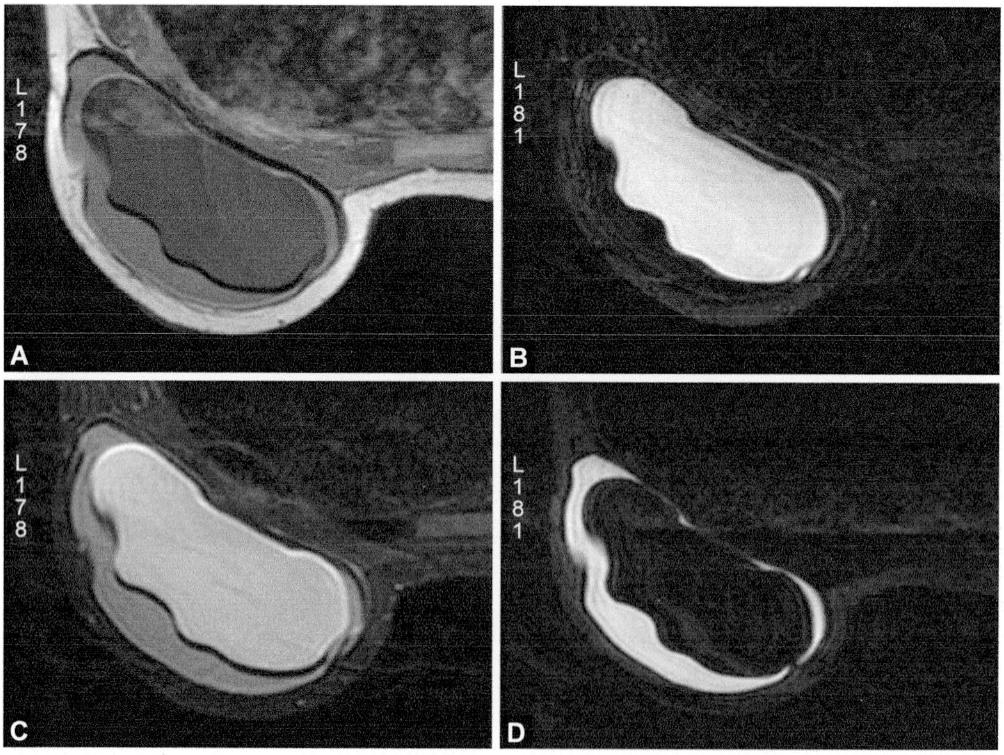

Figs. 10A to D: MRI—axial section of left breast showing (A) T1W; (B) Silicone-suppressed; (C) STIR and (D) Water-suppressed sequences with intact double chambered implants.

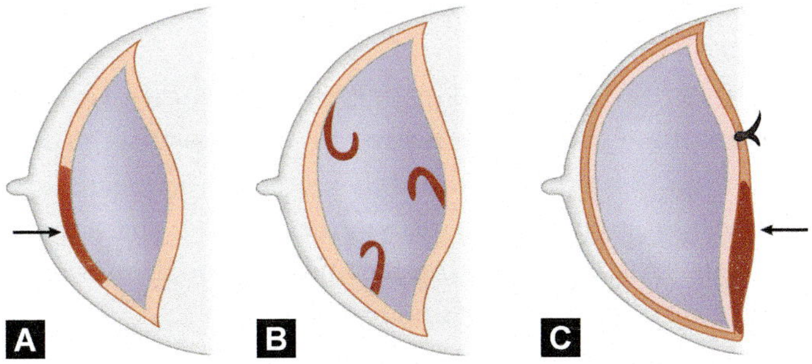

Figs. 11A to C: Variants of normal implants. (A) Peri-implant fluid (arrow); (B) Normal folds; (C) Thickening of fibrous capsule of implant (arrowhead) along with calcification (arrow).

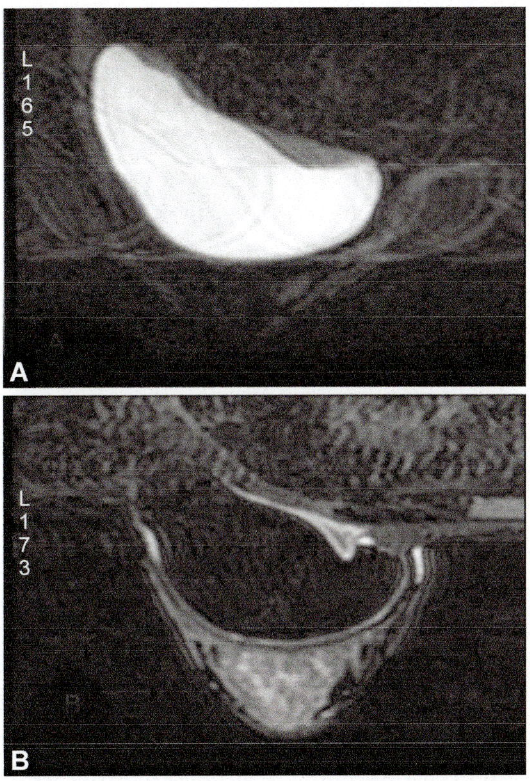

Figs. 12A and B: MRI of left breast in a patient with suspected implant rupture. (A) Axial water-suppressed: (B) Axial silicone-suppressed sequences show peri-implant fluid; however, there was no evidence of implant rupture.

It is seen as a series of parallel horizontal or curved echogenic lines extending beyond the interior of the implant and corresponds to ruptured elastomer. One should not confuse the stepladder sign with normal radial folds.

The sign of intracapsular rupture on MRI is "linguine sign", which is seen as multiple curvilinear low intensity lines in high signal intensity silicone gel. An uncollapsed silicone implant rupture is defined as a tear

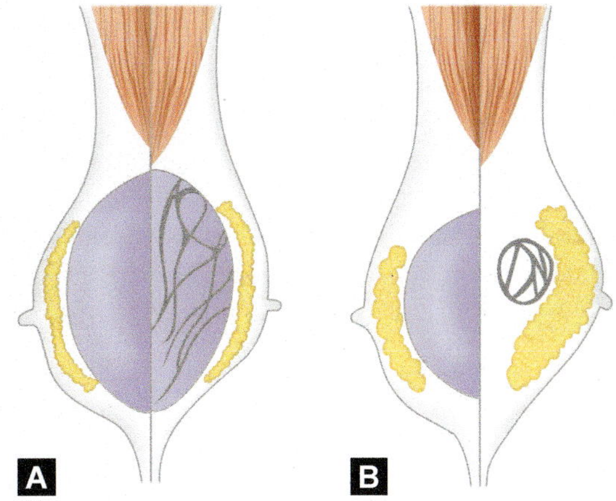

Figs. 13A and B: (A) Implant contracture in the left breast where the implant appears irregular, redundant and wrinkled; (B) Rupture of implant in left breast with residual collapsed, ruptured and wrinkled implant which has become small and partially calcified.

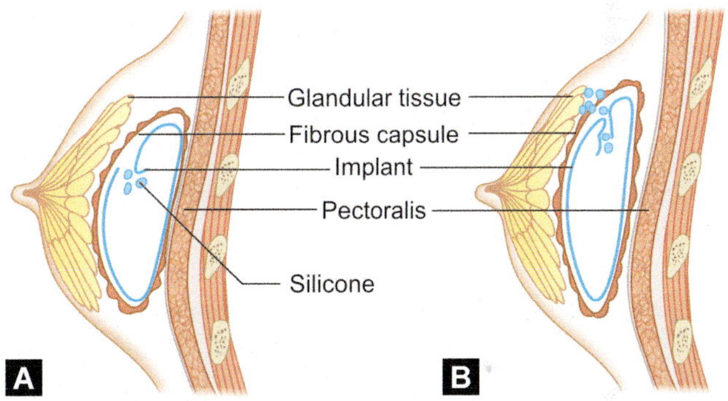

Figs. 14A and B: (A) Intracapsular rupture; (B) Extracapsular rupture. In intracapsular rupture, silicone is seen outside the implant shell but remains confined within the fibrous capsule. In extracapsular rupture, silicone is seen outside the fibrous capsule into the breast parenchyma. It may also be seen along the pectoralis muscle or within the axillary lymph nodes.

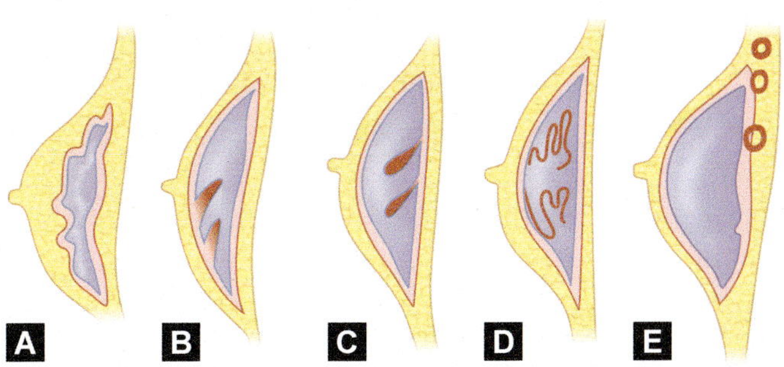

Figs. 15A to E: Signs of implant rupture on MRI: (A) Implant deformity; (B) Keyhole sign—small invagination of shell where the two membranes do not touch; (C) Teardrop sign—invagination of shell containing silicone droplet; (D) Linguine sign—collapsed implant shell seen as folded wavy lines within the silicone gel; (E) Free silicone and siliconoma—there is disruption of shell and fibrous capsule with free silicone in surrounding breast tissue.

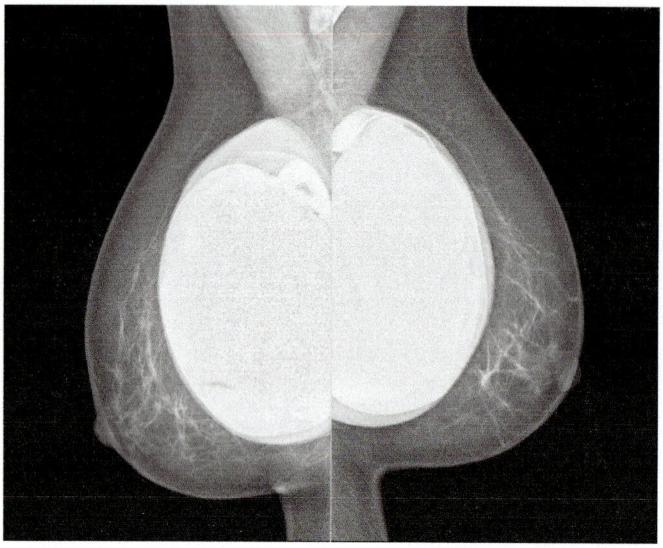

Fig. 16: Mammogram—MLO view of both breasts in a patient with breast implants shows radiolucent linear shadows, wrinkled, irregular and redundant appearance s/o intracapsular implant rupture. (MLO: mediolateral oblique.)

of the silicone implant shell and is considered an intracapsular rupture.

One should be aware of the phenomenon called "gel bleed" where there is microscopic silicone leakage through intact implant shell.[2] Therefore presence of silicone in regional lymph node may or may not be due to implant rupture but because of gel bleed. Ultrasound can show normal intact anechoic implant and silicone in lymph node (Figs. 18A to C).

On MRI, tear drop sign may be seen where there is entrapment of silicone inside a fold which is seen as an inverted tear (Figs. 18D and E). The signs of intracapsular rupture are "keyhole sign," "tear drop sign" and "linguine sign" (Figs. 19A to C); however, linguine sign is also seen in extracapsular rupture in some cases.

Extracapsular Rupture

Extracapsular rupture is relatively less common than intracapsular implant rupture. In extracapsular rupture, there is rupture of both implant shell and fibrous capsule and macroscopic silicone is seen beyond fibrous capsule. It is more easily detected on mammogram than intracapsular rupture. It shows radiopaque silicone in the breast parenchyma (Fig. 20), along the pectoralis muscle or within the axillary lymph node. The free silicone can be seen on both mammogram (Fig. 21A) and ultrasound (Fig. 21B).

The most useful sign of extracapsular rupture on ultrasound is the "echodense noise" or snowstorm appearance,[12] which represents diffusely increased echogenicity in breast parenchyma because of free silicone. There may also be a loss of normal implant parenchymal interface due to scattering of ultrasound beam.

On MRI, free silicone is seen in extracapsular rupture as focal areas of high signal intensity on silicone excited sequences (Figs. 22A to D). There may be false negative findings on MRI which may be due to ruptured noncollapsed elastomer located outside the implant, while keeping the homogeneous high signal intensity inside it. MRI confirms that there is also uncollapsed implant rupture which is seen as a focal silicone invagination between the inner shell and fibrous capsule called as "keyhole sign."

Rarely there may be multiple hypointense foci on water-suppressed sequence within the implant called "salad oil" sign and when this is seen then subtle signs of intracapsular rupture should be looked for.

Extracapsular rupture is relatively less common than intracapsular implant rupture and can show free silicone in peri-implant region on mammograms, on ultrasound and on MRI.

ADDITIONAL LESIONS IN BREAST IMPLANT EVALUATION

Sometimes additional findings may be seen in women with breast implants ranging from benign (Fig. 23A to G) to malignant pathology. The risk of breast cancer in women with breast implants is same as in other women. The sensitivity of mammography and ultrasound in breast cancer detection in women with implants may be reduced[13]; however, sensitivity of MRI remains the same. If ultrasound and mammogram are negative in a patient with a palpable finding, contrast-enhanced breast MRI is strongly recommended. It is also beneficial in the detection of recurrent breast cancer in patients with implant reconstructed breasts.

In conclusion, though mammography and ultrasound are useful modalities for initial evaluation of breast implants, MRI accurately assesses the type and integrity of implant along with other breast lesions in the patient.

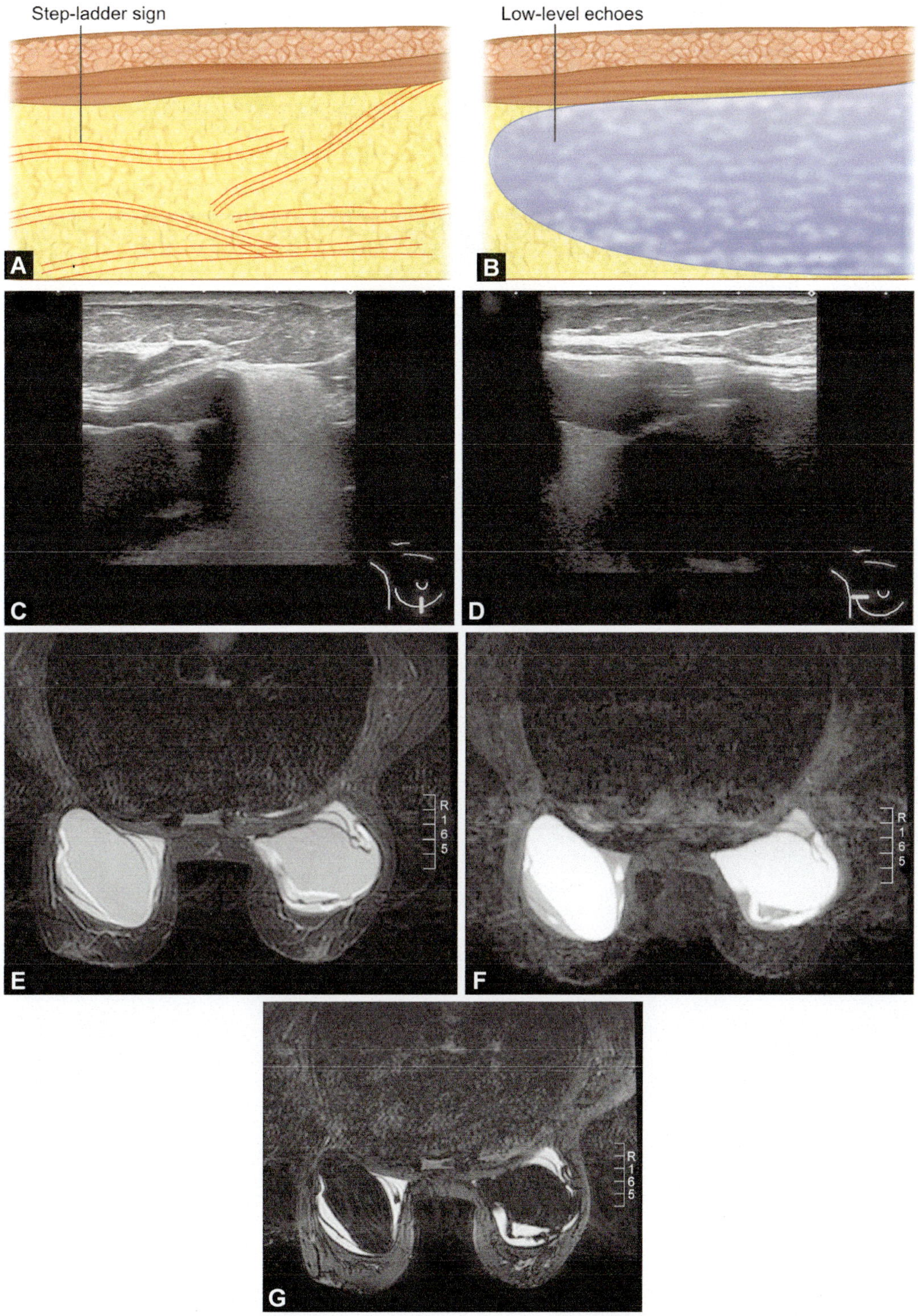

Figs. 17A to G: Line diagram showing ultrasound findings in intracapsular rupture. (A) Stacked echogenic lines corresponding to collapsed envelope of implant termed the "step-ladder" sign noted; (B) Low-level echoes in the implant; (C and D) Ultrasound of right breast in a patient with breast implant in lower and outer quadrant shows anechoic implant with echogenic area within suggestive of snow storm sign and step-ladder sign. A suspicion of implant rupture was considered and MRI of breast was done for further evaluation. MRI of both breasts in the same patient; (E) Axial STIR; (F) STIR, water sat and (G) Water sat, silicone-suppressed sequences show folded hypointense wavy lines "linguine sign" suggestive of intracapsular rupture of both breast implants.

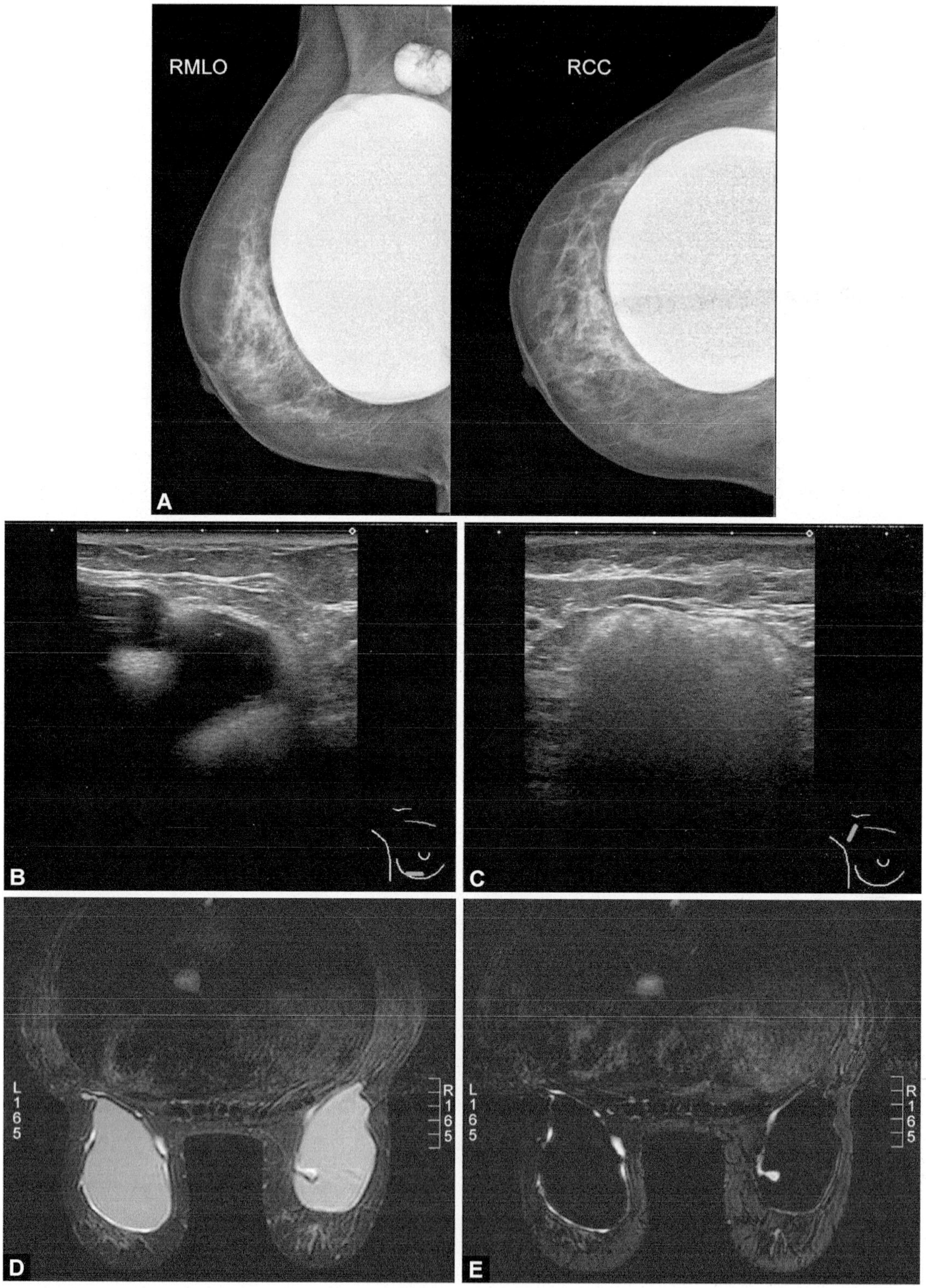

Figs. 18A to E: (A) Mammogram MLO and CC view of right breast in a 45-year-old female with breast implant shows silicone in axillary lymph node; (B and C) Ultrasound of the right breast in the same patient shows the anechoic implant with linear echogenic area within (C) Ultrasound of right axilla shows an echogenic area with posterior acoustic shadowing suggestive of lymph node with silicone; (D and E) MRI of right breast in the same patient shows "keyhole sign" on (D) STIR axial and (E) Silicone-suppressed sequence suggestive of intracapsular rupture. The left implant is intact. (CC: craniocaudal; MLO: mediolateral oblique.)

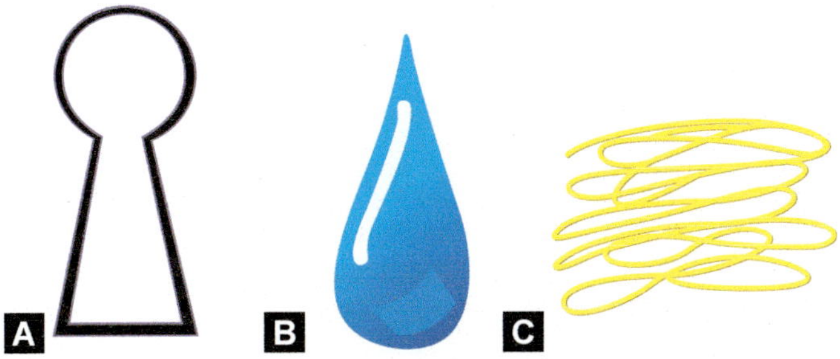

Figs. 19A to C: Diagrammatic representation of "named" signs of intracapsular rupture on MRI. (A) Keyhole sign; (B) Teardrop sign; (C) Linguine sign.

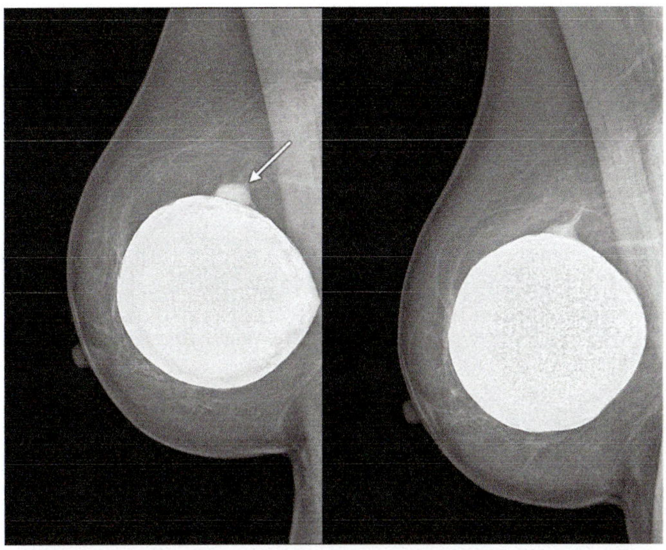

Fig. 20: Mammogram of right breast (MLO view) shows breast implant with a small radiopacity (arrow) in peri-implant region suggestive of extracapsular rupture of implant. (MLO: mediolateral oblique.)

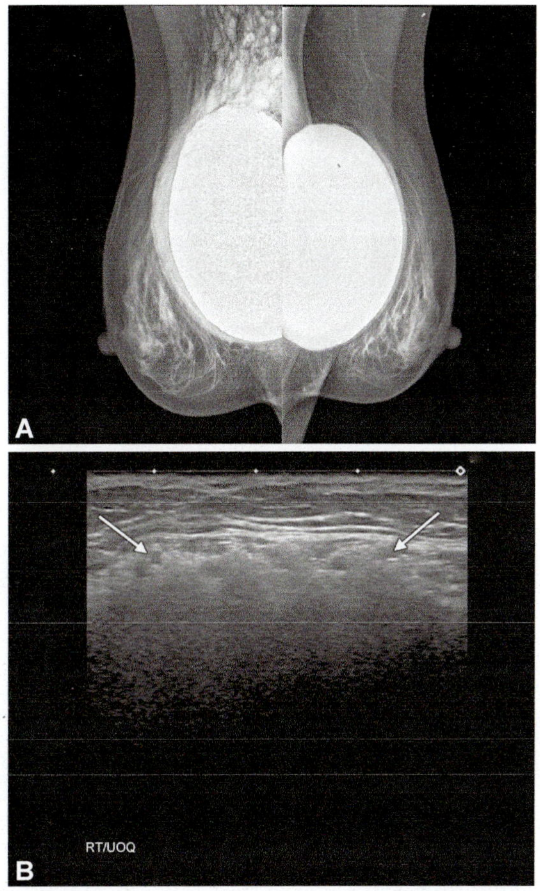

Figs. 21A and B: (A) Mammogram of both breasts in a 48-year-old female—MLO view show extracapsular rupture of right implant with free silicone in right upper and outer quadrant near the axillary region; (B) Ultrasound of right breast in the same patient in upper and outer quadrant shows multiple globules of silicone appearing as small anechoic structures (arrows) which are surrounded by extensive free silicone, which appears as echogenic area associated with dirty acoustic shadowing, consistent with snowstorm appearance. (MLO: mediolateral oblique.)

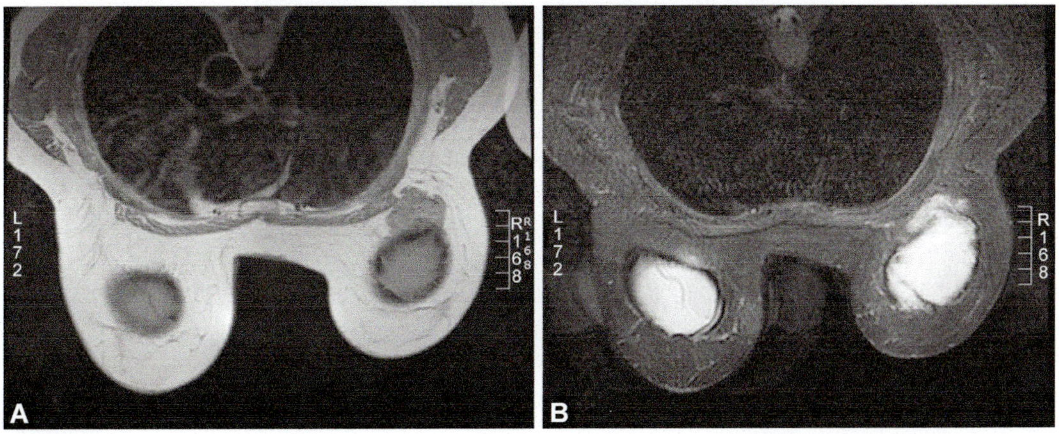

Figs. 22A and B: MRI of both breasts in a 42-year-old female with suspected implant rupture. (A) Axial T1W; (B) STIR fat-suppressed

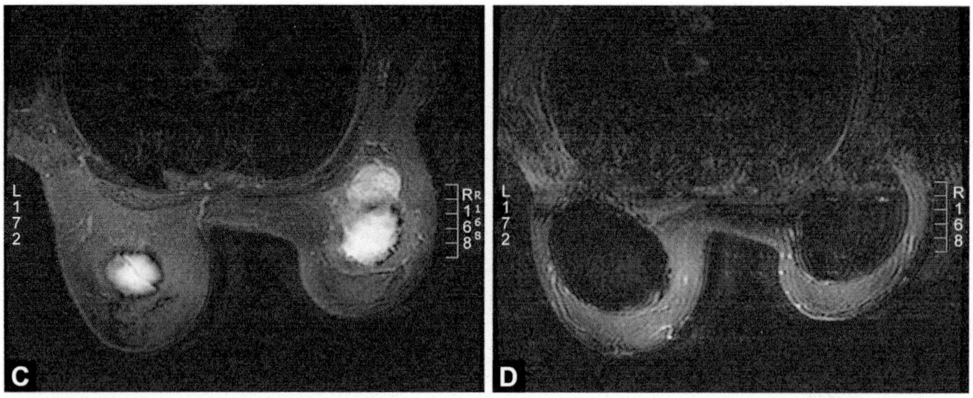

Figs. 22C and D: (C) Axial water-suppressed and (D) Axial silicone-suppressed sequences showed free silicone in posterolateral aspect of right breast suggestive of extracapsular implant rupture.

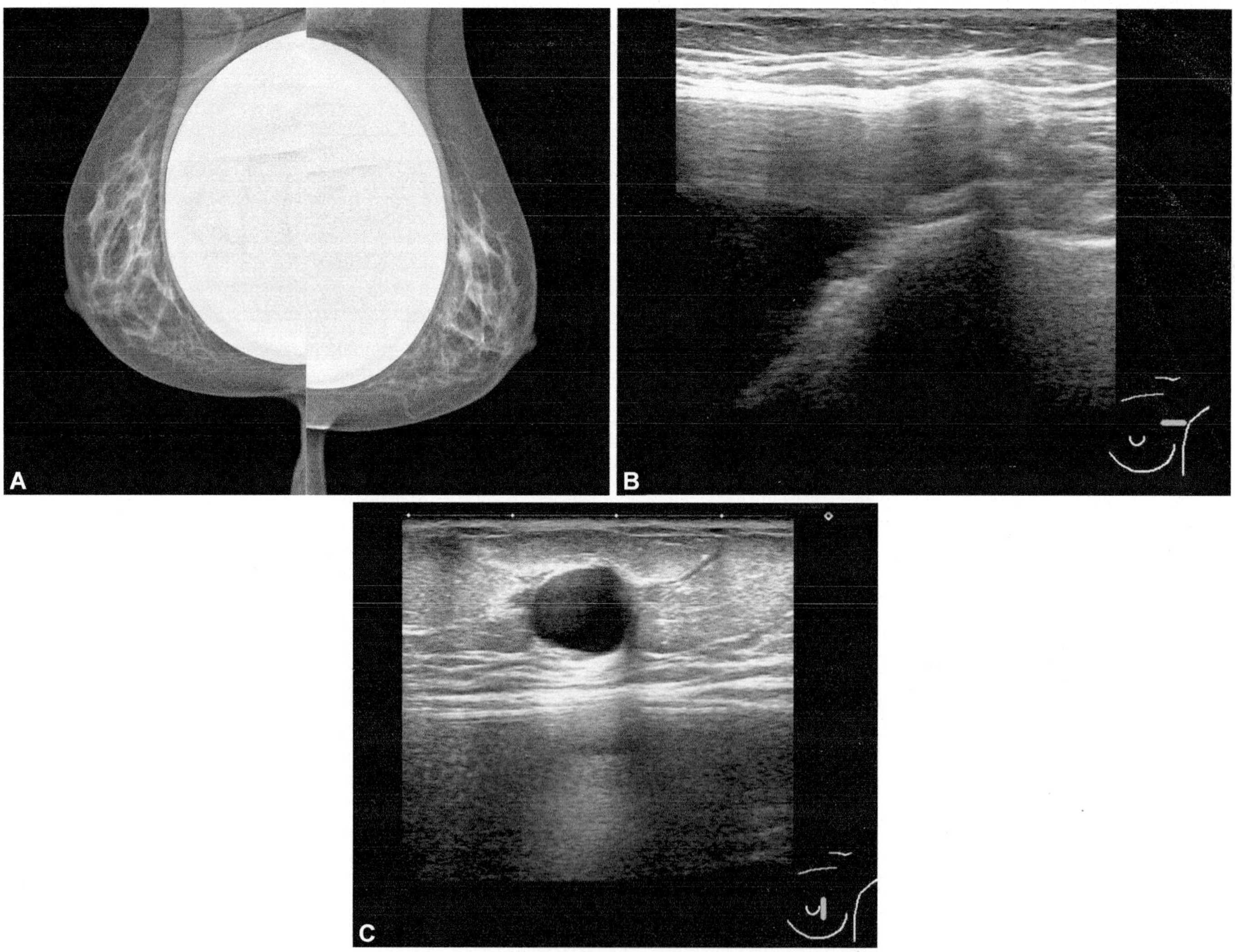

Figs. 23A to C: (A) Mammogram—MLO view of both breasts in a 46-year-old female shows submuscular breast implants on both sides; (B) Ultrasound of right breast shows normal anechoic implant while; (C) Ultrasound of left breast shows a small well-defined simple cyst with posterior acoustic enhancement in the lateral quadrant. MRI of left breast axial sections show a small well defined lesion which was

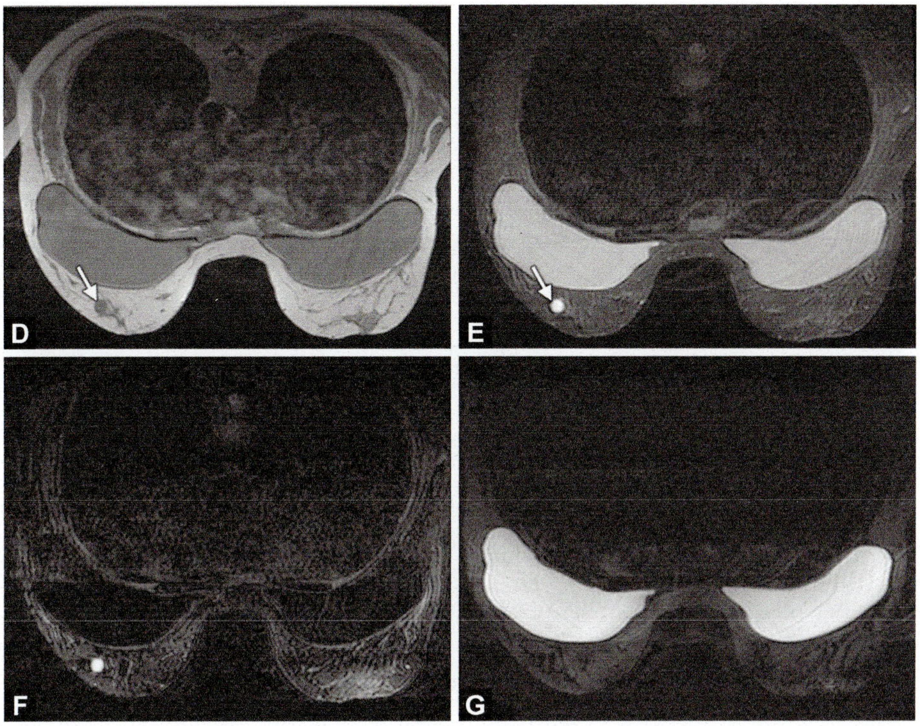

Figs. 23D to G: (D) hypointense on T1W and (E) hyperintense on STIR and (F) Silicone-suppressed sequence. The lesion is suppressed on; (G) Water-suppressed sequence suggestive of simple cyst. (MLO: mediolateral oblique.)

REFERENCES

1. Middleton MS, McNamara Jr MP. Breast implant classification with MR imaging correlation. Radiographics 2000;20:E1.
2. Yang N, Muradali D. The augmented breast: a pictorial review of the abnormal and unusual. AJR Am J Roentgenol 2011;196:W451-60.
3. Yasuo A, Ritsu A, Shinichiro K, et al. Silicone-selective multishot echo-planar imaging for rapid MRI survey of breast implants. Eur Radiol 2007;17:1875-8.
4. Herborn Cristoph U, Borut M, Daniel E, et al. Breast augmentation and reconstructive surgery: MR imaging of implant rupture and malignancy. Eur Radiol 2002;12:2198-206.
5. Eklund GW, Busby RC, Miller SH, et al. Improved imaging of the augmented breast. AJR Am J Roentgenol 1988;151:469-73.
6. Theophelis LG, Stevenson TR. Radiographic evidence of breast implant rupture. Plast Reconstr Surg 1986;78:673-5.
7. Baker JL, Bartels RJ, Douglas WM. Closed compression technique for rupturing a contracted capsule around a breast implant. Plast Reconstr Surg 1976;58:137-41.
8. Feliberti MC, Arrillaga A, Colon GA. Rupture of inflated breast implants in closed compression capsulotomy: case report. Plast Reconstr Surg 1977;59:848.
9. Andersen B, Hawtof D, Alani H, Kapetansky D. The diagnosis of ruptured breast implants. Plast Reconstr Surg 1989;84:903-7.
10. Juanpere S, Perez E, Huc O, et al. Imaging of breast implants—a pictorial review. Insights Imaging 2011;2:653-70.
11. Hölmich Lisbet R, Fryzek Jon P, Kim K, et al. The diagnosis of silicone breast-implant rupture clinical findings compared with findings at magnetic resonance imaging. Ann Plast Surg 2005;54:583-9.
12. Di Benedetto G, Sara C, Luca G, et al. Comparative study of breast implant rupture using mammography, sonography and magnetic resonance imaging: correlation with surgical findings. Breast J 2008;14:532-7.
13. Frank S, Mahdi R, Sherko K. Imaging in patients with breast implants—results of the First International Breast (Implant) Conference 2009. Insights Imaging 2010;1:93-7.

Breast Interventions

CHAPTER 9

9.1 Breast Interventions and Modalities Used for Imaging

INTRODUCTION

The diagnosis and management of breast diseases has changed significantly with the increase in number of biopsies and improvement in percutaneous breast biopsy techniques. This is because there are fewer complications, lower cost and faster recovery as compared to surgical biopsy. Ultrasonography (US), stereotaxy and MRI are the imaging modalities which are frequently used for guiding biopsies. Proper patient selection using an appropriate guidance modality with a correct and meticulous technique ensures good results.

ROLE OF RADIOLOGIST

The radiologist plays an important role in selecting the patient for breast biopsy which, upon the age of patient, comorbidities and risk factors. A close follow-up may sometimes be a better option in elderly patients. The next important step is selection of the modality for guidance, selection of lesion or area of architectural distortion or suspicious microcalcifications, needle selection and approach taken for accessing the lesion or area.

It is equally important to talk to the patient. The benefits, limitations and risks of procedure should be explained to patient.

INDICATIONS FOR BREAST BIOPSY

- BIRADS category 4 (4a, 4b and 4c) and BIRADS 5 lesions
- Suspicious microcalcifications
- Suspicious area of architectural distortion on mammogram
- Lesions that are "most probably benign"—BIRADS 3 (highly anxious patient v/s 6-month short-term follow-up).

PATIENT PREPARATION

It is important to be aware of any significant history like bleeding disorders, anticoagulant treatment, etc. Before starting any invasive procedure, an informed consent must be taken and documented.

The expected postprocedural complications and postprocedural care should also be told carefully.

ULTRASOUND GUIDANCE

Due to its dynamic nature, ease of maneuverability and constant visualization of needle, ultrasound is a very useful guidance modality.

Ultrasound guided interventions are safe procedures done regularly in a breast clinic. The most important thing to remember is that the lesion should be clearly visible on ultrasound. Another point to keep in mind is to avoid oblique path of needle as the breast flattens against the chest wall in supine position.

Using ultrasound guidance a parallel approach should be followed so that entire needle is visualized and position of tip can be monitored when the needle enters the lesion. Any risk of injury to deeper tissue is also minimized. It is a good practice to document the needle position during procedure and needle track after procedure.

- Fine needle aspiration cytology (FNAC)/Cyst aspiration
- Core needle biopsy (CNB)
- Hookwire localization for excision biopsies
- Vacuum-assisted biopsies/extractions.

FNAC/Cyst Aspiration

Simple cysts with anechoic component and imperceptible walls can be aspirated if they become painful or symptomatic. Contents are aspirated under guidance till the walls of the cyst are apposed.

Complicated cysts with low-level internal echoes can also be aspirated in a similar way if they become symptomatic or are enlarging in size. Their contents are usually discarded.

Complex cystic masses: These are defined as cysts with thick septa, thickened wall, intracystic mass or other discrete solid components. The solid component may be debris or pus or even a true mass with color flow within.[2]

Complex cystic mass with vascularity in solid portion: If there is a true solid component in the mass, then first aspiration should be done followed immediately by a biopsy of the residual portion because there may be a malignancy even if the aspirate does not show any malignant cells.[3,4]

Algorithm for complex cystic mass with no vascularity in solid portionc: This has been discussed in detail in the previous chapter.

Flowchart 1: Algorithm for complex cystic mass with no vascularity in solid portion

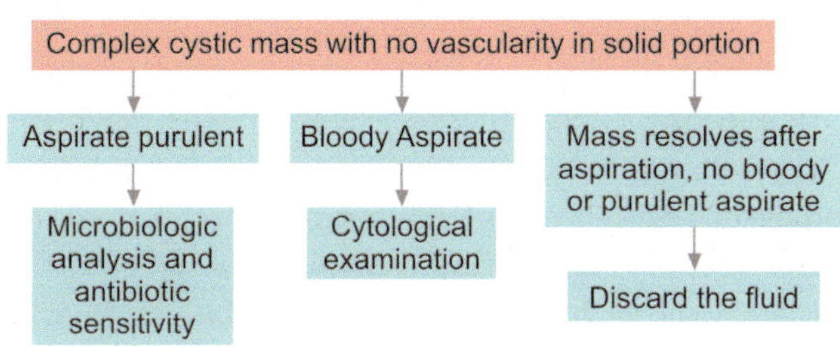

Hookwire for Presurgical Localization of Lesions

Hookwire localization is used to mark/localize nonpalpable lesions preoperatively so that the lesions can be accurately excised during surgery. It is a safe procedure but has a learning curve.

It is performed for both benign and suspicious lesions under ultrasound or mammography (stereotactic guidance).

If the lesion is visible on ultrasound, then ultrasound should be the modality used for guidance because of its dynamic status, ease of maneuverability and no radiation involved. On the other hand, stereotactic guidance is used in case of scar, focal asymmetry or suspicious micro calcification.

Indications for hookwire localization are:[5]

- Patients with a biopsy proven cancer
- Lesions with imaging vs pathological discordance at core needle biopsy (CNB)
- High-risk lesions such as atypical ductal hyperplasia, radial scar
- Where CNB is not an option or fails to provide a definitive histological diagnosis.

Hookwire with needle: This consists of a bevel tip needle with centimeters marking and wire inserted inside it (Figs. 1A to C). Variable needle lengths are available and can be chosen depending on the depth of the abnormality being localized in the breast (a 9 cm, 21 G needle is used commonly). The wire has a mark on it just outside the needle hub which tells the radiologist that the tip of the wire is within the needle during manipulation at the time of dislodging the wire. Since the tip of the wire is bent in the front in the shape of a hook, it is called a hookwire. A thickened palpable segment of the wire approximately 2 cm from the tip of the hook indicates its proximity to the tip of the wire for the benefit of the operating surgeon.

Procedure: One must choose a point on the skin with the shortest distance to the lesion while still approachable by ultrasound guidance. The area is then prepped with betadine solution. Under real-time ultrasound guidance and local anesthesia, the needle with hookwire is inserted using a parallel approach so that entire needle is visualized and position of advancing tip can be seen. Once the tip is well within the lesion, the needle tip is pushed further just beyond the lesion (up to 5 mm) to release the wire (Fig. 2). The position for release should be confirmed (tip should be within or just beyond lesion). Now wire is advanced slowly so that the hook opens. (Note: At this time, the mark on the wire outside the needle hub moves

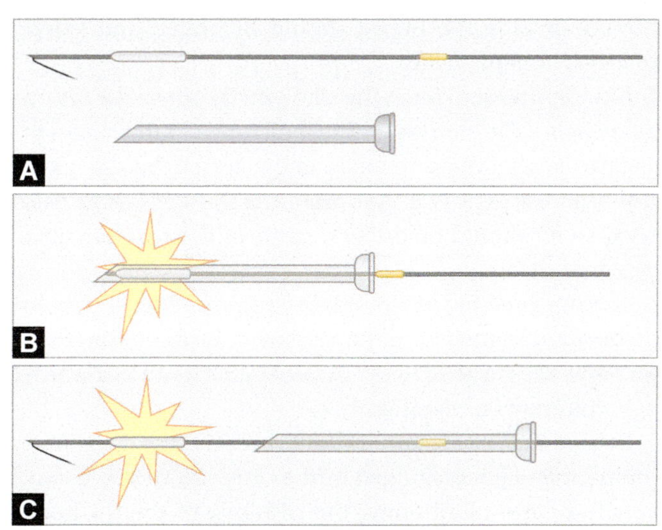

Figs. 1A to C: (A) Hookwire with needle; (B and C) Advancement and dislodgement of hookwire into the lesion.

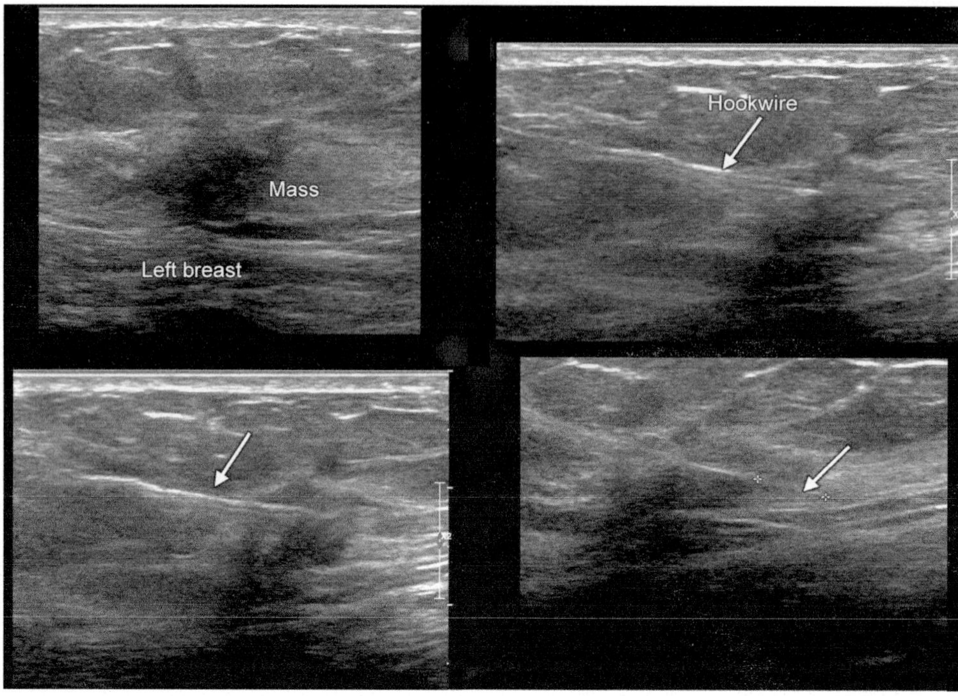

Fig. 2: Hookwire localization in a mass under ultrasound guidance where tip (arrow) of hookwire is seen just beyond the mass.

just inside the needle.) Once the hook is released it gets entangled in the breast tissue. This is confirmed it by pulling the wire gently and noting that the lesion is also pulled on ultrasound without the hook getting displaced. Now keeping the wire taut with one hand, the other hand is used to rotate the needle and withdraw it slowly. Care must be taken so as to not withdraw the wire along with the needle.

Once the procedure is complete, the portion of wire which is outside the breast should be coiled and safely fixed with help of plaster.

It is important to mark the skin exactly above the lesion and measure the shortest vertical distance to the lesion at this level, so that the surgeon is able to incise the skin closest to the lesion. A two-view mammogram (CC and true lateral view) should be done to confirm the wire position relative to lesion.

The distance of the tip of wire from the lesion should also be documented with the help of a free hand diagram. This helps the surgeon to avoid removing an unnecessarily large volume of tissue (Fig. 3).

Sometimes, especially in fatty breasts, the wire may overshoot and get dislodged further away from the lesion. In such a case, mentioning the distance of the tip/hook from the lesion and marking the lesion on the skin is even more important.

After the surgeon excises the lump, the specimen mammogram should be taken with wire in situ. This confirms whether the lesion is completely removed or not. Once the lesion is seen, its distance from margins should be measured. If any of the margin is inadequate, this information should be passed on to the surgeon so that clearance of margins can be done again. The specimen is then sent to pathology department for assessment.

Immersion ultrasound can be done for lesions which are seen on mammography and are localized on ultrasound.[6]

If performed properly, excision biopsy using preoperative hookwire localization is a safe and precise method. Once the hookwire is engaged and fixed in the tissue, it can only be removed by surgical intervention.

Potential problems associated with hookwire localization:

- Failure to excise the localized abnormality
- The hookwire may migrate and get dislodged from the lesion prior to surgery. This can be due to arm movement during patient transfer but is seen especially in fatty breast which provides poor grip for the hookwire
- Pneumothorax (rarely)
- Very rarely, fragments of wire are left in the surgical bed (as the result of accidental clipping or fragmentation of the wire). These may not cause harm as the

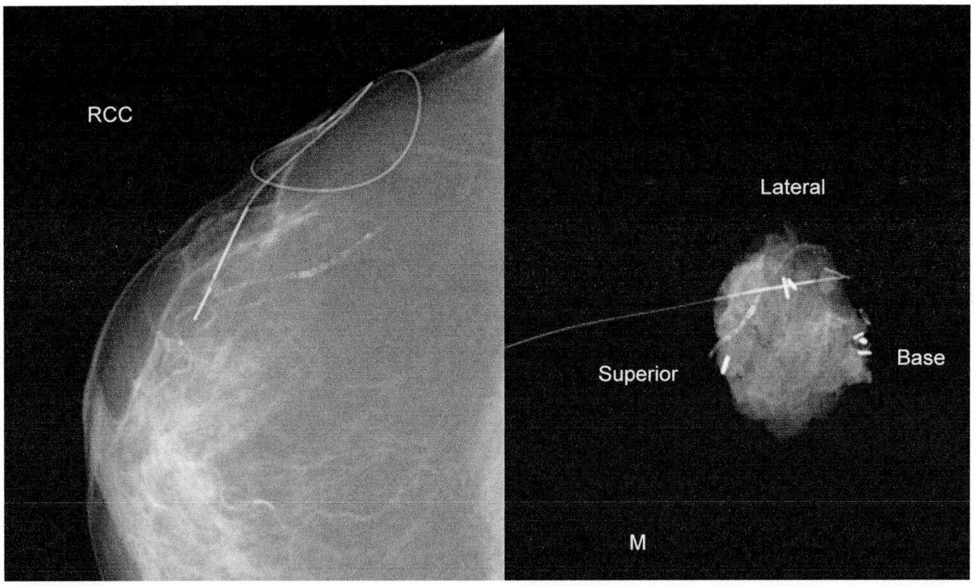

Fig. 3: Mammogram and specimen mammogram showing hookwire within the mass.

material used as same as in surgical clips and seldom require removal

For lesions which are located near the skin surface (<1 cm), a marker can be placed to localized the site of lesion and distance from skin surface to lesion should be documented.

Vacuum-assisted Breast Biopsy

Vacuum-assisted breast biopsy (VABB) is used both as a diagnostic and therapeutic method using ultrasound, mammogram or MRI guidance.[7] Since a large volume of tissue is extracted, repeat biopsies and sampling errors are reduced.

Diagnostic Indications

- Palpable or non-palpable lesions which are BIRADS category 3 and 4A
- Lesions smaller than 5 mm, mainly small stellate lesions which are difficult to remove with a standard core biopsy
- Solitary intraductal papillomas
- Clustered microcalcifications—biopsied under stereotactic guidance
- Used for suspicious microcalcification/architectural distortions

Therapeutic Indications

Complete removal of benign lesions <1 cm in diameter - a less expensive alternative to surgery.

Procedure

Once the approach and site of entry is selected, local anesthetic is infiltrated and a small incision is made using a surgical blade. After this, the probe is inserted in such a way so that it is just below the lesion or suspicious area. Its position is confirmed before the device is activated. A rotating cutting device cuts the tissue that is drawn in the probe by vacuum and collected in a tube attached to it. The probe is then rotated and multiple samples are taken till such time that sampling from the entire area is done.

Once the procedure is completed, a small clip (tissue marker) is inserted to mark the place from where the tissue was removed. A postmarker mammogram is taken in two orthogonal views.

In contrast to a standard core biopsy, there is no forward throw of the needle in VABB; hence, it can be used for lesions close to the nipple, the thoracic wall, the skin, or the axillary region. These are difficult locations but with experience, the retrieval of adequate samples from these lesions will be feasible.

Complications

Bleeding or pain during the procedure which can be controlled by compression.

- Postoperative pain
- Hematomas.

The patient is advised to bring any previous mammogram, ultrasound or MRI so that comparison can be done.

Vacuum-assisted biopsy causes little or no scarring on the skin/in the breast and takes less time as compared to surgical excision biopsy.

Precautions to be Taken on the Day of the Procedure

The patient should be advised not to put deodorant or talcum powder on the day of procedure if the procedure is under mammography guidance.

Postbiopsy markers: Clips or hydromarkers are extremely useful and are indicated in the following scenarios:

- If there is a risk that suspicious calcifications or lesion can no longer be visualized after biopsy
- Patients undergoing neoadjuvant chemotherapy to localize the original tumor bed in complete tumor response
- Patients with multiple lesions—most suspicious lesions should be marked
- Useful for correlation between various modalities.

After introduction of the marker, postmarker mammography should be performed in two orthogonal views to document marker position. The position of marker in relation to the biopsy site should also be mentioned in mammography report. These markers are titanium based and a have a hydrophilic component which swells up in coming in contact with breast tissue, fluid and get lodged. Their position can be confirmed on ultrasound where they are seen as linear echogenic foci. There are many options from various vendors available in market. With advancements in treatment options and type of surgery offered, there will be more and more use of these markers in future.

Stereotactic guidance: Stereotactic biopsy can be performed under analogue or digital mammography. The difference is in patient position (prone or supine) and in the way co-ordinates are calculated which is manual vs digital.

Stereotactic biopsy, also known as stereotactic core biopsy uses a computer and imaging performed in at least two planes to localize a target lesion (such as a tumor or microcalcifications in the breast) in three-dimensional space. Stereotactic core biopsy makes use of the underlying principle of parallax to determine the depth or "Z-dimension" of the target lesion.

Indications

- Solid suspicious mass seen only on mammogram with or without interval growth since previous mammogram
- An area of suspicious architectural distortion
- Suspicious microcalcifications
- Asymmetry associated with suspicious microcalcification, architectural distortion or focal skin thickening

Technique

A craniocaudal projection is taken initially compressing the breast with a small special paddle with a central "window." Once the lesion is identified in the first mammogram, two-additional projections are performed at +15 and -15°. After marking the center of the lesion, spatial co-ordinates *X*, *Y* and *Z* are calculated (Fig. 4).

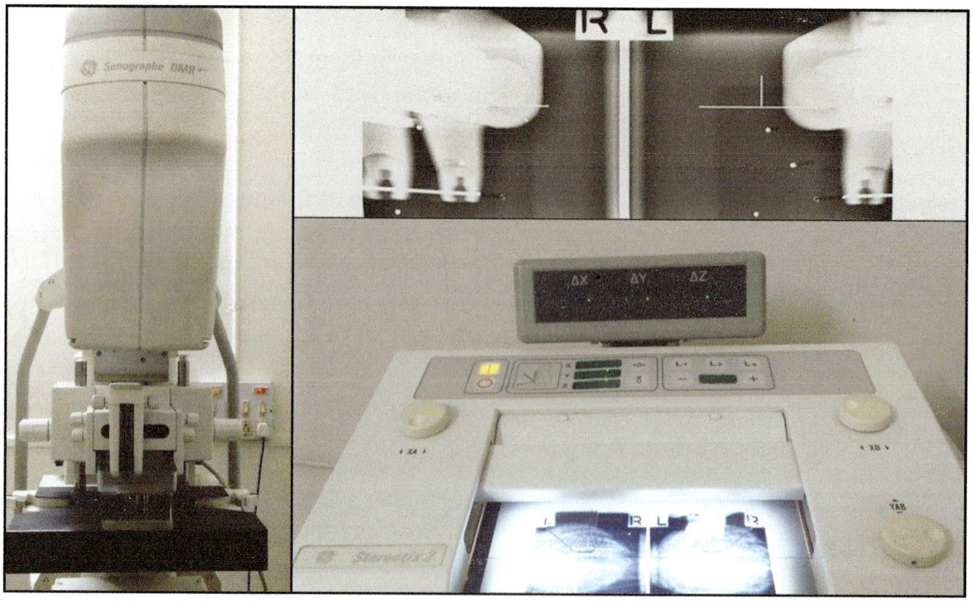

Fig. 4: Mammogram machine is shown with stereotactic biopsy set, calibration and 15° projections to calculate the *Z* co-ordinate.

The skin entry point is identified with the breast compressed lightly and local anesthetic is infiltrated. A small nick is then given with a surgical blade and biopsy needle is introduced. The position of the needle is then confirmed with further mammography projections and biopsy done.

Even after a false-negative stereotactically guided CNB, there are further follow-up recommendations so that cancer can be diagnosed timely. This depends on patient compliance and a robust system by which both patient and her referring doctor is informed of the appropriate follow-up.

REFERENCES

1. American College of Radiology. ACR BI-RADS ultrasound. In: ACR breast imaging reporting and data system, breast imaging atlas. Reston, VA: American College of Radiology; 2003.
2. Smith DN, Kaelin CM, Korbin CD, et al. Impalpable breast cysts: utility of cytologic examination of fluid obtained with radiologically guided aspiration. Radiology 1997;204:149-51.
3. Venta LA, Kim JP, Pelloski CE, Morrow M. Management of complex breast cysts. AJR Am J Roentgenol 1999;173:1331-6.
4. Berg WA. Image-guided breast biopsy and management of high-risk lesions. Radiol Clin North Am 2004;42:935-46.
5. Shetty M. Presurgical localization of breast abnormalities: an overview and analysis of 202 cases. Indian J Surg Oncol 2010;1:278-83.
6. Lee KY, Seo BK, Ann Y, et al. Immersion ultrasonography of excised non palpable breast lesion specimens after ultrasound-guided needle localization. Korean J Radiol 2008;9:312-9. doi: 10.3348/kjr.2008.9.4.312.
7. Park HL, Hong J. Vacuum-assisted breast biopsy for breast cancer. Gland Surg 20143:120-7.

9.2 Fine Needle Aspiration Cytology (FNAC) and Core Needle

INTRODUCTION

The diagnosis and management of breast cancer requires a team effort and involves the radiologist, pathologist and surgeon. Both FNAC and biopsy help in making a pathological diagnosis and have their limitations and advantages. Core needle biopsy (CNB) has a higher specificity and sensitivity in diagnosing benign and malignant breast lesions.[1]

In the Indian set-up, though core biopsy is now being done more frequently, some clinicians are still comfortable with FNAC.

FINE NEEDLE ASPIRATION CYTOLOGY

FNAC is easier to perform, takes less time and results depend on the technique & competence of the radiologist and adequacy of aspirate obtained. Usually a 22–23 Gauge needle is used to obtain the aspirate which is sent for cytological evaluation.

The average number of FNA passes recommended for adequate sampling of most palpable breast masses ranges from two to four, provided the smear is adequate.

The cytological interpretation of smears is dependent on the cytopathologist's experience and skills. Often smears are inadequate and multiple inconclusive FNAC reports necessitate a core needle biopsy or surgical excision biopsy.

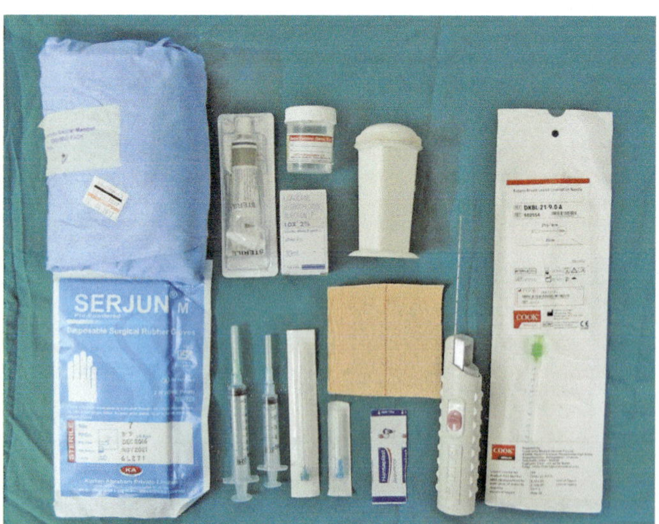

Fig. 1: Tray showing materials used while doing ultrasound guided FNAC or core needle biopsy. Materials in tray: Sterile glove, sterile drapes, sterile probe covers, sterile ultrasound gel, Lumbar puncture (LP) needle, core biopsy needle, 2% lignocaine, normal saline, leucoplast, scalpel blade, disposable syringe. (FNAC: fine needle aspiration cytology).

Indications

Though in India some surgeons still prefer FNAC, the scenario is changing gradually.

FNAC is indicated in:

- Smaller lesions which are superficially placed and close to skin, in patients with implants and for deep seated lesions situated close to chest wall which are difficult to reach
- In chest wall recurrences and to evaluate axillary lymph nodes before selecting the patients for sentinel lymph node biopsy.

Limitations

One of the limitations of FNAC is that it cannot distinguish between ductal carcinoma in situ (DCIS) and invasive cancers reliably and therefore cannot grade the malignancy cytologically. By definition invasion in the strictest sense is invasion through the basement membrane which cannot be reported with certainty on cytology.

The major limitation of FNAC however is in its inability to diagnose some benign or borderline breast lesions and their distinction from the malignant lesions. These lesions form the "true grey zone lesions" of the breast and include fibroepithelial lesions, fibrocystic disease, papillary lesions, radial scar and sclerosing adenosis.

The others in this category include flat epithelial atypia, atypical ductal hyperplasia, in-situ carcinoma, low-grade carcinoma and lobular carcinoma. Lobular carcinoma is commonly missed on FNAC due to high inadequacy rate and lower cellularity. The positive predictive value for suspicious lesions and high-risk lesions like atypical ductal hyperplasia is much lower for FNAC.

Westenend et al.[2] found that positive predictive value of FNAC for malignant lesions was similar to CNB (99%–100%), but when it came to suspicious and atypical lesions, the performance of FNAC was poor, especially for atypia. Therefore, the performance of CNB is better as compared to FNAC across various studies. FNAC is inadequate for non-palpable lesions and lesions <10 mm.[3] FNAC had an average success rate of 75%–90% for palpable and 34%–58% for non-palpable breast lesions, whereas success rates for CNB were 97% and 94%, respectively.[4]

There is a variable and often high rate of false negativity due to sampling error or error in interpretation of FNAC.

CORE NEEDLE BIOPSY

Indications

CNB is done for the definitive confirmation or exclusion of malignancy, which helps avoid un-necessary surgeries for definitive benign diseases. The specificity and positive predictive value of CNB is higher for suspicious lesions especially atypical lesions and fibroepithelial lesions.

In 20% of the patients with a diagnosis of DCIS by CNB, there is an invasive component found in the excised specimen which varies with the gauge of the needle used.[5] CNB reliably distinguishes between invasive lobular and invasive ductal carcinoma based on histological and immunohistochemistry features.

This preoperative differentiation is important for:

- Planning extent of the surgery if breast-conservative surgery is considered
- Considering neo adjuvant chemotherapy
- If invasive lobular carcinoma is diagnosed then contralateral MRI is required as there is high risk for contralateral cancer[6-8]

It is possible to do receptor studies (ER, PR and Her2 neu) on a specimen obtained by CNB and a proper preoperative assessment can be done, not possible with FNAC. The immune-histochemical and molecular tests are easily performed on CNB to determine additional prognostic and predictive markers and this is important as more patients are now being offered neoadjuvant chemotherapy.

Technique

A 14-G core biopsy needle with a 10 or 20-mm cutting lengths should be used for solid lesions visible on ultrasound (Fig. 2). The anesthetic agent (2% lignocaine) is infiltrated along the pathway of the needle up to the lesion. Access through the nipple–areolar complex should be avoided. With a blade, a 2–3-mm incision is a few cm away from the edge of the transducer, then the needle is inserted and advanced in a parallel to the probe and chest wall so that its entire length can be seen (Figs. 3 and 4) and risk of injury to deeper structures and pneumothorax is reduced (Figs. 5A to D).

The needle should be seen throughout the procedure till it reaches the lesion and fired just before the tip enters the mass. The needle track should be seen traversing through the mass when biopsy is taken.

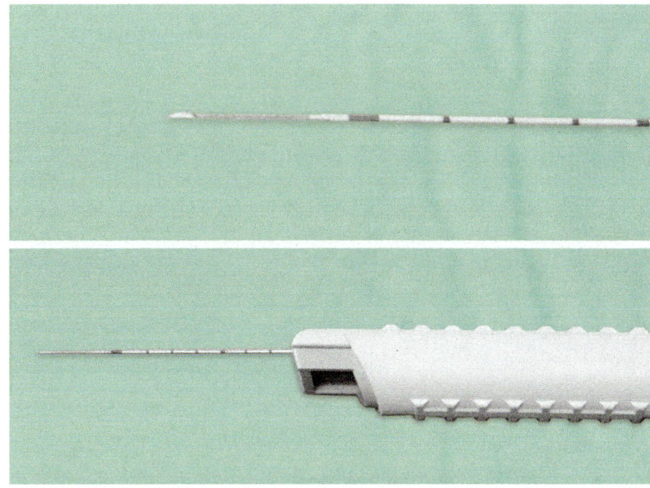

Fig. 2: Core biopsy needle showing the size of core obtained.

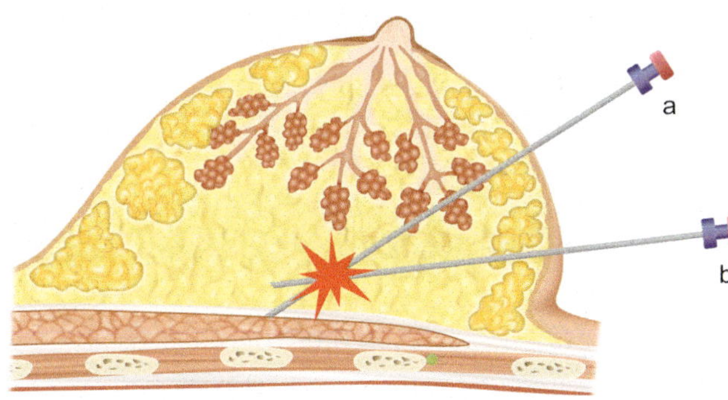

Fig. 3: (a) Wrong needle path; (b) Correct needle path which is parallel to chest wall.

The best possible route to avoid superficial vessels must be chosen to minimize bleeding. Also local compression should be given at biopsy site immediately after biopsy. The patient should be advised to restrict arm movements on the side in question and avoid strenuous exercise for 1–2 days.

Procedure-related Complications

- Vasovagal attack
- Bleeding or hematoma
- Infection
- Pneumothorax (very rare <1%)
- Needle seeding: Mechanical displacement of tumor cells along the needle track is common but these cells are not viable for a long time
- Possible need for rebiopsy due to inadequate sampling.

Lesions that Need Special Considerations

High-risk lesions: Atypical ductal hyperplasia, lobular carcinoma in situ, atypical papillomatosis and columnar

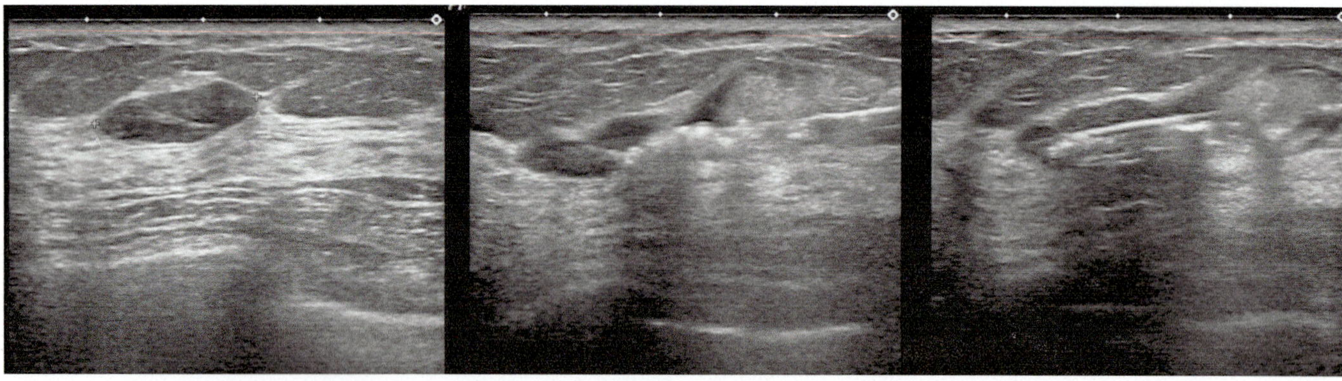

Fig. 4: Ultrasound showing needle positions while doing biopsy for fibroadenoma.

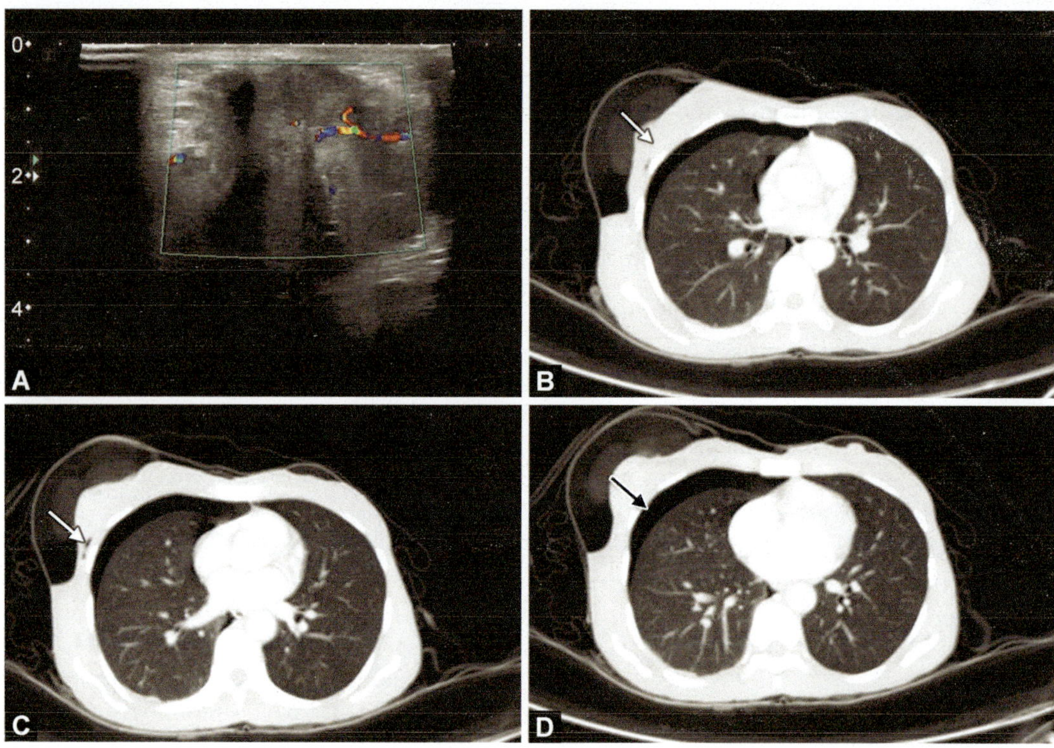

Figs. 5A to D: Ultrasound showing (A) Large breast mass with vascularity and (B to D) Pneumothorax caused due to biopsy of the breast mass. This is a rare complication which can be avoided by keeping the needle position parallel to chest wall.

cell lesions are accurately diagnosed on core needle biopsy. These are high-risk lesions and have an increased risk of invasive cancer on subsequent follow-up.

Papillary lesions: These lesions form a spectrum ranging from benign papilloma to papillary carcinoma. The overall accuracy of FNAC to predict benign from malignant papillary lesions is poor, especially for diagnosing malignant lesions.[7]

CNB has also got only a moderate accuracy in diagnosing papillary lesions with overlapping findings in papillary carcinoma in situ and papilloma; therefore, surgical **excision** is recommended.

Fibroepithelial lesions: These are a heterogeneous group ranging from fibroadenoma to phyllodes tumor which may be benign or malignant. Its challenging to distinguish between these two entities on FNAC as there are no universally accepted cytological criteria.[8] In fact, differentiation between these two entities is challenging even on preoperative core needle biopsy because of overlapping findings, and immunohistochemistry maybe helpful.[9] Phyllodes tumor is a heterogeneous group of tumors and both core needle biopsy and FNAC cannot grade them optimally. There are overlapping histopathological features amongst various subtypes and there may be transformation to a malignant subtype. A complete excision with an adequate margin is required to prevent recurrences.

Calcifications: CNB should be performed to assess suspicious microcalcifications.

POINTS TO REMEMBER

- All lesions with atypia on FNAC should be followed by CNB
- All benign lesions diagnosed on FNAC should be followed by CNB, if BIRADS score on imaging is discordant with benign FNAC findings
- All non-palpable breast lumps should undergo core needle biopsy.

FNAC is most accurate when experienced cytologists are available to immediately assess material adequacy, so that additional aspirations can be done. Overall, CNB has a higher sensitivity and specificity compared to FNAC.

In conclusion, there should be a judicious use of these techniques and diagnostic modalities in resource-limited settings. Parameters such as palpability and availability of an experienced cytopathologist should be taken into consideration before deciding on FNAC in selected cases.

REFERENCES

1. Ibrahim AE, Bateman AC, Theaker JM, et al. The role and histological classification of needle core biopsy in comparison with fine needle aspiration cytology in the preoperative assessment of impalpable breast lesions. J Clin Pathol 2001;54:121-5.
2. Westenend PJ, Sever AR, Beekman-De Volder HJ, et al. A comparison of aspiration cytology and core needle biopsy in the evaluation of breast lesions. Cancer 2001;93:146-50.
3. Barra AA, Gobbi H, de L Rezende CA, et al. A comparison of aspiration cytology and core needle biopsy according to tumor size of suspicious breast lesions. Diagn Cytopathol 2008;36:26-31.
4. Hukkinen K, Kivisaari L, Heikkila PS, et al. Unsuccessful preoperative biopsies, fine needle aspiration cytology or core needle biopsy, lead to increased costs in the diagnostic workup in breast cancer. Acta Oncol 2008;47:1037-45.
5. Rahka EA, El-Sayed ME, Reed J, et al. Screen-detected breast lesions with malignant needle core biopsy diagnoses and no malignancy identified in subsequent surgical excision specimens (potential false-positive diagnosis). Eur J Cancer 2009;45:1162-67.
6. Provenzano E, Pinder SE. Pre-operative diagnosis of breast cancer in screening: problems and pitfalls. Pathology 2009;41:3-17.
7. Michael CW, Buschmann B. Can true papillary neoplasms of breast and their mimickers be accurately classified by cytology?. Cancer 2002;96:92-100.
8. Putti TC, Pinder SE, Elston CW, et al. Breast pathology practice: most common problems in a consultation service. Histopathology 2005;47:445-57.
9. Jara-Lazaro AR, Akhilesh M, Thike AA, et al. Predictors of phyllodes tumours on core biopsy specimens of fibroepithelial neoplasms. Histopathology 2010;57:220-32.

9.3 Radiologic Pathologic Concordance and Discordance

INTRODUCTION

As breast imaging techniques continue to improve and more and more small cancers are detected, the radiologist's role is changing rapidly. His job is no longer restricted to categorizing lesions on imaging and deciding which lesion should be biopsied, but it extends even beyond that. He looks into radiologic pathologic correlation and whether the biopsy results are concordant or discordant with imaging findings. He also suggests management recommendations to the clinician, for example, whether the patient should go for surgical excision or a short interval follow-up.

There is an increase in image guided breast biopsies which are minimally invasive as compared to surgical biopsies. Approximately 86% of biopsies done in USA in 2004 were done using imaging guidance.[1] The success of an image-guided core needle breast biopsy not only depends on its technique but also postbiopsy management of the patient. There may be sampling error in spite of optimum technique leading to false-negative result which affects the patient management.[2]

Since there is a difference in radiology and pathology workflows, it leads to a lack of communication and discordance between radiology and pathology findings. The cases with discordant findings must be discussed to reach to a proper radiologic pathologic correlation so that such errors can be avoided. With improvement in communication of clinical information between radiologists and pathologists, discrepancies and errors can be reduced leading to a better diagnosis, patient treatment and reduction in cost.

ASSESSMENT OF PATIENT PRIOR TO BIOPSY

Before proceeding with the biopsy, the radiologist must review imaging features of the mass to be targeted so that correct categorization of mass prior to biopsy is ensured. Since in India we follow the BIRADS classification, the radiologist must put the case in the appropriate BIRADS category. The case may have been evaluated on multiple modalities; however, the most appropriate modality must be chosen for imaging guidance.

If suspicious microcalcifications detected on mammogram are biopsied, the radiologist has to ensure that the correct calcifications are sampled and a biopsy marker placed to mark the site. This will ensure the adequate sampling and guide any future procedures if there is need to excise residual calcifications. While performing biopsy under ultrasound, it is a good practice to document and store the image while obtaining the sample.[3] A good working relationship between the radiologist and pathologist goes a long way as the role of pathologist is to critically comment upon the quality and quantity of specimen obtained and effectively communicate it to the radiologist.

Improvement in radiologic-pathologic concordance will not only affect individual diagnosis but will also have an impact on population morbidity and mortality, thereby leading to an improvement in quality of cancer treatment.

CATEGORIES OF CONCORDANCE IN IMAGING-PATHOLOGY CORRELATION

The term concordance is used when pathological finding is able to explain the imaging features and discordance is used when pathological does not correlate with imaging features. There are five categories of concordance as suggested by Parikh and Tickman:[3]

1. Concordant malignancy
2. Discordant malignancy
3. Concordant benign
4. Discordant benign
5. Borderline or high risk.

1. **Concordant malignancy:** If a mass shows suspicious or malignant features on imaging, that is, BIRADS category 4 or 5, and core needle biopsy also confirms the finding, then it is concordant malignancy (Fig. 1). These findings should be communicated to the surgeon and further appropriate action should be taken.
2. **Discordant malignancy:** The mass appears benign on imaging (BIRADS 2 or 3) but is found to be malignant on core needle biopsy. This is a discordant malignancy

Table 1: Categories of concordance in imaging-pathology correlation.

Type	*Imaging*	*Pathology*
Concordant malignancy	Malignant (BIRADS 4 or 5)	Malignant
Discordant malignancy	Benign (BIRADS 2 or 3)	Malignant
Concordant benign	Benign (2 or 3)	Benign
Discordant benign	(BIRADS 4 or 5)	benign finding

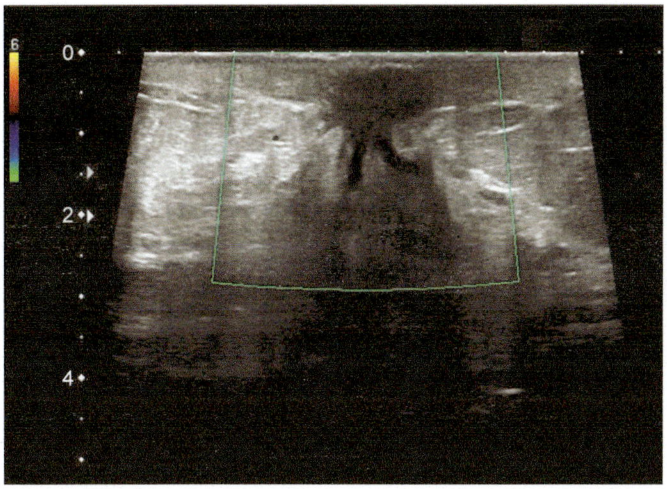

Fig. 1: Ultrasound in a 48-year-old female showing a hypoechoic mass with spiculations. Histopathology was s/o infiltrative ductal carcinoma—**concordant malignancy.**

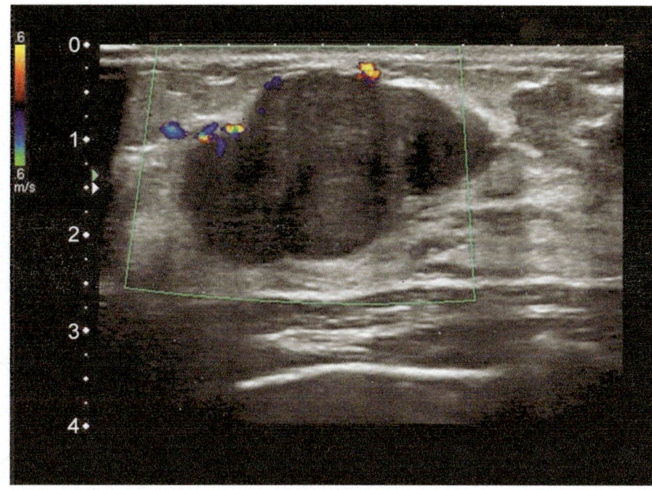

Fig. 2: Ultrasound in a 23-year-old female showing a well circumscribed hypoechoic mass with gentle lobulations. Histopathology was s/o fibroadenoma—**concordant benign.**

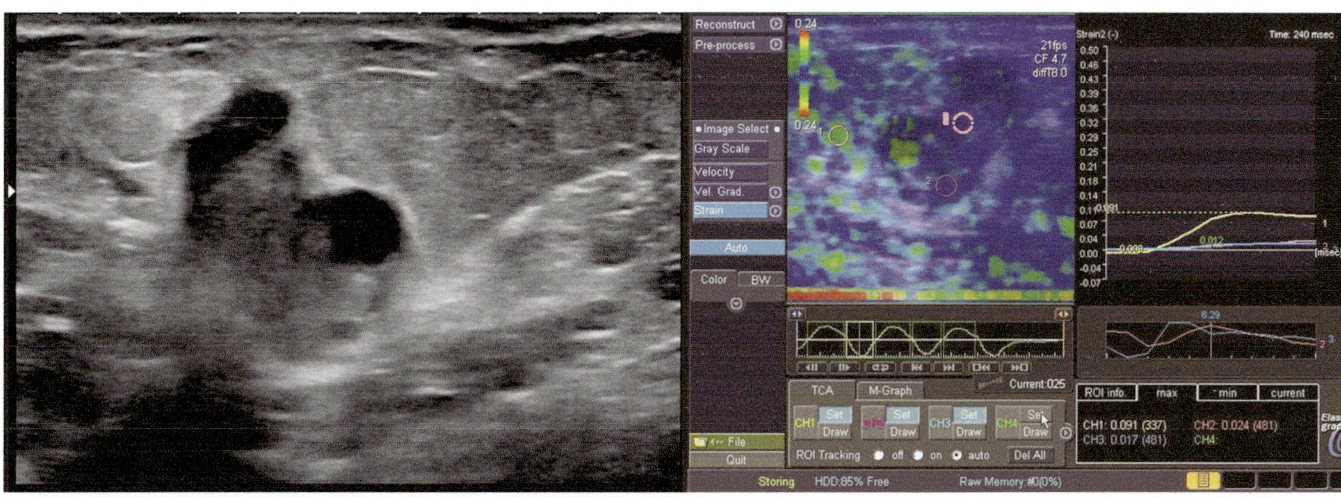

Fig. 3: Ultrasound in a 37-year-old female shows a heterogeneously isoechoic mass with anechoic component. Elastography shows high strain ratios. Histopathology was s/o sclerosing adenosis—**discordant benign.**

and has to be managed in a similar way as a concordant malignancy. This group includes circumscribed or benign appearing malignancies like medullary carcinoma and mucinous carcinoma. Others like high-grade invasive carcinoma, metastases and lymphoma can also have benign appearing features. The radiologist must convey the discordant result to pathologist so that a review can be done. At the same time, the radiologist must review the images once again to look for any missed associated features because of which the imaging findings were underestimated. The discrepancy between the radiology and pathology results must be discussed.

3. **Concordant benign:** This category includes those masses which are thought to be benign on imaging (BIRADS 2 or 3) and turn out to be benign on histopathology also (Fig. 2). Both the patient and clinician get reassurance and patient can be followed up till 2 years at 6 monthly intervals.
4. **Discordant benign:** Here, the mass is reported as malignant on imaging (BIRADS 4 or 5) but the pathologist reports it as a benign finding (Fig. 3). Benign masses that can appear as malignant on imaging include sclerosing adenosis, fat necrosis, postoperative scar, mastitis and diabetic mastopathy.

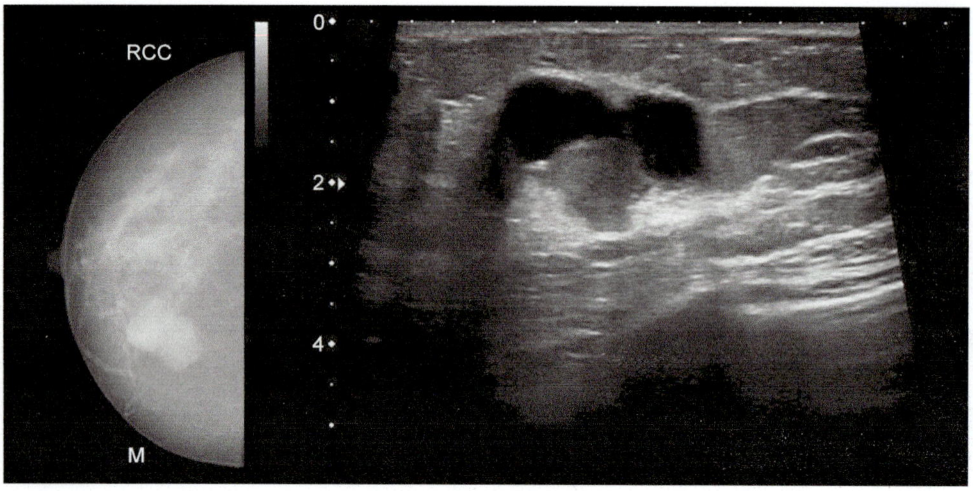

Fig. 4: Mammogram in a 49-year-old female shows a lobulated mass which appeared solid cystic on ultrasound. Histopathology was s/o intraductal papilloma—**borderline or high risk.**

The discordant lesions are extremely important and should immediately be communicated to the pathologist and a repeat biopsy should be recommended preferably excision biopsy since the first biopsy was not conclusive. It has been observed in literature that percutaneous biopsies gave up to 64% discordant results which were subsequently confirmed as cancer on surgical excision.[4] By using 14-G core biopsy needle under ultrasound guidance, the discordant lesions may have cancer in up to 50% cases.[5] These days vacuum assisted biopsy can be used as an alternative to surgical biopsy in discordant benign lesions.

5. **Borderline or high risk:** In this category, those lesions are included which are not malignant but have an increased life time risk of developing breast cancer. These include atypical ductal hyperplasia, radial sclerosing lesion, papillary lesion (Fig. 4) and possibly Phyllodes tumor. The management of patients in this category is still controversial and a case by case management is considered; however, a surgical biopsy is still recommended due to high risk.

REFERENCES

1. Vandromme MJ, Umphrey H, Krontiras H. Image guided methods for biopsy of suspicious breast lesions. J Surg Oncol 2011;103:299-305.
2. Youk JH, Kim EK, Kim MJ, Lee JY, Oh KK. Missed breast cancers at US-guided core needle biopsy: how to reduce them. Radiographics 2007;27:79-94.
3. Parikh J, Tickman R. Image-guided tissue sampling: where radiology meets pathology. Breast J 2005;11:403-9.
4. Liberman L. Percutaneous image-guided core breast biopsy. Radiol Clin North Am 2002;40:483-500.
5. Comstock CE. US-guided interventional procedures. In: Feig SA, ed. Syllabus: categorical course in diagnostic radiology breast imaging. Oak Brook, IL: Radiological Society of North America; 2005. pp. 155-68.

Uncommon Diseases of Breast

CHAPTER 10

10.1 The Paget Disease of Breast

INTRODUCTION

Paget disease of breast is an uncommon malignancy representing 1–3% cases of breast cancer[1] and was described by Sir James Paget in 1874.[2] It is associated with ductal carcinoma in situ (DCIS) and invasive malignancy in almost 80–90% cases.

CLINICAL FINDINGS

The common presentation is erythema, ulceration and eczematous changes in the nipple areolar region and sometimes there is a bloody nipple discharge.

Paget disease presents in fifth or sixth decade though it is also seen in adolescents.[3] It is more common in males as compared to females[4] and is usually unilateral.[5]

Sometimes the diagnosis is delayed as the patient is treated for eczema[6] and only a biopsy will establish the diagnosis.

The differential diagnosis includes allergic contact dermatitis, irritant dermatitis, lichen simplex chronicus and psoriasis.[7]

ETIOPATHOGENESIS

There are two important theories (Figs. 1A and B) that explain the possible pathogenesis of Paget disease.

Epidermotropic Theory

Since the Paget cells and underlying cancer share the same immune-histochemical profile, it is hypothesized that the malignant cells from DCIS migrate through lactiferous ducts and reach nipple areolar region.

Intraepidermal Transformation Theory

According to this theory, Paget cells arise from the epidermis of nipple by degeneration of existing cells or by in situ transformation.

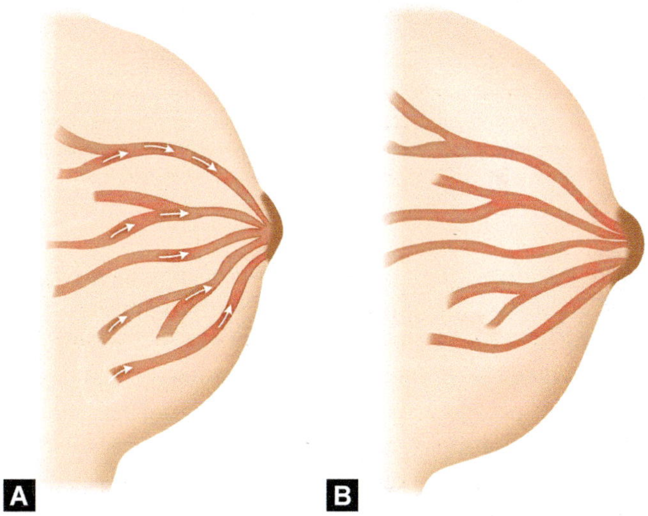

Figs. 1A and B: Pathogenesis of Paget disease of breast: (A) **Epidermotropic theory**: malignant cells from DCIS migrate through the lactiferous ducts and reach the nipple and areola; (B) **Intraepidermal transformation theory**: Paget cells arise from epidermis of nipple by degeneration of existing cells or by in situ transformation. (DCIS: ductal carcinoma in situ).

IMAGING FEATURES

Once the diagnosis of Paget disease is established on histopathology, the patient is referred for mammogram to rule out any underlying carcinoma or DCIS in breast. Mammogram and ultrasound may confirm the above findings, but if these are negative then a contrast enhanced magnetic resonance imaging (MRI) has to be done.

Mammography

The common mammographic findings noted in Pagets disease are skin thickening in the nipple areolar region, asymmetric density, nipple retraction, architectural distortion, pleomorphic calcifications (Fig. 2) or a discrete mass.

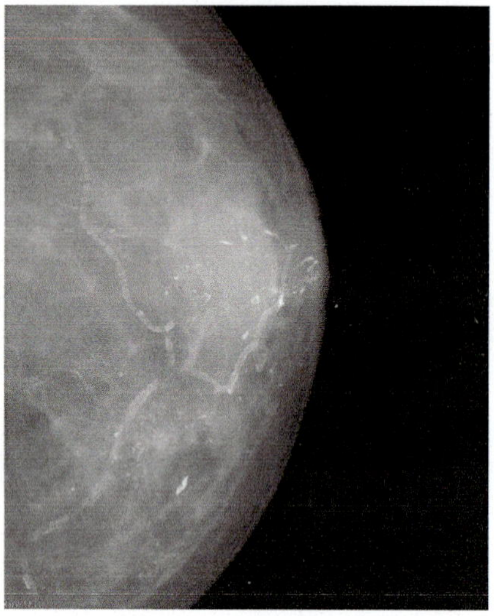

Fig. 2: A 48-year-old female presented with erythema and eczematous changes in the nipple areolar region of left breast and biopsy was s/o Paget disease. Mammogram of left breast showed linear pleomorphic calcifications s/o DCIS. (DCIS: ductal carcinoma in situ).

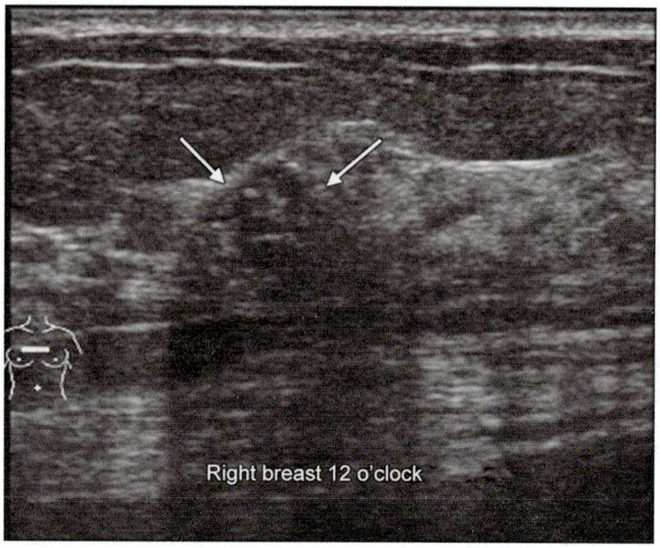

Fig. 3: Ultrasound in a proven case of Paget disease of nipple shows an ill-defined heterogeneous mass with multiple echogenic foci s/o microcalcifications.

The location of mass may vary and it may be close to nipple areolar region or away from it. Various studies have evaluated the role mammography in Paget disease, for example, Ikeda et al. found that approximately 50% cases of clinically proven Paget disease have a normal mammogram.[8] In a study by Muttark et al.,[9] a large number of clinically proven cases of Paget disease had invasive cancer and positive mammogram findings because of late presentation.

Ultrasound

Ultrasonography can show heterogeneous hypoechoic areas in breast parenchyma, or a discrete mass (Fig. 3) with or without calcifications and dilated ducts.

Magnetic Resonance Imaging

The MRI findings of Paget disease include enhancement and thickening in nipple areolar region, mass, DCIS showing enhancement or a combination of the above findings.

There may be absent, mild or intense enhancement in nipple areolar region[9] though asymmetric discoid or irregular enhancement[10] may also be seen. A study by Frei et al. compared preoperative mammography and MRI in Paget disease and concluded that underlying DCIS is diagnosed successfully on MRI.[11] Clinical and imaging findings complement each other in order to make an accurate diagnosis.[12]

MANAGEMENT

The treatment varies from resection of nipple areolar complex with or without local irradiation or mastectomy depending upon the presence of invasive component. If axillary lymph nodes are involved, an axillary dissection should also be done. Recurrence may occur if there is an in situ component along the nipple areolar region.[13]

CONCLUSION

Paget disease of breast is an uncommon malignancy that may have underlying DCIS or invasive cancer. The management depends upon the extent of involvement based on clinical and imaging findings.

REFERENCES

1. Ashikari R, Park K, Huvos AG, Urban JA. Paget's disease of the breast. Cancer 1970;26:680-5.
2. Paget J. On disease of the mammary areola preceding cancer of the mammary gland. St Bartholomews Hosp Rep 1874;10:87-9.
3. Martin VG, Pellettiere EV, Gress D, Miller AW. Paget's disease in an adolescent arising in a supernumerary nipple. J Cutan Pathol 1994;21:283-6.
4. O'Sullivan ST, McGreal GT, Lyons A, et al. Paget's disease of the breast in a man without underlying breast carcinoma. J Clin Pathol 1994;47:851-2.
5. Franceschini G, Masetti R, D'Ugo D, et al. Synchronous bilateral Paget's disease of the nipple associated with bilateral breast carcinoma. Breast J 2005;11:355-6.

6. Ward KA, Burton JL. Dermatologic diseases of the breast in young women. Clin Dermatol 1997;15: 45-52.
7. Lim HS, Feong SF, Lee FS, et al. Paget disease of the breast: mammographic, US and MR imaging findings with pathologic correlation. Radiographics 2011;31:1973-87.
8. Ikeda DM, Helvie MA, Frank TS, Chapel KL, Anderson IT. Paget disease of the nipple: radiologic-pathologic correlation. Radiology 1993;189: 89-94.
9. Muttarak M, Siriya B, Kongmebhol P, Chaiwun B, Sukhamwang N. Paget's disease of the breast: clinical, imaging and pathologic findings: a review of 16 patients. Biomed Imaging Interv J 2011;7: e16.
10. Da Costa D, Taddese A, Cure ML, et al. Common and unusual diseases of the nipple-areolar complex. Radiographics 2007;27:S65-77.
11. Frei KA, Bonel HM, Pelte MF, Hylton NM, Kinkel K. Paget disease of the breast: findings at magnetic resonance imaging and histopathologic correlation. Invest Radiol 2005;40:363-7.
12. Karakas C. Pagets disease of breast. J Carcinog 2011; 10:31.
13. Dixon AR, Galea MH, Ellis IO, Elston CW, Blamey RW. Paget's disease of the nipple. Br J Surg 1991;78:722-3.

10.2 Cystosarcoma Phyllodes

INTRODUCTION

Cystosarcoma phyllodes is an uncommon fibroepitheleal tumor of breast. The term phyllodes was used to describe cystic appearance and leaf-like growth pattern of the tumor. Its clinical, imaging and pathological features are similar to juvenile fibroadenoma and it has a potential for malignancy, recurrence and metastases.

CLINICAL FEATURES

Phyllodes tumors are seen in women between the age of 35 and 55 years.[1,2]

They present clinically as rapidly growing painless mass growing to a large size within weeks or months.

Histopathologically, they may range from benign to borderline or malignant[3] depending on histologic features such as stromal cellularity, infiltration at the tumor edge and mitotic activity.

IMAGING FEATURES

Mammogram

On mammogram, they are seen as large, circumscribed, lobulated dense masses of varying sizes either occupying a single quadrant of the breast or whole breast (Fig. 1A). There are no microcalcifications or architectural distortion. A radiolucent halo may be sometimes present. Calcification (typically coarse and plaque like) may be seen in a very small proportion of cases. No axillary lymphadenopathy is usually seen.

Ultrasound

It shows large, circumscribed, smooth walled heterogeneously hypoechoic masses (Fig. 1B) with or without cystic component. Fluid-filled elongated spaces or clefts in a large solid mass should raise a possibility of phyllodes tumor. Posterior acoustic shadowing may sometimes be seen. Vascularity may be present in the solid component of the mass.

Contrast-enhanced CT Scan

Contrast-enhanced CT scan (CECT) confirms the above findings with large enhancing heterogeneous masses showing cystic component in a few cases (Figs. 2A to C). Sometimes non-enhancing internal septations can be seen.

Magnetic Resonance Imaging

It can delineate the full tumor extent and potential satellite lesions before surgical excision is done. Phyllodes tumors are usually seen as oval, round or lobulated masses that are hypointense on T1 weighted images (T1W) and

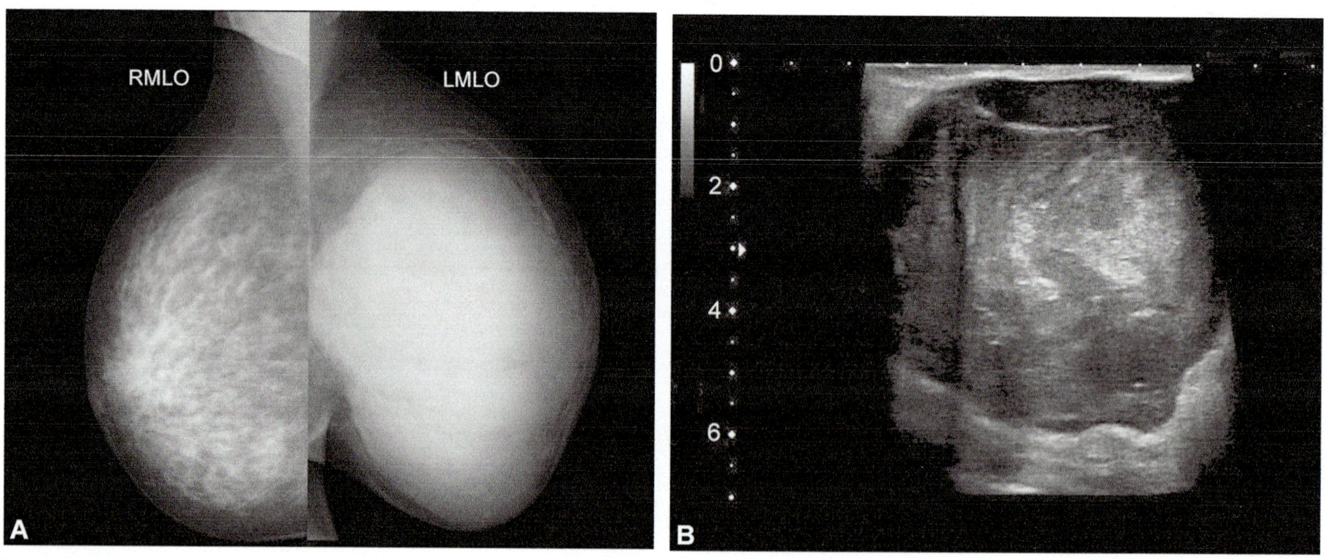

Figs. 1A and B: (A) Mammogram of left breast—MLO view in a 46-year-old female who presented with a rapidly growing mass showing a large mass occupying almost the whole of left breast; (B) Ultrasound showed a large heterogeneously hypoechoic mass with some lobulations. Histopathology was s/o benign phyllodes tumor (MLO: mediolateral oblique).

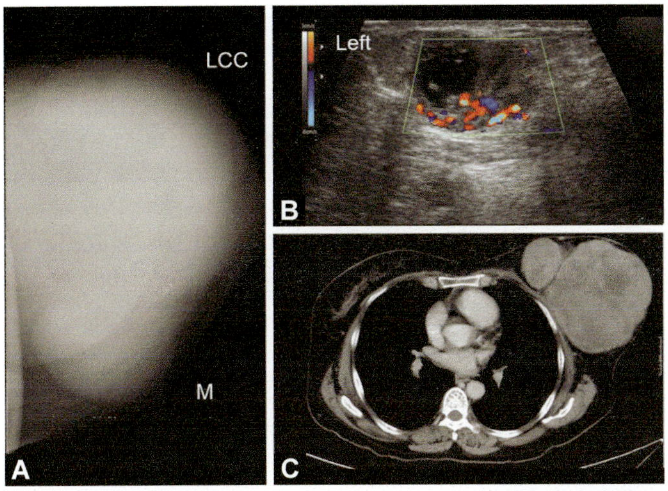

Figs. 2A to C: (A) Mammogram CC view of left breast in a 41-year-old woman shows a large mass with foci of macrocalcification; (B) Ultrasound shows a heterogeneous mass with increased vascularity and cystic areas within which is confirmed on (C) Contrast-enhanced CT scan; Histopathology confirmed the diagnosis of malignant phyllodes tumor with epithelioid leiomyosarcomatous differentiation. (CC: craniocaudal).

hyperintense on T2 weighted (T2W) and Short tau inversion recovery (STIR) images. They have circumscribed margins and enhanced heterogeneously. Malignant tumor shows a low ADC (Apparent deficient co-efficient) due to stromal hypercellularity.

DIFFERENTIAL DIAGNOSIS

The differential diagnosis of phyllodes tumor includes giant fibroadenoma, sarcoma, hamartoma, juvenile papillomatosis and large intraductal carcinomas with necrosis.

A giant fibroadenoma is a term used to describe a fibroadenoma measuring >5 cm in size and has similar imaging findings as phyllodes tumor on mammogram, ultrasound and MRI where non-enhancing internal septations are seen on T2W. It is often difficult to distinguish between phyllodes tumor and fibroadenoma on imaging and histopathology is required for confirmation. Larger lesions >4 cm should be excised as biopsy may not be representative.

Breast hamartoma (also known as a fibroadenolipoma) is composed of fat, fibrous and glandular tissue and imaging appearance depends upon the amount of each component and may cause a dilemma. These are seen as well-circumscribed, round-to-oval heterogeneous mass comprising both fat and soft-tissue densities (both radiolucent and radiodense components) with a thin capsule leading to a "breast within a breast" appearance.

Large malignant tumors with a large necrotic component also cause a diagnostic dilemma and should be considered in the differential diagnosis.

MANAGEMENT

The management of phyllodes tumor ranges from wide local excision for small tumors to simple mastectomy for large tumors. Both benign and malignant phyllodes tumors have a tendency to recur if not widely excised.

CONCLUSION

Large to moderately sized well-defined breast mass without microcalcifications, architectural distortion or lymphadenopathy on mammography is highly suggestive of phyllodes tumor.

Ultrasound shows heterogeneously hypoechoic mass with or without a cystic component that is confirmed on CT and MRI. Imaging cannot reliably distinguish between benign and malignant phyllodes.

REFERENCES

1. Salvadori B, Cusumano F, Del Bo R, et al. Surgical treatment of phyllodes tumors of the breast. Cancer 1989;63:2532-6.
2. Reinfuss M, Mitus J, Duda K, et al. The treatment and prognosis of patients with phyllodes tumor of the breast: an analysis of 170 cases. Cancer 1996;77:910-6.
3. Grabowski J, Salzsrein SL, Sadler GR, Blair SL. Malignant phyllodes tumors: a review of 752 cases. Am Surg 2007;73:967-9.

10.3 Lobular Carcinoma

INTRODUCTION

Invasive lobular cancer is the second most common cancer and a diagnostic challenge, because it is not easily seen on mammogram with a false negative rate ranging from 14 to 43%.[1]

It has a greater incidence of multifocal, multicentric and bilateral distribution; hence, imaging plays an important role in its diagnosis and management.

The term lobular was first coined by Foote and Stewart, in 1946, following their classic work on lobular carcinoma in situ in 1941.[2] They characterized it as small cells with round nuclei, void of tubule formation, invading the stroma and the ducts in a single file without destroying the surrounding architecture. Lobular cancers can be differentiated from ductal cancers by their unique architecture, cytology and immunohistochemistry.[3]

CLINICAL FEATURES

ILCs are difficult to diagnose because they do not form a discrete mass. They diffusely invade the normal tissue without destroying the anatomic structure or producing any desmoplastic reaction. Once they become clinically palpable, the size of the mass is larger with more advanced stage compared to IDC.[4]

IMAGING FEATURES

The higher false negative rate for the detection of ILC is attributed to its lack of desmoplastic reaction. A small percentage of palpable ILC can also be mammographically occult.[5] The mammographic sensitivity for the detection of ILC varies from 98% in women with fatty breasts to 30% in women with dense breasts.[6]

ILCs are seen on mammograms as spiculated (or stellate) or ill-defined masses, areas of architectural distortion and asymmetric densities (Figs. 1 and 2).[7] According to Tabar and Dean, the classic appearance of ILC is (1) spiculated mass that is seen as dense lines or spicules radiating from the mass (Fig. 3) and the length of the spicules

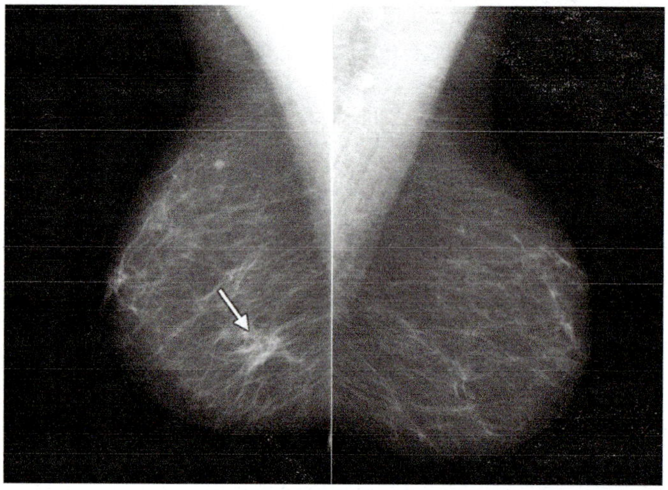

Fig. 1: Mammogram showing asymmetric density in MLO view of right breast which turned out to be an invasive lobular carcinoma on histopathology (MLO: mediolateral oblique).

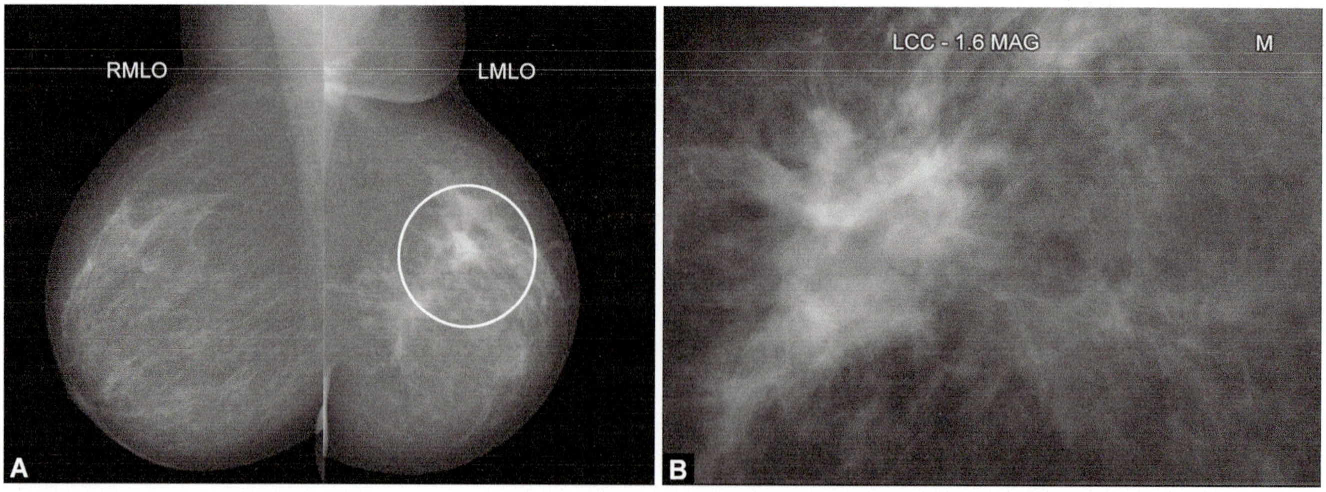

Figs. 2A and B: Asymmetric density and architectural distortion noted in MLO view and magnification view of left breast which on histopathology was s/o invasive lobular carcinoma.

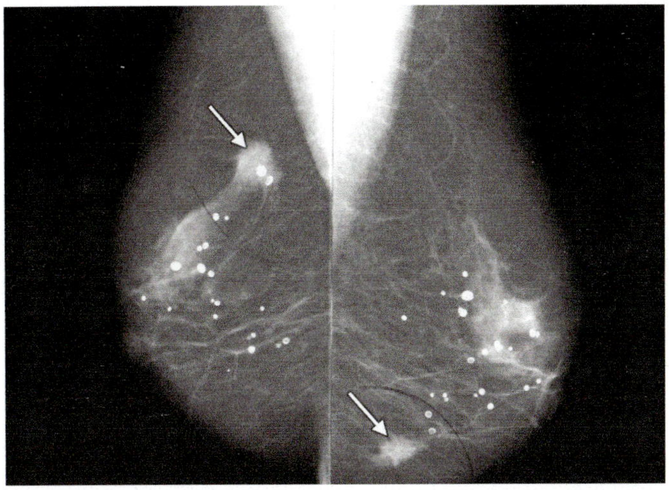

Fig. 3: Mammogram MLO view of both the breasts showing spiculated mass in upper quadrant of right breast and in lower quadrant of left breast. There are multiple diffuse benign calcifications also. Histopathology was s/o bilateral invasive lobular carcinoma. (MLO: mediolateral oblique).

increasing with the size of the lesion in the absence of a definite central mass. Skin retraction may be present. This was called a "white star" appearance in contrast to "black star" appearance of radial scar. Since these differences in appearances can be easily misinterpreted on mammograms, further assessment with focal magnification view and core biopsy is recommended. The spicules are because of pulling of Cooper ligaments toward the lesion, while absence of central mass is attributed to lack of desmoplastic reaction. (2) Another finding seen on mammogram is **architectural distortion** that is because of tissue's tethering. There is distortion of the parenchymal contour and absence of definite mass. (3) **Asymmetric density** is increase in density in one breast as compared to the same area in the contralateral breast.

The other causes of asymmetric density are: focal fibrosis, scar tissue, asymmetric involution or increase in fibroglandular growth because of hormonal activity. Asymmetric densities associated with ILC present as a subtle area of distortion and further assessment is required by focal compression views and mediolateral (ML) views.

Because of these subtle features, ILC is the most challenging abnormality to detect on mammograms. Additional mammographic views with focal compression and ML view may resolve the abnormality. However, focal compression may displace subtle distortions; this may be resolved by additional "rolled view" or by repeating the craniocaudal (CC) or ML oblique (MLO) views.

ILC is rarely associated with microcalcification or circumscribed masses. Microcalcifications in ILC have been associated with the presence of other variants such as pleomorphic lobular carcinoma in situ and other tumors such as ductal carcinoma in situ (DCIS) and IDC.[8]

ILCs tend to have a different appearance in different mammographic views. This phenomenon is also observed in radial scar lesions and in small breast cancers that may give rise to a benign diagnosis. In comparison, IDC have consistent appearance on both CC and MLO views. Many authors have concluded that ILC is better visualized on CC view than on MLO view because of better breast compression. On CC view, it is seen as a spiculated mass in contrast to architectural distortion or subtle density on MLO view.[9]

DIFFERENTIAL DIAGNOSIS

Mammogram

Mammographic features of ILC may mimic other benign or malignant lesions. Differential diagnosis includes:

- Summation artifact caused by overlapping of breast anatomy
- Fat necrosis due to previous breast surgery, trauma or infection
- Radial scars, sclerosing adenosis
- Other malignant lesions, for example, IDC, DCIS

A good clinical history will help exclude previous breast surgery, trauma or infection. Focal compression and ML views may help one to prove summation artefact by dispersing the overlapping tissue. The appearances of radial scars and sclerosing adenosis are difficult to differentiate from primary cancer; therefore, further assessment with core biopsy and detailed histological analysis is necessary.

Ultrasound

On ultrasound, it is commonly seen as an irregular, ill-defined hypoechoic mass with or without posterior acoustic shadowing. Ultrasound has the advantage of detecting any additional focal masses in the ipsilateral breast that may be occult on mammography.

Magnetic Resonance Imaging

On MRI, it is commonly seen as a spiculated or irregular mass. MRI is useful to look for multifocal or multicentric masses in the same breast or contralateral cancers.

These additional findings affect surgical management and help in deciding between breast conserving surgery and mastectomy.

Lehman et al.[10] recommend that any suspicious lesions detected by MRI should have "second-look" ultrasound and histopathological evaluation to decide appropriate surgical management.

MRI-guided biopsy is a useful tool but not widely available; therefore, mammography and ultrasound remain the principle biopsy methods.

Ultrasound and MRI may be the preferred imaging methods for cancers located deep in the breast and in the axilla, the areas that are not shown on mammography and may be helpful in assessing equivocal mammographic features.

CONCLUSION

The increase in the incidence of ILC is worrisome due to the difficulty in diagnosis with mammography; therefore, knowledge of its many radiographic features is very important. "To take full advantage of the capabilities of mammography, radiologists must search diligently not only for the typical features of malignancy but especially for the more subtle and indirect signs."

Familiarity with the multimodality imaging appearance and its underlying pathology can impact management of this subtle-yet-significant finding.

REFERENCES

1. Kim SH, Cha ES, Park CS, et al. Imaging features of invasive lobular carcinoma: comparison with invasive ductal carcinoma. Jpn J Radiol 2011;29(7):475-82.
2. Singhai R, Patil VW, Jaiswal SR, et al. E-Cadherin as a diagnostic biomarker in breast cancer. N Am J Med 2011;3(5):227-33.
3. Weigelt B, Geyer FC, Reis-Filho JS. Histological types of breast cancer: how special are they?. Mol Oncol 2010;4(3):192-208.
4. Arpino G, Bardou VJ, Clark GM, Elledge RM. Infiltrating lobular carcinoma of the breast: tumor characteristics and clinical outcome. Breast Cancer Res 2004;6(3):149-56.
5. Porter AJ, Evans EB, Foxcroft LM, Simpson PT, Lakhani SR. Mammographic and ultrasound features of invasive lobular carcinoma of the breast. J Med Imaging Radiat Oncol 2014;58(1):1-10.
6. Berg WA, Gutierrez L, Ness Aiver MS, et al. Diagnostic accuracy of mammography, clinical examination, US and MR imaging in preoperative assessment of breast cancer. Radiology 2004;233(3):830-49.
7. Lopez JK, Bassett LW. Invasive lobular carcinoma of the breast: spectrum of mammographic, US and MR imaging findings. Radiographics 2009;29(1):165-76.
8. Carder PJ, Shabaan A, Alizadeh Y, et al. Screen-detected pleomorphic lobular carcinoma in situ (PLCIS): risk of concurrent invasive malignancy following a core biopsy diagnosis. Histopathology 2010;57(3):472-8.
9. Garnett S, Wallis M, Morgan G. Do screen-detected lobular and ductal carcinoma present with different mammographic features?. BJR 2009;82(973):20-7.
10. Lehman CD, Gatsonis C, Kuhl CK, et al, MRI evaluation of the contralateral breast in women with recently diagnosed breast cancer. N Engl J Med 2007;356(13):1295-303.

10.4 Metaplastic Carcinoma

INTRODUCTION

Metaplastic breast cancer (MBC) is an uncommon invasive breast cancer having aggressive clinical presentation and a variety of distinct histologic types.

It accounts for <1% of all breast cancers.[1,2] This includes tumors in which adenocarcinoma is found to coexist with spindle cell, squamous, chondroid or bone-forming neoplastic cells.[3] Most metaplastic cancers are estrogen receptor (ER), progesterone receptor (PR) and Her2-*neu* negative.[4-6]

CLINICAL FEATURES

The age at presentation ranges from 48 to 59 years. It commonly presents as a rapidly growing mass and is larger than typical breast cancers. Axillary lymph nodal involvement is less frequent than standard invasive breast cancer.

IMAGING FEATURES

Mammography: Though there are varied appearances on mammogram that includes high-density masses with circumscribed, obscured (Fig. 1A), irregular and/or spiculated margins, it is seen commonly as a circumscribed round or oval mass resembling a fibroadenoma. The lesions are mostly non-calcified and whenever calcifications are present, they are of amorphous, coarse, punctate or pleomorphic types.

Ultrasound: It shows heterogeneous or hypoechoic solid mass or a mixed cystic and solid mass[7-9] often with posterior acoustic enhancement (Fig. 1B). The complex cystic nature is consistent with cystic degeneration and necrosis found on pathology specimen.

MRI: The lesion is irregular and shows intermediate to high signal on T2W sequence and isointense to hypointense signal on T1W imaging.

The incidence of stages III and IV disease at presentation is higher than IDC with an increased risk of local recurrence. It responds poorly to systemic chemotherapy. It has a larger tumor size at presentation, lower rates of axillary nodal involvement, higher rates of local

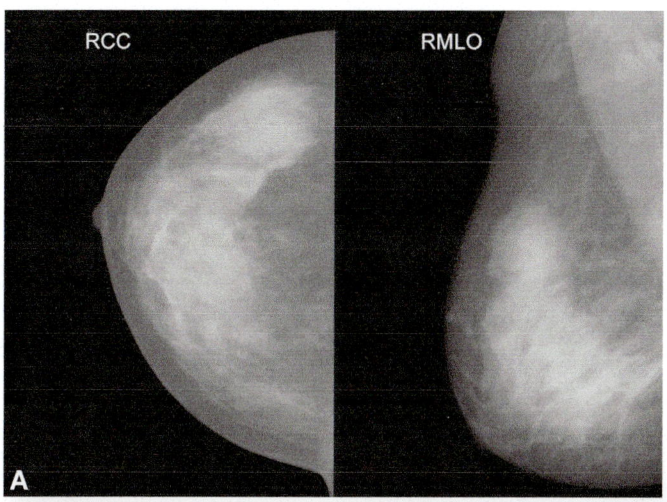

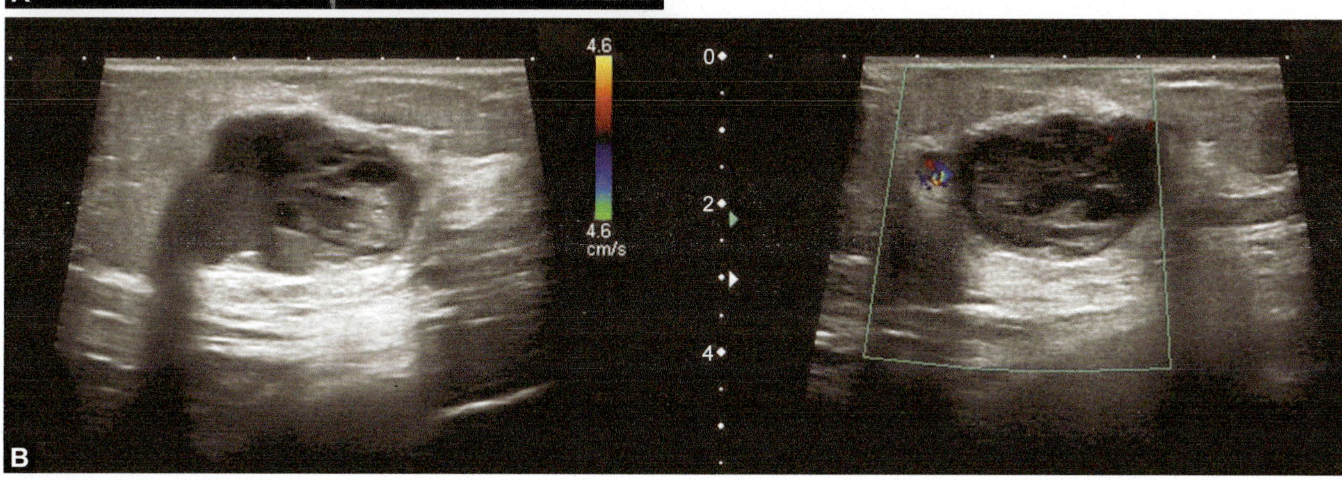

Figs. 1A and B: A 40-year-old woman presented with a palpable, non-tender right breast lump for one month. (A) Diagnostic mammogram of right breast with MLO and CC views shows a circumscribed mass with partially obscured margins in upper outer quadrant of right breast; (B) Ultrasound shows a complex cystic mass with posterior acoustic enhancement. Histopathology was s/o metaplastic carcinoma (MLO: mediolateral oblique, CC: craniocaudal).

reccurence and distant metastases, higher rates of ER, PR and Her2 negativity as well as a suboptimal response to systemic therapies when compared to other invasive breast cancers.

REFERENCES

1. Luini A, Aguilar M, Gatti G, et al. Metaplastic carcinoma of the breast, an unusual disease with worse prognosis: the experience of the European Institute of Oncology and review of the literature. Breast Cancer Res Treat 2007;101:349-53.
2. Tavassoli FA. Classification of metaplastic carcinomas of the breast. Pathol Annu 1992;27(Pt 2):89-119.
3. Rayson D, Adjei AA, Suman VJ, Wold LE, Ingle JN. Metaplastic breast cancer: prognosis and response to systemic therapy. Ann Oncol 1999;10(4):413-9.
4. Weigelt B, Kreike B, Reis-Filho JA. Metaplastic breast carcinomas are basal-like breast cancers: a genomic profiling analysis. Breast Cancer Res Treat 2009;117:273-80.
5. Tse GM, Tan PH, Putti TC, et al. Metaplastic carcinoma of the breast: a clinicopathological review. J Clin Pathol 2006;59:1079-83.
6. Al Sayed AD, El Weshi AN, Tulbah AM, et al. Metaplastic carcinoma of the breast clinical presentation, treatment results and prognostic factors. Acta Oncol 2006;45:188-95.
7. Yang WT, Hennessy B, Broglio K, et al. Imaging differences in metaplastic and invasive ductal carcinomas of the breast. Am J Roentgenol 2007;189:1288-92.
8. Shin HJ, Kim HH, Kim SM, et al. Imaging of metaplastic carcinoma with chondroid differentiation of the breast. Am J Roentgenol 2007;188:691-6.
9. Park JM, Han BK, Moon WK, et al. Metaplastic carcinoma of the breast: mammographic and sonographic findings. J Clin Ultrasound 2000;28:179-86.

10.5 Lymphoma

Primary lymphoma of breast is an uncommon disease accounting for 0.4–0.5% of breast cancers. In primary breast lymphoma, there is a malignant mass in breast with no evidence of lymphoma elsewhere in body except in regional lymph nodes draining the breast.

The median age of patients ranges from 60 to 65 years.[1] Bilateral breast involvement is seen in 11% of all primary breast lymphomas.[2] A single nodule is seen in 70% of cases of primary lymphoma, while multiple nodules can be seen in 9% cases. More than 80% of PBL (primary breast lymphoma) are B-cell lymphomas, mostly CD20+ with diffuse large B-cell lymphoma (DLBCL) as the most common histological diagnosis.

Non-Hodgkin lymphomas (NHL) are highly cellular lesions with no desmoplastic reaction. The NHL cells proliferate actively around the ducts and lobules. The prognosis for primary lymphoma is better than secondary lymphoma with 40–50% disease-free interval 4 years after local resection and radiotherapy.

IMAGING FINDINGS

Mammography: Findings are non-specific and may show circumscribed or partially circumscribed non-calcified mass. The mass is often quite large and may sometimes show microlobulations. There may be increased breast density with skin thickening with or without an underlying mass. This is because of inflammatory edema and lymphedema due to lymphatic obstruction. Bilateral axillary lymph nodes may be present (Figs. 1A and B).

Ultrasound: In patients with secondary breast involvement, there is bilateral axillary lymph node enlargement (Fig. 1C). In some cases of primary breast lymphoma, the mass may not be a lymph node or may represent a distorted lymph node. Many of these lymphomatous nodules are circumscribed and have a thin echogenic capsule. As they enlarge there is peritumoral inflammatory edema and a thick echogenic halo. They may be multilobulated with posterior acoustic enhancement. Some of the lymphomas can appear almost anechoic giving rise to a pseudocystic appearance. It is important to remember that ultrasound appearance is nonspecific and similar to any cellular lesion with very little desmoplastic reaction. They are usually hyper vascular on Doppler examination.

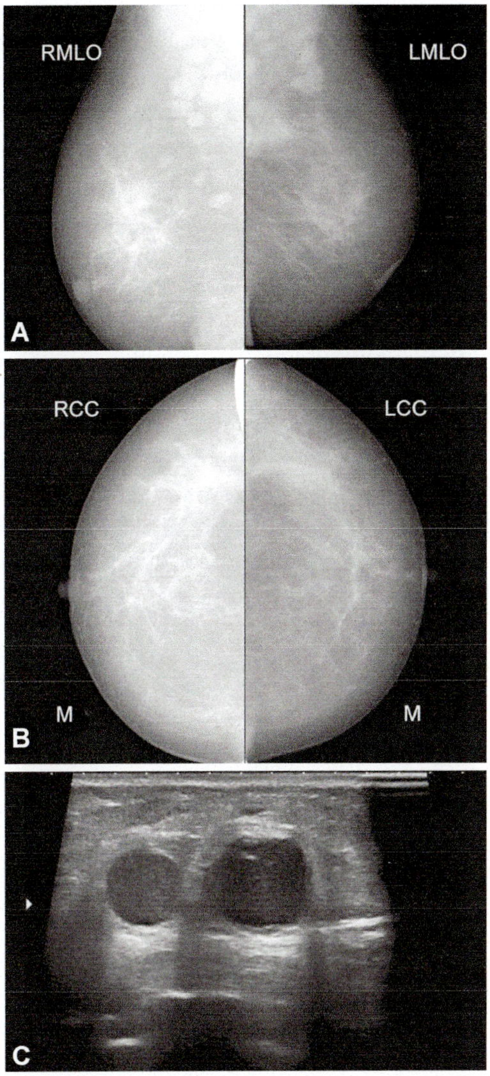

Figs. 1A to C: A 52-year-old female presented with lumps in left breast. She also had cervical and axillary lymphadenopathy. (A) Mammogram of both breasts MLO view shows multiple axillary lymph nodes on both the sides extending till the axillary tail on left; (B) CC views of both breast were normal; (C) Biopsy from axillary lymph nodes on both sides was s/o Non-Hodgkin's lymphoma (follicular type). The lymph node from axillary tail region was also s/o NHL. Specimen from breast showed extensively infarcted lymphomatous infiltration with adjacent fat necrosis (MLO: mediolateral oblique; NHL: non-hodgkins lymphomas).

REFERENCES

1. Jeanneret-Sozzi W, Taghian A, Epelbaum R, et al. Primary breast lymphoma: patient profile, outcome and prognostic factors. A multicentre Rare Cancer Network study. BMC Cancer 2008;8:86.
2. Ganjoo K, Advani R, Mariappan MR, McMillan A, Horning S. Non-hodgkin lymphoma of the breast. Cancer 2007;110:25-30.

10.6 Angiosarcoma

Angiosarcoma is a rare (0.4%) soft-tissue tumor of the breast that occurs in both a primary form[1] without a known precursor and a secondary form that has been associated with a history of irradiated breast tissue. With the increasing use of breast conservation therapy for breast cancer, postirradiation angiosarcoma has increased. Both primary and secondary angiosarcomas may present with bruise-like skin discoloration, which may delay the diagnosis.

Primary angiosarcoma tends to occur in younger women in third to fourth decades, while secondary forms occur in elderly women[2] in sixth decade.

The tumors tend to be usually cutaneous or subcutaneous in location. Radiologic findings are often non-specific and may appear completely normal in one-third of cases with primary angiosarcoma. They often appear as irregular masses on mammograms. Differential diagnosis of this rare tumor includes benign hemangioma, phyllodes sarcoma, stromal sarcoma, metaplastic carcinoma, fibrosarcoma and liposarcoma.

The prognosis is usually poor because of the high rates of local recurrence and early development of metastasis. Surgery is the principal mode of treatment for primary angiosarcoma of the breast and generally consists of a total mastectomy. The prognosis for patients with primary angiosarcoma depends on the tumor grade. Metastases to the contralateral breast also have been reported.[3]

REFERENCES

1. Yang WT, Hennessy BT, Dryden MJ, Valero V, Hunt KK, Krishnamurthy S. Mammary angiosarcomas: imaging findings in 24 patients. Radiology 2007; 242:725-34.
2. Brenn T, Fletcher CD. Postradiation vascular proliferations: an increasing problem. Histopathology 2006; 48: 106-14
3. Donnell RM, Rosen PP, Lieberman PH, et al. Angiosarcoma and other vascular tumors of the breast. Am J Surg Pathol 1981;5:629-42.

10.7 Pseudoangiomatous Stromal Hyperplasia

Pseudoangiomatous stromal hyperplasia (PASH) is the benign myofibroblastic proliferation of stromal cells.[1] It is a common incidental finding on breast biopsies. It is seen in premenopausal and perimenopausal women.

Etiology is incompletely elucidated, but hormonal influence has been demonstrated. Microscopically, PASH consists of a network of slit-like spaces lined by myofibroblasts that resemble vascular spaces. The intervening stroma consists of collagen.

These lesions are progesterone receptor-positive and demonstrate similar features to intralobular stroma (versus interlobular stroma, which is not hormonally sensitive) during the luteal phase of the menstrual cycle.

It presents clinically as a large, circumscribed palpable mass. On mammography, it is seen as a circumscribed or partly circumscribed mass typically lacking calcification. It can be mammographically occult also. Ultrasound shows a heterogeneously hypoechoic mass resembling a fibroadenoma. Contrast-enhanced MRI may show clumped non-mass-like regions of persistent enhancement.

REFERENCE

1. Bowman E, Oprea G, Okoli J, Gundry K, Rizzo M, Gabram-Mendola S et al: Pseudoangiomatous stromal hyperplasia (PASH) of the breast: a series of 24 patients.Send to Breast J. 2012 May-Jun;18(3):242-7. doi: 10.1111/j.1524-4741.2012.01230.x2.
2. SS Jaunoo, S Thrush, P Dunn: Pseudoangiomatous stromal hyperplasia (PASH): A brief review; International Journal of Surgery Volume 9, Issue 1, 2011, Pages 20-22

10.8 Mondor Disease

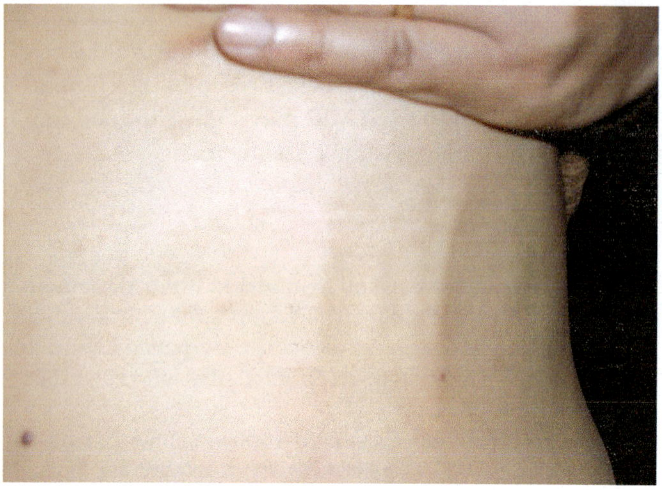

Figs. 1: A middle-aged woman presented with pain and tenderness in the inframammary region on left side. Prominent linear cord-like structure with erythema was seen s/o Mondor disease that is a rare condition due to thrombophlebitis of the superficial veins of the breast.

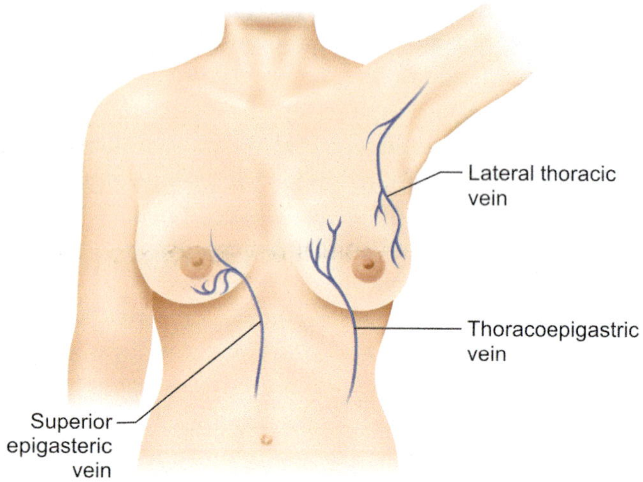

Fig. 2: Thoracoepigastric and/or lateral thoracic veins involved in Modor disease.

Mondor disease is a rare benign breast condition characterized by thrombophlebitis of the subcutaneous veins of the breast and anterior chest wall (Fig. 1). The patient may present clinically with a painful cord-like mass in breast with overlying skin erythema. It most commonly affects the thoracoepigastric and/or lateral thoracic veins towards the upper outer quadrant (Fig. 2).

IMAGING

Mammography may be normal or may show a superficial, dilated, tubular density corresponding to the mass. On ultrasound, a tubular anechoic or isoechoic structure with multiple areas of narrowing is noted giving a beaded appearance suggestive of a thrombosed a superficial vein. Low-level internal echoes within denote the thrombus. No color flow is seen on Doppler examination. It is a benign self-limiting condition with recanalization of thrombosed vein resolving the clinical symptoms. Mondor disease[1] is a rare entity and usually limits itself in a few weeks. It is hard to establish its real prevalence due to this self-limiting condition. Etiology is usually trauma or idiopathic.

REFERENCE

1. Huseyin Kadioglu,* Şeyma Yildiz, Yeliz Emine Ersoy, Serap Yücel and Mahmut Müslümanoğlu: An unusual case caused by a common reason: Mondor's disease by oral contraceptives: Int J Surg Case Rep. 2013; 4(10): 855-857.

Breast Cancer Screening

CHAPTER 11

INTRODUCTION

Breast cancer is the commonest cancer in women and leading cause of death among women all over the world, both in developed and developing countries.[1] A screening test is carried out in the asymptomatic population with an intention of detecting early disease, ideally, at such a stage that it can improve treatment outcome and reduce mortality. It should have a low false-negative rate so that early cancers are not missed and have a low false-positive rate so that the patient is not subjected to un-necessary investigations and treatment. The test should be inexpensive, available for large segments of populations and reproducible. Randomized controlled trials (RCTs) have demonstrated that screening mammography in women 40–74 years of age decreases deaths from breast cancer.

BREAST CANCER IN INDIA

In India, breast cancer is rapidly increasing, especially in the urban population. If detected early, it is treatable. However,

It is unfortunate that even today, the lack of awareness about the disease and the social stigma attached to it avert patients from consulting doctors while still in the early stage, leading to late diagnosis and increase in cancer-related suffering and death. The **GLOBOCAN Project 2012** that provided contemporary estimates of the incidence, prevalence and mortality of major cancers in 184 countries revealed some startling data: about 1.4 lakh new cases of breast cancer are diagnosed each year in India with a 50% mortality rate, that is, approximately 70,000 women—or 1 in every 2 patients—die due to the disease. In contrast, of the 2.4 lakh new cases detected each year in USA, approximately 43,000 prove fatal, which is 1 in 6 cases. It is worth noting that there is no organized breast cancer screening program in India and we have a disproportionately higher mortality rate of breast cancer compared to those in the developed world. Hence, there is a need for culturally appropriate breast cancer education and intervention strategies. It is time we look at the feasibility of breast screening in India and decide what kind of breast screening India can afford and is ready for. It has been said that for a low-resource country like India, implementation of mammography for screening is challenging as it requires extensive resources and quality control; hence, low cost alternatives like clinical breast examination (CBE) or breast self-examination should be explored on a larger basis.

Breast Cancer Screening in India

The government of India in 2016 has made it mandatory for screening for oral cancer, breast cancer and cancer of cervix for above 30 years of age and has identified 100 districts to begin with.

In addition, there are already opportunistic screening, institution-based screening and mobile outreach programs in various parts of the country which have been running for some time now. As the level of awareness amongst the people increases, the number of such programmes will also increase.

The Women's Cancer Initiative had launched its first mobile screening van in partnership with Department Of Preventive Oncology, Tata Memorial Hospital, Mumbai for early detection of breast, cervix and oral cancer in 2009. In this program, free screening was offered to women from lower socioeconomic status in regions within and around Mumbai.

Asha Jyoti: Women's healthcare mobile outreach program launched the first mobile unit in Chandigarh to work with marginalized women in 2013. The school of public health in post-graduate institute of medical research had helped in providing community education and sensitized women with the idea of screening tests, provided education about the signs and symptoms of breast cancer, cervical cancer and osteoporosis before the program was launched.

Breast cancer screening drive was launched in Pune in 2016 by Tata Trust and Prashanthi Mission in association with Swasth India which aims to target 2.3 lakh women in

Pune. It has state-of-the-art mobile vans equipped with mammography units and colposcopy equipment to detect early breast cancer and cancer of cervix.

So, one can see that there are positive steps taken both by the government and private organizations to detect early breast cancers.

STATUS OF BREAST CANCER SCREENING AROUND THE WORLD

Mammography has been used for detecting early breast cancer in many countries all over the world for a long time and is found to decrease mortality.[2,3] There are different recommendations used in different countries, especially with regard to age and the frequency of screening.

United Kingdom: National Health Service Breast Screening Program (NHS BSP)

This program was introduced in 1988, for 50–64-year olds, following the recommendations of the Forrest Committee.

The program was set up using the Swedish Two-County Study RCT as the performance yardstick. In the initial years, recommendation was single-view mammography and single read. Two-view mammography was introduced for screening as a policy in 1995. This led to higher cancer detection rate both in situ cancer and small invasive cancers (<10 mm).

The age for screening was extended from 64 to 70 years in 2000.

By the year 2005, two-view mammography had started and almost 1.3 million women from the age group of 50–70 years were screened. A total of 75% of these women were invited. By using two-view mammography, the cancer detection rate increased by 25%.

Present Status

The NHS breast screening program conducts screening for women between 50 and 70 years every 3 years by invitation. It is mandatory to be registered with general practitioner (GP) to receive the invitations. At present, the age range is extended from 47 to 73 years.

Interval cancers: A significant number of interval cancers appear in the second/third year of screening. These led to interval cancer meets where units were expected to look at interval cancers and classify them. This evaluation caused an increased workload leading to a shortage of radiologists and led to introduction of radiographer-led film reading, ultrasound and biopsies. The concept of assistant practitioners was also introduced to perform mammography and read mammography films.

The NHS breast screening program was started in 1988. Its benefits so far have been that breast cancer is detected at early stage, mastectomy rates have come down and a large number of these women receive chemotherapy and hormonal therapy.

Now, the NHS is providing an option of informed choice to these women by way of information booklets which discuss both the limitation and importance of breast screening. It's a robust program which is improving both technically and clinically day by day.

Breast Cancer Screening in USA

The American Cancer Society laid down the guidelines for screening. Later on, U.S. Preventive Services Task Force (USPSTF), an independent government agency, brought some changes in its policy in 2009. It emphasizes on a more personalized screening system with an opportunity for women to discuss the potential benefits and risks of screening mammography with clinicians before going ahead with it.

Current Recommendations of American Cancer Society and USPSTF

The various categories are divided based on age and risk category.

Women aged 40–49 with average risk:

- **American Cancer Society (2015):**
  - Women aged 40–44 years should have the choice to start annual breast cancer screening with mammogram if they wish to do so. The risks of screening as well as the potential benefits should be considered
  - Women aged 45–49 years should get mammogram every year
- **US Preventive Services Task Force:**
  - The decision to start screening mammography in women prior to age 50 years should be an individual one. Women who place a higher value on the potential benefit than the potential harms may choose to begin biennial screening between the ages of 40 and 49 years

Women aged 50–74 with average risk:

- **American Cancer Society (2015):**
  - Women aged 50–54 years should get mammogram every year

- Women aged 55 years and older should switch to mammogram every 2 years or have the choice to continue yearly screening
- **U.S. Preventive Services Task Force (USPSTF) recommendations(2016):**
  - Biennial screening mammography is recommended.

Women aged 75 or older with average risk:

- **American Cancer Society:**
  - Screening should continue as long as a woman is in good health and is expected to live 10 years more or longer
- **USPSTF:**
  - Current evidence is insufficient to assess the balance of benefits and harms of screening mammography in women aged 75 years or older

Women with dense breasts:

- **American Cancer Society:**
  - There is not enough evidence to make a recommendation for or against yearly magnetic resonance imaging (MRI) screening
- **USPSTF:**
  - Current evidence is insufficient to assess the balance of benefits and harms of adjunctive screening for breast cancer using breast ultrasonography, MRI, digital breast tomosynthesis (DBT) or other methods in women identified to have dense breasts on an otherwise negative screening mammogram

Women at higher than average risk:

- **American Cancer Society:**
  - Women who are at high risk for breast cancer based on certain factors (such as having a parent, sibling or child with a BRCA 1 or BRCA2 gene mutation) should get an MRI and a mammogram every year
- **USPSTF:**
  - Women with a parent, sibling or child with breast cancer are at higher risk for breast cancer and thus may benefit more than average-risk women from beginning screening in their 40s

Breast Cancer Screening Program in European Union

Breast cancer prevention is a major public health goal in the European Union and therefore breast cancer screening programs are in place in nearly all European Union countries. These had started as sporadic or opportunistic screening programs covering different sections of population with a goal for nationwide coverage. There were considerable differences in target population coverage, age at which screening started and in the techniques deployed.[4]

Western Europe has the highest incidence of breast cancer in the world.[5]

Breast cancer screening was first started in Sweden but had a lot of variability. In women from 50 to 74 years age group, mammogram was done once in 2 years. In almost 60% of the country women from 40 to 49 years were invited for mammogram once in 18 months.

Austria was the first European Union Member State to implement a breast cancer screening program with opportunistic screening in 1974. Mammography was offered to all women >40 years old[6] and nationwide screening began as recent as 2007. The last member state to begin screening is Bulgaria which started screening in 2011. Clinical breast examination is an integral part of first-level screening in French screening program.[7]

In 2003 the European Commission recommended population-based screening for women aged 50–69 years; in 2007 programs based on council indications were active or were being organized in 22 states. Most of the countries in the European Union now have a nation-wide, population-based screening program based on mammography (film screen and/or digital mammography) as per data given in 2014.

Breast Cancer Screening in Australia

In Australia, the screening program is called "Breast screen Australia," in which women between 50 and 74 years of age are invited every 2 years. Once the patients complete their treatment, they are advised to have follow-up mammogram annually. Some states permit the return of these women to the regular screening program 5 years after their diagnosis while other states don't.

Singapore Breast Screening Program

The Singapore national breast screening program, Breast Screen Singapore (BSS), was set up in 2002 under the Health Promotion Board (HPB) to raise public awareness, encourage early detection of breast cancer and reduce mortality. It is the only publicly funded national breast screening program in Asia. It enrolls women aged 50–64 for screening every 2 years. Screening can be done at the hospital and polyclinics under BSS. BSS hotlines help women book appointments for screening mammogram. HPB subsidizes the cost of the mammogram under HPB's Screen for Life program.

After the mammogram is done on the screening date, the result's letter is received within 3–4 weeks; there is no medical report or X-ray films provided as the reading results are recorded in the BSS system.

If the results are normal, monthly breast self-examination and regular screening once every 2 years is recommended.

If the results are abnormal or show changes, result letters with instructions to book an appointment at the recommended hospital assessment center are sent and further evaluations, such as additional mammograms, ultrasounds, tomosynthesis (3D mammography) and needle biopsies, may be performed on the assessment day.

The Singapore Cancer Society (SCS), which officially opened its mammogram facility in 2015, will pay for the screening fee for an initial period of 3 years, after which it will be reviewed to see if it should be extended.

Breast Cancer Screening in China

Chinese Ministry of Health along with Chinese Anti-Cancer Association (CACA) is leading a screening program since 2009 combining CBE, mammography and ultrasound and recruiting women in the age group of 35–69 years.

If there are positive findings on ultrasound, a mammogram and biopsy are done.

Once this initial 3-year program was completed, another program was launched in 2012 which was the second-generation screening program in which the age of women was modified.

Breast Cancer Screening in Middle East Countries

Kuwait

It has a nation-wide organized breast screening program launched in 2014 and provides high-quality breast screening services for target women aged 40–69 years. It issues recall notices for screening by SMSs and notifies women of their screening results. It facilitates those women with abnormal screens to move through the diagnostic tests and arrange any additional imaging or tissue diagnosis.

Qatar

Their breast cancer screening program was launched in 2016 and is currently offered by Primary Health-Care Corporation (PHCC). It is recommended that women begin regular breast cancer screening from the age of 45 till 69 once in 3 years. Eligible patients register is provided by Ministry of Healthcare Qatar and invitation system is based on screening call center. Cases for further investigation are evaluated under umbrella of Hamad Medical Corporation (HMC).

CONCLUSION

In conclusion, we can see that almost all the countries are running breast screening programs for early detection of breast cancer. Though there are a lot of controversies about the need for breast cancer screening using mammography, it has been effective in detecting early breast cancer.

As the incidence of breast cancer is increasing in developing countries, some form of breast cancer screening is required. This can be in the form of breast self-examination, CBE or mammographic screening which can be institution based. This would depend upon the resources available.

It is important for women to be breast aware and told the importance of early detection of breast cancer in which media can play an important role.

REFERENCES

1. Forbes JF. The incidence of breast cancer: the global burden, public health considerations. Semin Oncol 1997;24(Suppl 1): S1-20-35.
2. Swedish Organised Service Screening Evaluation Group. Reduction in breast cancer mortality from organized service screening with mammography: 1. Further confirmation with extended data. Cancer Epidemiol Biomarkers Prev 2006;15:45-51.
3. Duffy SW, Tabar L, Chen HH, et al. The impact of organized mammography service screening on breast carcinoma mortality in seven Swedish counties. Cancer 2002;95: 458-69.
4. Altobelli E, Lattanzi A. Breast cancer in European Union: an update of screening programmes as of March 2014 (Review). Int J Oncol 2014;45:1785-92.
5. Ferlay J, Shin HR, Bray F, Forman D, Mathers C, Parkin DM editors. GLOBOCAN 2008: cancer incidence and mortality worldwide. IARC Cancerbase No, 10. International Agency for Research on Cancer, Lyon, 2010.
6. Vutuc C, Waldhoer T, Haidinger G. Breast cancer trends: opportunistic screening in Austria versus controlled screening in Finland and Sweden. Eur J Cancer Prev 2006;15:343-6.
7. International Cancer Screening Network. Breast cancer screening programs in 26 ICSN countries, 2012: organization, policies and program reach. Atlanta: International Cancer Screening Network. http://appliedresearch.cancer.gov/icsn/breast/screening.html [Accessed Nov 23 2013]

Miscellaneous

CHAPTER 12

12.1 Positron Emission Tomography (PET) in Breast Malignancy

INTRODUCTION

Positron emission tomography (PET) is a noninvasive imaging technique by which metabolic or functional assessment is done to differentiate between normal tissue, benign and malignant lesions.

It is more sensitive than conventional nuclear medicine techniques like single positron emission computed tomography (SPECT). PET is usually a whole-body examination. Normal breast tissue shows diffuse low-level physiologic activity. Focal, intense breast activity requires further evaluation.

PET works on the principle that tumor cells in most types of tumors show increased glucose metabolism.

There is a high rate of glycolysis in tumor cells under aerobic conditions. In PET CT, FDG (^{18}F-fluorodeoxyglucose) is used, which is an analog of glucose. Its metabolism is similar to glucose and the tumor cells show increased uptake. PET imaging detects the γ rays from the positron-emitting isotopes.

PET focuses more on the contrast between the normal tissue and tumor, rather than on spatial resolution.

INDICATIONS

The indications of PET in breast cancer are:

- Preoperative staging and metastatic workup to help in treatment planning
- PET is the second best modality in detecting a mammographically and sonographically occult primary tumor, only next to magnetic resonance mammography (MRM). PET is recommended in all patients with axillary lymph node metastasis in which primary tumor could not be localized
- PET can also detect axillary, supraclavicular and infraclavicular lymph-node metastases
- PET helps in identifying intramammary metastases from other primary tumors of thyroid and kidney
- PET helps in evaluating the response of tumor to chemotherapy, radiotherapy and postsurgical recurrence.

Invasive lobular carcinoma is generally less metabolically active than infiltrating ductal carcinoma (IDC) and is less likely to be detected by PET.

Low-grade tumors that do not show tracer uptake are likely to be missed on PET scans. Another disadvantage of PET is that the increased uptake of radiotracer is not limited to tumors but also infectious and inflammatory lesions in proportion to their glucose metabolism.

^{99m}Tc-sestamibi and ^{18}F-fluorodeoxyglucose (FDG) PET have a limitation of a poor resolution; therefore, breast-specific γ imaging (BSGI) and positron emission mammography (PEM) have been developed, which shows a high resolution.

PEM is done on a high-resolution PET scanner with a small field of view and once acquisition is taken after an hour of intravenous injection of ^{18}F-FDG. Primary breast tumors show variable uptake.

SUGGESTED READING

1. Eric L. Rosen,MD, William B. Eubank, MD, David A. Mankoff, MD, PhD: FDG PET, PET/CT and Breast Cancer Imaging;RadioGraphics 2007; 27:S215–S229.
2. Sang Kyu Yang, MD, Nariya Cho, MD and Woo Kyung Moon, MD:The Role of PET/CT for Evaluating Breast Cancer: Korean J Radiol. 2007 Sep-Oct; 8(5): 429–37.

12.2 Breast-specific γ Imaging

INTRODUCTION

In breast-specific γ imaging (BSGI), high-resolution images are obtained with a detector resolution of 3 mm after intravenous administration of either ^{99m}Tc-sestamibi or ^{99m}Tc-tetrofosmin.

MECHANISM

The two main mechanisms that are responsible for increased radiotracer uptake are

- The radiotracers ^{99m}Tc-sestamibi or ^{99m}Tc-tetrofosmin bind predominantly to the mitochondria in cells. The tumor cells are highly proliferative with increased number of mitochondria, hence the increased uptake
- The neoangiogenesis in tumor leads to increased delivery of the radiotracer to the cancerous cells

Since it is a functional technique, density of breast tissue, breast implants and scars from previous surgery are not a hindrance to the image quality in BSGI.

TECHNIQUE

Scintimammography uses a general purpose γ camera to acquire images after intravenous injection of radiotracer, though the image quality is not as good as mammography. A high-resolution small field γ camera is used and craniocaudal and mediolateral views are taken.

INDICATIONS

- Detection of malignancy in denser breasts of young women, in whom mammography may not help
- Detection of subcentimetric and nonpalpable breast malignancy

The disadvantages of this technique are:

- Fibrocystic changes, fibroadenomas may show false-positive results
- Lesions close to the chest wall, deep in the breast tissue may be missed by the technique
- Radiation exposure is higher than in mammography.

Dual-phase imaging is a technique used in BSGI to help differentiate between benign and malignant lesion where the lesions are imaged at two different points of time after injection of contrast. It is based on the hypothesis that malignant lesions retain radiotracer for a longer duration than benign lesions.

SUGGESTED READING

1. Lauren R. Rechtman, Megan J. Lenihan, Jennifer H. Lieberman, Christine B. Teal, Jessica Torrente, Jocelyn A. Rapelyea et al:Breast-Specific Gamma Imaging for the Detection of Breast Cancer in Dense Versus Nondense Breasts:American Journal of Roentgenology. 2014;202: 293-298. 10.2214/AJR.13.11585
2. Rachel F. Brem, Angelique C. Floerke, Jocelyn A. Rapelyea, Christine Teal, Tricia Kelly, Vivek Mathur: Breast Specific gamma imaging as an adjunct modality for diagnosis of breast cancer: Radiology; june 2008, volume 247(3).

12.3 Thermography

INTRODUCTION

The basic principle of thermography is that increase in skin temperature is an indication of underlying pathology. Accurate spot temperature readings can be done by thermocouples, thermistors or radiometers.

The intensity of radiation depends on the temperature and the frequency (wavelength) of the electromagnetic radiation.

This technique determines the intensity of radiation produced by biological structures. Both infrared and microwave thermography are used in the detection of temperatures of inner biological structures.

The electromagnetic radiation produced by various physical bodies is measured by microwave radiometry which delineates the depth of lesion because of greater wavelength and less tissue absorption.

The ability to produce heat (i.e. thermogenicity) in breast cancer is directly proportional to its doubling time. The heat produced by a malignant lesion has to travel a path before reaching the skin surface, which may lead to false-negative results. This technique is not accurate for detecting small or deep seated cancers and should not be used as a stand alone technique.

FURTHER READING

1. Zhu A, Lee D, Shim H. Metabolic PET imaging in cancer detection and therapy response. Semin Oncol 2011;38(1): 55-69.
2. Vercher-Conejero JL, Pelegrí-Martinez L, Lopez-Aznar D, Cózar-Santiago M del P. Positron emission tomography in breast cancer. Diagnostics 2015;5(1):61-83.
3. Eric L. Rosen, William B. Eubank and David A. MankofRadioGraphics 2007 27:suppl_1, S215-S229 FDG PET, PET/CT and Breast Cancer Imaging.
4. Clinical usefulness of breast-specific gamma imaging as an adjunct modality to mammography for diagnosis of breast cancer: a systemic review and meta-analysis. Eur J Nucl Med Mol Imaging February 2013;40(3):450-63.
5. A comparative study of breast-specific gamma imaging with the conventional imaging modality in breast cancer patients with dense breasts. Ann Nucl Med December 2012; 26(10):823-9.
6. Diagnostic performance of breast-specific gamma imaging (BSGI) for breast cancer: usefulness of dual-phase imaging with ^{99m}Tc-sestamibi. Nucl Med Mol Imaging March 2013; 47(1):18-26.
7. Baltag O, Banarescu A, Costandache D, Rau M. Ojica S. Microwaves and infrared thermography—applications in early breast cancer detection. In: Vlad S, Ciupa RV, Nicu AI, editors. International conference on advancements of medicine and health care through technology. IFMBE Proceedings, vol 26. Berlin, Heidelberg: Springer; 2009.

Self-evaluation Based on Case Discussions

CHAPTER 13

INTRODUCTION

The cases are organized into three levels: 1, 2, and 3 based on difficulty of interpretation and/or the rarity of the lesion presented. The selection of cases is entirely random and the aim is to interpret the findings following a pattern based approach. It's not just the specific diagnosis but the quality of the differential diagnosis and the inclusion of appropriate options which is equally important.

The best way to go through these cases is to look at the images, answer the questions and then turn the page for the answers.

Level 1: These are cases which the young radiologists and residents should have relatively little difficulty in identifying. In fact, these are mainly based on technique and positioning.

Level 2: This consists of cases that require more study but most people should get into identifying the salient features and get their differential diagnoses.

Level 3: This is the challenging section. Most radiologists will be able to mention entities in the differential diagnoses of these cases, but it may not hit the target all the times. These cases are really designed to whet one's appetite for further reading on these entities and to test one's wits.

LEVEL 1

CASE 1

History: A 45-year-old asymptomatic woman underwent a screening mammogram. Craniocaudal views of both sides are shown (Figs. 1 and 2).

1. What is the abnormality in Figure 1?
2. What is the remedial measure taken in Figure 2?

Answer

Motion unsharpness due to inadequate compression.

Comments: Proper compression of breast while doing a mammogram is essential not only for maintaining image quality but also for reducing patient dose. It reduces breast thickness, provides uniform density, improves contrast by decreasing scatter radiation and decreases the likelihood of motion unsharpness. If the image is not sharp and clear, there are chances of missing microcalcifications.

CASE 2

History: A 51-year-old female presented with history of right breast lump for 6 months. (Figs. 3 and 4).

1. What are the standard views done on mammogram?
2. The mass is not seen on one of the standard views (Fig. 3). Why?
3. Which view would you advise next and how is it done?

Answers

1. The standard mammogram views are craniocaudal and mediolateral oblique views.
2. The mass is not seen on CC view. Sometimes, when the mass in present in the deeper and outermost portion of breast, it may not be included or covered in the standard CC view.

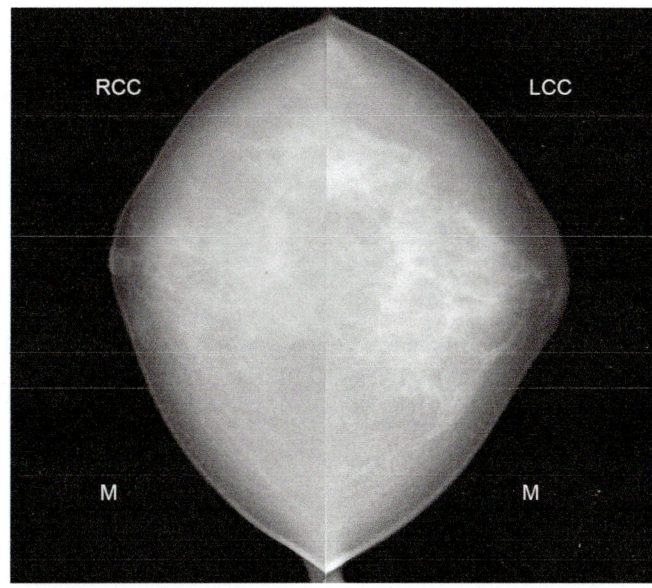

Fig. 2: CC view with adequate compression and sharp images.

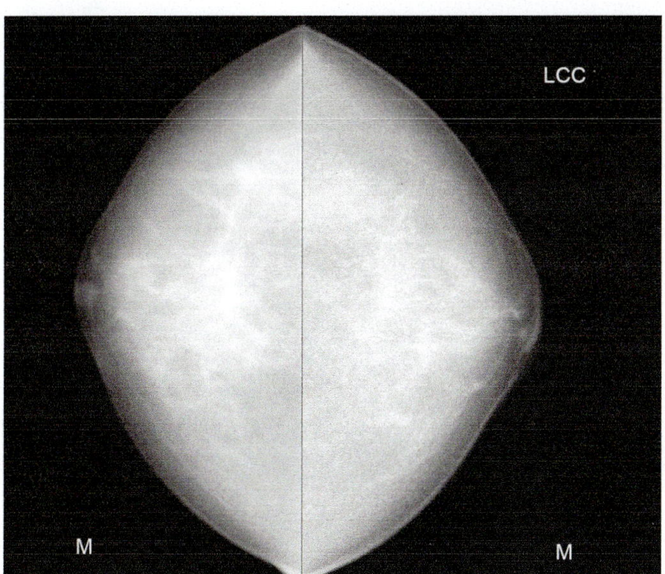

Fig. 1: Cranio-caudal view of both breast showing motion unsharpness.

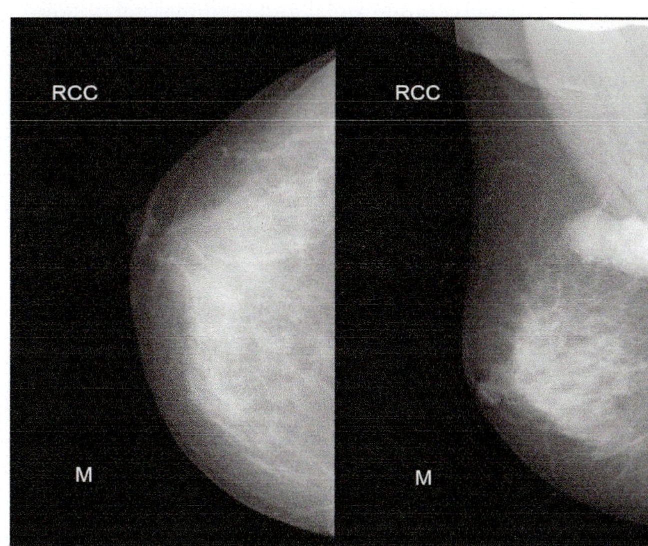

Fig. 3: Standard Cranio-caudal and Medio-lateral oblique views are shown where mass in seen only on MLO view.

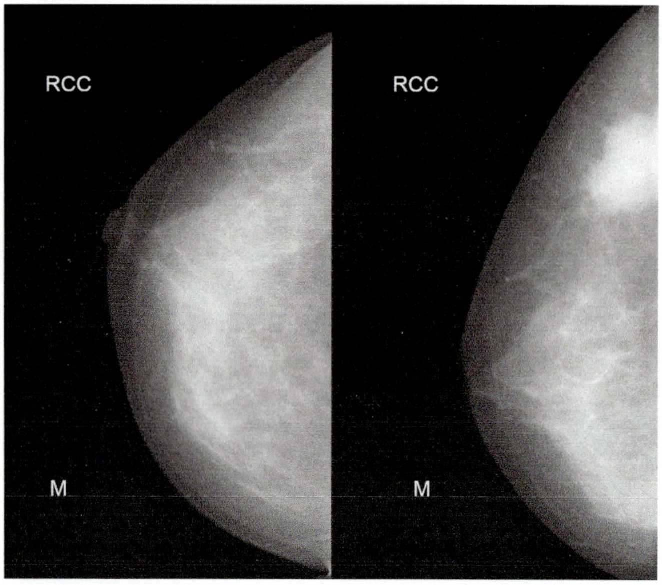

Fig. 4: Laterally extended CC view is done to include the lateral most aspect of breast so that mass is adequately covered.

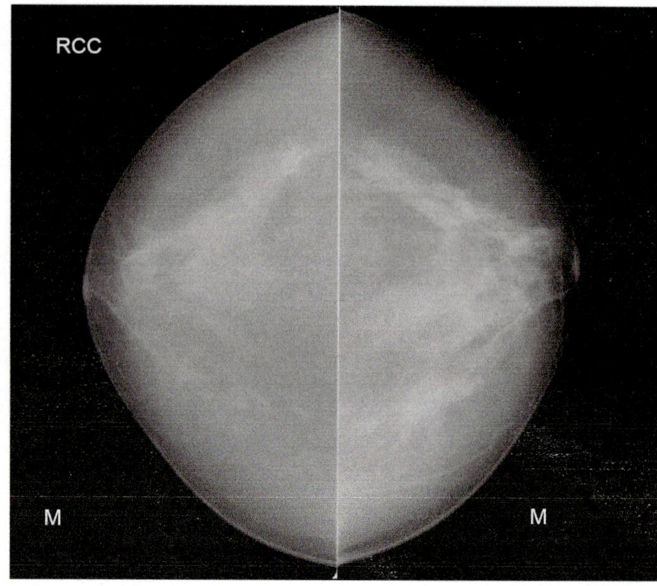

Fig. 5: CC view on the right side shows a small irregular focal mass in lateral quadrant.

3. In these patients, **laterally extended craniocaudal view** should be done (Fig. 4). The positioning for this view is begun in a similar way as for a standard CC view but after elevating the inframammary fold, the patient is rotated in such a way that the lateral aspect of breast is positioned on cassette holder. If shoulder comes on the way of positioning, then a 5° lateral tube angle should be used without pushing down the shoulder. It is important to remember that both the shoulders should remain at the same level.

Comments: Though craniocaudal and mediolateral oblique views are standard views, there are additional views which may be needed based on the location of mass. These include extended (laterally/medially) craniocaudal view, laterolateral view, axillary tail view and cleavage view (also called valley view).

CASE 3

History: A 61-year-old female underwent screening mammogram of both breasts. CC view of both breasts is shown (Fig. 5).

1. Is there any abnormality in the mammogram?
2. What additional view will you suggest and what are its advantages?
3. What role does ultrasound have?

Answers

1. There is a focal asymmetric density/mass in lateral quadrant of right breast.
2. Magnification view should be done which provides a better assessment. In this case the magnification view (Fig. 6) showed spiculated margins of mass.

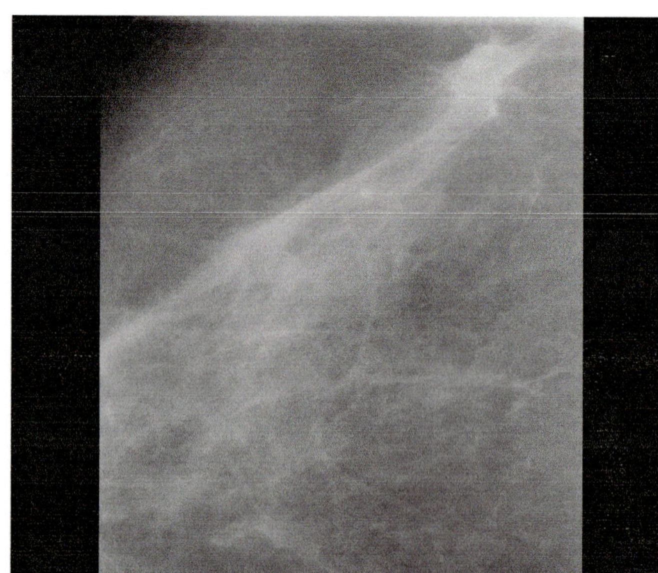

Fig. 6: Magnification view shows the spiculated margins of the mass clearly.

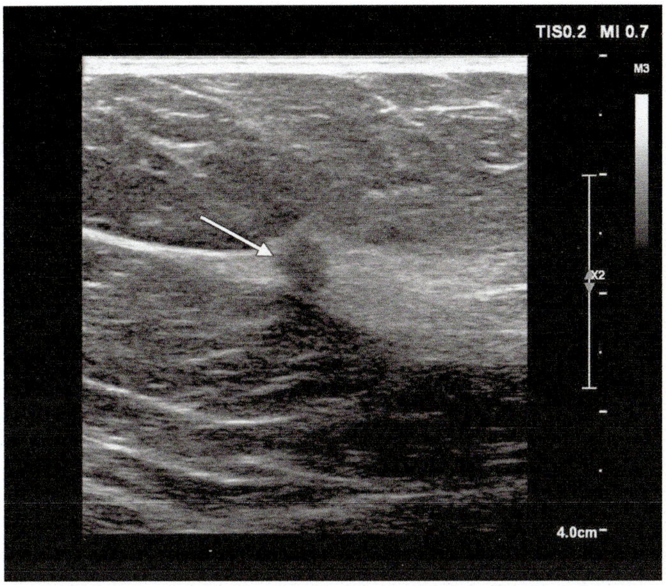

Fig. 7: Targeted ultrasound showed a taller than wide mass with irregular margins.

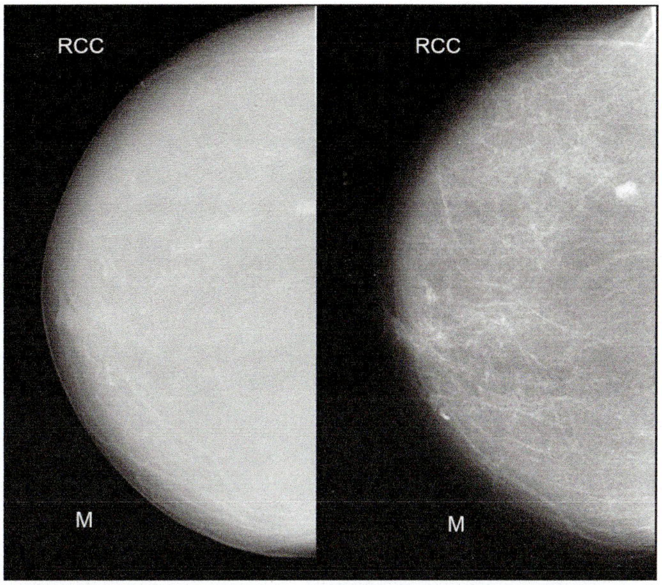

Fig. 8: CC view shows indequately included mass in retroglandular region which is better included in the second image (on lifting and pulling the breast).

3. Targeted ultrasound in the region of interest showed a hypoechoic mass with irregular margins which was antiparallel to the skin surface (Fig. 7).

Ultrasound guided wire localization was done followed by wide local excision. Histopathology was suggestive of invasive ductal carcinoma.

Comments: Magnification views are often used to evaluate microcalcifications and small masses which may indicate a small cancer. The margins of a masses are better appreciated on magnification, while in case of microcalcifications, their morphology and number can be seen well. In this case ultrasound also confirmed the findings.

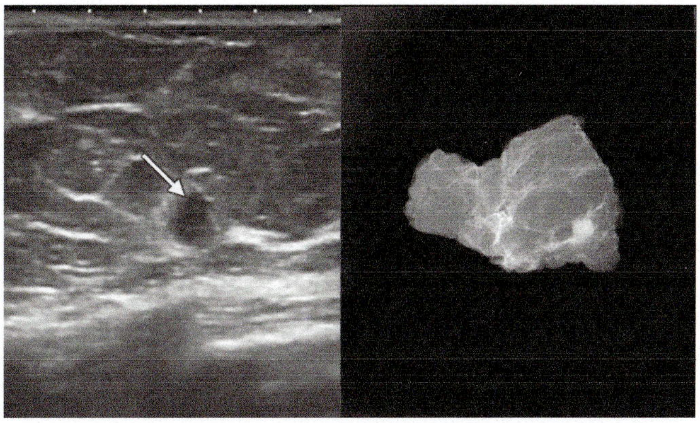

Fig. 9: Targeted ultrasound through the region of interest shows malignant mass which was confirmed on resected specimen.

CASE 4

History: A 57-year-old asymptomatic female underwent a routine mammogram. Craniocaudal views of breast are shown (Fig. 8).

1. Where is the abnormality?
2. Did repeat view help and in what way ? What instructions should be given to the radiographer?
3. What does ultrasound show in this case (Fig. 9)?
4. What is the significance of mass in this region on cranio-caudal view (Fig. 10)

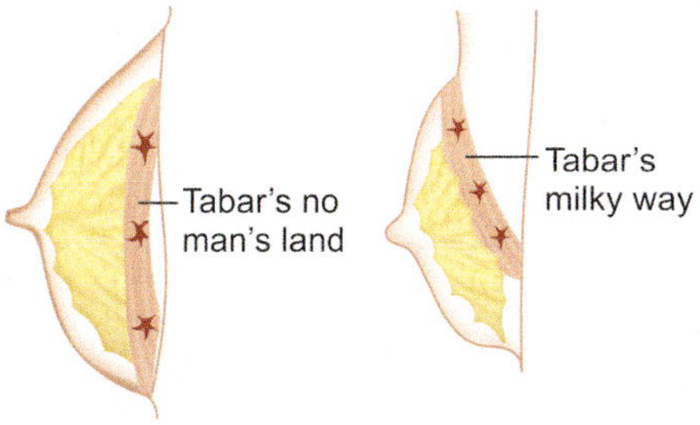

Fig. 10: Line diagram showing Tabar's no man's land and milky way in CC view and MLO view respectively.

Answers

1. A circumscribed mass is seen in the right breast in the retroglandular space.
2. Yes, repeat view has to be taken as the posterior most part of breast is not included adequately and portion of the mass is cutoff. The radiographer has to be instructed to lift and pull the breast so that the posterior most portion of breast is included.
3. Ultrasound helps in demonstrating the morphology of mass which helps in categorizing it into BI-RADS. Other than that, in masses which are non-palpable as in this case, biopsy and wire localization can be done under ultrasound guidance.
4. The retroglandular region on CC view is important (Fig. 10) because according to Tabar, it is one of the forbidden, check or review areas requiring special attention since cancers are common here.

Comments: Optimum positioning is extremely important in mammography; hence, a trained technologist is required. The definition "forbidden areas" is based on the incidence and distribution of cancer or interval cancers identified in screening with clusters in the axillary tail and inframammary fold on the MLO view and centrally and in the medial portions of the breast on CC view.

The gland-fat interface and the edge of the glandular tissue should be looked at properly and edge should be concave. There should not be any convex bulge or pulling in of tissue (tent sign) or straight lines.

The retroareolar region is also important. It is not compressed adequately and there is superimposition of ducts, vessels and fibrous tissue. Since there is a rich network of lymphatics located here, there is faster spread of cancer from this location.

Areas requiring special attention according to Tabar are

- **On craniocaudal view:**
  - The medial half of the breast
  - "No man's land" (the retroglandular space) behind the glandular tissue
- **On mediolateral oblique view:**
  - The "milky way" (retromammary fat): a 3-4-cm-wide band parallel to edge of pectoral muscle
  - Retroareolar region.

CASE 5

History: This 55 years old female underwent her routine screening mammogram. CC and MLO view of left breast are shown (Fig. 11). A convex density is seen in the posterior third of the left CC view. No suspicious lesion was seen on the MLO view.

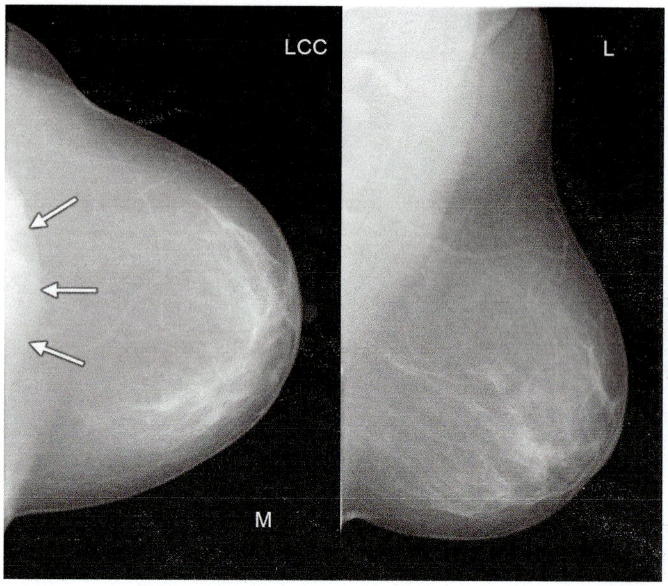

Fig. 11: CC view shows a convex density in the retro-glandular region.

1. What is this?
2. Is it desirable to position the breast in such a way that the pectoralis is included on the CC view?
3. Can this be a mass?

Answers

1. This is a portion of the pectoralis muscle. The pectoralis muscle lies posterior to the breast, forming the only part of the chest wall that is visualized on the mammogram
2. It is important to position the breast as deeply as possible to include the posterior most portion of breast. If pectoralis is seen on CC view, one can be confident that all the posterior breast tissue is included
3. This is a portion of the pectoralis muscle rather than a breast mass because no mass is seen on the MLO view. The pectoralis muscle may have a convex anterior margin to such an extent that it appears like a mass.

Comments: Pectoralis muscle is a valuable tool in recognizing the adequacy of positioning. It should be seen on the MLO view up to the level of the nipple and should have a convex anterior margin.

On the CC view, some of the pectoralis muscle can be seen along the posterior aspect of the breast in approximately 25% of patients. When it is seen, one is confident that the breast tissue is completely included since the pectoralis is the most posterior structure that can be seen on the mammogram.

Care must be taken to recognize the pectoralis muscle and yet, not miss a possible mass at the edge of the film. If not sure, spot compression view may help to more completely evaluate the pectoralis.

CASE 6

History: A 65-year-old woman with lump in left breast underwent mammogram (Fig. 12) followed by ultrasound of left breast (Fig. 13).

1. What is the location of mass on mammogram?
2. What will be the corresponding clock position on ultrasound?
3. What is BI-RADS category and recommendation?

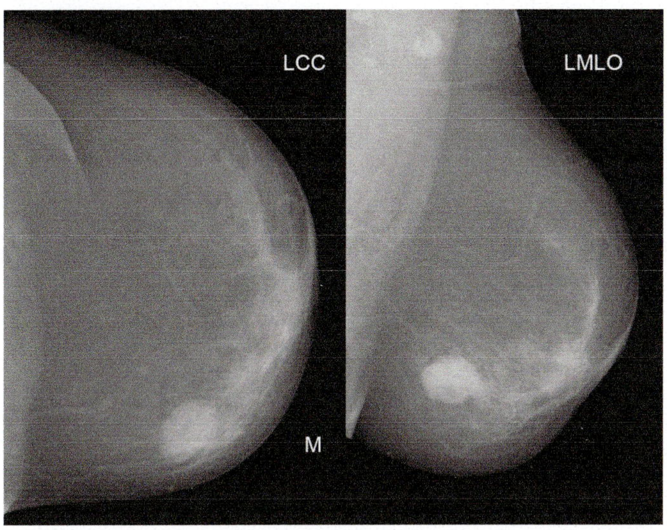

Fig. 12: CC and MLO view show a mass with irregular margins in lower inner quadrant of left breast.

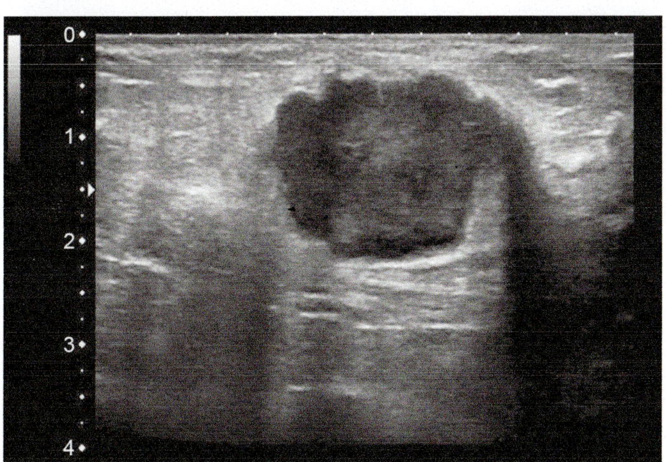

Fig. 13: Ultrasound of left breast showed a, hypoechoic mass with irregular margins and microlobulations.

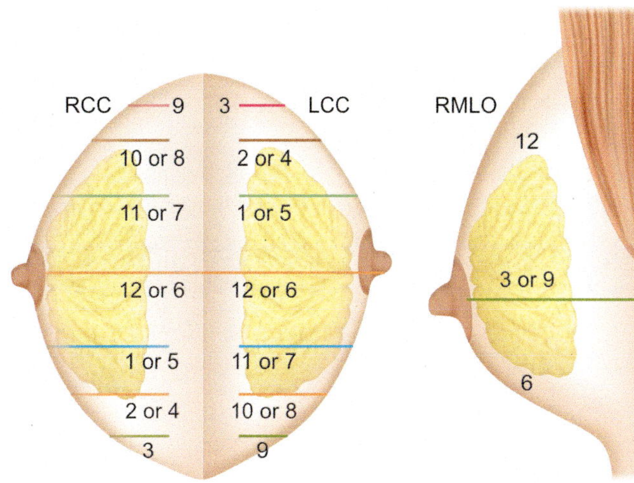

Fig. 14: showing the corresponding clock position of the left breast mass which is at 6 to 7 'o clock position.

Answers

1. The mass is located at inferomedial quadrant of left breast on mammogram
2. The corresponding clock position on ultrasound is 7–8 o'clock
3. The mass is circumscribed has high density and shows microlobulated margins on mammogram. On ultrasound, the mass is hypoechoic and shows microlobulations—BI-RADS category 4c. A core needle biopsy is recommended for further evaluation

The final histopathological diagnosis was invasive ductal carcinoma.

Comments: It is important to estimate the expected clock position of mass on ultrasound by looking at the mammogram especially when there are multiple masses or if one of the mass is suspicious and needs a biopsy. These findings should be mentioned clearly in the mammogram report for future follow-ups.

CASE 7

History: A 47-year-old woman underwent wide local excision for a left breast lump 2 weeks ago in a peripheral setup. Since histopathology showed invasive ductal carcinoma, patient was referred for a mammogram to look for residual lesion. The patient did not have any preoperative mammogram or ultrasound films for comparison.

1. What are the findings on mammogram? What is your interpretation?
2. Does ultrasound have a role?

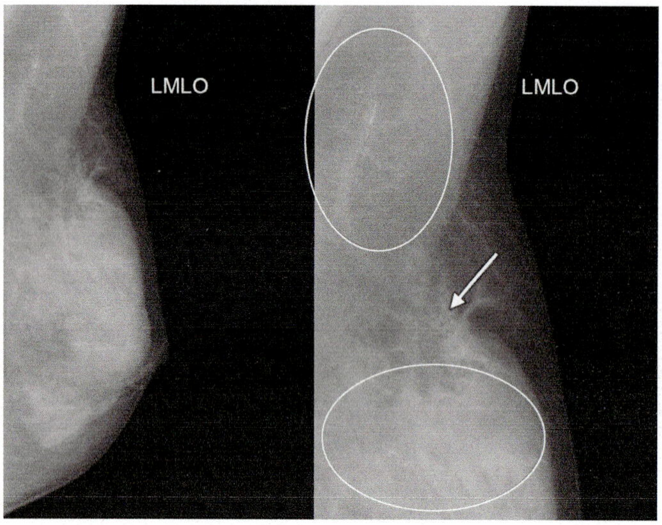

Fig. 15: MLO view shows architectural distortion in upper quadrant of left breast with linear radio-opacities along the pectoralis muscle and in upper quadrant (circled in white).

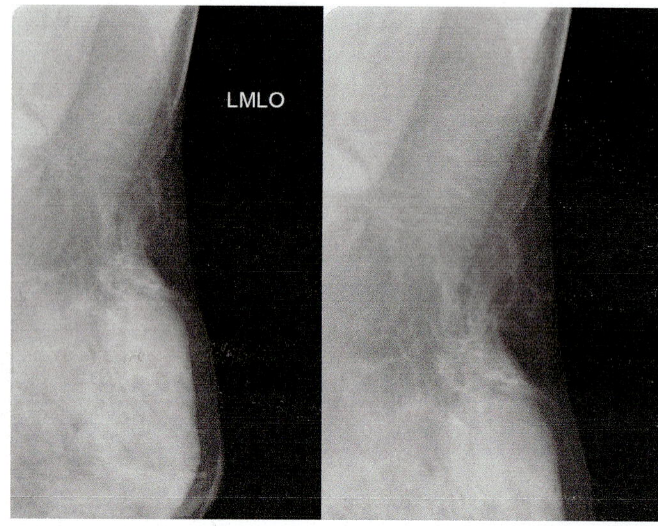

Fig. 16: A repeat MLO view after cleaning the site was normal.

Answers

1. There is architectural deformity in upper quadrant of left breast. Also there are linear radiopacities along the pectoralis muscle and in upper quadrant (circled in white in Fig. 15).

   It is important to note that this finding does not fit in to a fine linear or fine pleomorphic malignant calcification or any other kind of a benign calcification. This may have been produced by something from outside—artifact. In this case, it was due to marks left on the skin by the adhesive plaster at the surgical site which was not cleaned properly and had dust deposition over a period of time. A repeat mammogram done after cleaning the area confirms the same (Fig. 16).
2. Yes. Ultrasound can help in showing the postoperative changes like seroma, skin thickening, scar, etc. and if there is a residual lesion at the operative site.

Comments: It is important to know the details of the surgery done before reporting the mammogram in a postoperative breast. The radiographer should be vigilant and note local findings while doing a mammogram and inform the reporting radiologist. It is still not uncommon in the Indian scenario to find a patient undergoing a lumpectomy without adequate preoperative imaging and when histopathology suggests a malignancy, then the patient is referred for a mammogram to rule out a residual lesion at a higher centre.

Such cases can prove to be challenging for beginners especially if they have failed to notice subtle findings.

CASE 8

History: A 57-year-old female underwent mammogram for a palpable mass in left breast. Mammogram (MLO and CC view) are shown in Figure 17.

1. What is the breast density as per ACR?
2. Where is the mass located?
3. Describe the mass using BI-RADS lexicon
4. What is the BI-RADS category?
5. Is there any incidental finding seen?

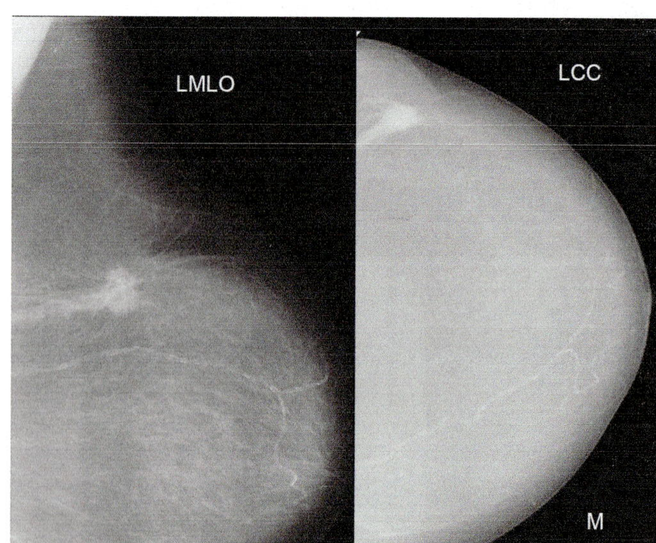

Fig. 17: An irregular, high density mass with spiculated margins is seen in upper outer quadrant of left breast.

Answers

1. The breast is almost entirely fatty.

According to ACR, breast density is divided into four categories:

   a. Breast is almost entirely fatty.
   b. Scattered area of fibroglandular tissue.
   c. Heterogeneously dense tissue which may obscures small masses.
   d. Extremely dense breast, which lowers the sensitivity of the mammograms.

2. The mass is located in upper outer quadrant of left breast.
3. An irregular high-density mass with spiculated margins is seen.
4. BI-RADS category 5.
5. Yes. There is vascular calcification which is benign calcification-BI-RADS category 2.

CASE 9

History: A 65-year-old female underwent routine mammogram of both breasts. MLO and CC views are shown Fig. 18 and Fig. 19.

1. Is there any abnormality in mammogram? Yes/No.
2. Describe the mammogram findings
3. What is the additional view taken?
4. What are the differential diagnoses?
5. Describe the ultrasound findings
6. What is BI-RADS category and recommendations?

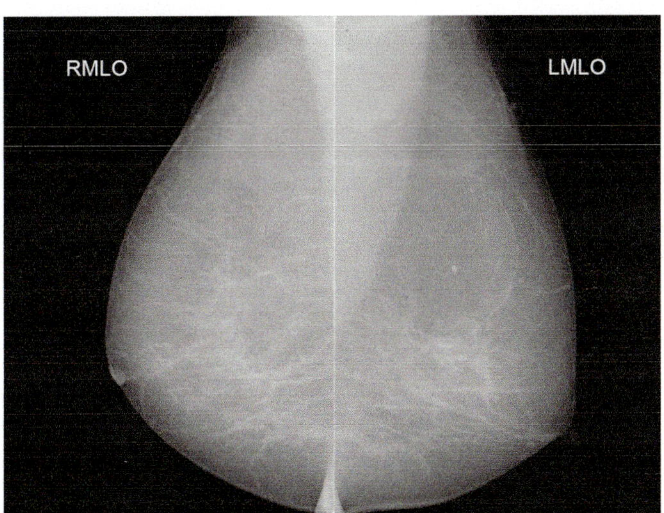

Fig. 18: A well circumscribed , encapsulated fat density mass is seen in superior quadrant—MLO view of left breast with two foci of macro-calcifications.

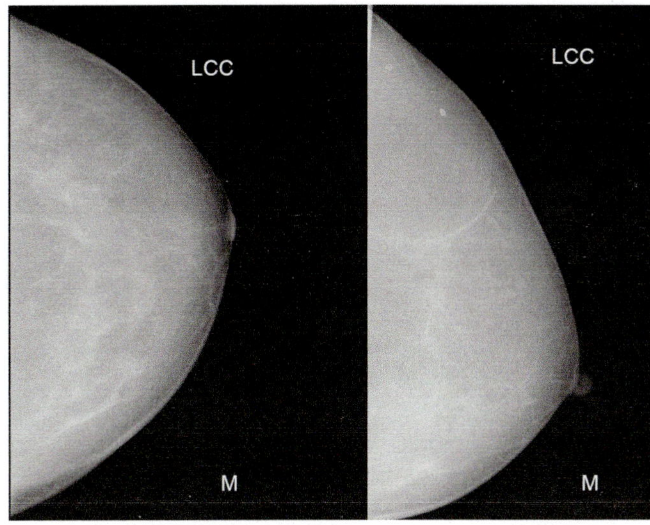

Fig. 19: The mass was not covered in routine CC view but seen in lateral quadrant in exaggerated CC view.

Answers

1. Yes. There is abnormality in left breast
2. A circumscribed, encapsulated fat density mass is seen in upper outer quadrant-MLO view of left breast with two foci of macrocalcifications. The mass is not covered in CC view
3. Since the mass was not covered in CC view, an laterally extended CC view was taken (Fig. 19) which showed the mass laterally in better visualisation.
4. The differential diagnosis for fat containing masses includes lipoma, fibroadenolipoma or hamartoma, fat necrosis and galactoceles.
5. Ultrasound shows a circumscribed, fat echogenicity mass with thin linear septae like structures and has an echogenic capsule (arrows) (Fig. 20).
6. BI-RADS category 2—benign findings

Comments: Fat containing masses are definitely benign and do not require biopsy for confirmation. These include lipomas, hamartomas, fat necrosis and galactoceles.

Lipomas are benign fat containing masses and are sometimes difficult to distinguish from normal fatty tissue in the breast. These are slow-growing masses and are more commonly seen in postmenopausal women. They have a thin fibrous pseudocapsule surrounding the mass which may require a spot compression magnification view to be demonstrated.

Fibroadenolipomas or hamartomas are due to benign proliferation of fibrous, glandular and fatty tissue in different proportions. They are also described as having a

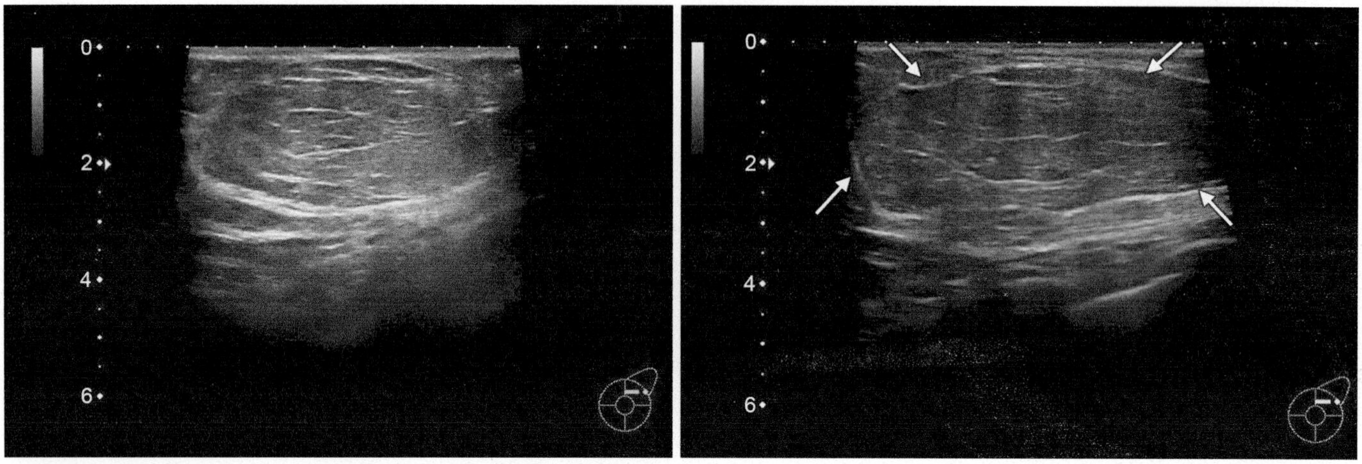

Fig. 20: Ultrasound shows a circumscribed, fat echogenicity mass with thin linear septae like structures with echogenic capsule (arrows).

"breast within a breast" appearance. On mammogram, they are seen as circumscribed mixed density masses surrounded by a thin capsule.

Fat necrosis is commonly seen as a small circumscribed lucent mass with a rim calcification in post-traumatic breast or in patients with history of breast conservative surgery.

LEVEL 2

CASE 1

History: A 51-year-old female got a routine mammogram done. Craniocaudal view of left breast showed a circumscribed dense focal asymmetry along the posterior medial edge of the breast which was not seen on MLO view (Fig. 1).

1. What is this?
2. Does the patient require further work up?
3. Is this unilateral craniocaudal or bilateral?

Answers

1. A circumscribed dense focal asymmetry was noted on the craniocaudal view. This is sternalis muscle which is a thin slip of muscle running longitudinally along the medial border of the sternum. The sternalis, when present, lies just anterior to the medial margin of the pectoralis muscle
2. This is a normal variant hence no further work up is required
3. Sternalis muscle is more often seen unilaterally

Final diagnosis: sternalis muscle

A similar case showing sternalis muscle (Fig. 2). Line diagram (Fig. 3).

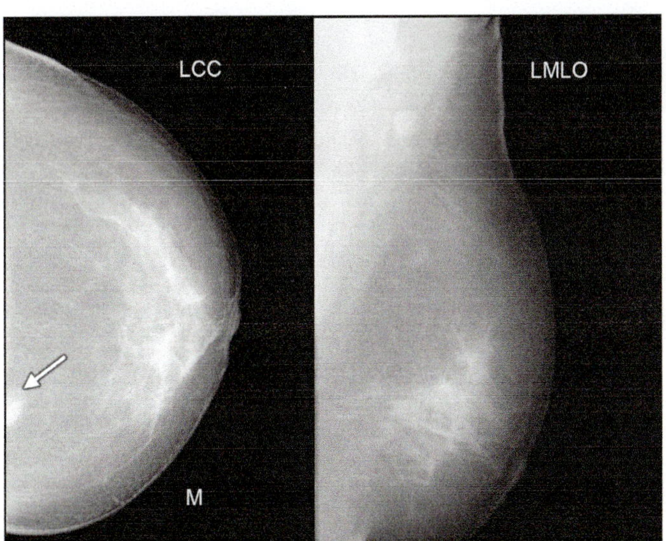

Fig. 1: CC view shows a circumscribed dense focal density (arrow) not seen on MLO view.

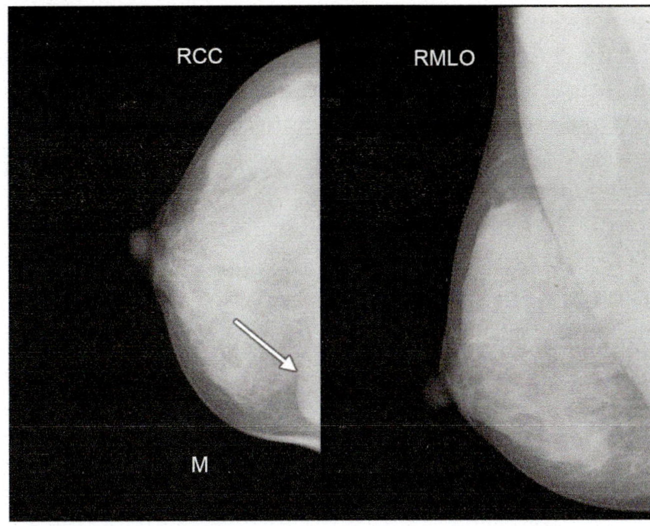

Fig. 2: CC view in another case where a similar density is noted as an incidental finding (arrow).

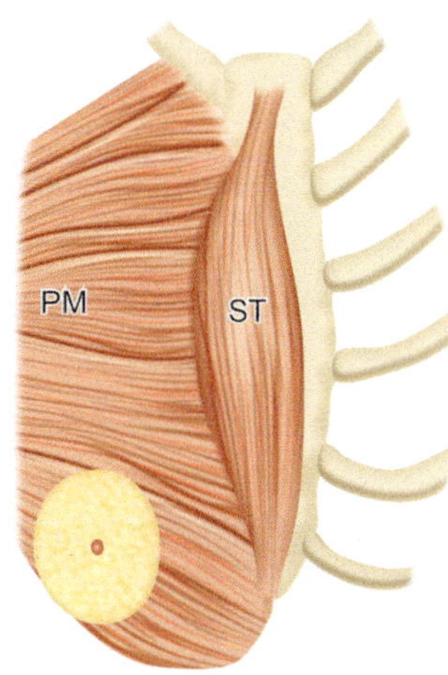

Fig. 3: Line diagram showing ST-sternalis muscle and PM- Pectoralis major muscle.

Comments: It is important to be aware of this finding where a small soft-tissue density (1–2 cm) is seen on the medial aspect on craniocaudal view abutting the chest wall. The sternalis muscle ranges in appearance from a round mass to a flame shaped mass. This finding is not seen on the ML or MLO view.

Knowledge of this normal variant is important so that unnecessary biopsies and additional workups are avoided.

CASE 2

History: A 52-year-old female who underwent breast conservation therapy for right breast got her follow-up mammogram (Figs. 4 and 5) after one year of surgery. Ultrasound of surgical site is also shown (Fig. 6).

1. What are the mammogram findings? What is your diagnosis?
2. Does ultrasound help in this case?
3. What BI-RADS category would you assign?

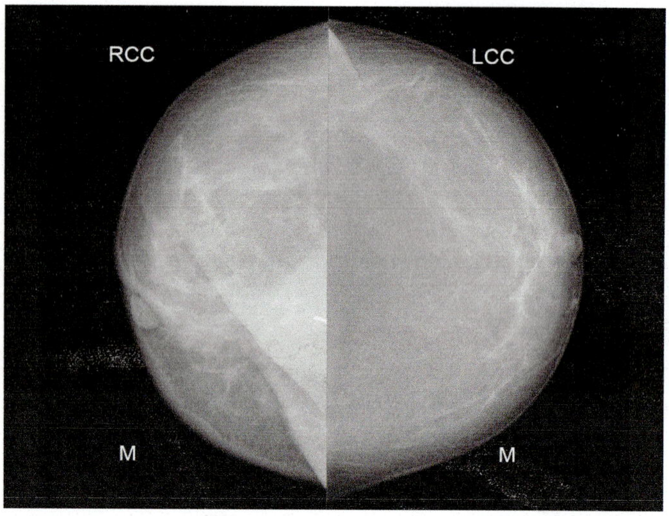

Fig. 4: CC view on right side shows diffuse increase in breast density with skin fold , architectural distortion and increased skin thickness.

Answers

1. There is diffuse increase in right breast density with skin folds, architectural distortion and increased skin thickness. There is also a focal density seen at the surgical site adjacent to the surgical staples in both views which represents a seroma.
2. Yes. Ultrasound shows a circumscribed cystic collection with a small echogenic nodule at the surgical site. This was a seroma and confirmed the mammogram findings. Seroma has varied appearance on ultrasound and should not be mistaken for a mass. Ultrasound is useful not just in confirming the diagnosis of seroma but is also useful in looking for any residual or recurrent mass.
3. BI-RADS category 2 is assigned to postoperative changes in breast.

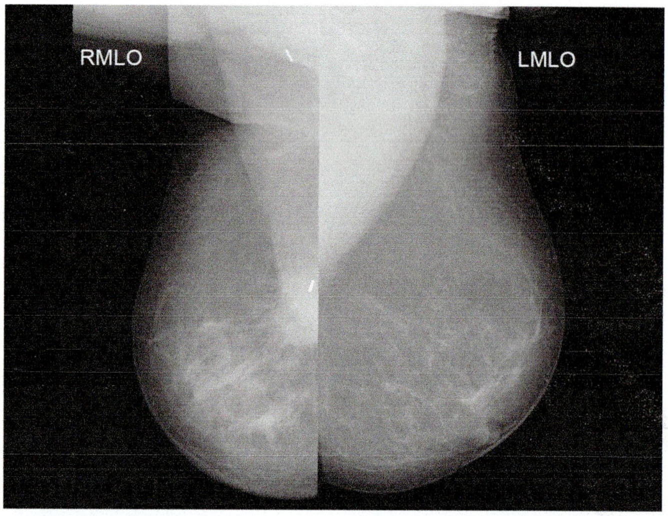

Fig. 5: Right MLO view also a focal density seen at the surgical site adjacent to the surgical staples.

Final diagnosis: breast conservative therapy changes with seroma formation

Comments: Mammograms with post-breast conservative therapy changes are challenging to read especially for budding radiologists because of changes in normal appearance of breast and increased breast density, architectural distortion due to surgery and radiotherapy. It is important to know what constitutes a normal finding and which finding

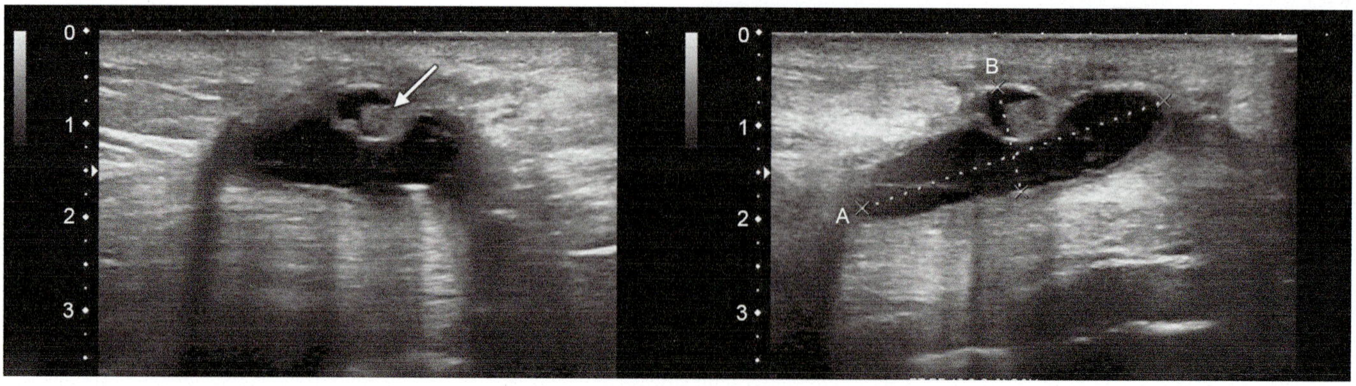

Fig. 6: Ultrasound of right breast shows a circumscribed cystic collection with a small echogenic nodule at the surgical site s/o seroma.

requires an action. Seroma has various appearances on ultrasound ranging from anechoic or cystic mass with or without septations to a hypoechoic heterogeneous mass.

Stabilization is defined as the lack of interval change on two successive studies. After stabilization has been achieved, a new mass, new microcalcifications, architectural distortion or an area of increased soft-tissue density at the lumpectomy site should be investigated for possible tumor recurrence.

CASE 3

History: A 42-year-old female presented with complaint of lump in left breast and underwent mammogram (Fig. 7) followed by ultrasound examination (Fig. 8).

1. Describe the mammogram
2. Does ultrasound help in making a diagnosis?
3. What is the BI-RADS category?

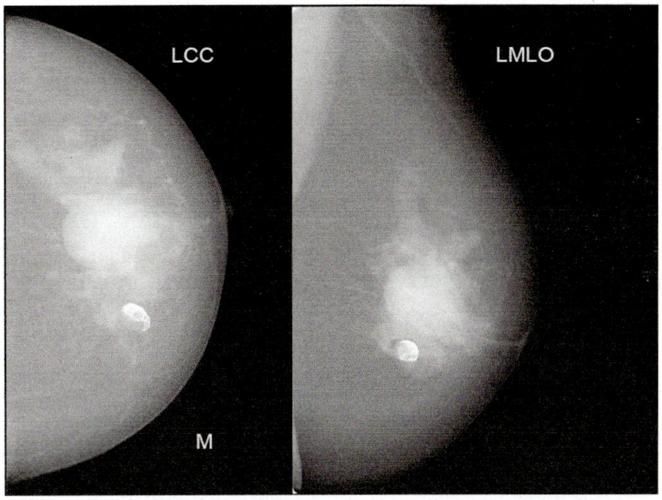

Fig. 7: Mammogram of left breast shows a circumscribed mass in retro-areolar region with obscured anterior margins, partially calcified oval mass infero-medially and a few small soft tissue densities.

Answers

1. Mammogram of left breast shows a circumscribed mass in retroareolar region with obscured anterior margins. The posterior margins appear smooth. A partially calcified oval mass is seen inferomedial to the above-mentioned mass. In addition, there are a few overlapping soft tissue densities in upper outer quadrant
2. Yes. Ultrasound helps in confirming the consistency of the mass, whether it is cystic or solid. In this case, a large cyst was seen with thick septa within and a few internal echoes suggestive of complicated cyst. In addition there was an echogenic focus with posterior acoustic shadowing due to a partially calcified cyst which was noted on mammogram. Calcification in involuting fibroadenoma is more coarse, larger and popcorn like. A few other subcentimeter simple cysts were also seen
3. BI-RADS category 2

Final diagnosis: cysts in left breast one of them is partially calcified—BI-RADS category 2

Comments: Cysts are one of the commonest incidentally detected findings on ultrasound. One has to differentiate between simple cyst, complicated cyst and complex

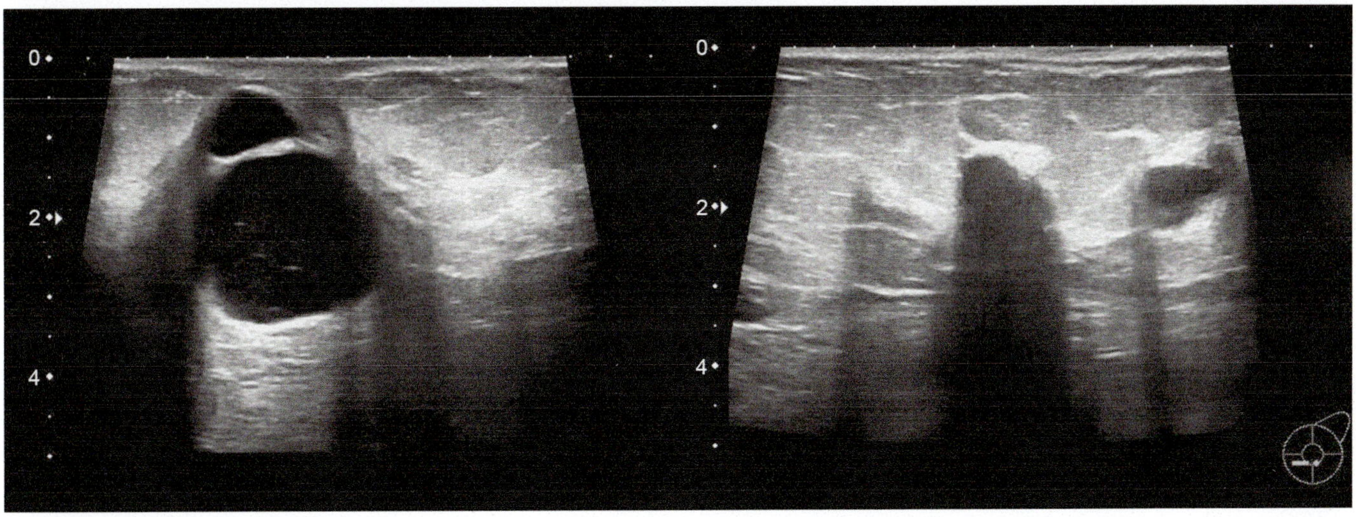

Fig. 8: Ultrasound shows a large cyst with thick septa and a few echoes s/o complicated cyst. In addition other cysts and a partially calcified cyst seen with posterior acoustic shadowing.

cysts as the management differs. Often the simple cysts and complex cysts are left alone unless they are getting enlarged, painful or symptomatic. In such cases depending on the local policy of the department, they are aspirated completely under ultrasound guidance till their walls are apposed. The complex cysts have both solid and cystic components and their management differs. (Please refer to chapter on cysts.)

CASE 4

History: A 64-year-old female presented with thickening in left breast and pain on and off for 6 months. Mammogram of both breasts (Figs. 9 and 10) was done followed by ultrasound (Fig. 11).

1. What are the mammogram findings?
2. Describe the ultrasound finding.

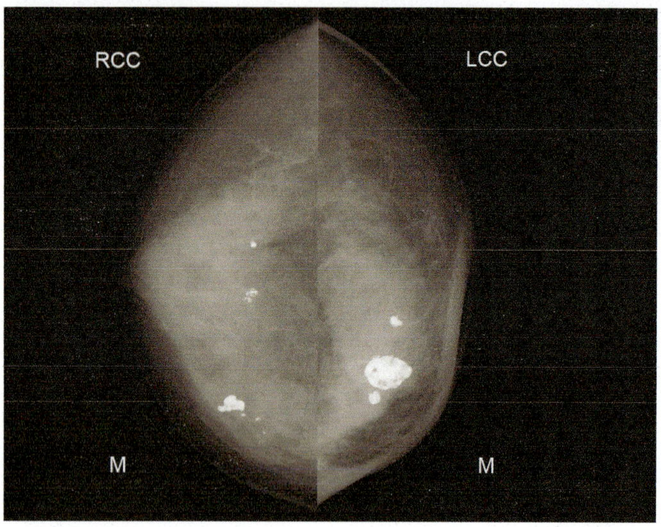

Fig. 9: CC view showed multiple calcified nodules/masses in varying sizes in the lower inner quadrant of both breasts with focal asymmetry in left breast, skin thickening and adjacent architectural distortion.

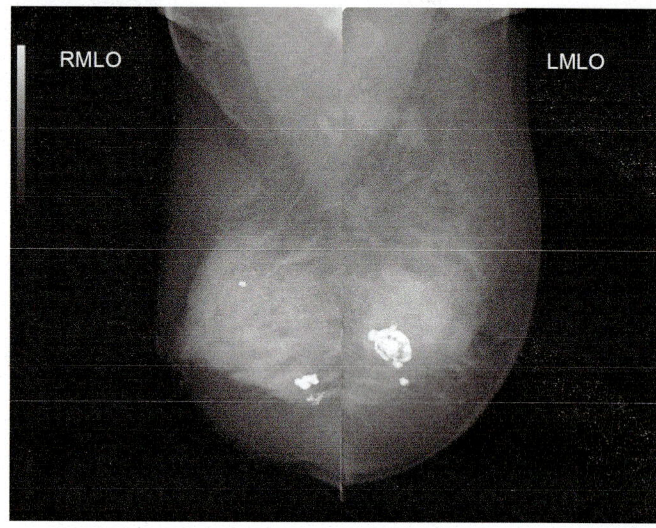

Fig. 10: MLO view of both breasts showed multiple calcified nodules/masses in the lower inner quadrant of both breasts. Focal asymmetry with adjacent architectural distortion, skin thickening and enlarged axillary lymph nodes with loss of fatty hilum are seen in the left breast.

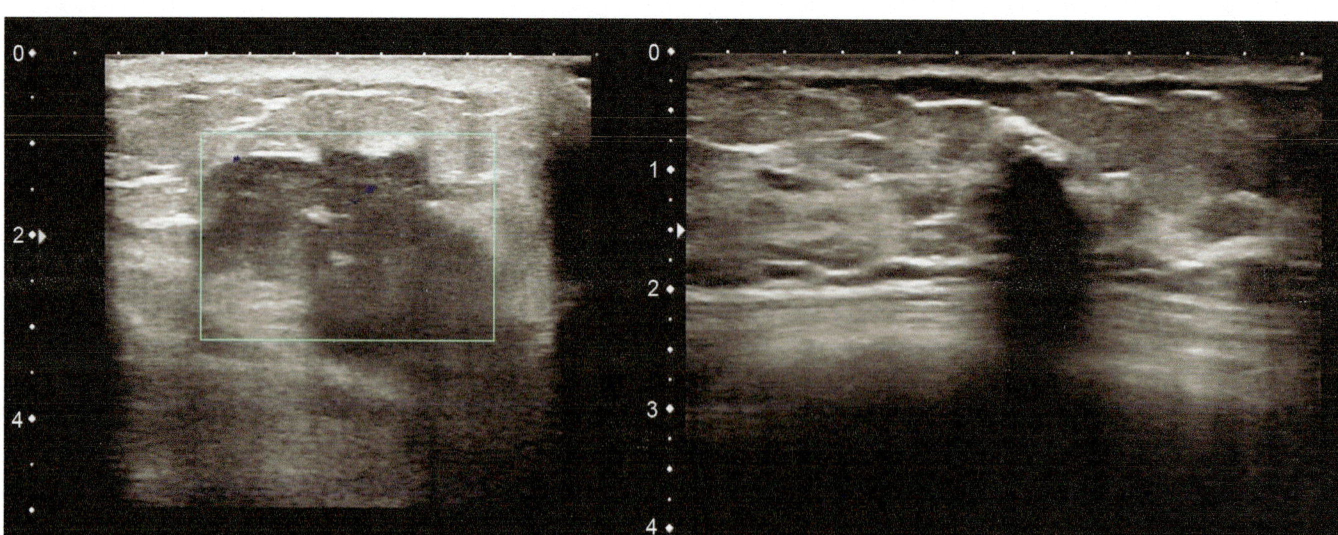

Fig. 11: Ultrasound of left breast shows an irregular hypoechoic mass at 9 'o clock position with another mass with dense posterior acoustic shadowing adjacent to it s/o calcification.

Answers

1. Both breasts are composed of heterogeneously dense parenchyma.

   There are multiple-calcified nodules/masses in varying sizes in the lower inner quadrant of both breasts. In addition, the left breast shows focal asymmetry in the lower inner quadrant in the posterior third with adjacent architectural distortion and overlying periareolar skin thickening. Enlarged axillary lymph nodes with loss of fatty hila are also seen on left.
2. Ultrasound of left breast shows an irregular hypoechoic mass at 9 o'clock position. An mass having area of dense posterior acoustic shadowing was seen adjacent to it s/o calcification

   Biopsy from the left breast mass and FNAC from left axillary lymph nodes were done. Histopathology was s/o invasive ductal carcinoma with lymph node metastases.

Final diagnosis: invasive ductal carcinoma with metastatic axillary lymph nodes along with involuting fibroadenomas in both breasts

Comments: It is important to see the mammograms carefully especially when multiple findings are present so that the important findings requiring further evaluation are not missed. It is essential to read the mammogram in a systematic manner in order to achieve this and take appropriate action.

CASE 5

History: A 66-year-old male presented with complaint of swelling in both breasts for last 6 months and was referred for ultrasound.

1. What are the ultrasound findings?
2. What is your diagnosis?
3. Do you want to elicit any specific history?

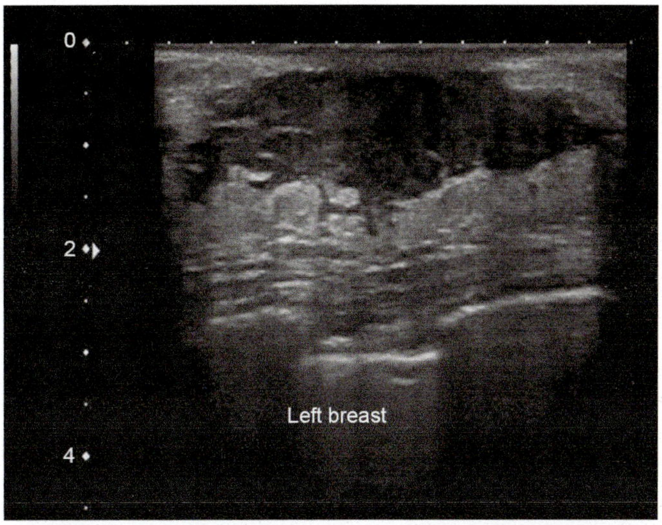

Fig. 12: A triangular hypoechoic retro areolar mass with finger-like projections is seen extending from the nipple into the surrounding tissue.

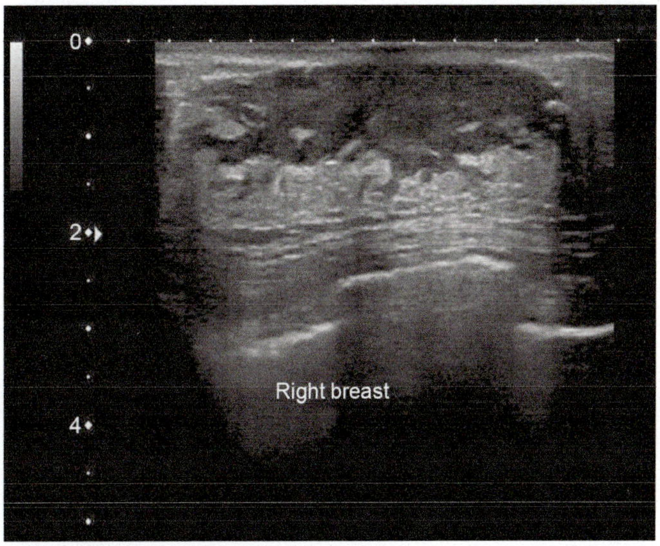

Fig. 13: A triangular hypoechoic retro areolar mass with finger-like projections is seen extending from the nipple into the surrounding tissue.

Answers

1. Ultrasound of both breasts shows similar findings. A triangular hypoechoic retroareolar mass with finger-like projections is seen extending from the nipple into the surrounding tissue (Fig. 12 and Fig. 13). There was no vascularity.
2. Gynecomastia—dendritic pattern.
3. A detailed drug history is important as drugs like cimetidine, thiazide diuretics, antihypertensives, antidepressants and steroids can cause bilateral gynecomastia. It is also essential to take history of cirrhosis, hyperthyroidism and chronic renal disease.

Final diagnosis: gynecomastia—dendritic pattern

Comments: Gynecomastia may be physiological or pathological. Three patterns are recognized on both imaging and histopathology: nodular, dendritic and diffuse. Knowledge of its various imaging features is important to prevent a misdiagnosis of malignancy.

CASE 6

History: A 45-year-old female presented with complaint of lump in left breast which was progressively enlarging for last 4 months. On clinical examination, the lump was firm to hard in consistency. The patient underwent a mammogram (Fig. 14) followed by ultrasound (Figs. 15 and 16).

1. Describe the mammogram findings
2. What are the ultrasound findings?
3. What BI-RADS category will you assign?
4. What are the differential diagnosis?

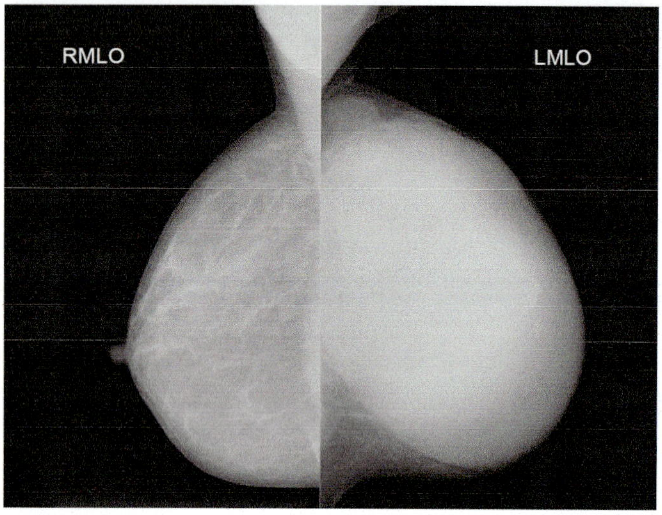

Fig. 14: MLO view of left breast shows a large, circumscribed mass occupying almost the whole breast with a large calcific focus within.

Answers

1. Mammogram of left breast MLO view shows a large, circumscribed mass occupying almost the whole left breast. There is a large calcific focus within. A few line artifacts are also seen.
2. Ultrasound shows a large, circumscribed heterogeneously hypoechoic mass with a circumscribed hyperechoic area within s/o fatty component. Vascularity was seen on Doppler. Ultrasound using a high-resolution transducer showed a few anechoic clefts within. There was no axillary lymphadenopathy.
3. BI-RADS category 4B
4. Differential diagnosis: Phyllodes tumor, giant fibroadenoma, metaplastic carcinoma
   Patient underwent simple mastectomy.

Final diagnosis: malignant phyllodes with liposarcomatous differentiation

Comments: Cystosarcoma phyllodes is a rare fibroepithelial tumor of the breast, accounting for 0.4%–1% of all breast tumors. It shares clinical, pathologic and imaging features with giant fibroadenoma and demonstrates a wide spectrum of biologic behavior having potential for invasive growth, recurrence, or metastasis. A phyllodes tumor may be considered benign, borderline or malignant depending on histologic features including stromal cellularity, infiltration at the tumor edge and mitotic activity. Surgery is the mainstay of treatment and includes wide local excision and simple mastectomy.

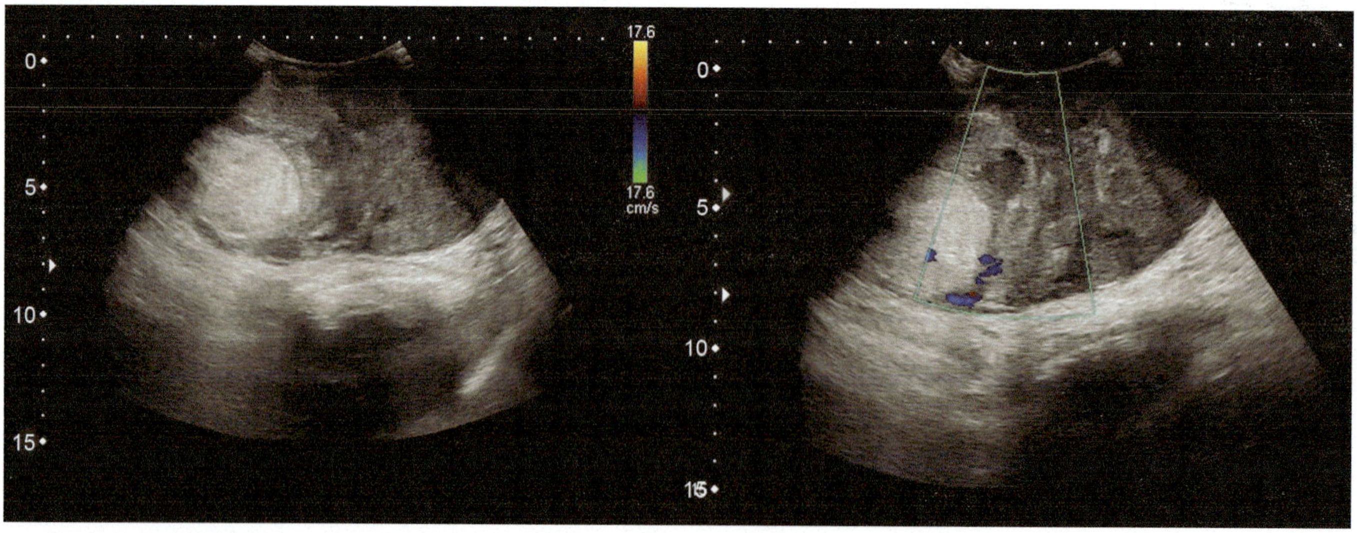

Fig. 15: Ultrasound of left breast shows a large, circumscribed heterogeneously hypoechoic mass with a circumscribed hyperechoic area within s/o fatty component. Minimal vascularity noted.

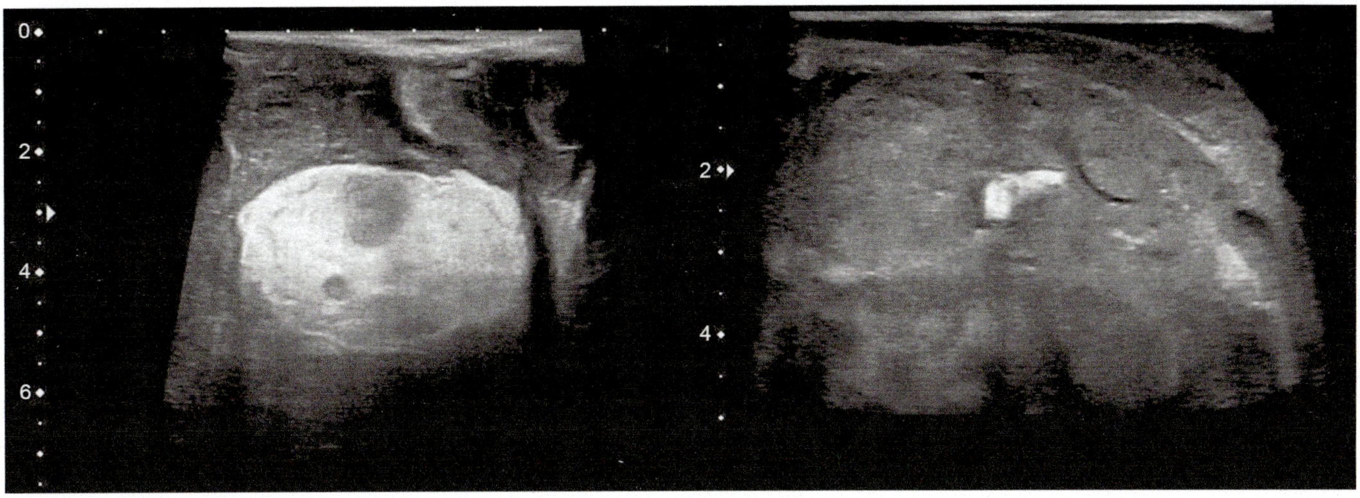

Fig. 16: High resolution ultrasound cofirmed the same findings with fluid cleft within.

CASE 7

History: A 52-year-old female got her routine screening mammogram. Mediolateral oblique and craniocaudal views of left breast are shown in Figure 17.

1. What is the breast density as per ACR?
2. What are the mammogram findings (Fig. 17)?
3. What BI-RADS category would you assign?
4. What is the diagnosis?

Answers

1. The breast density as per ACR is—heterogeneously dense.

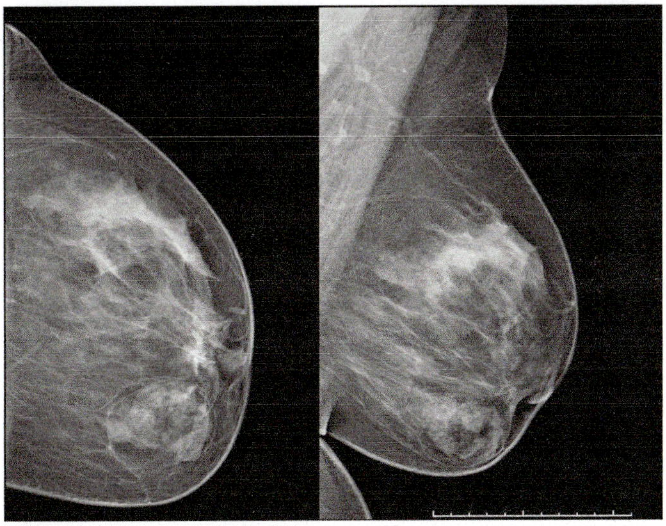

Fig. 17: Mammogram of left breast showed a heterogenous mass with lucent and dense fibrous tissue and a subtle capsule in lower inner quadrant.

2. Mammogram—MLO and CC view of left breast show a round, circumscribed mass of mixed density in lower inner quadrant. No architectural distortion or calcification is seen
3. BI-RADS category 2
4. Hamartoma or fibroadenolipoma of breast

Final diagnosis: breast hamartoma

Comments: Breast hamartoma is a benign tumor presenting as a soft-mobile lump. They are detected incidentally on imaging. On mammogram they are seen as heterogeneous mass with dense fibrous tissue and thin capsule. This leads to a breast within breast appearance on ultrasound where mixed adipose tissue and fibrous tissue are seen with an echogenic thin capsule.

CASE 8

History: A 28-year-old female presented with lump in left breast for 1 month duration. Ultrasound images are shown in Figure 18.

1. Describe the ultrasound findings
2. What is BI-RADS category?

Answers

1. Ultrasound shows a circumscribed heterogeneously hypoechoic mass with smooth margins It also has multiple echogenic foci and a small cystic component. The mass shows posterior acoustic enhancement
2. BI-RADS category 3

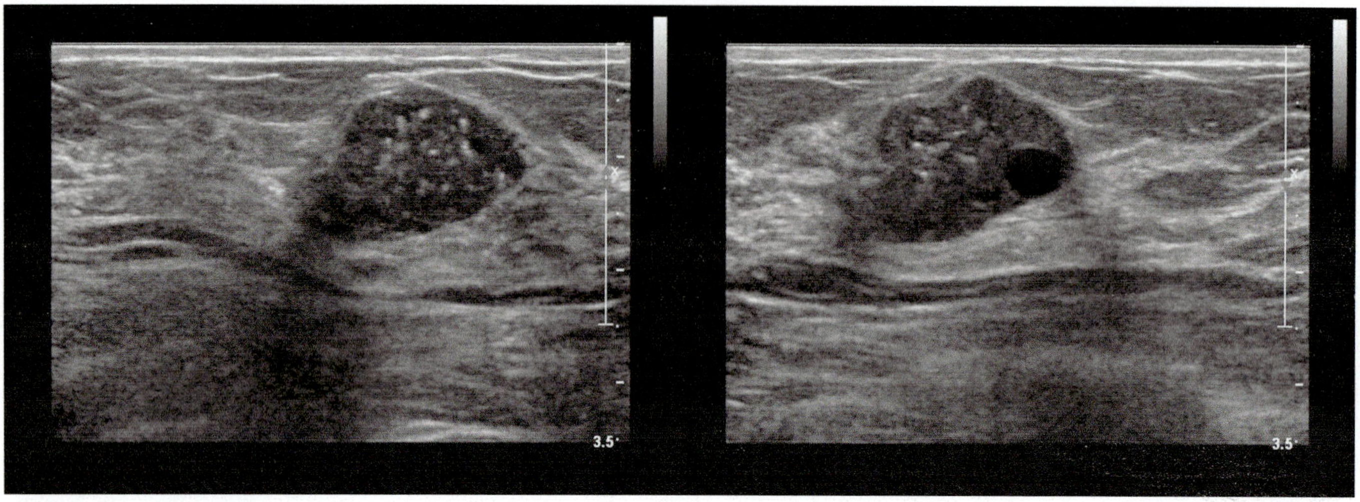

Fig. 18: Ultrasound shows a circumscribed heterogeneously hypoechoic mass with multiple echogenic foci, cystic component and posterior acoustic enhancement.

Final diagnosis: tubular adenoma of breast

Comments: Tubular adenomas of breast (also known as a pure adenoma of the breast) are extremely rare benign breast lesions typically found in young women. They are almost unknown in postmenopausal women. They have a variable appearance on mammogram where they are seen as non-calcified, round or oval masses with circumscribed or obscured margins.

Since they are seen in young women, primary imaging is almost always with ultrasound. The ultrasound findings overlap with fibroadenoma and differentiation is impossible. They are seen as circumscribed hypo-echoic lesions. Posterior acoustic enhancement may be seen.

CASE 9

History: A 52-year-old female underwent mammogram for lumpy feeling and pain in both breasts. Mammogram—Left MLO and CC views are shown (Fig. 19). She had undergone ultrasound of both breasts 2 years back which was reported as fibrocystic disease with multiple cysts in varying sizes in both breasts. No old ultrasound or mammogram images were available for comparison.

1. What are the mammogram findings?
2. Ultrasound at two different positions of left breast is shown (Fig. 20). Does it give any additional information?
3. What is combined BI-RADS and recommendation?

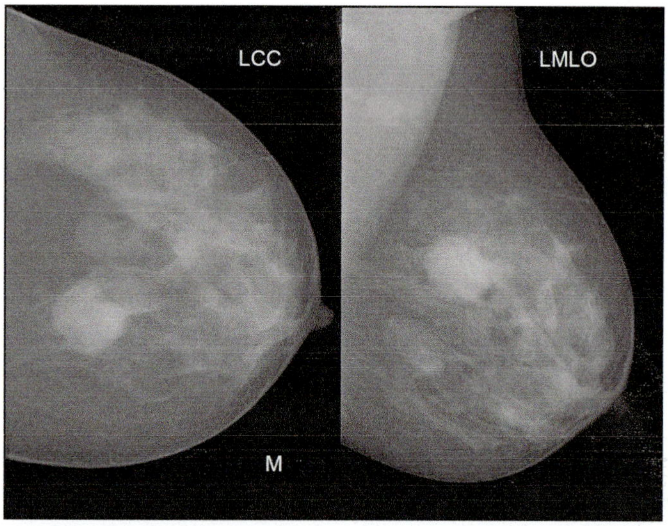

Fig. 19: Mammogram of left breast shows an equal density oval mass in nipple axis in the posterior third. Another round denser mass with irregular margins is seen supero-medial to it.

Answers

1. Mammogram of left breast shows an equal density oval mass in central part of the breast. Another dense mass with irregular margins is seen supero-medial to it. Since the patient gives a history of fibrocystic disease, the low density mass may represent a cyst while the mass with higher density needs additional imaging to categorize it. In a diagnostic setup, it is better to do additional imaging at the same sitting and give a final BI-RADS rather than giving BI-RADS 0

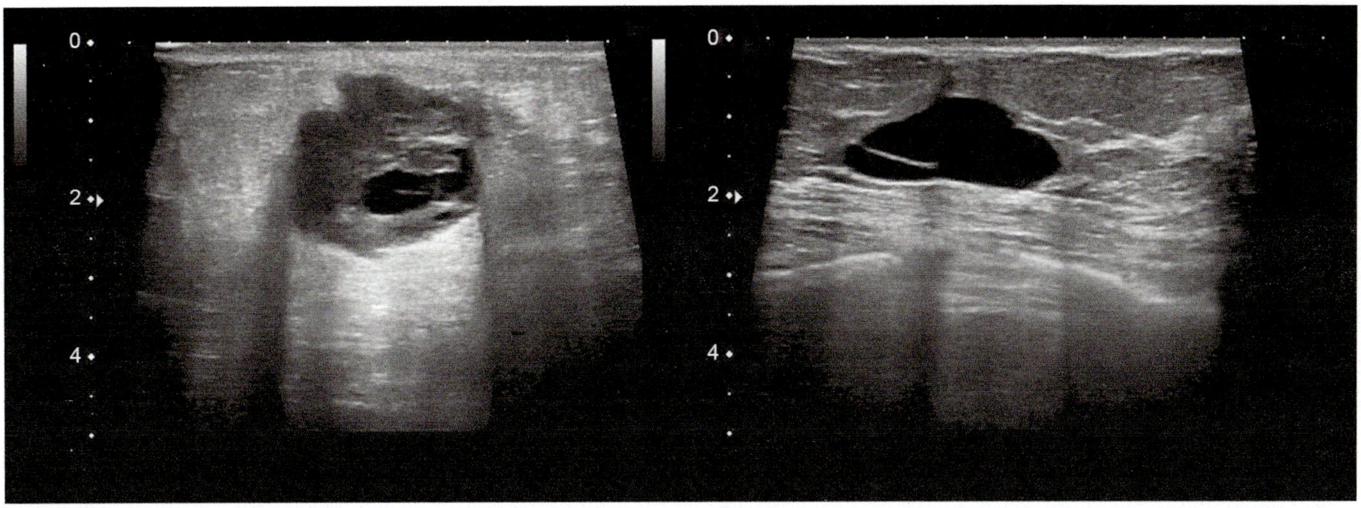

Fig. 20: Targeted ultrasound through the region of interest showed a heterogeneous mass with irregular margins and cystic component which appears suspicious. The other mass is a cyst with septation.

2. Ultrasound definitely gives additional information. There is a heterogeneous mass with irregular margins and cystic component which appears suspicious. The other mass is a cyst with septation.
3. The suspicious mass is assigned a BI-RADS category 4C and a biopsy is recommended

The patient underwent ultrasound guided biopsy. **Final diagnosis: infiltrative ductal carcinoma SBR grade 2**

Comments: Fibrocystic disease was a background finding in this patient. Fibrocystic disease is a benign entity generally showing multiple cysts in both breast in which some of the cysts may show septae or low level echoes. In this case, the suspicious lesion was an incidental finding amidst all these cysts; hence, it is important to assess the patient carefully so as not to miss any important findings. In this case, ultrasound differentiates the mass easily.

CASE 10

History: A 45-year-old female presented with a lump in left breast for last 4 months which was rapidly increasing (Fig. 21) in size. There was no history of pain or fever.

1. Describe the mammogram findings
2. What are the ultrasound findings (Fig. 22)?
3. What is the BI-RADS category?
4. What are the differential diagnoses?

Answers

1. Mammogram—MLO and CC view show a large, circumscribed mass occupying almost the whole left breast. There is skin thickening but no axillary lymph nodes are seen (Fig. 21).
2. Ultrasound of left breast shows a circumscribed, heterogeneously hypoechoic mass occupying all four quadrants. Vascularity was seen on color Doppler.
3. BI-RADS category 4B

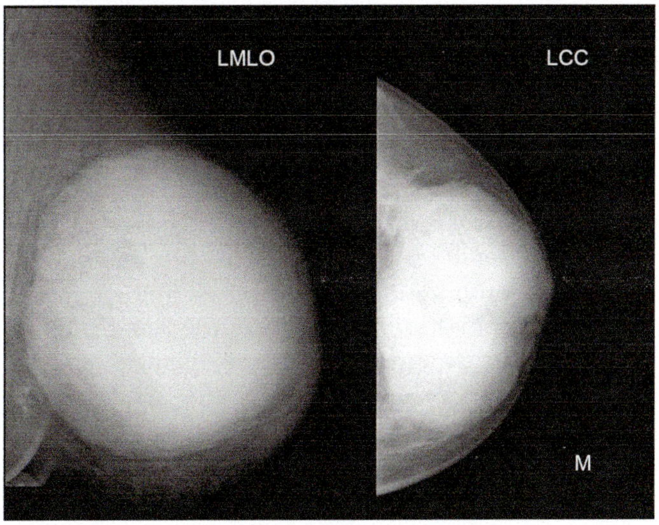

Fig. 21: MLO and CC view of left breast show a large, circumscribed mass occupying almost the whole breast with overlying skin thickening.

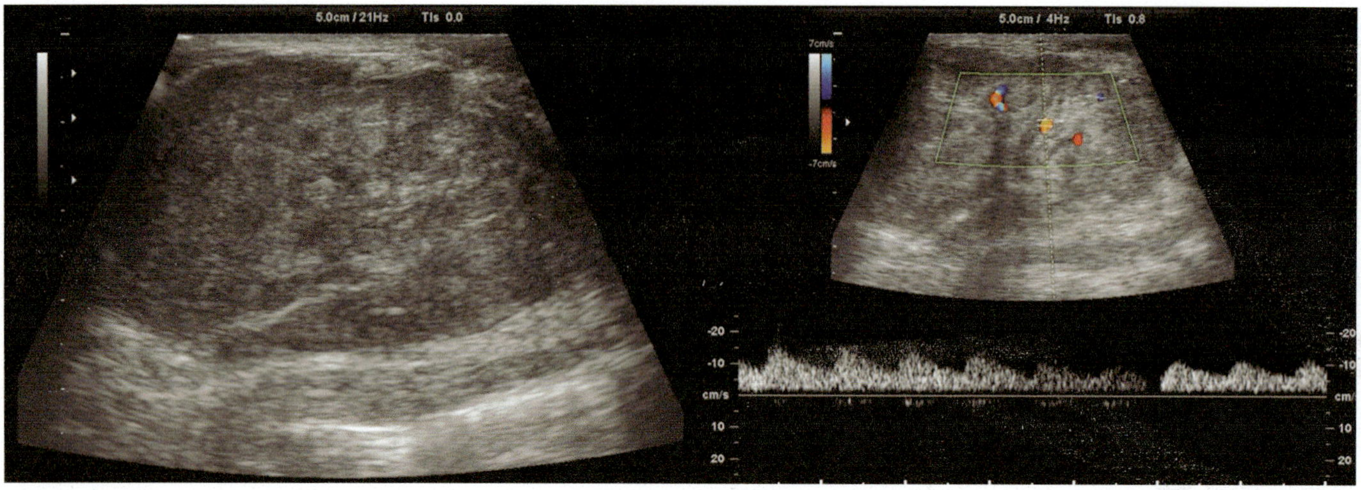

Fig. 22: Ultrasound of left breast shows a large circumscribed, heterogeneously hypoechoic mass with increased vascularity and arterial waveforms.

4. The differential diagnosis includes phyllodes tumor and metaplastic carcinoma.

Patient underwent simple mastectomy.

Final diagnosis: benign phyllodes tumor of breast

Comments: Phyllodes tumors usually occur in women from the age of 35–55 years. They often present clinically as rapidly growing discrete, palpable masses growing within weeks or months and can occupy more than one quadrant. On mammogram large, circumscribed, lobulated dense masses in varying sizes are seen either occupying a single quadrant of the breast or whole breast. Ultrasound shows large, circumscribed heterogeneously hypoechoic masses with or without cystic component. Fluid-filled, elongated spaces or clefts in a large solid mass should raise a possibility of phyllodes tumor.

CASE 11

History: A 62-year-old female presented with complaint of bilateral breast lumps for 6–8 months. She noticed one lump initially in one breast and after two months the second lump was felt in the other breast. The lumps were firm to hard in consistency on clinical examination. Mammogram of both breasts MLO and CC view were done followed by ultrasound (Figs. 23 to 25).

1. Describe mammogram findings
2. What is the breast density?
3. What are the ultrasound findings?
4. What is BI-RADS category?

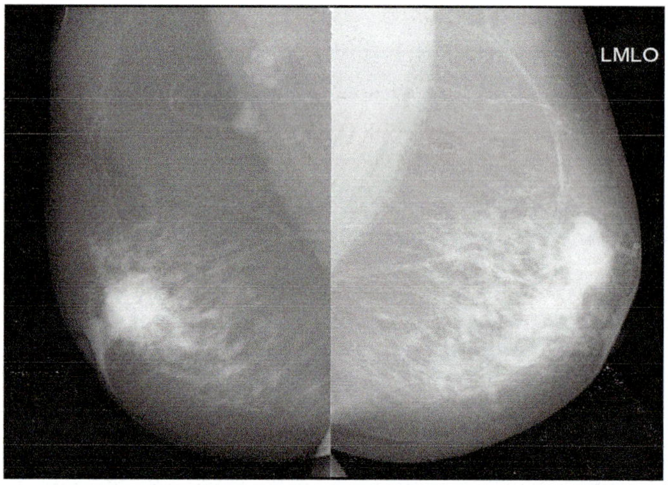

Fig. 23: Mammogram of both breasts—MLO view shows mass on both sides having partially obscured and irregular margins.

Answers

1. Mammogram of right breast shows an irregular mass with spiculated margins in retroareolar region causing nipple retraction. Another mass with irregular margins is seen in the upper outer quadrant in the anterior third of left breast.
2. The breast density is category B (ACR)—scattered fibro glandular density
3. Targeted ultrasound in right breast shows an irregular, microlobulated hypoechoic mass in the retroareolar region. A similar mass is seen in left breast in 2 o'clock position (Fig. 25).
4. BI-RADS category 5

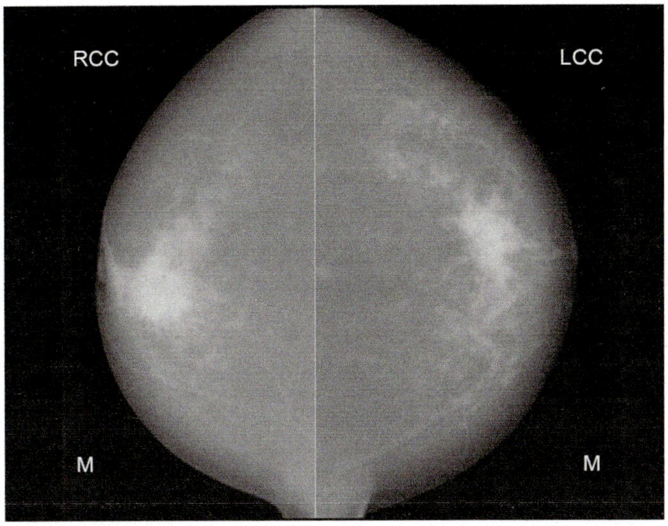

Fig. 24: Mammogram of right breast—CC view shows a mass with irregular margins in retro-areolar region causing nipple retraction. Another similar mass with irregular margins is seen in left breast.

The patient underwent core biopsy from both breast and histopathological diagnosis was invasive ductal carcinoma. Bilateral modified radical mastectomy was done.

Final diagnosis: Bilateral invasive ductal breast carcinoma

Comments: Bilateral breast cancers are not uncommon in contemporary breast clinics. The cancer which develops later can be either synchronous or metachronous. Synchronous breast cancers are defined as two tumors diagnosed with in an interval of 6 months and a second cancer diagnosed after 6 months is labeled as metachronous breast cancer.

The second cancer in bilateral cancers is diagnosed at an early stage than the index cancer. This is why screening is important for both the breasts so that cancer in contralateral breast can be detected early. Many of these cancers are estrogen dependent and seen in older age.

Bilateral cancers are common in women whose index cancer is lobular carcinoma, the first cancer is diagnosed at young age and BRCA mutations and these are risk factors.

CASE 12

History: A 49-year-old female presented with a lump in left breast and underwent lumpectomy in a peripheral setup without presurgical ultrasound or mammogram. The postoperative histopathological diagnosis was invasive ductal carcinoma. Therefore, the patient was referred to a tertiary center for further management. MLO view and magnification view of left breast are shown (Fig. 26) along with targeted ultrasound of region of interest (Fig. 27).

1. What are the mammogram findings in left breast?
2. What are the ultrasound findings?
3. What is the BI-RADS category?
4. What would you suggest and recommend to the surgeon?

Answers

1. Mammogram of left breast (MLO view) shows postoperative changes in the form of volume loss, architectural deformity and increased skin thickening along the nipple areolar region. In addition two small spiculated masses are seen in the axillary tail of left breast which are appreciated on magnification view.

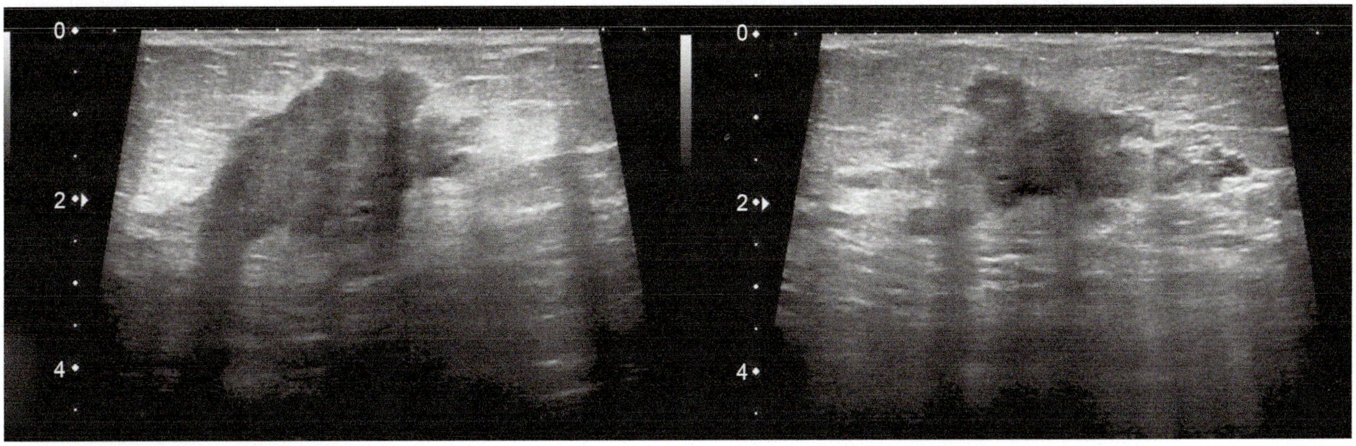

Fig. 25: Targeted ultrasound in the region of interest in right breast shows an irregular hypoechoic mass in retroareolar region having microlobulations. A similar mass is seen in left breast in 2 o'clock position.

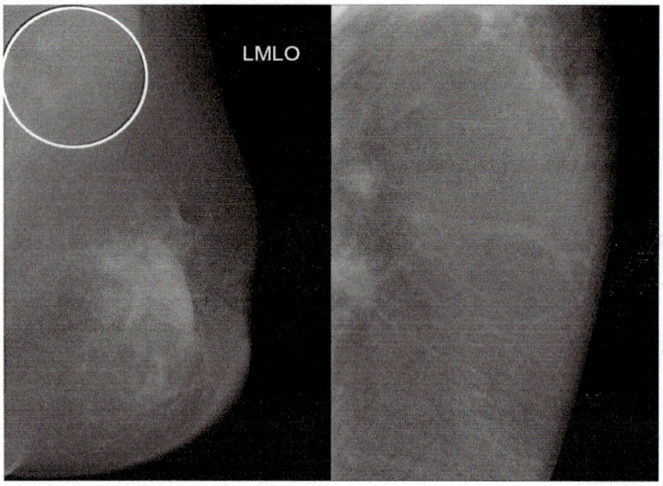

Fig. 26: Mammogram of left breast (MLO view) shows postoperative changes in the form of volume loss, architectural deformity with two small spiculated masses in the axillary tail region (white circle) better appreciated on Magnification view.

2. Targeted ultrasound shows postoperative changes in the form of increased skin thickness and surrounding echogenic fat. A circumscribed anechoic cystic mass is seen at 12–1 o'clock position of left breast s/o seroma. Two small hypoechoic lesions with irregular margins and dense posterior acoustic shadowing were seen in axillary tail of left breast.
3. BI-RADS category 5.
4. The masses in the axillary region could represent residual lymph node masses which are highly suggestive of malignancy and require biopsy for confirmation.

The patient underwent are excision and axillary clearance. Histopathology confirmed metastatic lymph nodes. There was no residual malignant mass in the breast.

Final diagnosis: postoperative case of malignant breast mass showing seroma with residual metastatic axillary lymph nodes

Comments: Sometimes the patient is referred for mammogram after surgery and no previous mammograms or ultrasound films are available for comparison. In such cases, it is pertinent to ask the histopathological report of previous surgery. If the report shows malignant findings then signs of residual malignancy are what the radiologist has to look for and if it is present, the treating clinician has to be informed so that proper management can be done.

CASE 13

History: A 21-year-old female presented with complaint of multiple lumps in both breasts for 4 months. The lumps were painless and were mobile on palpation. Ultrasound of both breasts was done (Figs. 28 to 31).

1. Describe the ultrasound findings
2. What is BI-RADS category?
3. What is the type of vascularity seen in these masses?

Answers

1. There are multiple horizontally oriented, mildly heterogeneous hypoechoic masses with smooth undulations. One of the masses shows vascularity.
2. BI-RADS category 3—Fibroadenomas
3. The type of vascularity seen in fibroadenoma is as follows:
   a. Feeding vessels: These are vessels which extend form the normal breast tissue into fibroadenoma
   b. Vessels in the capsule of fibroadenoma
   c. Vessels located in the septae of fibroadenoma

Final diagnosis: Multiple fibroadenomas.

Comments: Fibroadenomas are benign tumors frequently seen in young woman between 20 and 30 years of age and are composed of stromal and epithelial elements. On

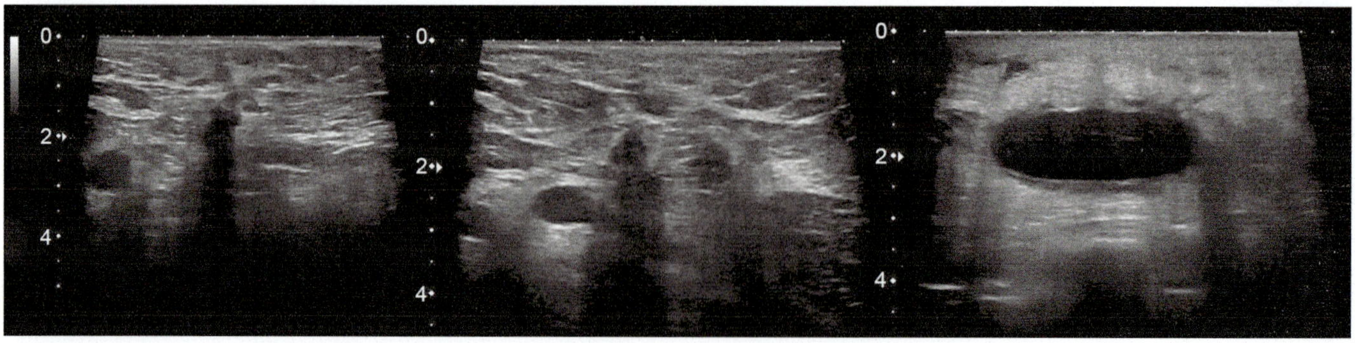

Fig. 27: Targeted ultrasound through axillary tail region of left breast shows two small hypoechoic lesions with irregular margins and posterior acoustic shadowing. In addition a seroma was seen at 12 to 1 o' clock position of left breast.

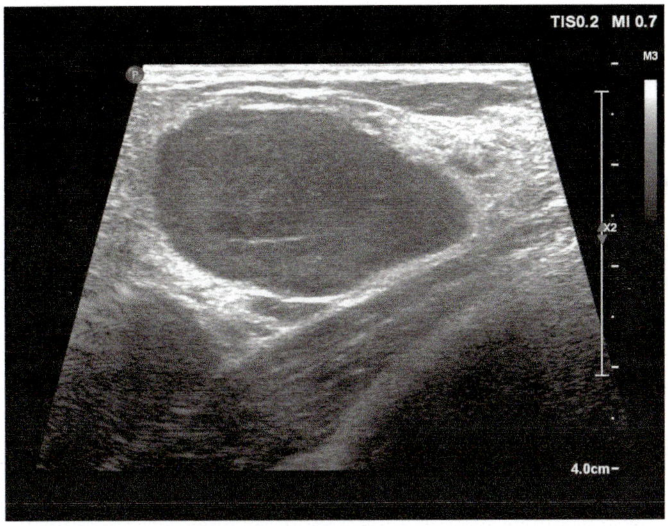

Fig. 28: Ultrasound of left breast shows a horizontally oriented, hypoechoic mass with smooth undulations.

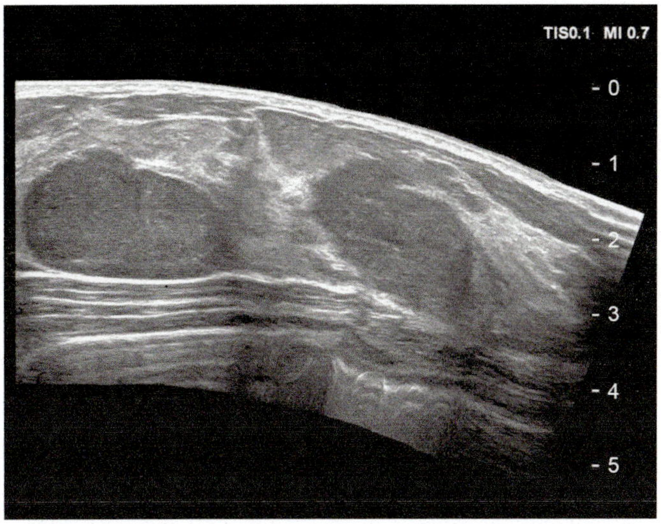

Fig. 30: Ultrasound of left breast with extended field of view showed two circumscribed hypoechoic masses one after the other.

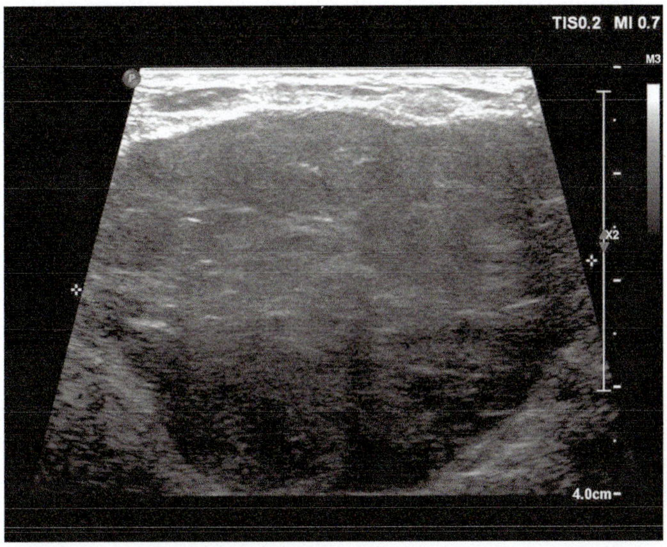

Fig. 29: Ultrasound of right breast shows a horizontally oriented, heterogenously hypoechoic mass.

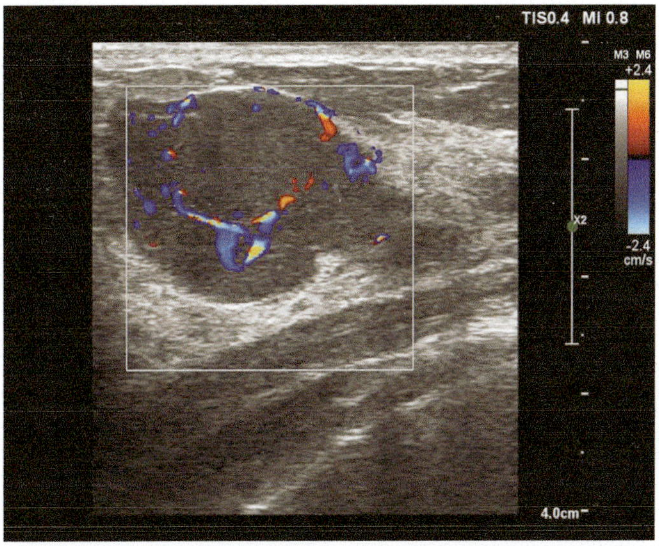

Fig. 31: Ultrasound showing Feeding vessels and capsular vessels into the fibroadenoma.

mammograms, they are seen as circumscribed, equal density masses having smooth margins and macrolobulations. They can be multiple and bilateral.

There is an increased risk of cancer in complex and multiple fibroadenomas which is twice higher than in patients without fibroadenomas.

On ultrasound, fibroadenomas have variable appearances ranging from homogeneous hypoechoic to heterogeneous hypoechoic masses with or without vascularity. The vascularity can be peripheral or central or both. In malignancy, there are radially aligned external vessels and the number of internal vessels are more than external. Marginal or peripheral vessels are more commonly seen in benign lesions.

CASE 14

History: 1. A 54-year-old female presented with complaint of rapidly growing lump in left breast. Her mammogram is shown in Figure 32.

1. What is the breast density?
2. What are the findings on mammogram?
3. What is BI-RADS category?

Answers

1. The breast shows scattered fibroglandular tissue-B category (ACR).
2. A large circumscribed mass is seen in retroareolar region of right breast with pleomorphic calcifications and obscured margins at places. There is overlying skin thickening and nipple retraction. The mass is extending up to the posterior third of the breast and is infiltrating the pectoralis major muscle
3. BI-RADS category 5

The patient underwent modified radical mastectomy on right side.

Final diagnosis: BI-RADS 5 mass with pectoralis muscle invasion

Comments: Assessment of pectoralis muscle invasion is important for treatment planning for breast cancer which can be suspected on mammogram. Some studies have used MRI for evaluation of pectoralis muscle and showed that enhancement of the pectoralis muscle correlates well with muscle invasion with a few potential pitfalls. Disruption of the fat plane between tumor and muscle, without muscle enhancement, might not indicate tumor involvement of the pectoralis muscle. Although pectoralis muscle involvement alone does not change the clinical breast cancer stage, it is important to include this information in radiology reports because it will alter surgical management.

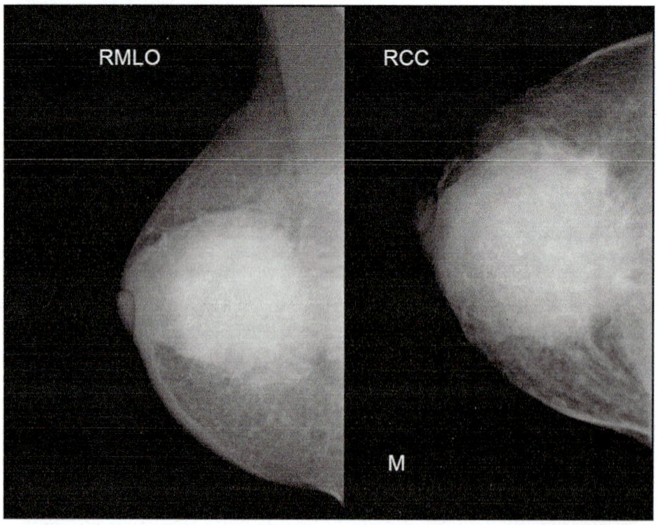

Fig. 32: Mammogram of right breast—MLO and CC view show a large circumscribed mass in retro areolar region with pleomorphic calcifications exteding into retroglandular region and abutting/infiltrating pectoralis muscle.

CASE 15

History: A 48-year-old female presented with complaint of lump in right breast. She underwent mammogram (Fig. 33) and ultrasound (Fig. 34).

1. What is breast density on mammogram?
2. Describe the mammogram findings. What kind of calcification is seen in cysts on mammogram?
3. What are the ultrasound findings?
4. What is BI-RADS category?

Answers

1. The breast density on mammogram is scattered fibroglandular tissue—B category (ACR).
2. Mammogram—MLO and CC view of right breast show multiple, circumscribed, round masses with a lucent halo in a few of them. The halo sign is commonly seen in benign lesions like cysts. On mammogram, rim calcifications are commonly seen in cysts. When there is dependent calcium layering within breast cysts it is seen as "tea cup" or "crescent-shaped" calcifications on a true lateral (LM or ML) view.
3. Ultrasound shows multiple circumscribed round and lobulated cystic masses adjacent to each other. There

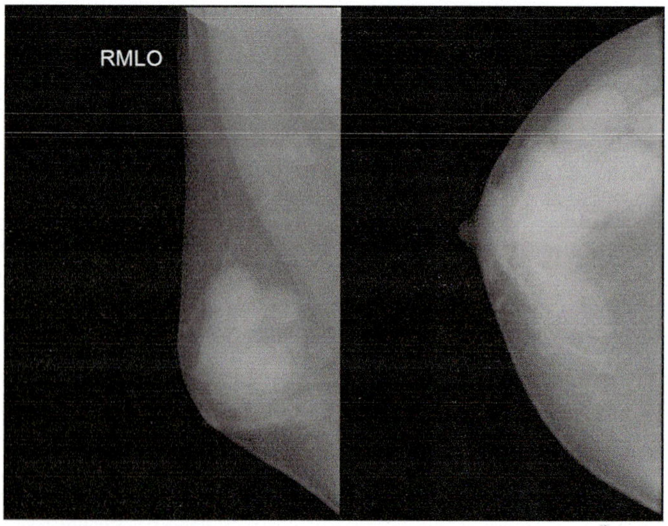

Fig. 33: Mammogram of right breast—MLO and CC view show multiple, circumscribed, round masses with a lucent halo in a few of them.

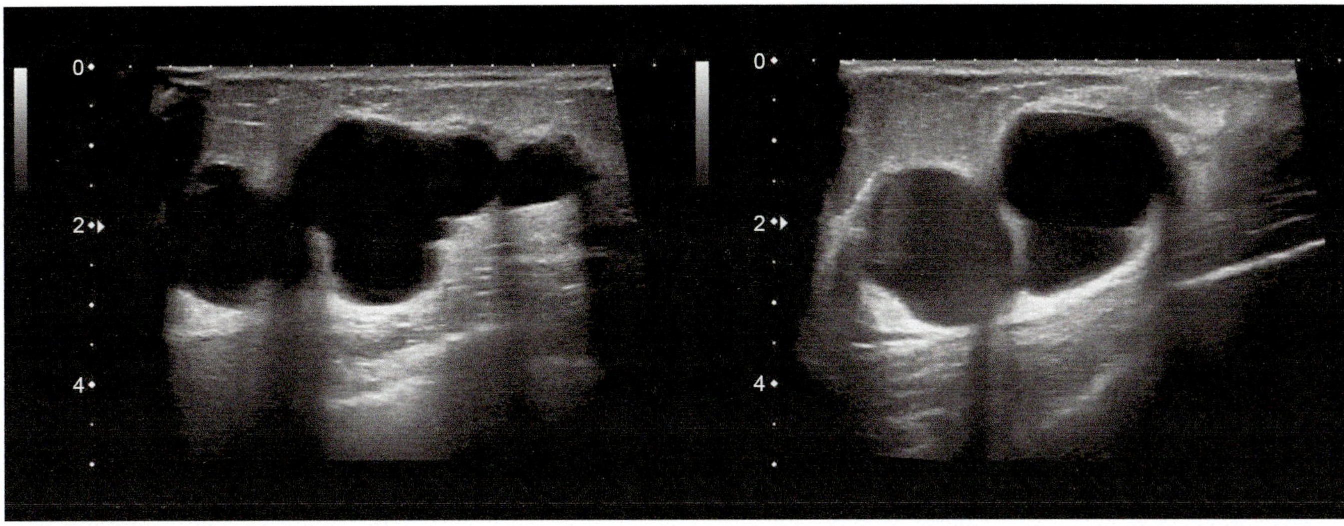

Fig. 34: Ultrasound shows multiple circumscribed round and lobulated cystic masses some of them are intercommunicating with each other. No calcification or debris seen.

are no septations or internal echoes within which means that there is no ultrasound evidence of complicated cysts

4. BI-RADS category 2

Final diagnosis: Multiple simple breast cysts

Comments: Simple cysts are one of the most common benign breast masses and do not require any treatment unless they become symptomatic due to increase in size or when they get infected when aspiration has to be done. Milk of calcium is found much more frequently in small breast cysts.

When a cyst is seen on ultrasound, it is important to comment if it is a simple cyst, complicated cyst or complex cyst as management differs for complex cystic lesions.

CASE 16

History: A 46-year-old female underwent lumpectomy in left breast for a cyst following ultrasound findings in a peripheral setup (preoperative ultrasound images are not available). The postsurgical histopathology findings showed evidence of malignancy. She was then referred for mammogram and further management to a tertiary care hospital.

Mammogram and ultrasound images are shown in Figures 35 and 36.

1. What is the breast density?
2. What is one positive finding do you see? Which view would you suggest?
3. Describe the ultrasound features.

Answers

1. The breasts are extremely dense—D category (ACR).
2. There is pleomorphic microcalcification grouped well depicted on magnification view which shows the morphology of calcifications clearly (shown within black circle).
3. Ultrasound shows a fluid collection which is s/o seroma.

Final diagnosis: malignant microcalcifications

Comments: For a 46-year-old woman, it is important to note that mammogram should have been done, followed

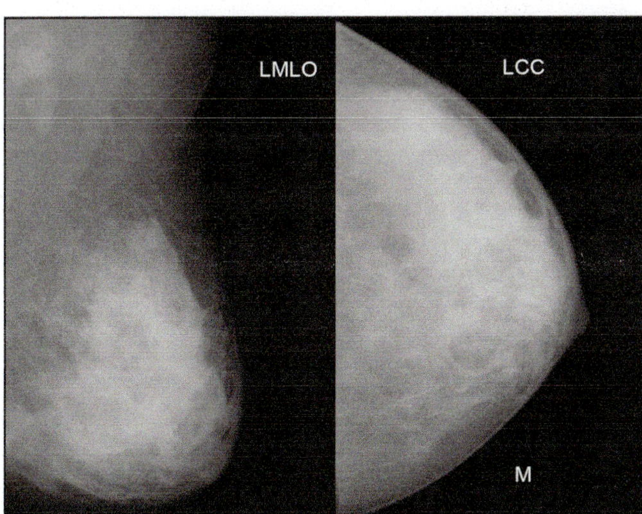

Fig. 35: Mammogram of left breast—MLO and CC view show subtle pleomorphic calcification.

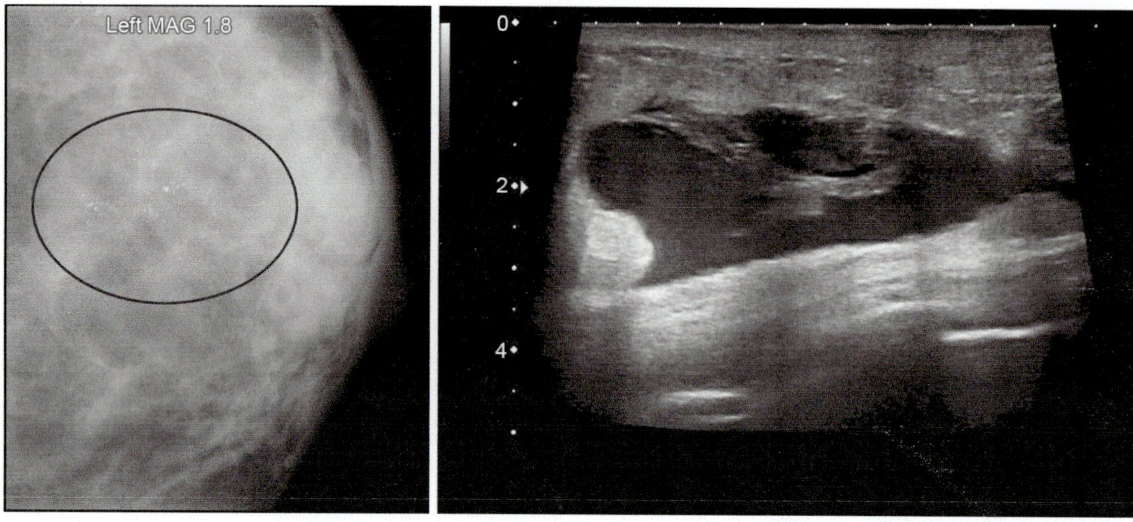

Fig. 36: Magnification view through the region of interest confirmed the microcalcification while ultrasound showed a circumscribed collection s/o seroma from postoperative site.

by ultrasound if required. Mammogram is the modality of choice to show microcalcifications which can be benign, suspicious or malignant and these can be missed on ultrasound. In fact ductal carcinoma in situ is detected on mammogram and on mammogram only.

This lady was operated based on ultrasound findings only where only the cyst was seen and lumpectomy was done leaving behind the malignant microcalcifications which were not detected on ultrasound. The onus is up to the radiologists to make both the clinician and patient aware of the appropriate radiological investigation patient must undergo depending upon her age and clinical findings.

CASE 17

History: A 48-year-old female had undergone breast conservative surgery for a malignant mass in right breast and follow-up annual mammogram was done. Mammogram craniocaudal view is shown in Figure 37.

1. Describe the mammogram findings
2. What is your diagnosis?
3. What is the BI-RADS category?

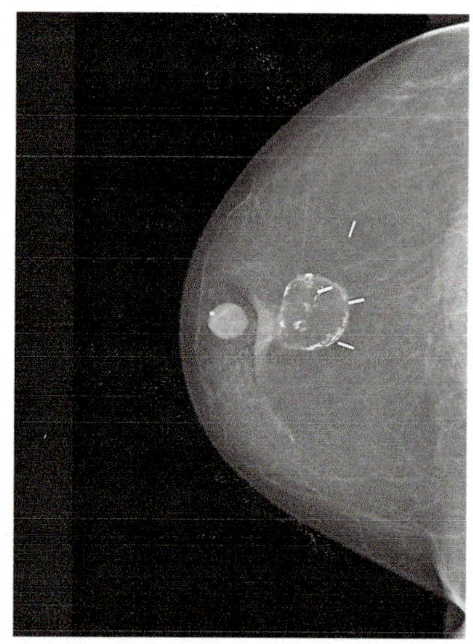

Fig. 37: Mammogram CC view in a conservatively treated breast shows a circumscribed lucent cyst with rim calcification s/o fat necrosis.

Answers

1. Postoperative changes are seen in the form of architectural deformity, surgical staples and nipple retraction. In addition, there is a circumscribed fat-density mass at the surgical site having a rim calcifications.
2. Fat necrosis
3. BI-RADS category 2

Final diagnosis: Fat necrosis following breast conservative surgery.

Comments: Fat necrosis is a benign non-suppurative inflammatory process of adipose tissue seen in post-traumatic breast or in patients with history of breast surgery. Its imaging appearances on mammogram depend upon the stage of evolution. In early stages, it is seen as a soft-tissue density mass with partial halo, while in later stages, it is seen as a small circumscribed lucent mass with a rim calcification. Presence of fatty tissue in breast mass is usually a sign of benignity and no further assessment is required.

CASE 18

History: A 55-year-old female underwent routine mammogram. Mammogram of right breast—MLO and CC view are shown in Figure 38.

1. Describe the mammogram findings
2. What is BI-RADS category?
3. What is BI-RADS recommendation?

Answers

1. There is a high-density mass in the nipple axis with irregular margins and comet tail and grouped pleomorphic microcalcifications.
2. BI-RADS category 5
3. Biopsy should be done to establish the diagnosis.

Final diagnosis: malignant mass with microcalcifications

Comments: Biopsy showed invasive ductal carcinoma.

Mammography is the modality of choice to detect suspicious or malignant microcalcifications including fine pleomorphic, fine branching and coarse heterogeneous. Sometimes, the malignant masses appear circumscribed, but one should look for areas of irregular margins, comet tail sign, lobulations or suspicious calcifications which can be present in these masses. With the use of high resolution transducers these microcalcifications can also be seen within the mass on ultrasound as tiny echogenic foci with or without posterior acoustic shadowing.

CASE 19

History: A 55-year-old female presented with lump in right breast for 6 months that was painless and hard on palpation. Mammogram MLO and CC view are shown (Fig. 39).

1. What are the mammogram findings?
2. Describe the findings in axilla
3. What is the BI-RADS category?

Answers

1. An irregular mass is seen in upper outer quadrant of right breast with spiculations and obscured margins at places. There is surrounding architectural deformity; however, no microcalcifications are present. Multiple enlarged axillary lymph nodes were seen either.
2. Multiple lobulated and a few round lymph nodes are present in the axilla some of them show loss of fatty hilum.
3. BI-RADS category 5

Biopsy from the breast mass and axilla showed invasive ductal carcinoma with metastatic lymphadenopathy.

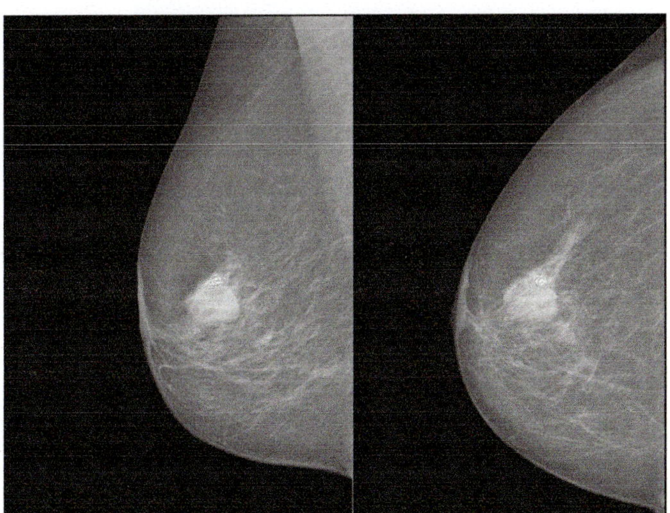

Fig. 38: Mammogram of right breast—MLO and CC view show a high-density mass in the central part with irregular margins, comet tail and grouped pleomorphic microcalcifications.

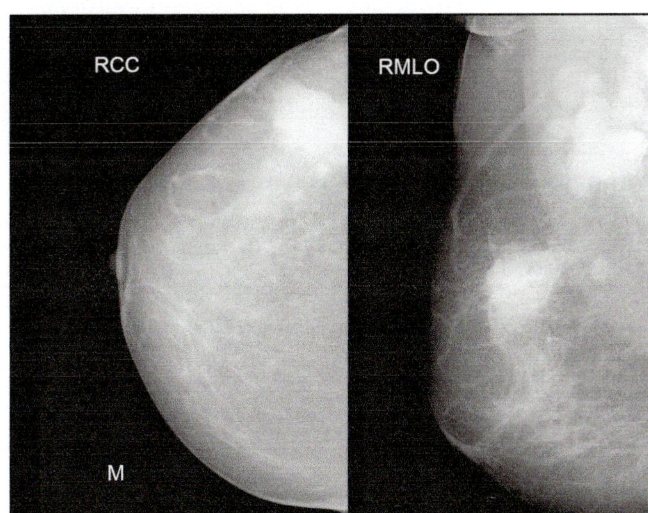

Fig. 39: Mammogram of right breast: CC and MLO view show an irregular mass in upper outer quadrant with spiculations and obscured margins. Multiple enlarged axillary lymphnodes were also seen.

Patient underwent right mastectomy with axillary clearance followed by radiotherapy and chemotherapy.

Final diagnosis: malignant mass with metastatic lymphadenopathy

Comments: Whenever there are axillary lymph nodes on mammogram in the presence of a suspicious mass in breast, they should always be commented upon. One should look for shape, size, loss of fatty hilum, margins and microcalcifications. An ultrasound should be done and morphology of lymph nodes along with their level can be commented upon as some surgeons are more comfortable with ultrasound findings. This helps the treating surgeon to decide the course of treatment.

CASE 20

History: A 51-year-old female had a lumpectomy for a benign mass in left breast 2 years back. She felt a thickening in left breast in upper quadrant and underwent a mammography. Craniocaudal view of both breasts and MLO view of left breast are shown in Figures 40 and 41, respectively.

1. What is the breast density as per ACR.
2. Describe the mammogram findings
3. What is the BI-RADS category?

Answers

1. The breast density is category B—scattered fibroglandular tissue.
2. There is an asymmetry in lateral part on craniocaudal view of left breast with skin thickening. MLO view shows a focal asymmetry with pleomorphic microcalcification in the posterior third near axillary tail region. Targeted ultrasound of this area showed a heterogeneous area, no obvious mass was seen.
3. The finding on mammogram in left breast appears suspicious for malignancy hence BI-RADS category 4 is assigned.

Final diagnosis: malignancy arising in scar tissue at the surgical site

Comments: Patient underwent an excision biopsy with wide local excision. Histopathology showed invasive ductal carcinoma SBR grade II and tubular carcinoma with foci of microglandular adenosis like arising in scar. Although malignancy arising in scar tissue is not common, this case stresses the importance of obtaining prior surgical history. The operative site should be looked at carefully for scar tissue and for any other significant changes compared to previous mammogram. In addition focused ultrasound of the surgical site should be done to look for any positive findings.

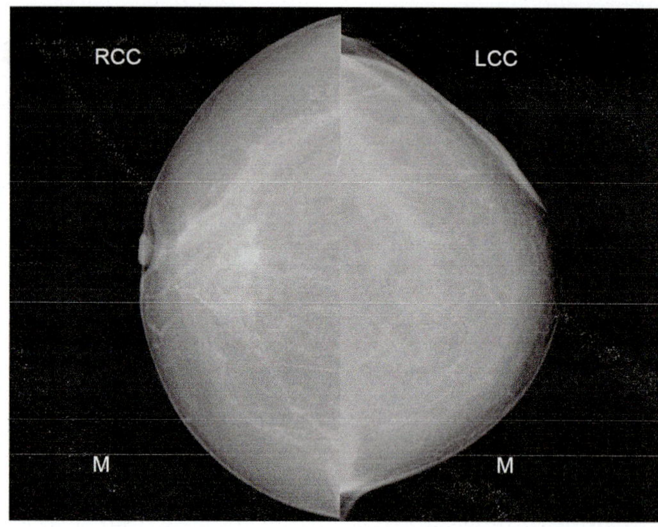

Fig. 40: Mammogram CC view of left breast shows skin thickening in lateral quadrant.

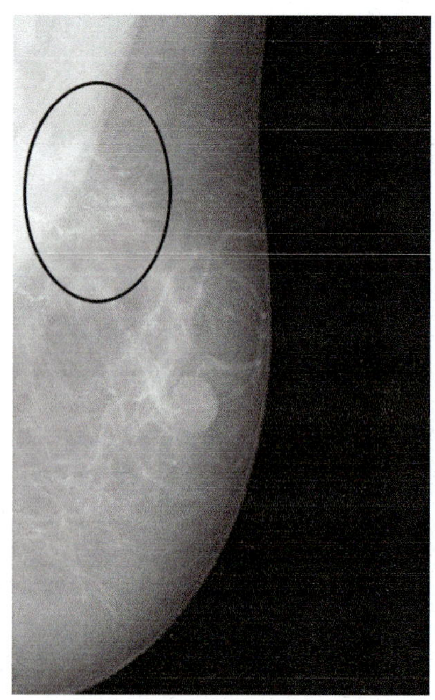

Fig. 41: Mammogram MLO view of left breast shows a focal asymmetry with pleomorphic microcalcification.

LEVEL 3

CASE 1

History: A 60-year-old female underwent a screening mammogram of both breasts. Figure 1 shows mammogram of left breast, CC and MLO views.

1. What are the findings on mammogram?
2. Are there any additional views which are useful in such a case?

Answer

Mammogram of left breast showed multiple cutaneous nodules in the nipple areolar complex and along the rest of the cutaneous surface of the left breast showing incomplete border sign. This patient was a known case of neurofibromatosis and the nodules represented multiple neurofibromas.

Additional view which are useful are tangential view in such a case to show the origin from the skin surface.

Final diagnosis: multiple neurofibromas in left breast

Comments: Medical devices, scars and nevus on the skin may create pseudomasses; hence, the patients' skin should be examined properly by the radiographer and a note made on the mammogram requisition form. A proper history from the patient is always very useful.

Normally the skin lesions have air surrounding them but they can have a complicated look if ointment is applied by the patients.

A tangential view or use of a BB marker can help in differentiating skin lesion from a breast mass on mammogram.

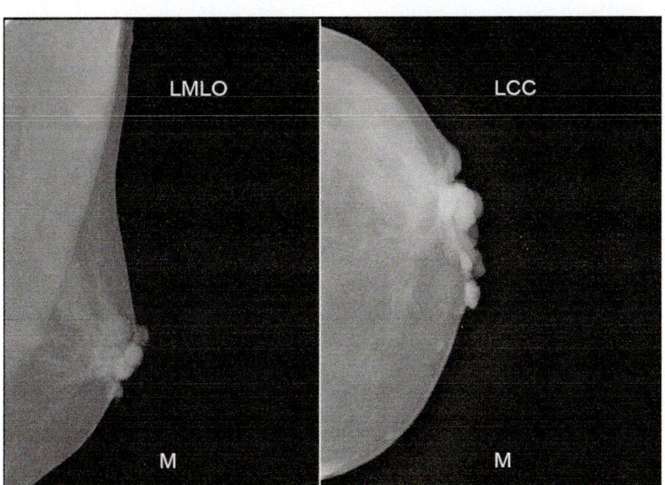

Fig. 1: Mammogram of left breast showed multiple cutaneous soft tissue densities in the nipple areolar complex and along the rest of the cutaneous surface of the left breast showing incomplete border sign.

CASE 2

History: A 37-year-old female was referred for mammogram and ultrasound of breast with a complaint of a palpable, painless left breast lump for three months.

1. Mammogram of both breasts-craniocaudal (CC) views are shown (Fig. 2). Describe the mammogram findings.
2. Which special ultrasound view is shown in Figure 3 and what are its advantages?
3. What are the ultrasound findings?

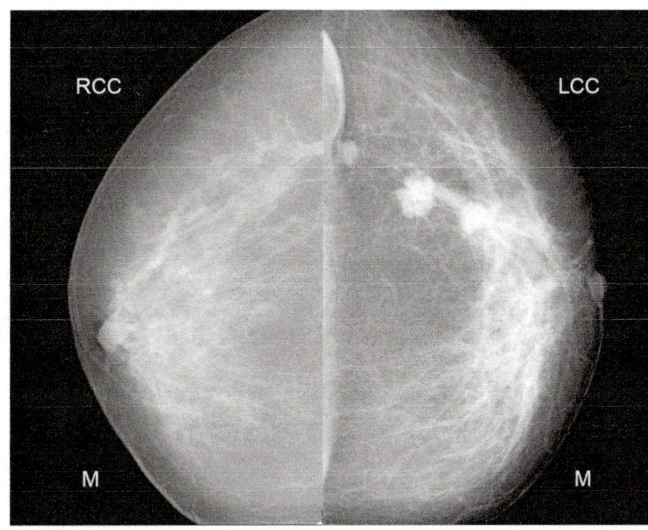

Fig. 2: Mammogram of left breast—CC view showed multiple masses as described in text suspicious of multifocality.

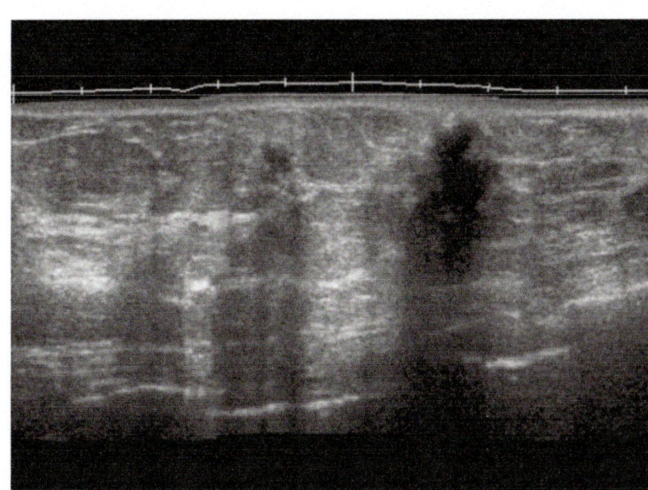

Fig. 3: Ultrasound of left breast—Panoramic view showed the multiple masses and their distance from each another.

Answers

1. Mammogram of left breast—CC view shows a spiculated dense mass lesion in the middle third in lateral quadrant. Another smaller irregular rounded dense mass is demonstrated in the anterior third of same quadrant. There is also a circumscribed dense oval focal asymmetry/mass in the posterior third in the same quadrant. Multifocality is highly suspicious.
2. Ultrasound of left breast—panoramic view is shown in Figure 2. The advantage of panoramic view is that it shows the relationship of the mass/masses with rest of the breast parenchyma. It is especially useful in multiple masses to assess the distance between the masses to differentiate between multicentric and multifocal masses.
3. Ultrasound of left breast confirmed the above findings and shows both round and irregular hypoechoic masses with posterior acoustic shadowing. In addition, a smaller hypoechoic mass was also seen.

Ultrasound guided biopsy showed features of mixed carcinoma. Histopathology from the bigger nodule was suggestive of mixed carcinoma: invasive ductal carcinoma NOS SBR II with micropapillary area and cribriform invasive carcinoma.

Histopathology from smaller nodules was suggestive of invasive mucinous carcinoma with invasive ductal carcinoma—SBR grade II.

The patient underwent quadrantectomy.

Final diagnosis: multifocal malignancy

Comments:

Multifocal and multicentric tumors

The presence of two or more foci of cancer within the same breast quadrant is defined as multifocal, while the presence of two or more foci of cancer in different quadrants of the same breast and separated by >5 cm of normal breast tissue is defined as multicentric.

Multifocal cancers occur in 10–12% of patients. A synchronous contralateral tumor occurs within 3–12 months of diagnosis of initial tumor. Approximately 52% of the cases with multifocal and multicentric masses have axillary node involvement. These patients have an increased tumor load and an aggressive breast cancer. Multifocal cancers are more common than multicentric cancers.

CASE 3

History: A 52-year-old female underwent conservation surgery of left breast 2 years ago for invasive ductal carcinoma. She was on regular follow-up and underwent annual mammogram examinations.

1. Mammogram of left breast-CC and MLO views are shown in Figure 4:
   a. An irregular mass is seen. True/False
   b. A circumscribed mass is seen. True/False
   c. Postoperative changes are seen. True/False
2. Ultrasound of left breast in the region of interest revealed (Figs. 5 and 6):
   a. A circumscribed heterogeneously hypoechoic mass with an anechoic rim. True/False
   b. An irregular hypoechoic mass. True/False
3. Is biopsy indicated in this case? Yes/No
4. If answer to above question is "yes," please indicate the site from which biopsy is taken:
   a. From the circumscribed heterogeneous lesion. Yes/No
   b. From the irregular mass. Yes/No
5. What is your diagnosis?
   a. Seroma
   b. Recurrence
   c. Both

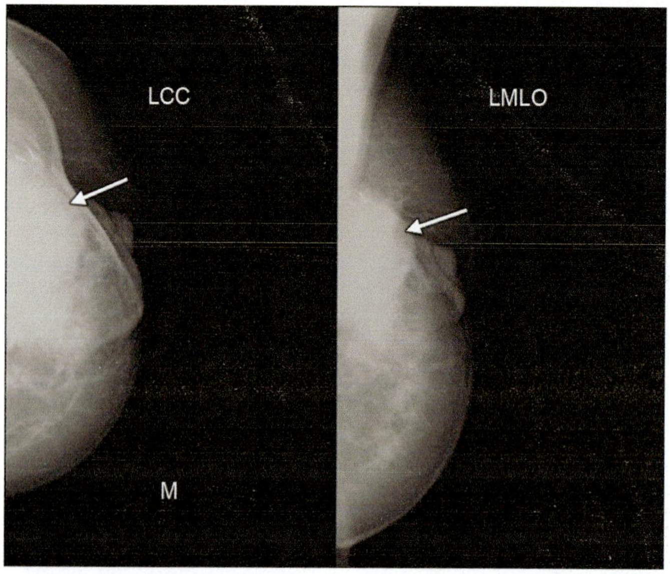

Fig. 4: Mammogram of left breast—CC and MLO view show postoperative changes in the form of skin fold and surgical staples at the surgical site with a circumscribed mass (arrow) s/o seroma.

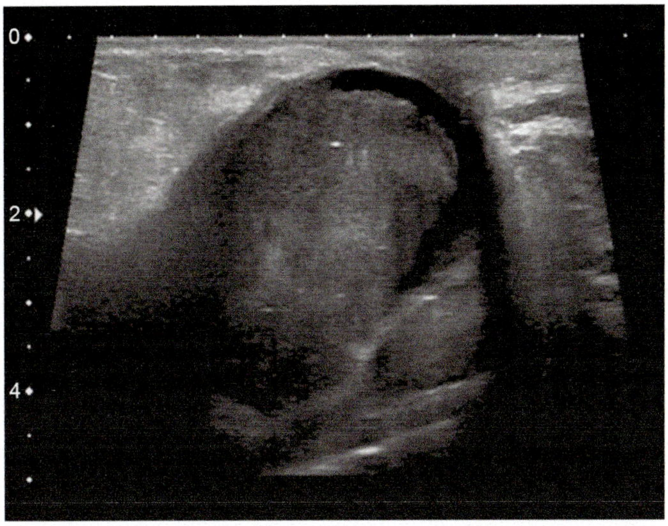

Fig. 5: Targeted ultrasound through the region of interest confirmed a large circumscribed heterogeneous lesion with anechoic rim-seroma.

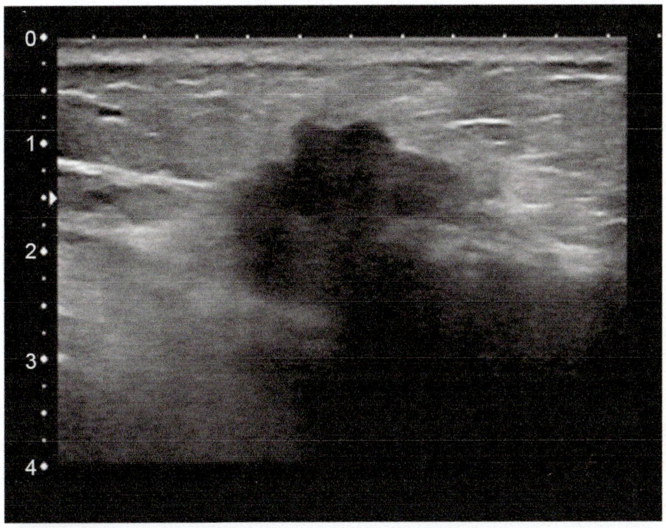

Fig. 6: Ultrasound also showed a suspicious irregular hypoechoic mass noted adjacent to the seroma.

Answers

1. a. False, b. True, c. True
2. a. True, b. True
3. Yes
4. a. No, b. Yes
5. c.

Findings: Mammogram of left breast—CC and MLO view shows postoperative changes in the form of skin fold and surgical staples at the surgical site with a circumscribed mass (arrow) s/o seroma (Fig. 4). The patient underwent a targeted ultrasound of the region of interest which confirmed the same and showed a large circumscribed heterogeneous lesion with anechoic rim (Figs. 5 and 6). In addition, an irregular hypoechoic mass was noted adjacent to the seroma. Since this was a new lesion which was not mentioned in earlier reports, a possibility of recurrence was considered and the patient underwent ultrasound-guided core needle biopsy from this mass. Histopathology was s/o invasive ductal carcinoma. Therefore, the patient had a recurrent malignant mass at surgical site. Mammogram had shown increased breast density due to seroma.

The patient underwent mastectomy and axillary clearance.

Final diagnosis: recurrence in conservatively treated breast with seroma

Comments: The reporting of postoperative mammograms is a challenge especially for the budding radiologist and has a learning curve. In a conservatively treated breast, it is always better to compare serial mammograms, so that any changes from previous films are not missed.

On mammogram, seromas are usually seen as oval or round mass at the surgical site with surrounding architectural deformity. The ultrasound appearances of seroma include a circumscribed anechoic collection, collection with thick wall or septations or with mural nodule, a hypoechoic lesion or a cystic lesion showing an echogenic mesh like appearance, which may reduce in size over a period of time or may persist for a few years.

The signs of recurrence on mammogram include relative increase in asymmetry or skin thickening or edema, enlarging mass or appearance of pleomorphic calcifications near the tumor site.

CASE 4

History: A 32-year-old female in her postpartum period presented to the emergency triage with a complaint of breathlessness. She gave a history of a rapidly progressive painless lump in left breast for last 4 months. She underwent CXR and ultrasound of left breast (Figs. 7 and 8).

1. Looking at the chest X-ray, answer the following:
   a. The left breast shadow is enlarged. True/False
   b. There is rib destruction on the left side. True/False
   c. A nodular opacity is seen in right lung. True/False
2. What are the findings on ultrasound of left breast?
   a. A large complex cystic mass is seen. True/False
   b. A complicated cyst is seen. True/False

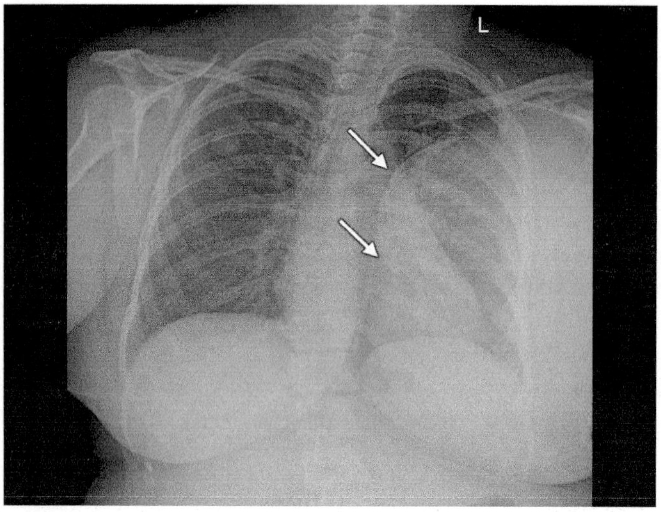

Fig. 7: CXR PA view showed enlarged left breast shadow (arrows) and a nodular opacity in right lung.

   c. Multiple septations are seen in cystic component. True/False

3. What are the differential diagnoses based on ultrasound findings?
4. What BI-RADS category would you assign to it?
5. Does Chest X-ray give additional information?
6. What are the findings on MRI of chest?

Answers

1. a. True, b. False, c. True
2. a. True, b. False, c. True
3. The differential diagnosis includes: Phyllodes tumor, metaplastic carcinoma
4. BI-RADS 4B
5. Yes, chest X-ray shows nodular opacity in right lung s/o metastases
6. MRI of chest T2W sequence with and without fat suppression shows a complex cystic mass in left breast with a large hyperintense cystic component. There are metastatic nodules in both lungs. In addition there is involvement of anterior pericardium (Fig. 9).

Final diagnosis: metaplastic carcinoma of breast with lung metastases and involvement of the anterior pericardium

Comments: This mass was so large that it did not fit into the breast coil hence MRI of the thorax had to be done. Metaplastic carcinoma is a rare malignancy (0.25–1%) characterized by mixture of epithelial and mesenchymal components histologically. It is commonly seen in postmenopausal women.

It has variable features on imaging with mammography showing high-density mass with circumscribed, obscured, irregular or spiculated margins.

On ultrasound, a circumscribed or irregular heterogeneously hypoechoic solid mass may be seen. Sometimes a mixed solid cystic mass is noted with microlobulated or indistinct margins. This tumor commonly metastasizes to lungs and bones. When a cystic component is present, phyllodes tumor should be considered as a differential diagnosis.

The predictors affecting poor outcome in metaplastic carcinoma are skin invasion, younger age (<39 years of age) at presentation and squamous cell carcinoma in the lymph nodes.

This patient died after two months of starting chemotherapy.

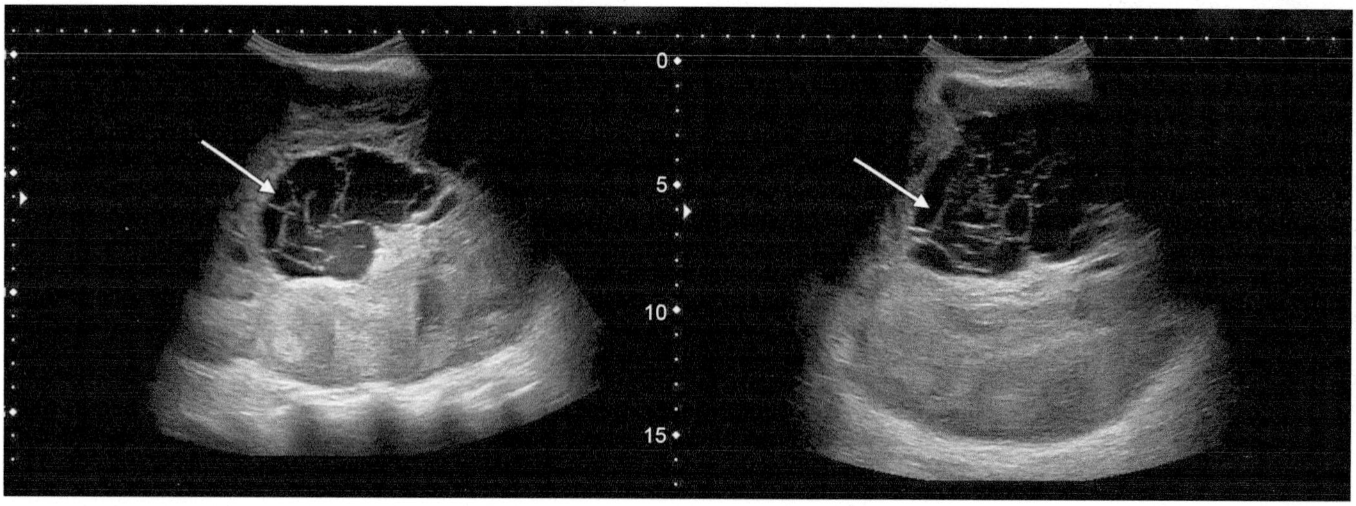

Fig. 8: Ultrasound showed a large circumscribed complex cystic mass with multiple septations and a large solid component.

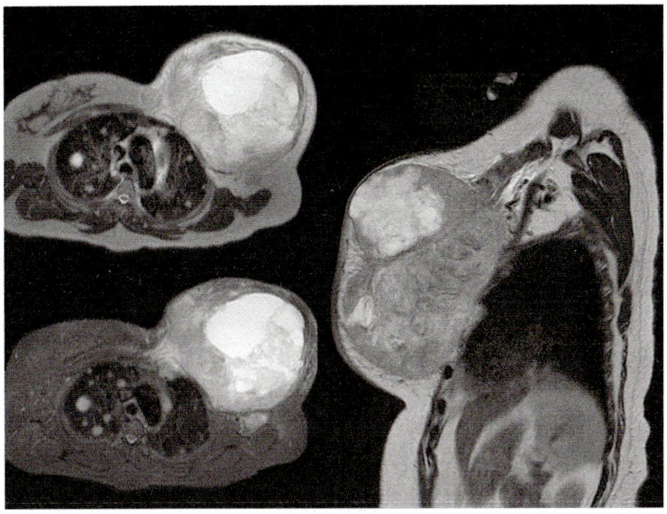

Fig. 9: MRI of chest T2W with and without fat suppression shows a complex cystic mass in left breast with metastatic nodules in both lungs and anterior pericardium involvement.

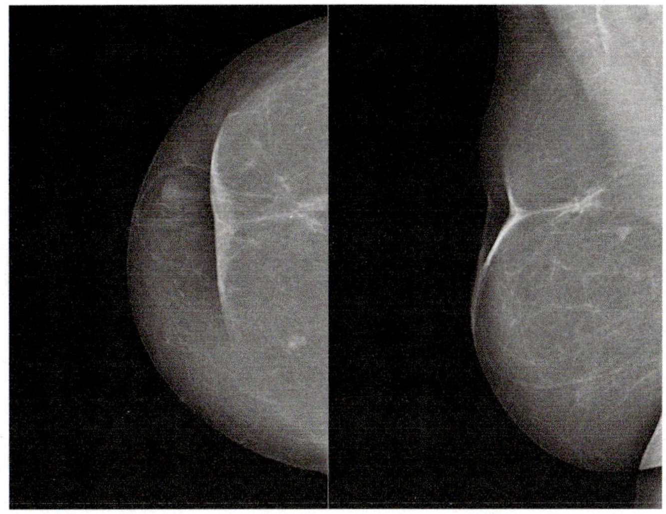

Fig. 10: Mammogram of right breast—CC and MLO view show post surgical changes along with focal asymmetry in upper inner quadrant.

CASE 5

History: A 66-year-old female underwent wide local excision 10 years back for a malignant mass in the right breast. She was on regular imaging follow-up. Her present screening mammogram showed a small irregular mass in the right breast (Fig. 10).

1. Describe the mammogram findings.
2. How does ultrasound (Fig. 11) help in this case?
3. What is the importance of postbiopsy marker and post marker mammogram (Fig. 12)?
4. What are the commonly used postbiopsy markers?

Answers

1. Mammogram shows postsurgical changes in the right breast in the form of scar, architectural deformity, skin retraction and skin thickening. In addition, there is a small focal asymmetry in the upper inner quadrant of right breast which is a new finding as it was not seen in the previous mammogram
2. Ultrasound helped in confirming the above mass which was hypoechoic, had irregular margins and measured 4.5 mm × 5 mm in size. A core needle biopsy was done under ultrasound guidance and postbiopsy

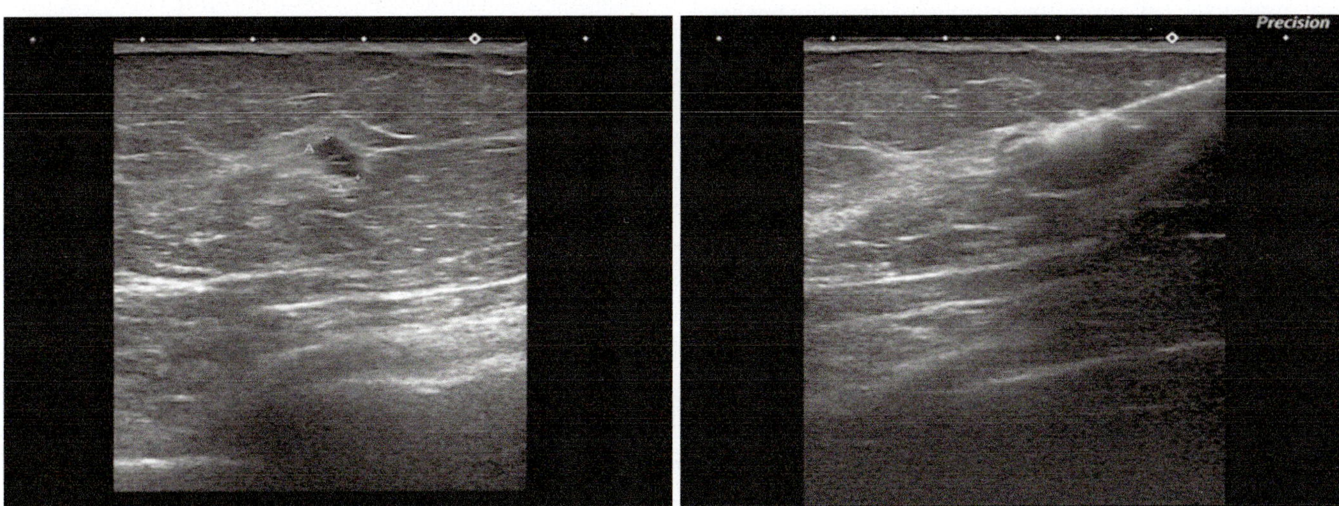

Fig. 11: Ultrasound confirmed the mass which was hypoechoic, had irregular margins and measured 4.5 mm × 5 mm in size from which a core needle biopsy was done.

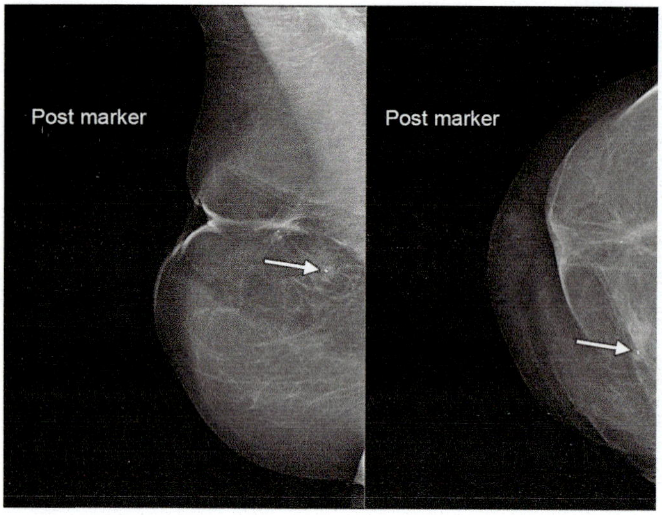

Fig. 12: Post-biopsy marker mammogram showed that the area in question has been assessed.

marker was introduced. Histopathology showed adequate sampling and was s/o inflammatory changes with no e/o residual neoplasia

3. The postbiopsy marker is introduced to show that the area in question has been assessed and evaluated adequately. Postbiopsy mammogram should be taken in two orthogonal views to confirm the area from the biopsy is taken and should be clearly mentioned in the report.
4. The commonly used markers are titanium based with hydrophilic component which swells up and gets lodged after coming in contact with breast tissue and fluid at the biopsy site. These come in various shapes and can be identified on ultrasound.

Final diagnosis: inflammatory changes following breast conservative surgery

Comments: It is important to remember that all masses in postsurgical breast may not be malignant but would require a biopsy to establish the diagnosis. The use of postbiopsy marker in a case like this where the mass is very small is important especially for future follow-ups. This woman should be put on a mammography and ultrasound follow-up till 5 years.

The use of postbiopsy markers is increasing and picking up in our country. These are especially useful when there is a risk that suspicious calcifications or mass can no longer be visualized after biopsy.

These are extremely useful in patients undergoing neoadjuvant chemotherapy to localize the original tumor bed in complete tumor response to treatment. They can also be used in patients with multiple masses to mark the most suspicious lesion. In cases where the biopsy results are benign and patient is kept on follow-up, radiologist assessing the patient is reassured that the area in question has been adequately assessed.

CASE 6

History: A 30-year-old female presented with history of low backache for one year which had increased for last 6 months with radiation to both lower limbs. She underwent a CECT MRI of thoracolumbar and lumbosacral spine (Figs. 13A to F).

She also complaint of a lump in left breast which she noticed 20 days back and which she felt was growing in size. Ultrasound of left breast is shown (Fig. 14).

1. Describe the MRI findings.
2. What is the diagnosis based on MRI findings?
3. What are the findings seen on ultrasound and what would you advise?

Answers

1. (A) T1W pre contrast sagittal, (B–D) postcontrast T1W sagittal and axial, (E) T2W sagittal and (F) STIR sagittal MRI images.

MRI of spine shows reduced height of body of T12 and L4 vertebrae.

There is an ill-defined altered signal intensity marrow lesion involving T12 vertebral body which is hypointense on T1W sequence, heterogeneously hyperintense on T2 and STIR sequence with heterogeneous post contrast enhancement on post contrast study. In addition, there is enhancing extradural soft-tissue component along the anterior and posterior aspect at this level causing cord compression.

L4 vertebra shows similar signal changes involving posterior elements causing spinal canal stenosis. A lesion showing post contrast enhancement is noted involving left sacral ala.

2. MRI findings are s/o vertebral metastases at multiple levels with cord compression.
3. Ultrasound of left breast shows multiple, circumscribed, heterogeneously hypoechoic masses with echogenic margins and two of them show vascularity on color Doppler. Ultrasound guided biopsy should be done from the breast mass showing vascularity.

The patient underwent ultrasound guided core biopsy from left breast mass with immunohistochemistry assessment. The diagnosis was non-Hodgkin lymphoma of large cell type-non alk 1 expressing.

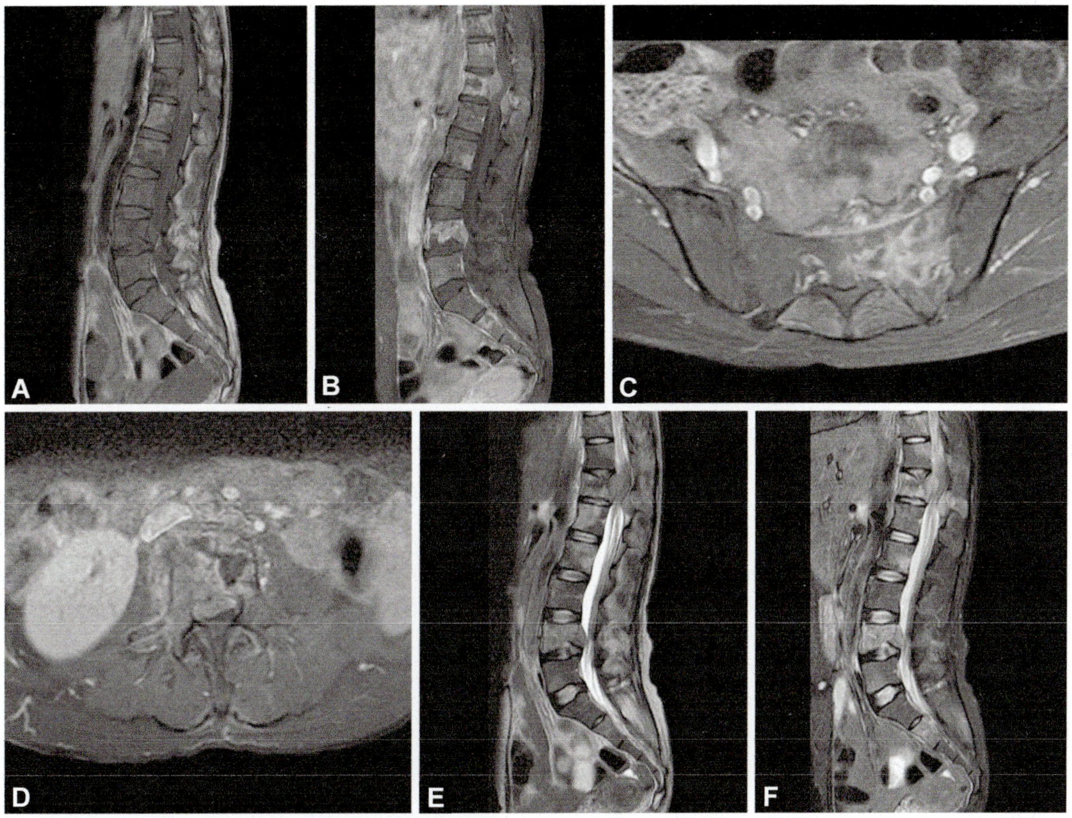

Fig. 13: (A) T1W pre contrast sagittal, (B–D) postcontrast T1W sagittal and axial, (E) T2W sagittal and (F) STIR sagittal MRI images. MRI of spine shows reduced height of body of T12 and L4 vertebrae. There is ill-defined altered signal intensity marrow lesion involving T12 vertebral body which is hypointense on T1W, heterogeneously hyperintense on T2W and STIR sequence with heterogeneous post contrast enhancement on post contrast study. There is enhancing extradural soft-tissue component along the anterior and posterior aspect at this level causing cord compression.

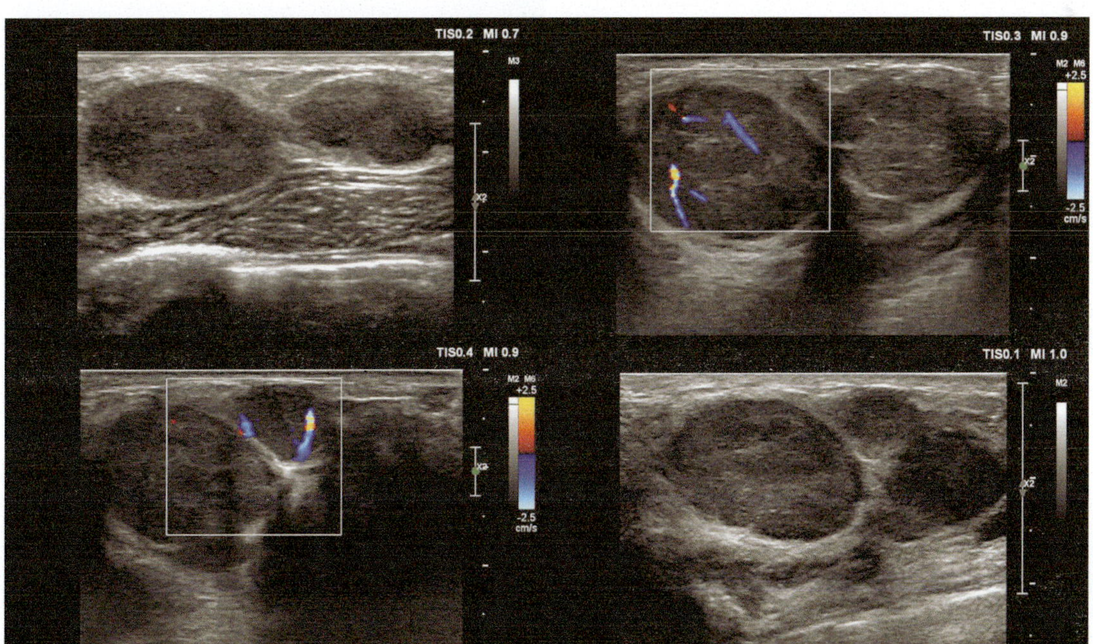

Fig. 14: Ultrasound of left breast shows multiple, circumscribed, heterogeneously hypoechoic masses with echogenic margins and increased vascularity.

PET-CT was done for metastatic work up which showed active disease in left breast and left level 2 axillary lymph nodes. Active disease was seen in both lobes of liver and in vertebrae at multiple levels.

Final diagnosis: non-Hodgkin lymphoma of anaplastic large cell type-non alk 1 expressing in left breast with liver and skeletal metastases. The patient was started on CHOP regime

Comments: Non-Hodgkin lymphoma (NHL) is a highly cellular lesion with no desmoplastic reaction. The NHL cells proliferate actively around the ducts and lobules. The prognosis for primary lymphoma is better than secondary lymphoma with 40%–50% disease free interval 4 years after local resection and radiotherapy.

In patients with secondary breast involvement, there are bilateral axillary lymph node enlargements. The number of intra mammary lesions is commonly higher in secondary than in primary lymphoma. Many of these lymphomatous nodules are circumscribed and have a thin echogenic capsule on ultrasound. They may show homogeneously hypoechoic or heterogeneously mixed hypo- to hyperechoic appearance. They may be multilobulated with posterior acoustic enhancement. Some of the lymphomas can be almost anechoic giving rise to a pseudocystic appearance. As they enlarge, there is peritumoral inflammatory edema and a thick echogenic halo. It is important to remember that ultrasound appearance is non-specific and similar to any cellular lesion with very little desmoplastic reaction. They are usually hypervascular on Doppler examination.

Biopsy followed by immunohistochemistry should be done to establish the diagnosis.

CASE 7

History: A 47-year-old female presented with a lump in left breast along with a history of seropurulent nipple discharge on and off for 4 months. There was no history of associated fever. On examination, nipple retraction was seen on both sides. There was no history of nipple discharge on right side.

She underwent mammogram of both breasts followed by ultrasound.

1. Describe the mammogram findings (Fig. 15).
2. Assign a BI-RADS category on mammogram.
3. Ultrasound of left breast (Fig. 16) reveals:

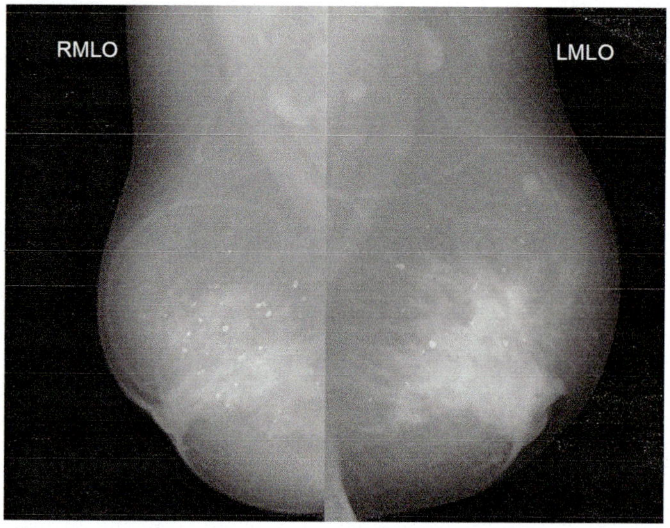

Fig. 15: Mammogram showed asymmetric density in retroareolar region of left breast and nipple retraction on both the sides (left>right) with scattered macrocalcifications bilaterally.

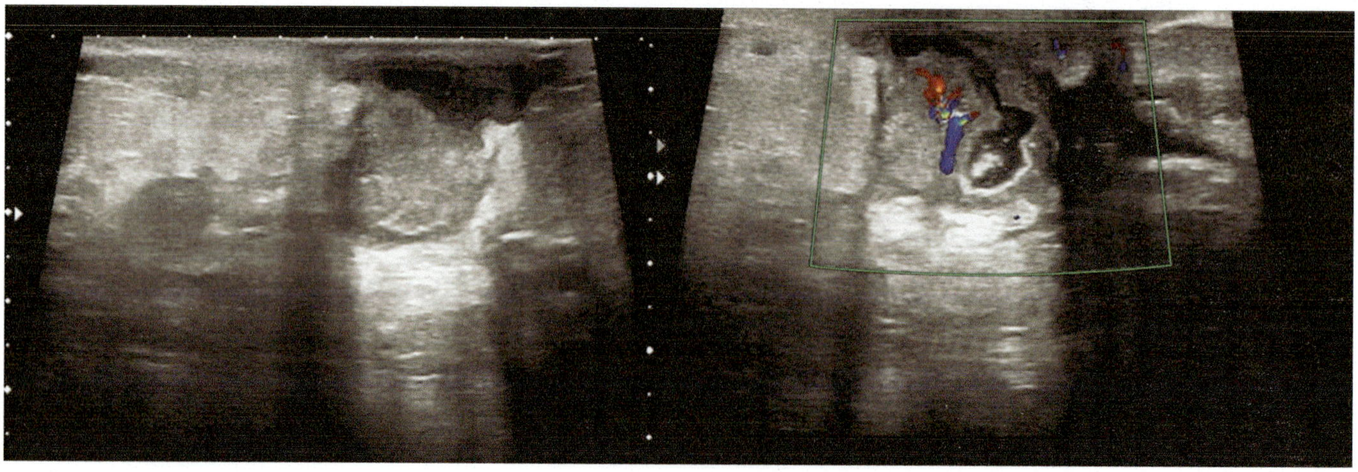

Fig. 16: Ultrasound of left breast reveals complex cystic mass in retro-areolar region with vascularity in solid portion.

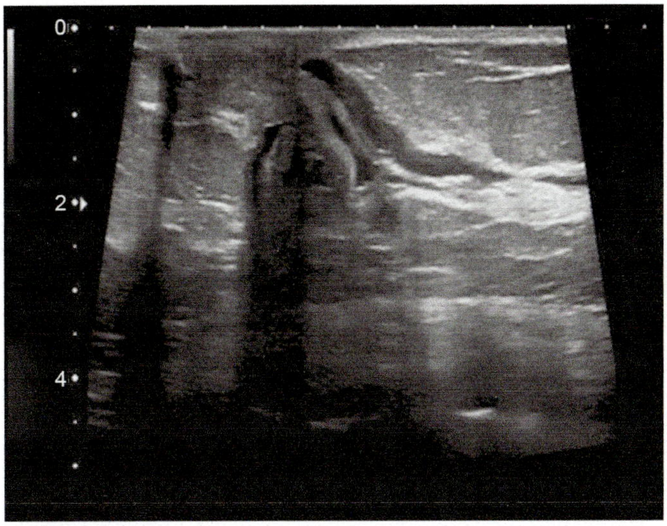

Fig. 17: Ultrasound of right breast showed dilated duct filled with echogenic material in retroareolar region which was seen extending up to the nipple.

   a. Complex cystic mass with vascularity in solid portion. True/False
   b. Complicated cyst. True/False
4. Describe the ultrasound findings in right breast (Fig. 17).
5. What is the combined ultrasound and mammogram BI-RADS category? What would you like to do next?

Answers

1. Mammogram showed asymmetric density in retroareolar region of left breast and nipple retraction on both the sides (more on left). There are scattered macrocalcifications in both breasts
2. Mammogram findings are s/o BI-RADS category 3
3. a. True, b. False
4. Ultrasound of right breast showed dilated duct filled with echogenic material in retroareolar region which was seen extending up to the nipple
5. A combined mammogram and ultrasound BI-RADS is 4A. A core needle biopsy should be done from the left breast mass

The biopsy showed chronic lobulitis with granulomatous inflammation, giant cells and epitheloid cells. Caseous necrosis was absent and the giant cells were morphologically of foreign body type and Langerhans's type. These features were s/o granulomatous mastitis.

Final diagnosis: idiopathic granulomatous mastitis

Comments: Idiopathic granulomatous mastitis is a chronic inflammatory disease common in young parous women of child bearing age.

It presents clinically with a palpable lump (firm to hard in consistency), mastalgia, erythema or swelling in breast. There is a tendency to involve the subareolar region. Although it is seen globally, a higher racial predilection in Hispanic and Asian women is recognized.

Imaging: On mammogram, there may be asymmetric density, architectural distortion, diffuse increase in breast density, skin thickening and sometimes macrocalcifications. These macrocalcifications may be due to chronic inflammatory pathology or chronic mastitis.

Ultrasound has variable appearances ranging from parenchymal heterogeneity, irregular hypoechoic masses with or without hypoechoic tract extending to skin surface, abscess formation and skin thickening.

It is difficult to differentiate idiopathic granulomatous mastitis from other infective and inflammatory pathologies like fungal infections, tuberculosis and also from malignancy; hence, biopsy should be done to confirm the diagnosis. Histopathology shows non-necrotizing granulomatous inflammation of lobules without evidence of any microorganisms.

CASE 8

History: A 57-year-old female underwent a screening mammogram. Mammogram of right breast—MLO and CC view are shown (Fig. 18).

1. What are the mammogram findings?
2. What should be done next?
3. What is the purpose of screening mammogram?

Answers

1. Mammogram of right breast shows fatty breast with scattered areas of fibroglandular tissue. A small dense mass/focal asymmetry is seen in the posterior third of right breast. There are no suspicious microcalcifications.
2. Ultrasound of right breast was done to localize the mass. Since no mass was seen on ultrasound, hence a stereotactic biopsy was done (Fig. 19) followed by postmarker mammogram (Fig. 20). Histopathology showed invasive lobular carcinoma grade 2 and high-grade DCIS (cribriform and comedo pattern of growth). ER, PR receptor status was positive and Her 2 nu was negative.
3. Breast screening is done to so that small invasive cancers are detected in early part of natural history.

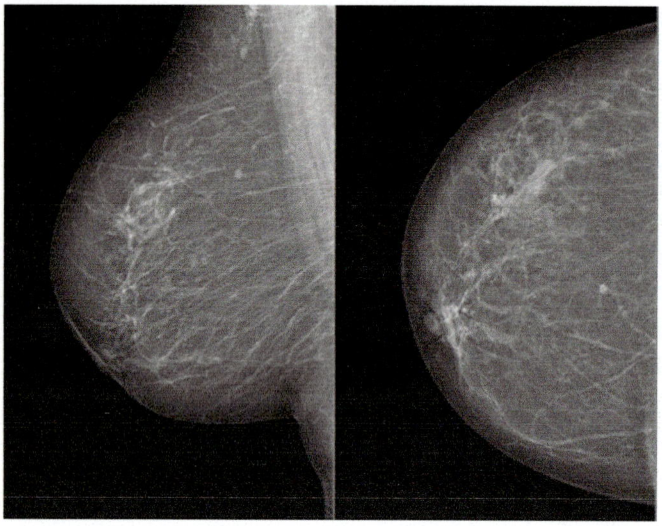

Fig. 18: Mammogram of right breast—MLO and CC view shows a small dense mass in the posterior third of right breast.

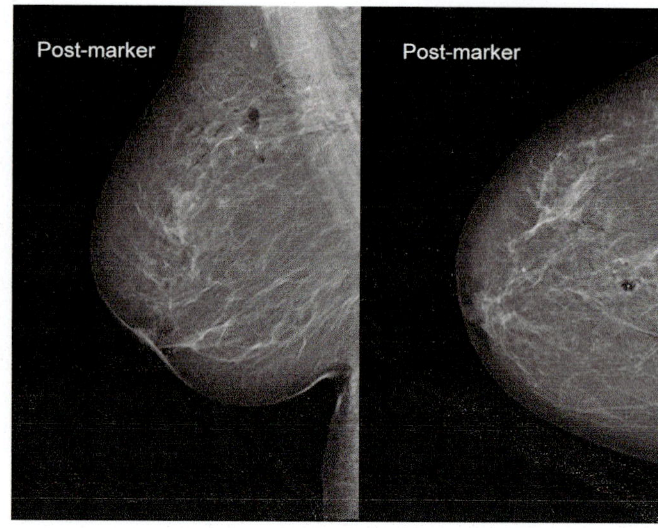

Fig. 20: Post marker mammogram after stereotactic biopsy.

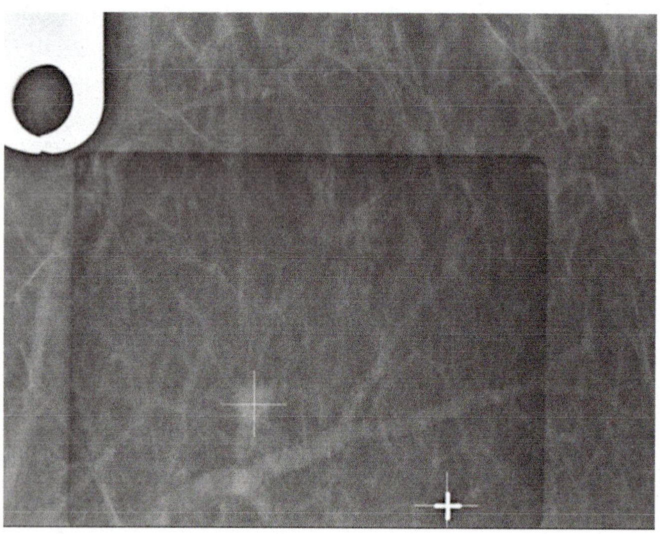

Fig. 19: Stereotactic biopsy was done as mass was not seen on ultrasound.

Final diagnosis: Invasive lobular carcinoma.

Comments: Breast screening detects a wide range of cancers ranging from low-grade DCIS to large high-grade invasive cancer.

Masses are easier to visualize in a fatty breast because of difference in density. In this case, since histopathological diagnosis was lobular cancer, hence MRI of the breast should be done to look for multifocal disease or contralateral cancer.

Many low-grade cancers which are detected at screening may never present clinically or be life threatening. On the other hand, some of these cancers may dedifferentiate over a period of time into aggressive cancers or less differentiated cancers and therefore, if they are detected at screening, they can be removed. In this way, breast cancer mortality can be reduced.

CASE 9

History: A 66-year-old female, a nurse by profession, incidentally detected a lump in right breast a few days after a fall which produced bruises on the breast.

1. Mammogram—MLO view of right breast is shown (Fig. 21):
   a. A circumscribed high-density mass with smooth margins is seen in right breast with a small portion of irregularity. True/False
   b. There are microcalcifications within the mass. True/False
2. Ultrasound of the right breast (Fig. 22) shows:
   a. Complex cystic mass with solid and cystic components. True/False
   b. Complicated cyst. True/False
3. Elastography of the lesion was done and strain ratios were obtained (Fig. 23):
   a. Only high strain index is seen. True/False
   b. Both high and low strain index are seen. True/False
4. What is the BI-RADS category?

Answers

1. (a) True, (b) False
2. (a) True, (b) False

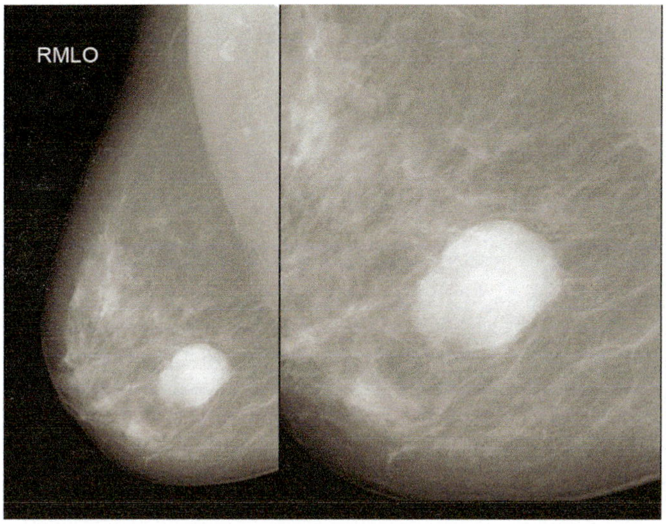

Fig. 21: Mammogram of right breast shows a circumscribed mass with mildly irregular margin at places.

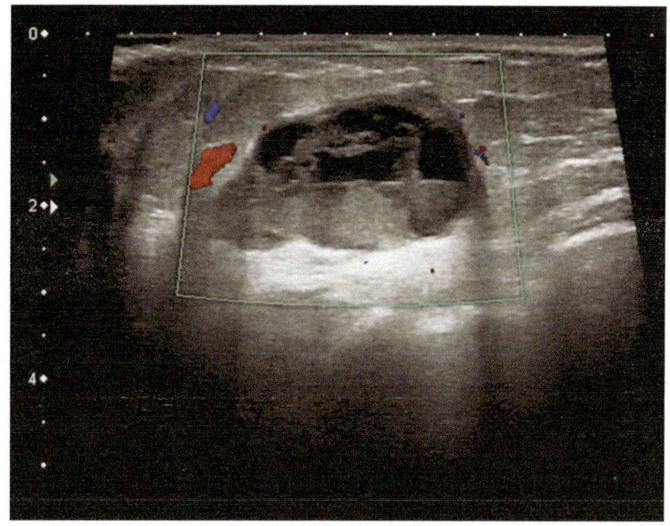

Fig. 22: Ultrasound of the right breast shows a complex cystic mass with solid and cystic components.

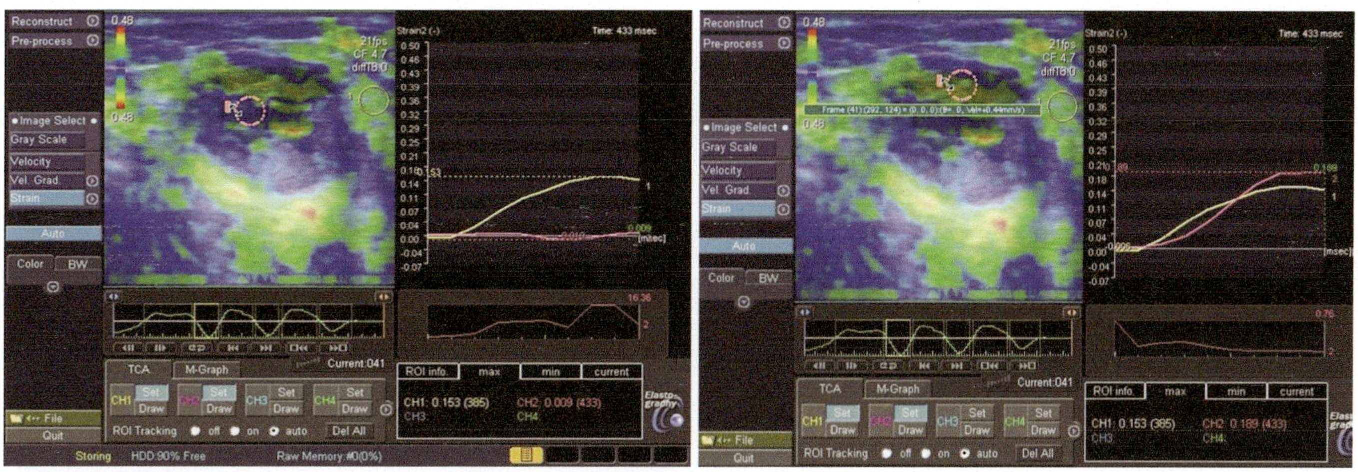

Fig. 23: Elastography showed both high and low strain ratios within the mass.

3. (a) False, (b) True
4. BI-RADS 4C

Mammography of the right breast—MLO view shows a circumscribed high-density mass in the inferior quadrant of right breast. The margins of mass are smooth throughout except a small portion showing mild irregularity. There is no architectural deformity and no microcalcifications are seen.

Ultrasound of right breast showed a complex cystic mass with solid and cystic components and thick septations. Posterior acoustic enhancement is seen.

Strain elastography showed both high and low values of strain index.

Based on mammogram and ultrasound findings a BI-RADS category of 4B is assigned (moderate suspicion of malignancy) with an advise for core needle biopsy.

The patient underwent an excision biopsy which showed features s/o mixed carcinoma—mucinous carcinoma with invasive ductal carcinoma.

Final diagnosis: mucinous carcinoma

Comments:

Mucinous carcinoma: Occurs in older women and has a prevalence of 1%–7% among women who are 75 years or older.

It presents clinically as a soft mass and is divided histologically into two broad types: (1) pure mucinous (approximately in 2% cases) and (2) mixed mucinous which contains areas of mucinous carcinoma with invasive ductal carcinoma. It has a favorable prognosis due to a lower incidence of lymph nodal metastases.

On mammography, it is commonly seen as a circumscribed low density mass with partially faded or obscured margins. Ultrasound shows mixed echogenicity mass with solid and cystic components. Posterior acoustic enhancement is common.

Almost all mucinous carcinomas are estrogen and/or progesterone-receptor positive, which means that hormonal therapy is likely to be an effective treatment.

CASE 10

History: A 50-year-old female presented with complaint of bloody nipple discharge from right side and sticky watery discharge from left nipple for 8 months. Clinical examination revealed bilateral nipple retraction; however, no mass was palpable.

Mammogram of both breasts was done (Figs. 24 and 25) followed by ultrasound (Figs. 26 and 27).

1. What are the mammogram findings?
2. Describe the ultrasound findings in both breasts

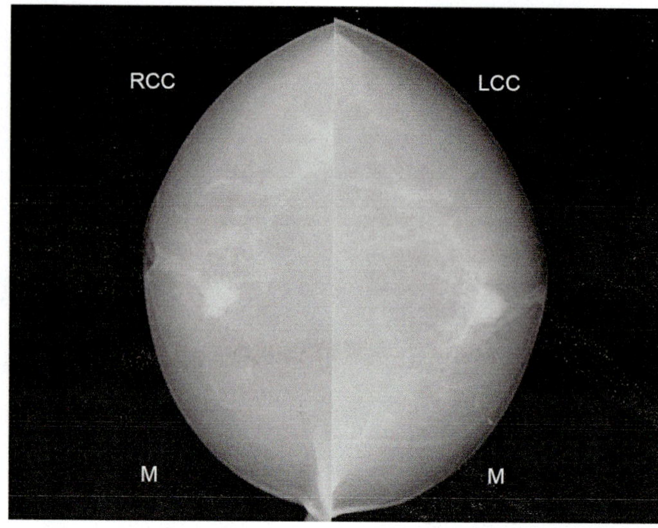

Fig. 24: Mammogram of both breasts CC view shows a circumscribed mass in the retroareolar region of both breasts with nipple retraction and a linear density extending from the nipple towards the mass.

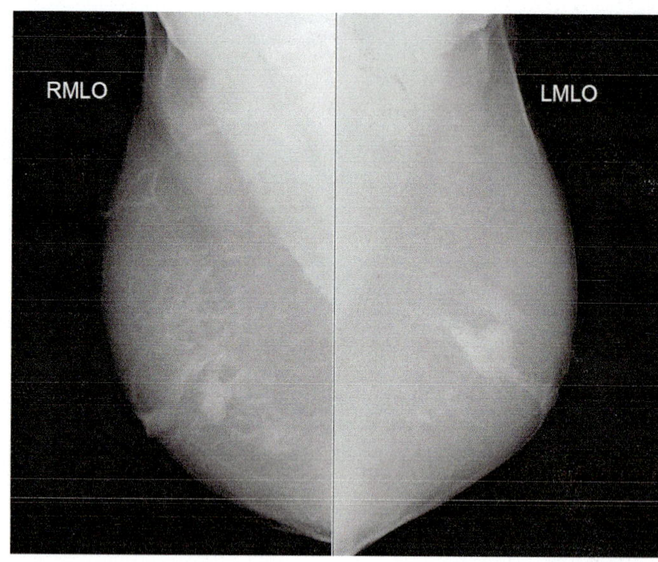

Fig. 25: Mammogram of both breasts MLO view shows a circumscribed mass in the retroareolar region of both breasts with nipple retraction.

Answers

1. Mammogram of right breast shows a circumscribed mass in the retroareolar region with nipple retraction and a linear density extending from the nipple towards the mass. No suspicious microcalcifications are seen. Mammogram of left breast shows a similar looking mass in retroareolar region with partially obscured margins.
2. Ultrasound of right breast showed a circumscribed intraductal mass (arrow) in retroareolar region with dilated duct extending up to the nipple. Ultrasound of left breast showed a cystic mass in retroareolar region with a round mural nodule within. There was no vascularity within

   The patient underwent bilateral excision biopsy.

Final diagnosis:

a. **Histopathology from right breast showed fibrocystic disease with intraductal papilloma having a fibrovascular core**
b. **Histopathology from left breast showed fibrocystic disease with adenosis**

Comments: Papillomas are the commonest benign intraductal epithelial tumors and have a characteristic frond like structure with a central fibrovascular core. They may be asymptomatic or present with serosanguinous discharge. They can be seen as circumscribed solid nodules or mural-based nodules within a dilated duct. On color Doppler imaging, flow may be detected within the papilloma arising from a vascular feeding pedicle. Earlier, conventional ductography used to be done to confirm the above findings wherein the duct was cannulated after identifying the pore from where the discharge was oozing

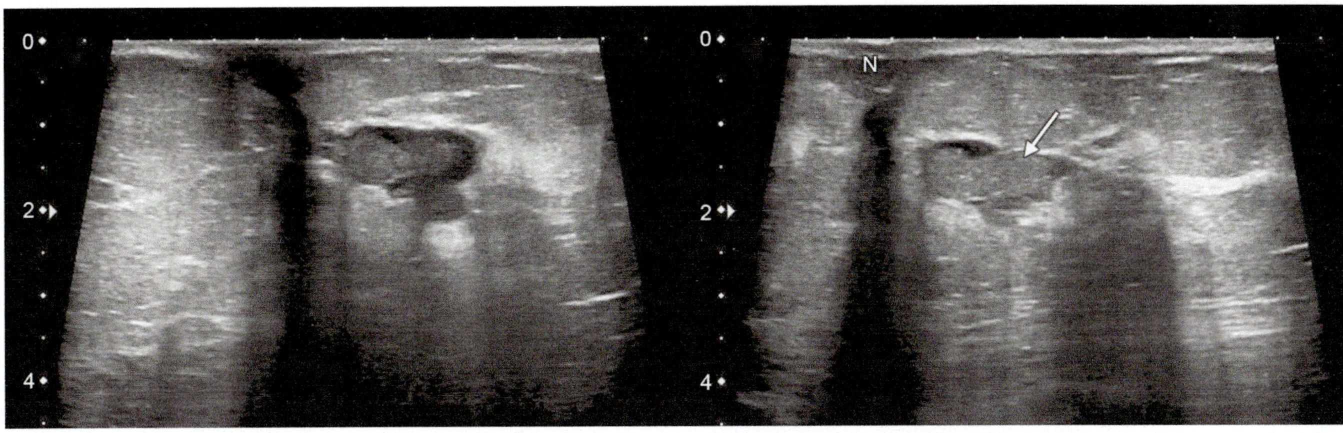

Fig. 26: Ultrasound of right breast showed a circumscribed intraductal mass (arrow) in retroareolar region.

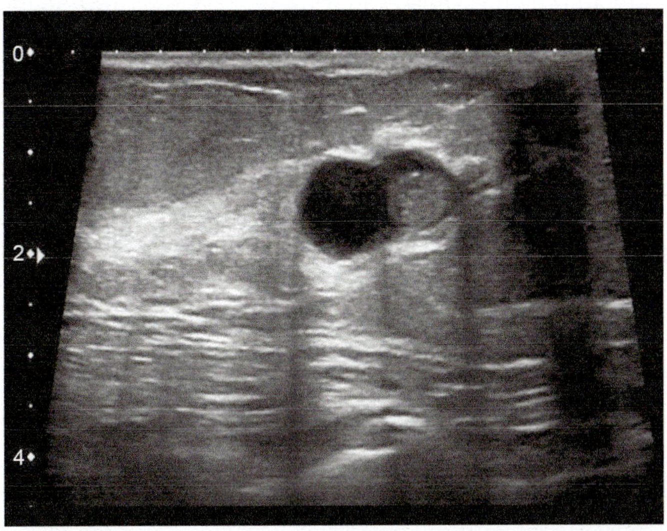

Fig. 27: Ultrasound of left breast showed a cystic mass in retroareolar region with a round mural nodule within.

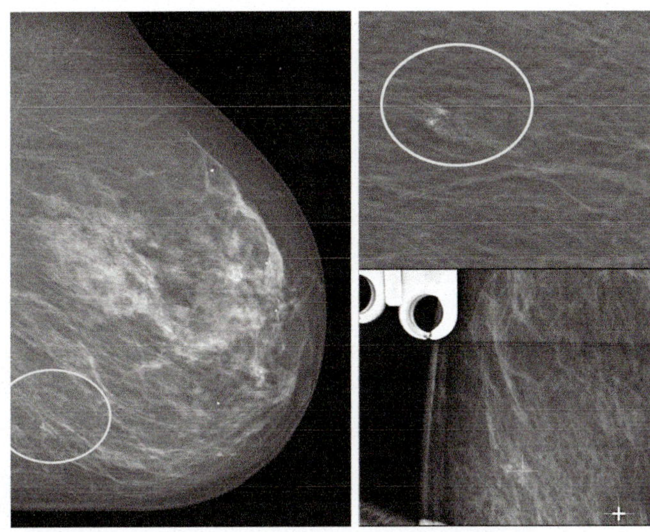

Fig. 28: Mammogram of left breast—MLO and magnification view showed grouped microcalcifications.

out. Contrast was then injected which opacified the duct while intraductal mass was seen as a filling defect.

CASE 11

History: A 56-year-old female came for screening mammogram. Mammogram with magnification view is shown in Figure 28. Vacuum-assisted biopsy was done (Fig. 29).

1. What are the mammogram findings?
2. Describe the magnification view

Answers

1. Mammogram showed grouped microcalcification in MLO view in inferior aspect (Fig. 28). No mass is seen.
2. Magnification view showed the morphology of calcifications clearly. The calcifications are coarse, heterogeneous and grouped in appearance.

Vacuum-assisted breast biopsy using VACORA was done and calcium is seen on Faxitron specimen mammogram (Fig. 29) which showed coarse heterogeneous calcifications.

Histopathology showed intermediate nuclear grade ductal carcinoma in situ with a cribriform growth pattern and extensive microcalcification. There also appears to be a focus of comedo necrosis. Elsewhere, there is fibroelastosis with entrapped tubules suggestive of a radial scar. There is no evidence of invasive neoplasia.

Final diagnosis: intermediate nuclear grade ductal carcinoma in situ with a cribriform growth pattern

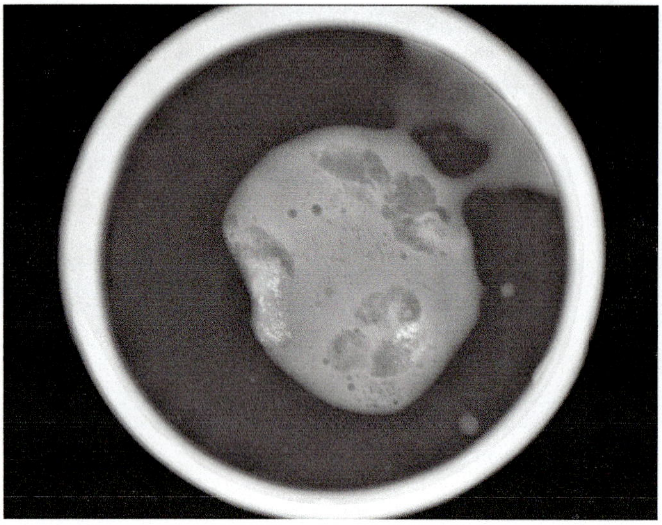

Fig. 29: Vacuum-assisted breast biopsy using VACORA showed coarse heterogeneous calcifications.

Comments: Vacuum-assisted breast biopsy using VACORA is a percutaneous large core biopsy procedure where a portable hand held device with a 10-G needle is used under stereotactic guidance to perform breast biopsies and lesion extractions. Faxitron is used to see if calcifications are retrieved.

On mammography, DCIS can be seen as pleomorphic calcifications which are present in a linear fashion or in a group.

In DCIS, histologically there is proliferation of malignant epithelial cells in the TDLU with no invasion beyond the basement membrane.

At least 10–20% are non-calcified and can be mammographically occult. These are seen on MR mammogram as clumped, non-mass like enhancement in a ductal, linear, segmental or regional distribution.

CASE 12

History: A 46-year-old female underwent routine mammogram examination. Mammogram of both breasts—MLO views (Fig. 30) are shown followed by ultrasound (Fig. 31). Since she also complained of abdominal distension and breathlessness, CECT thorax and abdomen were also done (Figs. 32 and 33).

1. Describe the mammogram findings.
2. What does ultrasound show?
3. Does CECT thorax give additional information?
4. What findings does CECT Abdomen show?

Answers

1. Mammogram of both breasts—MLO view shows normal breast parenchyma on both sides. There is a lobulated mass with calcific foci in the right axillary tail.

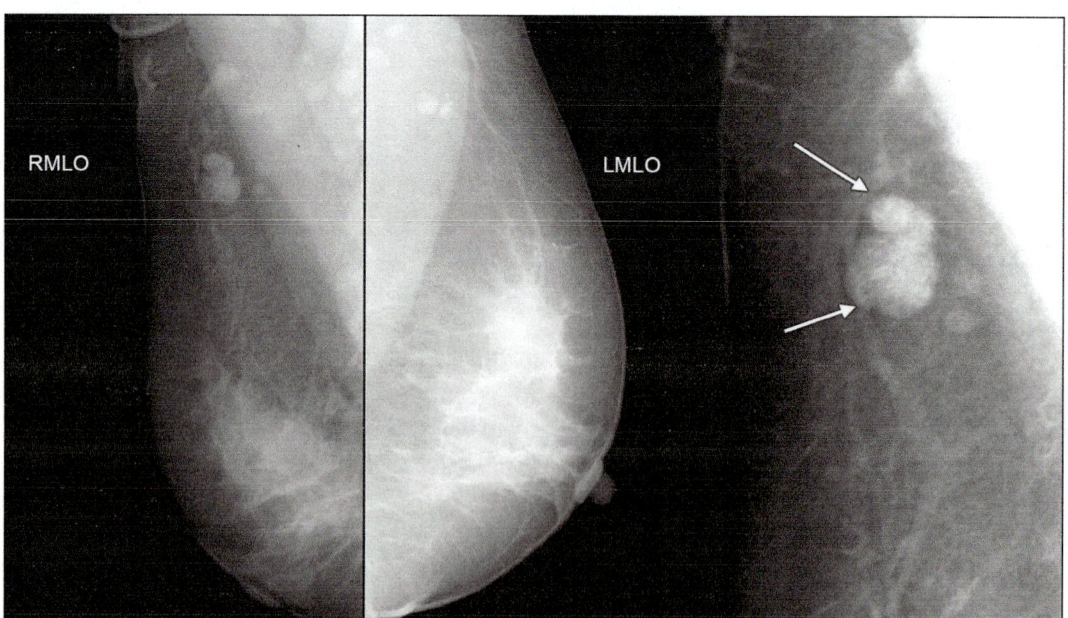

Fig. 30: Mammogram of both breasts—MLO view shows normal breast parenchyma on both sides. There is a lobulated mass seen near the axillary tail region on the right side with calcific foci.

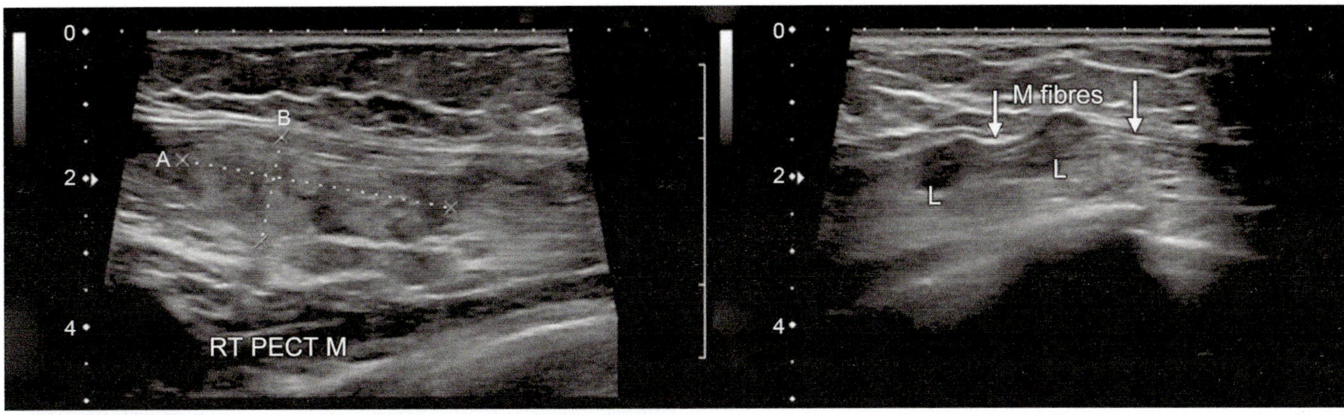

Fig. 31: Targeted ultrasound in the region of interest shows a circumscribed, lobulated heterogeneous lesion along the right pectoralis muscle.

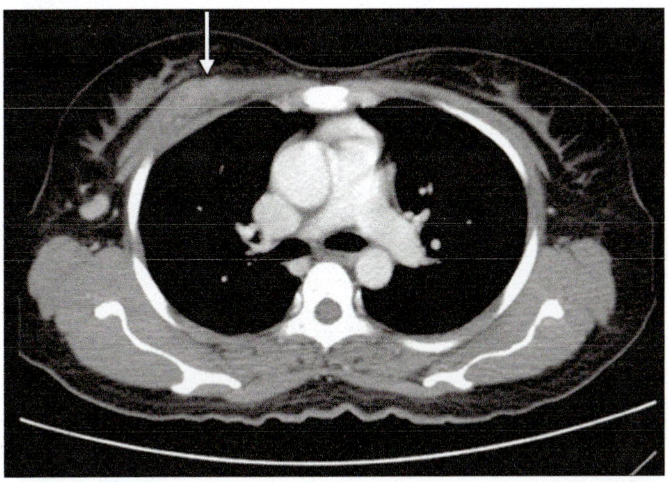

Fig. 32: CECT Thorax shows a heterogeneous lesion along the right pectoralis muscle.

2. Targeted ultrasound in the region of interest shows a circumscribed, lobulated heterogeneous lesion along the right pectoralis muscle.
3. Yes. CECT thorax shows a heterogeneous lesion along the right pectoralis muscle.
4. CECT abdomen shows bilateral solid cystic ovarian masses with ascites.

The patient underwent biopsy from the lesion along the right pectoralis muscle which showed metastatic tumor deposit. Ascitic fluid showed malignant cells. Biopsy from adnexal masses showed papillary cystadenocarcinoma of both ovaries.

Final diagnosis: bilateral papillary cystadenocarcinoma of both ovaries with metastatic deposit along the right pectoralis muscle

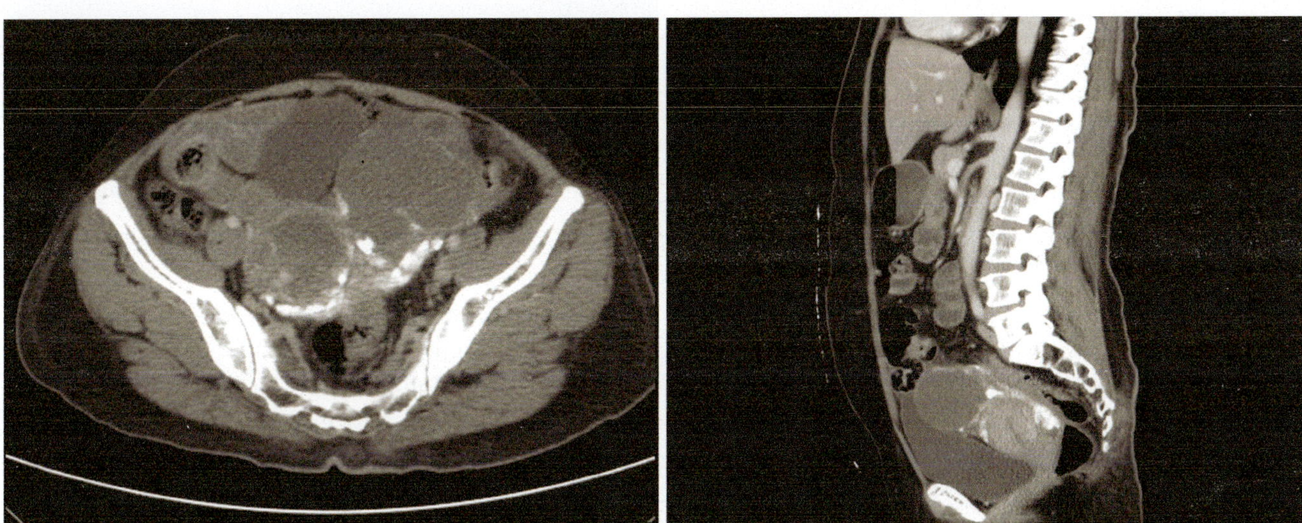

Fig. 33: CECT abdomen shows bilateral solid cystic ovarian masses with ascites.

Comments: Distant tumor metastases in ovarian cancer patients in striated muscles are extremely rare. This case shows incidental finding of metastases in muscle which was asymptomatic.

CASE 13

History: A 55-year-old female underwent breast conservative surgery for malignancy in left breast a year ago. She presented a year later with a palpable right axillary lymph node. Postsurgical mammogram (Fig. 34) of both breasts and mammogram after 1 year (Fig. 35) are shown.

1. What are the findings in mammogram shown in Figure 34?
2. What are the findings shown in mammogram in Figure 35?
3. Does magnification view help (Fig. 36)?
4. What is the important learning point in this case?

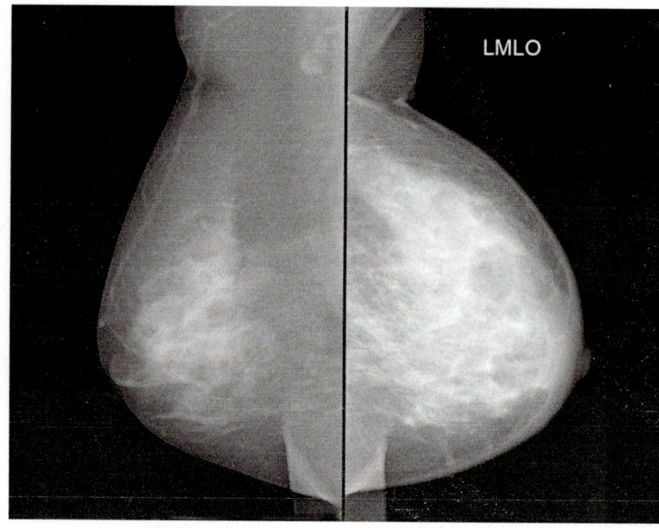

Fig. 34: Mammogram of both breast—MLO view showed breast conservative surgery changes in left breast in the form of skin thickening, architectural deformity, surgical clips an increased breast density. Right MLO view is normal.

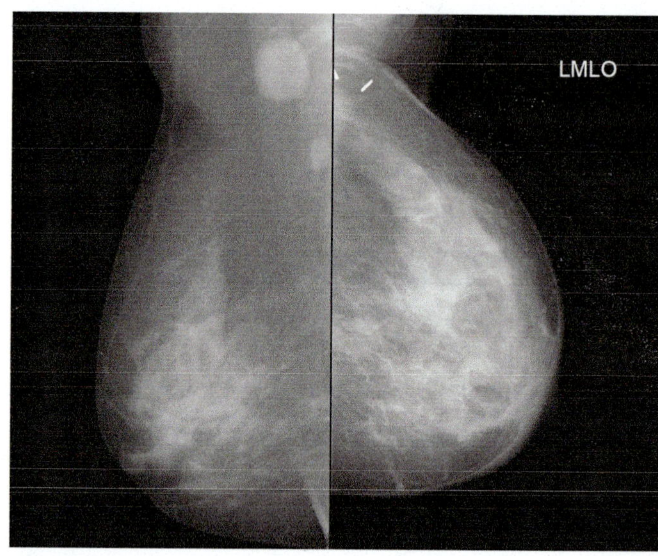

Fig. 35: Mammogram of right breast showed a grouped microcalcifications with enlarged right axillary lymph node.

Answers

1. Mammogram of both breast—MLO view showed breast conservative surgery changes in left breast in the form of skin thickening, architectural deformity, surgical clips an increased breast density. Right breast is normal.
2. Mammogram in Figure 35 showed a grouped microcalcifications with enlarged right axillary lymph node having loss of fatty hilum. FNAC from lymph node showed malignant changes.
3. Yes. Magnification view showed the microcalcification more clearly. The size, number and morphology could be appreciated better.
4. The important learning point in this case that in postsurgical cases, it is not just important to look at the postop mammogram but also the normal breast to look for any new findings like mass, microcalcifications, lymph nodes, etc. One must always develop a habit of comparing serial mammograms to pick up any new findings.

Final diagnosis: a new malignancy in contralateral breast—metachronous cancer

Comments: Breast cancer survivors are at higher risk for getting another breast cancer. Breast cancer may come back after treatment—sometimes years later. This is called a recurrence. Recurrence can be local (in the same breast or in the mastectomy scar), regional (in nearby lymph nodes) or in a distant area.

Cancer that is found in the opposite breast is not a recurrence—it is a new cancer that requires its own treatment. Survival rates are much better when any second breast cancer is detected early. It is important to have regular follow-up mammograms.

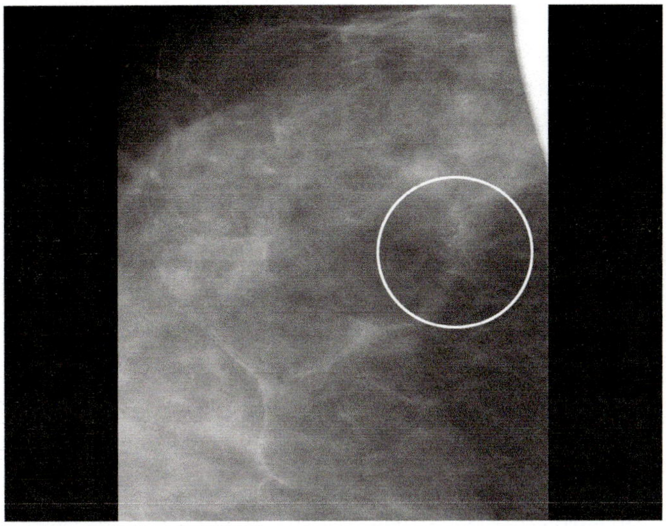

Fig. 36: Magnification view showed the microcalcification more clearly.

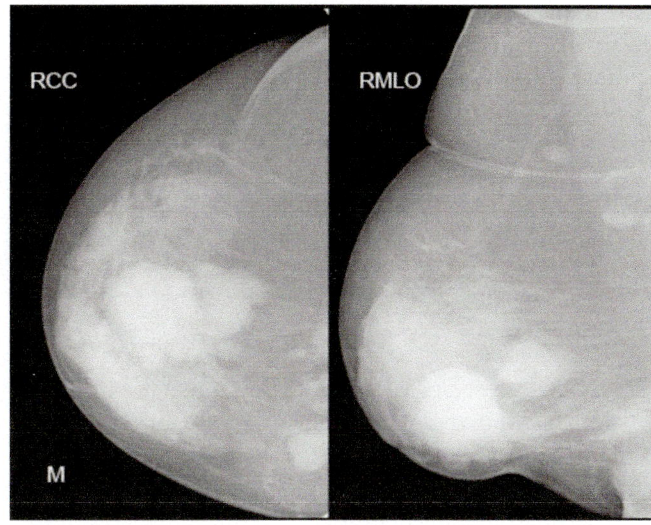

Fig. 37: Mammogram of right breast—MLO and CC view shows multiple, well-circumscribed masses.

CASE 14

History: A 64-year-old female presented with rapidly growing lump with focal puckering in right breast. Mammogram and ultrasound were done. Mammogram—MLO and CC view (Fig. 37) and ultrasound of right breast are shown (Fig. 38).

1. Describe the mammogram findings
2. What are the ultrasound findings?
3. What is BI-RADS category?

Answers

1. Mammogram of right breast—MLO and CC view showed multiple, circumscribed masses with a few microlobulation in lower inner quadrant, in the middle and posterior third of right breast. Normal axillary lymph nodes are present (maintained fatty hilum).
2. Ultrasound of right breast showed multiple solid cystic masses with low level echoes. The solid components showed increased vascularity.
3. BI-RADS 5.

Biopsy was taken from the solid component followed by aspiration which showed features of invasive ductal carcinoma. Patient underwent right modified radical mastectomy. Histopathology was suggestive of invasive ductal carcinoma with solid and papillary variants.

Final diagnosis: invasive ductal carcinoma with solid and papillary variant with DCIS

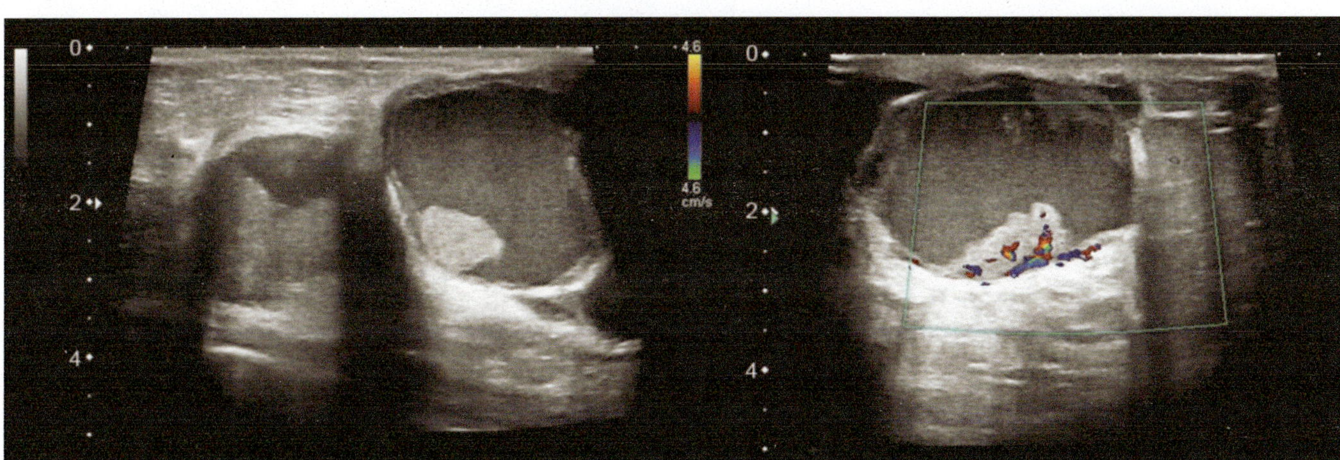

Fig. 38: Ultrasound of right breast showed multiple solid cystic masses with low level echoes and solid component showing increased vascularity.

Comments: The invasive papillary cancers are rare tumors seen in elderly women. The name comes from papillary projections or small finger like projections. On ultrasound, they are generally seen as cystic masses with a solid component. The histologic discrimination of the papillary tumors (benign or malignant) is based on the presence or the absence of the myoepithelial component and such tumors are classified as solid papillary carcinomas.

CASE 15

History: A 52-year-old female presented with lump in right retroareolar region. There was no history of nipple discharge. Mammogram of right breast and targeted ultrasound of right breast are shown (Fig. 39).

1. Describe the mammogram findings
2. What does ultrasound show?
3. What is BI-RADS category?

Answers

1. Mammogram of right breast—MLO view showed an irregular mass with spiculated margins in retroareolar region causing nipple retraction. A few axillary lymph nodes with lucent fatty hilum were seen.
2. Targeted ultrasound showed hypoechoic mass. Minimal vascularity was noted.
3. BI-RADS category 5.

Patient underwent a guided core needle biopsy which showed benign spindle cell lesion suggestive of fibromatosis. The histopathology and immunohistochemistry were suggestive of adenomyoepithelioma. No cellular atypia or necrosis were seen.

Final diagnosis: Adenomyoepithelioma of breast.

Comments: There was discordance between radiological and pathological findings in this case—discordant benign. The mass looked malignant on imaging; therefore, the patient underwent core needle biopsy and then excision biopsy which showed adenomyoepithelioma (AME) of breast. This is a relatively rare, benign tumor that has a **spectrum** of disordered epithelial-myoepithelial proliferations. In our case, it showed features of benign mass with no features of atypia.

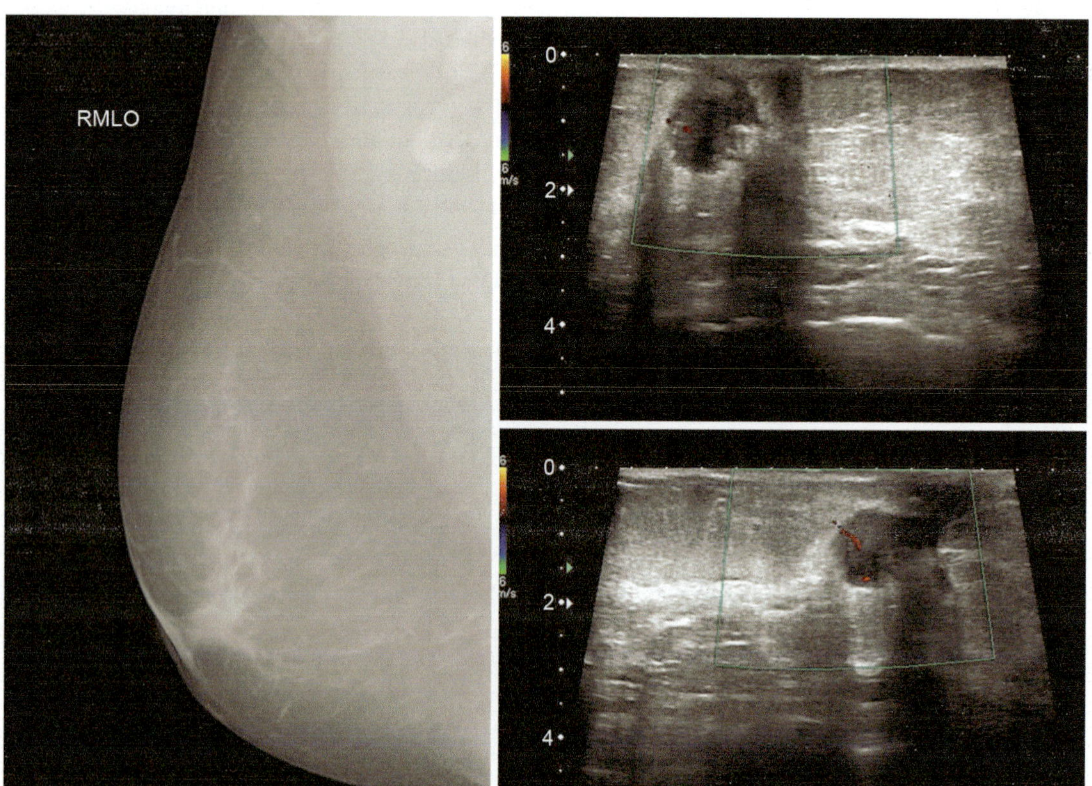

Fig. 39: Mammogram of right breast—MLO view and targeted ultrasound showed an irregular mass with spiculated margins in retroareolar region causing nipple retraction.

Because of the morphologic heterogeneity of this tumor, misinterpretation on a needle biopsy may occur. Recognition of biphasic cellular elements and the overall architecture of the tumor in combination with immunohistochemistry are important when diagnosing these tumors. Papillary architecture is seen in most tumors and therefore, AME is considered to be a variant of intraductal papilloma.

Although most tumors are benign, local recurrences malignant transformations and metastases have been reported. Cases with significant cytologic atypia, necrosis and brisk mitotic rates raise the likelihood that the lesion is malignant and therefore should be mentioned in pathology report. In these cases, complete excision with adequate margins is recommended to decrease the potential for recurrence and metastasis.

CASE 16

History: A 53-year-old lady had undergone right mastectomy 5 years ago for invasive ductal carcinoma. She came for her annual mammogram (Fig. 40) of left breast which showed a new finding. Targeted ultrasound (Fig. 41) was also done. Her previous mammogram done 1 year ago is also shown (Fig. 42) which was normal.

1. What are the mammogram findings in the recent mammogram?
2. Is it important compare with previous findings?
3. Did ultrasound help in this case? Describe the ultrasound findings

Answers

1. The most recent mammogram (Fig. 40) showed a focal asymmetry in upper outer quadrant of left breast (marked in white)
2. The new finding was not seen in previous mammogram (Fig. 42) done one year ago. This makes it significant. This is the reason that comparison with previous mammogram is important especially in a patient with a known malignancy in the contralateral breast
3. Yes. Ultrasound helped in this case (Fig. 41) as it showed a small hypoechoic mass in region of interest at 2–3 o'clock position which on elastography showed raised TLR.

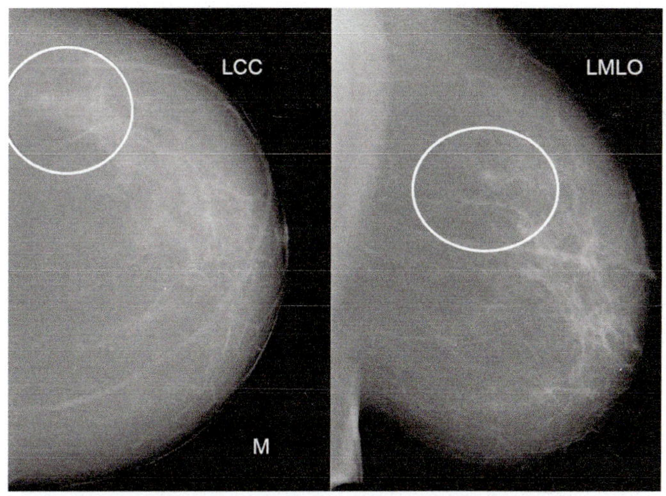

Fig. 40: Mammogram of left breast—CC and MLO view showed a focal asymmetry in upper outer quadrant (circled in white).

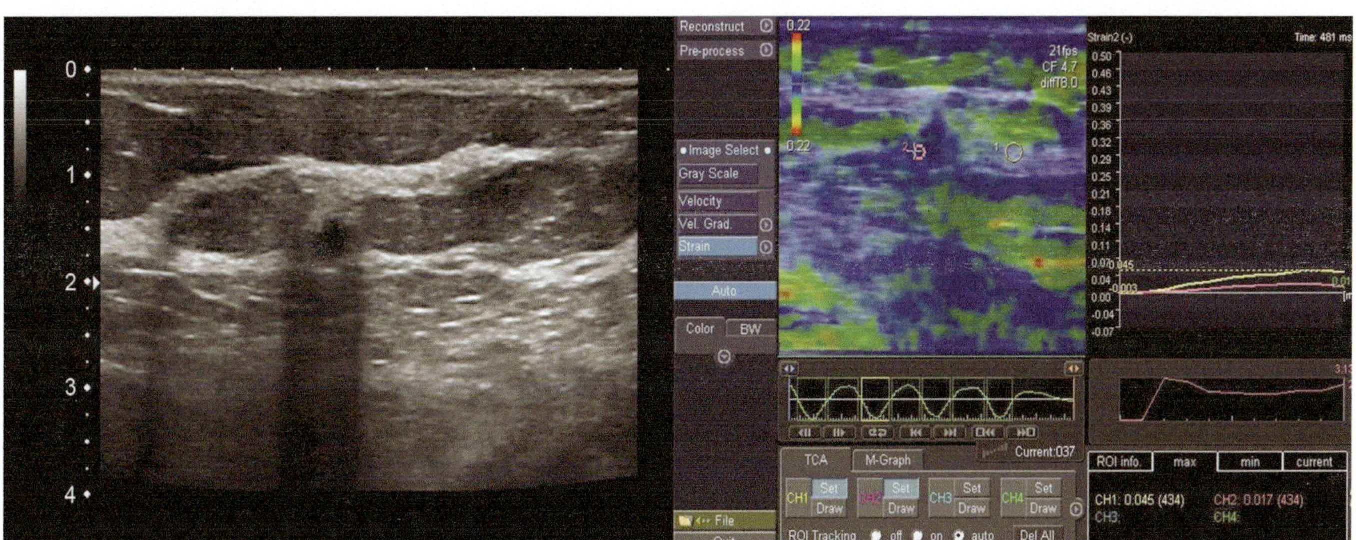

Fig. 41: Ultrasound showed a small hypoechoic mass in region of interest at 2–3 o'clock position which on elastography showed raised TLR values.

Ultrasound guided core needle biopsy was done which was s/o invasive ductal carcinoma. The patient underwent modified radical mastectomy which showed features of DCIS (high grade) with microinvasion.

Final diagnosis: DCIS (high grade) with microinvasion

Comments: The risk of a breast cancer survivor developing a second breast cancer is much higher than the risk of a comparable healthy woman developing a first breast cancer. Therefore, role of imaging is important and one has to be cautious while reporting mammogram in these patients. Any new finding compared to previous mammogram should be considered significant and appropriate measures should be taken. In this case, the patient was very apprehensive because of diagnosis of a second cancer and wanted to undergo mastectomy.

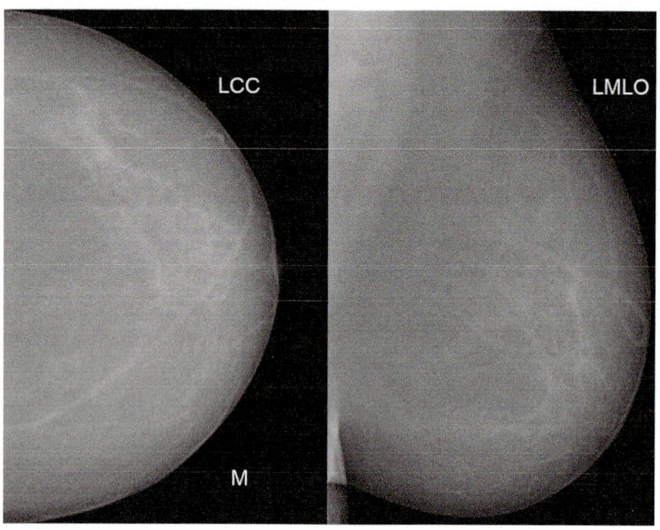

Fig. 42: Mammogram of left breast done one year ago was normal.

CASE 17

History: A 48-year-old female with breast implants came for her routine mammogram (Figs. 43 and 44) followed by ultrasound of breast.

1. Describe the mammogram findings.
2. Does ultrasound show additional findings?
3. What would you do next?

Answers

1. Mammogram of both breasts—MLO and CC view show subglandular implants. Visualized breast parenchyma appears normal.
2. Yes. Ultrasound of left breast shows a round, hypoechoic mass with irregular margin in one aspect without posterior acoustic enhancement measuring 6 × 5.5 mm. The mass is situated at 12 o'clock position close to the implant.
   The right breast parenchyma is normal.
   Implants in both breasts appear normal.
3. The mass in left breast appears suspicious hence ultrasound guided biopsy should be done.

Ultrasound guided biopsy from the hypoechoic mass was done and histopathology was s/o lobular carcinoma.

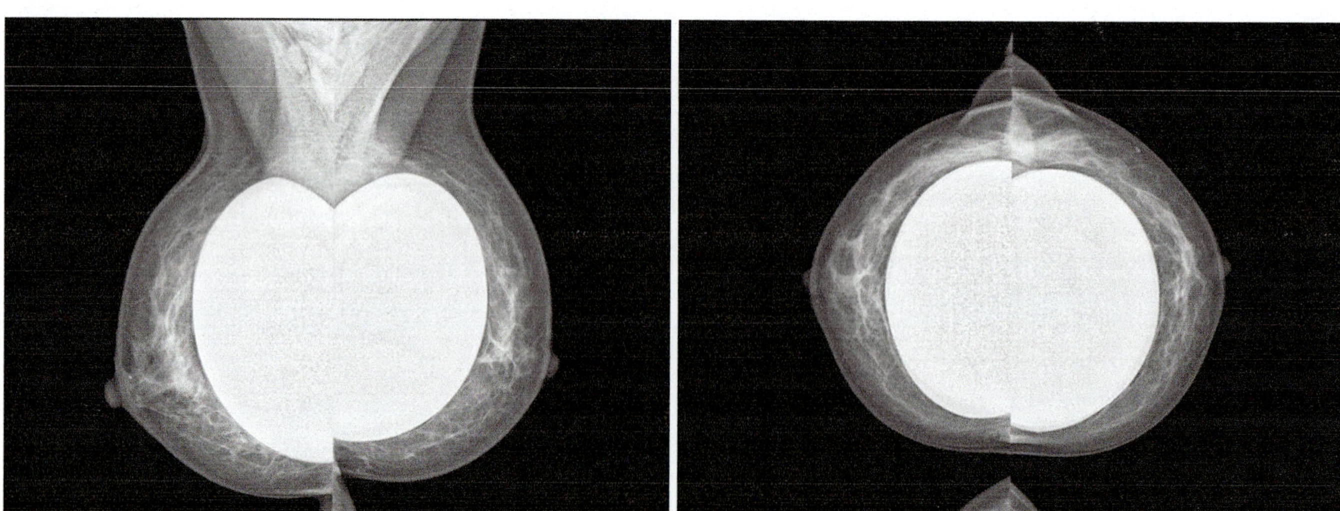

Fig. 43: Mammogram of both breasts—MLO and CC views showed subglandular implants.

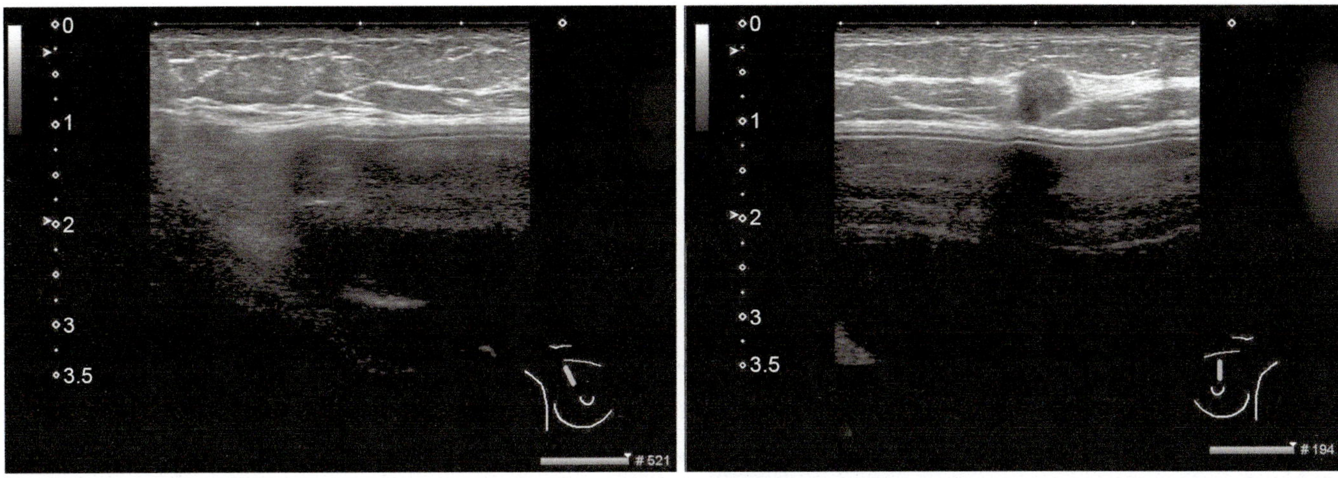

Fig. 44: Ultrasound of left breast showed a round, hypoechoic mass close to the anterior aspect of implant.

Final diagnosis: Lobular carcinoma in a woman with breast implants.

Comments: The presence of the implant may impair the ability of mammography or ultrasound for cancer detection. A correlation between physical examination and mammography findings should be first done. Any palpable abnormality can then be subjected to an ultrasound or contrast-enhanced MRI. MRI is especially useful in the detection of small cancers which may go undetected on mammography.

Suspicious findings should be further evaluated with biopsy. While doing biopsy in a patient with breast implants, one has to be careful as to not cause rupture of the implant.

There can be other benign or malignant lesions in patients with implants which are diagnosed incidentally. Though there are no known associations of lobular carcinoma and breast implants, a case of recurrent invasive lobular carcinoma presenting as a ruptured breast implant has been reported in literature.

Women with breast implants have a very low but increased risk of developing anaplastic large cell lymphoma compared to women who do not have breast implants.

CASE 18

History: A 52-year-old female presented with swelling in right breast. There was no pain and no history of fever. Mammogram of both breasts was done followed by targeted ultrasound of right breast (Figs. 45 to 47).

1. Describe the mammogram findings.
2. Does ultrasound help in making a diagnosis?
3. What is the diagnosis?
4. What are the extra-mammary pathologies you can diagnose on ultrasound?

Answers

1. Mammogram of both breasts—MLO view showed that the right pectoralis muscle is prominent as compared to left side with a low density mass within, displacing the margins of the muscle anteriorly. The same is confirmed on CC view. There is no mass within both breasts.
2. Yes. Ultrasound showed that there is a hypoechoic mass located within pectoralis muscle with a thin rim

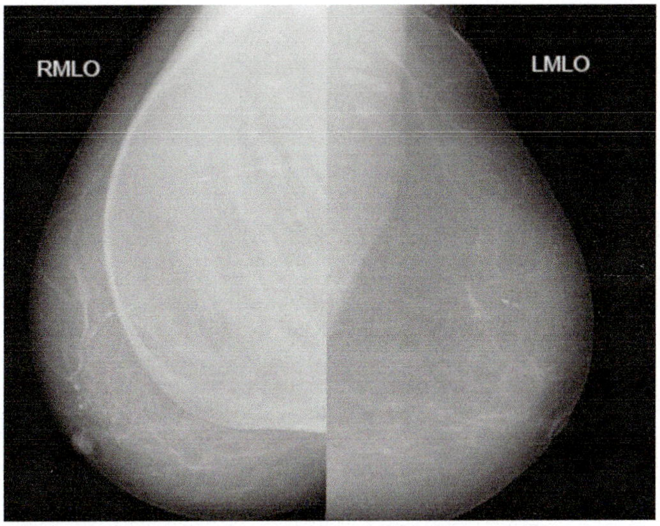

Fig. 45: Mammogram of both breasts—MLO view showed that the right pectoralis muscle is prominent compared to left side with a low density mass within.

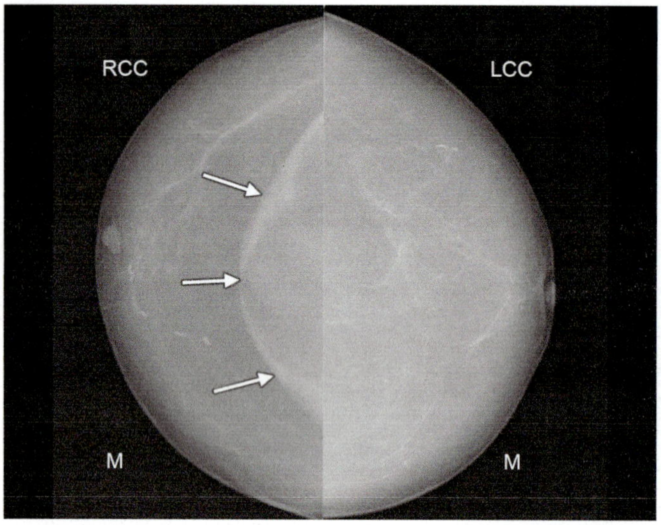

Fig. 46: Mammogram of both breasts—CC view confirmed the findings noted on MLO view.

of anterior and posterior fibers diverging because of mass. The mass is separate from breast parenchyma.

3. Intramuscular lipoma within the pectoralis muscle.
4. The extramammary pathologies that can be diagnosed on ultrasound are chest wall lesions which displace the breast tissue anteriorly. These include inflammatory pathologies like tubercular abscess, lipomas, hemangioma and chest wall metastatic lesions.

Comments: Lipomas are common benign tumors which are composed of adipocytes in subcutaneous tissues. They can arise from the muscle (intramuscular) or between muscles (intermuscular). The intramuscular lipomas commonly arise from skeletal muscles of thigh or shoulder. Lipomas arising from pectoralis are rare and clinically appear as a breast mass.

CASE 19

History: A 54-year-old male presented with painless lump in left breast since 5 months. Mammograms—MLO and CC view of both breast (Figs. 48 and 49) were done followed by targeted ultrasound of left breast (Fig. 50).

1. Describe the mammogram findings
2. What are the ultrasound findings?
3. Which type of cancer is rare in males?

Answers

1. Mammogram of left breast shows a circumscribed, round to oval, retroareolar mass causing nipple retraction. There are no microcalcifications present.
2. Ultrasound showed a circumscribed, hypoechoic, taller than wide mass in retroareolar region. No vascularity was seen.
3. Since there are very few lobules in male breast, lobular carcinoma is rare in males.

Biopsy was done from the mass which came as invasive ductal carcinoma.

Final diagnosis: invasive ductal carcinoma in male breast.

Comments: Carcinoma is rare in the male breast compared to females, accounting for 0.7% of all male cancers. All

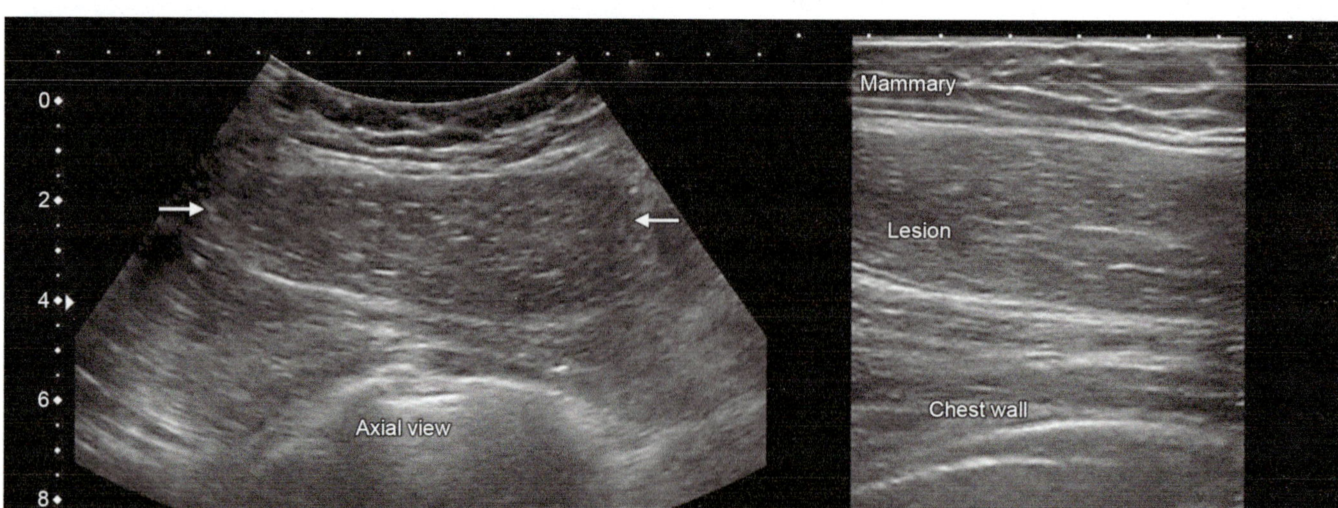

Fig. 47: Ultrasound showed that there is a hypoechoic mass located within pectoralis muscle.

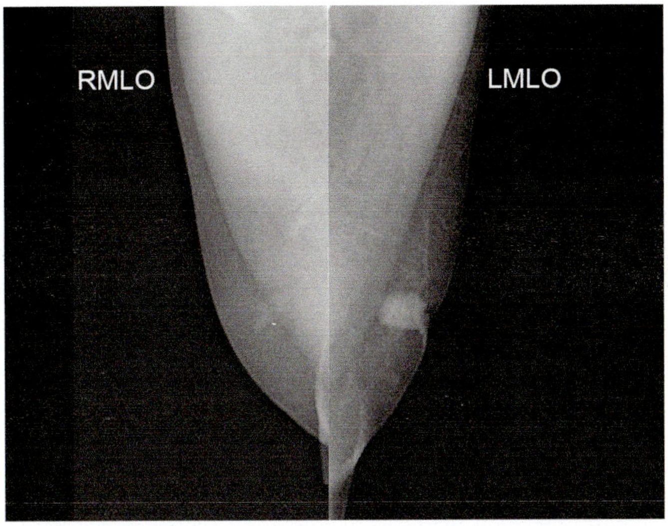

Fig. 48: Mammogram of both breast—left MLO view showed a circumscribed, round to oval, retroareolar mass causing nipple retraction.

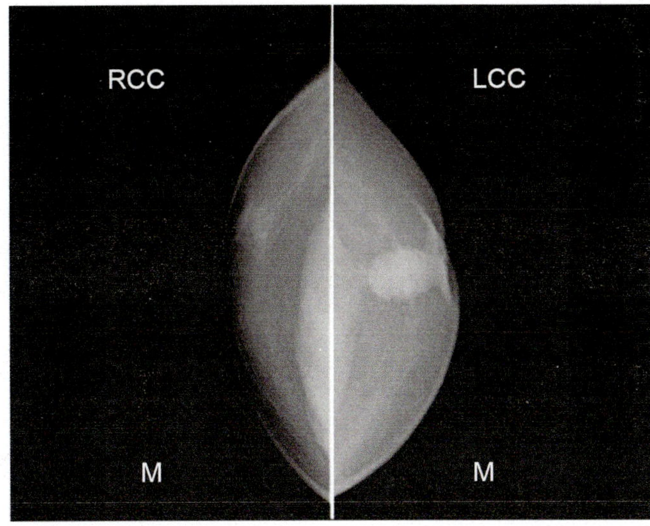

Fig. 49: Mammogram of both breasts—left CC view showed the same findings as in MLO view.

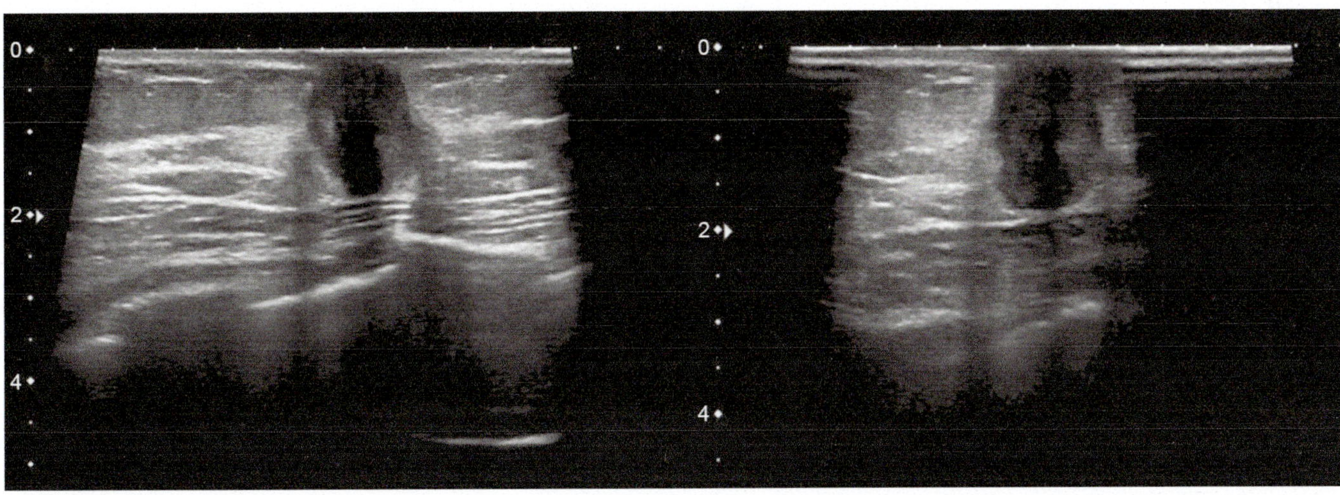

Fig. 50: Ultrasound showed a circumscribed, heterogenously hypoechoic, taller than wide mass in retroareolar region.

circumscribed masses in males should raise a high index of suspicion for carcinoma and all cysts should be rigorously imaged to exclude an intracystic neoplasm. Very often the masses are eccentric, lobulated or circumscribed but may also be spiculated. Nipple retraction may be present. Biopsy has to be done to establish the diagnosis. Please note that gynecomastia should not be confused with carcinoma.

Index

Page numbers followed by *f* refer to figure, *fc* refer to flowchart, and *t* refer to table

C

D

M

N